AF251855

# Control of Cardiac Arrhythmias by Lengthening Repolarization

Edited by

## Bramah N. Singh, M.D., D. Phil., F.R.C.P.

*Professor of Medicine*
*University of California Los Angeles*
*School of Medicine*
*and*
*Wadsworth VA Medical Center*
*Los Angeles, California*

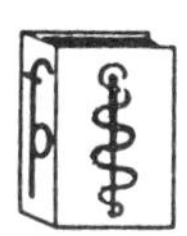

*Futura Publishing Company*
*Mount Kisco, New York*
*1988*

Library of Congress Cataloging-in-Publication Data

Control of cardiac arrhythmias by lengthening repolarization.

Includes bibliographies and index.
1. Arrhythmia—Chemotherapy.  2. Myocardial depressants.
I. Singh, B. N. (Bramah N.). [DNLM: 1. Anti-Arrhythmia
Agents—pharamacodynamics.  2.  Anti-Arrhythmia Agents—
therapeutic use.  3. Arrhythmia—drug therapy.  4. Heart
Conduction System—drug effects.  WG 330 C764]
RC685.A65C593   1988            616.1′28061          87-46001
ISBN 0-87993-316-X

Copyright 1988
Futura Publishing Company, Inc.


Published by
Futura Publishing Company, Inc.
P.O. Box 330, 295 Main Street
Mount Kisco, New York 10549

L.C. No.: 87-46001
ISBN No.: 0-87993-316-X



Printed in the United States of America

# CONTRIBUTORS


**Anderson, Jeffrey L., M.D.,** Associate Professor of Medicine, University of Utah, Salt Lake City, Utah.

**Atkinson, Arthur J., Jr., M.D., Ph.D.,** Professor of Medicine and Pharmacology, Northwestern University School of Medicine, Chicago, Illinois

**Brugada, Pedro, M.D.,** Department of Cardiology, Annadal Hospital, Maastricht, The Netherlands

**Davidson, Charles, M.D.,** Clinical Cardiac Electrophysiology Laboratory, Section of Cardiology, Department of Medicine, Northwestern University Medical School, Chicago, Illinois

**Dunnington, Catherine, R.N., M.D.,** Clinical Cardiac Electrophysiology Laboratory, Section of Cardiology, Department of Medicine, Northwestern University Medical School, Chicago, Illinois

**Feld, Gregory K., M.D.,** Assistant Professor of Medicine, UCLA School of Medicine and Wadsworth VA Medical Center, Los Angeles, California

**Gilmour, Robert F., Jr., Ph.D.,** Krannert Institute of Cardiology, The Department of Medicine, Indiana University School of Medicine, Indianapolis, Indiana

**Heger, James, J., M.D.,** Associate Professor of Medicine, Krannert Institute of Cardiology, Indiana University School of Medicine, Indianapolis, Indiana

**Hershman, Jerome M., M.D.,** Professor of Medicine and Endocrinology, UCLA School of Medicine, and Wadsworth VA Medical Center, Los Angeles, California

**Josephson, Martin A., M.D.,** Associate Professor of Medicine, UCLA School of Medicine and Wadsworth VA Medical Center, Los Angeles, California

**Kannan, Ram, Ph.D.,** Adjunct Associate Professor of Medicine, UCLA School of Medicine and Wadsworth VA Medical Center, Los Angeles, California

**Kates, Robert E., Ph.D.,** Associate Professor of Medicine, University of Stanford School of Medicine, Palo Alto, California

**Kehoe, Richard, M.D.,** Assistant Professor of Medicine, Clinical Cardiac Electrophysiology Laboratory, Section of Cardiology, Department of Medicine, Northwestern University Medical School, Chicago, Illinois

**Klein, Lawrence S., M.D.,** Assistant Professor of Medicine, Krannert Institute of Cardiology, Indiana University School of Medicine, Indianapolis, Indiana

**Lesch, Michael, M.D.,** Professor of Medicine, Clinical Cardiac Electrophysiology Laboratory Section of Cardiology, Department of Medicine, Northwestern University Medical School, Chicago, Illinois

**Locati, Emanuela, M.D.,** Unita'di Studio dell Aritmie, Centro di Fisiologia Clinica e Ipertensione, Ospedale Maggiore e Istituto di Clinica Medica Generale Universita'di, Milano, Italy

**Lucchesi, Benedict, R., M.D., Ph.D.,** Professor of Pharmacology, The University of Michigan Medical School, Ann Arbor, Michigan

**Lynch, Joseph, J., Ph.D.,** Assistant Research Scientist, The University of Michigan Medical School, Department of Pharmacology, Ann Arbor, Michigan

**Marcus, Frank I., M.D.,** Professor of Medicine, University of Arizona School of Medicine, Tuscon, Arizona

**Mattioni, Thomas, M.D.,** Clinical Cardiac Electrophysiology Laboratory, Section of Cardiology, Department of Medicine, Northwestern University Medical School, Chicago, Illinois

**Miles, William, M., M.D.,** Assistant Professor of Medicine, Krannert Institute of Cardiology, Indiana University School of Medicine, Indianapolis, Indiana

**Mostow, Nelson, D., M.D.,** Assistant Professor of Medicine, Case Western Reserve University, School of Medicine, Cleveland, Ohio

**Nademanee, Koonlawee, M.D.,** Associate Professor of Medicine, UCLA School of Medicine, and Wadsworth VA Medical Center, Los Angeles, California

**Parker, Michelle, R.N., M.S.,** Clinical Cardiac Electrophysiology Laboratory, Section of Cardiology, Department of Medicine, Northwestern University Medical School, Chicago, Illinois

**Piergies, Antoni, A., M.D.,** Clinical Pharmacology Center, Departments of Medicine and Pharmacology, Northwestern University Medical School, Chicago, Illinois

**Platou, Eivind, S., M.D., Ph.D.,** Medical Department, Cardiology Section, Ullevaal Hospital, Oslo, Norway

**Prystowsky, Eric, N., M.D.,** Professor of Medicine, Duke University School of Medicine, Durham, North Carolina

**Rakita, Louis, M.D.,** Professor of Medicine, Cleveland General Hospital and Case Western Reserve University, School of Medicine, Cleveland, Ohio

**Refsum, Helge, M.D., Ph.D.,** Professor of Medical Physiology, Institute of Medical Biology, University of Trømso, Tromsø, Norway

**Rieders, Daniel, M.D.,** Cardiology Fellow, Wadsworth VA Medical Center, Los Angeles, California

**Roden, Dan, M., M.D.,** Associate Professor of Medicine and Pharmacology, University of Vanderbilt School of Medicine, Nashville, Tennessee

**Ruo, Tseun, Ih, Ph.D.,** Clinical Pharmacology Center, Departments of Medicine and Pharmacology, Northwestern University Medical School, Chicago, Illinois

**Sarmiento, Joseph, M.D.,** Clinical Cardiac Electrophysiology Laboratory, Section of Cardiology, Department of Medicine, Northwestern University Medical School, Chicago, Illinois

**Schwartz, Peter, J., M.D.,** Professor of Medicine, University of Milan, School of Medicine, Milan, Italy

**Silver, Mitchell, D., M.D.,** San Francisco General Hospital, UCSF School of Medicine, San Francisco, California

**Singh, Bramah N., M.D., D. Phil., F.R.C.P.,** Professor of Medicine, UCLA School of Medicine, and Wadsworth VA Medical Center, Los Angeles, California

**Stevenson, William, M.D.,** Assistant Professor of Medicine, Director Clinical Electrophysiology, UCLA School of Medicine, Los Angeles, California

**Sung, Ruey, J., M.D.,** Professor of Medicine, San Francisco General Hospital, UCSF School of Medicine, San Francisco, California

**Vaughan Williams, E.M., M.D., D.Sc., F.R.C.P.,** University of Oxford and Hartford College, Oxford, England

**Weiss, James, M.D.,** Associate Professor of Medicine, UCLA School of Medicine, Los Angeles, California

**Wellens, Hein, J., M.D.,** Professor of Medicine, University of Linburg, Maastricht, The Netherlands

**Wit, Andrew, L., Ph.D.,** Professor of Pharmacology, Columbia University School of Medicine, New York, New York

**Zheutlin, Terry, M.D.,** Clinical Cardiac Electrophysiology Laboratory, Section of Cardiology, Department of Medicine, Northwestern University Medical School, Chicago, Illinois

**Zipes, Douglas, P., M.D.,** Professor of Medicine, Krannert Institute of Cardiology, Indiana University School of Medicine, Indianapolis, Indiana

# Foreword

In spite of a dramatic decline in cardiovascular deaths over the past two decades, sudden cardiac events kill over 350,000 Americans each year. These acute arrhythmias are the most common cause of death in ischemic heart disease but also account for a substantial proportion of deaths from primary myocardial disease and end-stage valvular diseases. Thus far the role of antiarrhythmic agents in preventing sudden death is unproven, however, some important new data on amiodorone is reported in this text. As more is learned about the mechanism of rhythm disorders, the difficulties with pharmacological therapy become increasingly obvious. Not only are there a variety of mechanisms for arrhythmias, including several forms of enhanced automaticity, early and delayed afterdepolarizations, and other forms of continuous electrical activity, but the mechanism for ventricular tachycardia and fibrillation may be quite different at various stages of the disease. The mechanisms early in acute myocardial infarction seem to be quite different from those after the first few hours. These difficulties are compounded further by the limitations of clinical electrophysiology to accurately define the nature of arrhythmias in a significant number of patients. It is clear that programmed stimulation may not be definitive in characterization of mechanisms in many patients.

It is not surprising that the use of antiarrhythmic agents in patients has been largely empiric. In spite of the ability to classify antiarrhythmic drugs and to define the mechanisms of their action in isolated muscle preparations or Purkinje fibers, the relevance of these effects and the impact on the human heart during disease can only be deduced by actual clinical trials. In the course of these trials, the search continues for an ideal antiarrhythmic agent. Such a drug would be highly effective against life-threatening arrhythmias, with little or no systemic side effects, and no important cardiac hemodynamic or arrhythmogenic properties.

In this text Dr. Singh and colleagues have provided important additional insights into the search for such an antiarrhythmic agent. Emphasis is placed upon the effects of lengthened repolarization in the control of cardiac arrhythmias. This is done on a background in which diverse mechanisms for cardiac arrhythmias are lucidly reviewed. The discussion provides additional insight by focusing on Class III agents and the features that make each of them unique. Although cardiologists and electrophysiologists have been concerned about prolongation of the QT interval as an ominous portent of torsades de pointes, several authors in this text emphasize that prolongation of repolarization may be beneficial providing that the prolongation is uniform and arises in association with a lengthening of the refractory period of cardiac tissue without a depression of conduction. Moreover, as Dr. Singh points out, prolongation of repolarization might be expected to increase contractile force as a result of continued activation of the myofibrillar apparatus. When QT interval prolongation occurs as a consequence of delayed intraventricular conduction and is associated with dispersion of recovery, electrolyte disturbances, or further drug interactions, the results can be catastrophic. However, a homogeneous prolongation of the refractory period may be quite effective in obliterating reentrant rhythms and decreasing the ventricular response to an increased rate of stimulation. Drawing attention to the role of repolarization has several benefits. It emphasizes the potential for the importance of a class of antiarrhythmic agents that would uniquely and effectively produce this electrophysiological result. It allows an explanation of such curious phenomena as the antiarrhythmic effect of metabolic products such as N-acetylprocainamide (NAPA). In addition, it provides some rationale for drug combinations that might not otherwise be envisioned.

Unfortunately, the two drugs of this group that have been approved for use in the United States have remarkably complex mechanisms of action. Bretylium has profound effects to initially release norepinephrine and to produce sympathetic ganglionic blockade. Amiodorone has effects on thyroid metabolism in addition to its direct electrophysiological effects. In both cases side effects and complexities of administration are important limiting features in the use of these drugs. At the same time, they have clearly focused attention on the potential importance of lengthening repolarization and added to our understanding of arrhythmias and their treatment.

Dr. Singh and his colleagues have provided a very useful analysis of agents that have an important Class III effect. The potential of this approach should stimulate the search for additional drugs that feature Class III effects. Indeed, it is conceivable that a combination of a Class III agent and a Class I agent may have substantial synergistic benefit but the relative magnitude of such effects that might be optimal for arrhythmia control remains to be determined. The final analysis still depends critically on the careful assessment of one or more pharmacological agents in humans. As our understanding of the natural history of human arrhythmia unfolds, it is entirely conceivable that the agent or agents used will be modified in the course of the natural history of cardiac disease in each patient. Dr. Singh and his colleagues have added considerably to the conceptual framework by which this process evolves.

**Kenneth I. Shine, M.D.**
Professor of Medicine and Dean, UCLA School of Medicine, Los Angeles, California
Past President of the American Heart Association

# Preface

It has long been known that quinidine exerts two major electrophysiological actions: slowing of conduction and prolongation of repolarization. Both properties lead to a lengthening of the refractory period, a basis for the control of cardiac arrhythmias. In the development of pharmacological approaches to the therapy of arrhythmias, the initial focus was essentially on slowing conduction. Subsequently, however, compounds that selectively slow conduction and those that prolong repolarization have become available. The "discovery" that an isolated lengthening of repolarization independently of depolarization, might be antiarrhythmic was serendipitous. In 1970 it was found that the beta-blocker sotalol (MJ 1999) markedly prolonged the refractory period by selectively lengthening cardiac repolarization. In experimental animals, the compound exerted a potent antiarrhythmic action. Such an action was designated a new class of antiarrhythmic mechanism. This so-called Class III action was later found to be a property of a large number of chemically heterogeneous compounds—sotalol and its isomers, bretylium, n-acetylprocainamide, melperone, and, above all, amiodarone. Interest in this class of agents, stemming from the unusually potent clinical effects of amiodarone, has burgeoned in recent years. It is becoming increasingly apparent that, as a group, the so-called Class III agents have minimal negative inotropic effects and low arrhythmogenic potential, but potent antiarrhythmic and especially antifibrillatory properties. However, lengthening of repolarization per se may not be the key to the potent clinical effects. Perhaps the way in which this parameter is modulated by hormonal and autonomic influences is of crucial significance. The purpose of this text is to critically review the evolving new information on the control of cardiac arrhythmias by lengthening repolarization.

Cellular electrophysiological mechanisms of cardiac arrhythmias are described by Wit, and their relevance to clinical mechanisms are reviewed by Zipes and Gilmour. These ideas form the background to my own discussion of how antiarrhythmic drugs are thought to work and why it is felt that prolonging repolarization is a desirable antiarrhythmic mechanism. Schwartz outlines his unrivaled experience with the long QT interval syndromes and indicates under what circumstances prolonged repolarization is not an antiarrhythmic mechanism but constitutes an arrhythmogenic substrate. This is followed by chapters on hemodynamic (Josephson and Singh) and pharmacokinetic (Kates, Kannan, and Singh) properties of Class III agents. A series of chapters on the electrophysiological effects and evolving clinical roles of the major Class III agents follows. The properties of sotalol, reflecting UCLA-Wadsworth experience in ventricular arrhythmias, are discussed by Nademanee and Singh, and the experimental basis for the antifibrillatory and antiarrhythmic actions of sotalol and its optical isomers is discussed by Lucchesi and Lynch. The next three chapters deal with N-acetylprocainamide. The pharmacological basis of its antiarrhythmic actions is discussed by Feld and Singh, pharmacokinetics by Atkinson and his colleagues, and clinical antiarrhythmic effects by Sung and Silver. The significance of the Class III antiarrhythmic effects of adrenergic-neurone blocking agents is discussed at length by Anderson, that of the neuroleptic agent, melperone, by Refsum and Platou. This is followed by a series of chapters on amiodarone based in part on data acquired at Wadsworth-UCLA Medical Centers on the topics of electropharmacological properties (Singh), thyroid hormone metabolism (Hershman), and the management of supraventricular tachycardias (Stevenson and his colleagues). The experience in Maastricht on the use of amiodarone in the Wolff-Parkinson-White syndrome is critically discussed by Wellens and Brugada. Heger and his colleagues compare the effects of amiodarone to the broad-spectrum Class I agent propafenone in patients with ventricular tachycardia and fibrillation. The controversial roles of programmed electrical stimulation and of ambulatory ECG monitoring as predictors of long-term response to amiodarone in the case of sustained ventricular tachyarrhythmias are explored by Kehoe and his associates. The UCLA-Wadsworth experience with amiodarone in the survivors of out-of-hospital sudden deaths presented by Nademanee and his colleagues emphasizes the potential of the drug for curtailing arrhythmic deaths. This is placed in perspective by Rakita and Mostow who consider the side effects profile of the drug, while the large potential of amiodarone to induce drug interactions is discussed by Marcus. The propensity of Class III agents to induce arrhythmogenic effects is discussed by Roden with a particular emphasis on likely mechanisms in comparison to the effects of Class I agents. Finally, Vaughan Williams, drawing on a life-time of preoccupation with the fundamental mechanisms of antiarrhythmic actions, presents a critique of the concept of the control of cardiac dysrhythmias by selectively prolonging repolarization. He provides directions for the future.

It is hoped that this book will provide further impetus for continuing experimental and clinical research towards a better understanding of what appears to be a novel pharmacological approach for a reduction in morbidity and mortality from cardiac arrhythmias.

**Bramah N. Singh, M.D.**

**Acknowledgments:** I would like to thank Lawrence Kimble and Francesca Frederick for their secretarial support throughout the course of the preparation of this book. Special thanks also go to the contributors to this monograph and to Mr. Steven Korn and his staff at Futura Publishing Company for making the path to print so smooth. Finally, I am deeply indebted to my wife, Roshni, and my children, Pramil, Nalini, and Sanjiv, for their continuous love, support, and encouragement.

# CONTENTS

Contents                                                                    xix

Chapter 1

# Cellular Electrophysiological Mechanisms of Cardiac Arrhythmias

Andrew L. Wit

Cardiac arrhythmias result from abnormalities in the rate, regularity, or site of origin of the cardiac impulse or a disturbance in the conduction of the impulse that alters the normal sequence of activation of atria and ventricles.[1] Arrhythmias thus result from abnormalities in the initiation of impulses or in conduction of these impulses through the heart.[2,3] Such alterations in impulse initiation or conduction are readily apparent in recordings of extracellular signals from the heart, in the form of the electrocardiogram. However, the recording of transmembrane electrical events of individual myocardial cells with microelectrodes has provided that information necessary for understanding the mechanisms responsible for arrhythmias. Although arrhythmias may have many different pathological causes, in the final analysis, all arrhythmias are a consequence of critical alterations in cellular electrophysiology.

## Arrhythmias Caused by Abnormal Impulse Initiation

Abnormalities of impulse initiation are an important cause of arrhythmias. The term *impulse initiation* is used to indicate that an electrical impulse can arise in a single cell or group of closely coupled cells through depolarization of the cell membrane because

From: *Control of Cardiac Arrhythmias by Lengthening Repolarization*, edited by Bramah N. Singh, MD, Futura Publishing Company Inc., Mount Kisco, NY, © 1988.

of localized changes in the ionic currents that flow across the membranes of single cells. There are two major causes for the impulse initiation that may result in arrhythmias: automaticity and triggered activity. Each has its own unique cellular mechanism resulting in membrane depolarization. Automaticity is the result of spontaneous (diastolic) phase 4 depolarization that can occur de novo, whereas triggered activity is caused by afterdepolarizations that require a preceding action potential for their induction. These different cellular mechanisms are predicted to result in arrhythmias that have very different characteristics in their mode of onset, their rate, and their response to interventions, such as external pacemakers and drugs.

## Automaticity—Normal and Abnormal

It is convenient to subdivide automaticity into normal and abnormal. Normal automaticity is found in the primary pacemaker of the heart, the sinus node as well as in certain subsidiary or latent pacemakers, which can become the pacemaker if the function of the sinus node is compromised. Impulse initiation is a normal property of these latent pacemakers. Abnormal automaticity occurs only in cardiac cells after major changes in their transmembrane potentials, whether the result of experimental interventions or pathology. This property is not confined to a specific latent pacemaker but may occur anywhere in the heart.

The cause of normal automaticity in the sinus node is a spontaneous decline in the transmembrane potential during diastole, referred to as *phase 4* or *diastolic depolarization* (Fig. 1). When the depolarization reaches threshold potential a spontaneous action potential (impulse) is initiated. Diastolic depolarization results from the gradual turning on of an inward current, called $i_f$, that is activated after repolarization of the action potential.[4,5] It is likely that a significant fraction of this membrane current is carried by Na[4,5] but activation of the slow inward Ca current also may contribute to the pacemaker depolarization.[6]

The intrinsic rate at which sinus node pacemaker cells initiate impulses is determined by the interplay of three factors: (1) the maximum diastolic potential; (2) the threshold potential; and (3) the rate or slope of phase 4 depolarization (Fig. 1). The last is related to the properties of the pacemaker current.[7] A change in any one of these factors will alter the time required for phase 4 depolarization to carry the membrane potential from its maximum diastol-

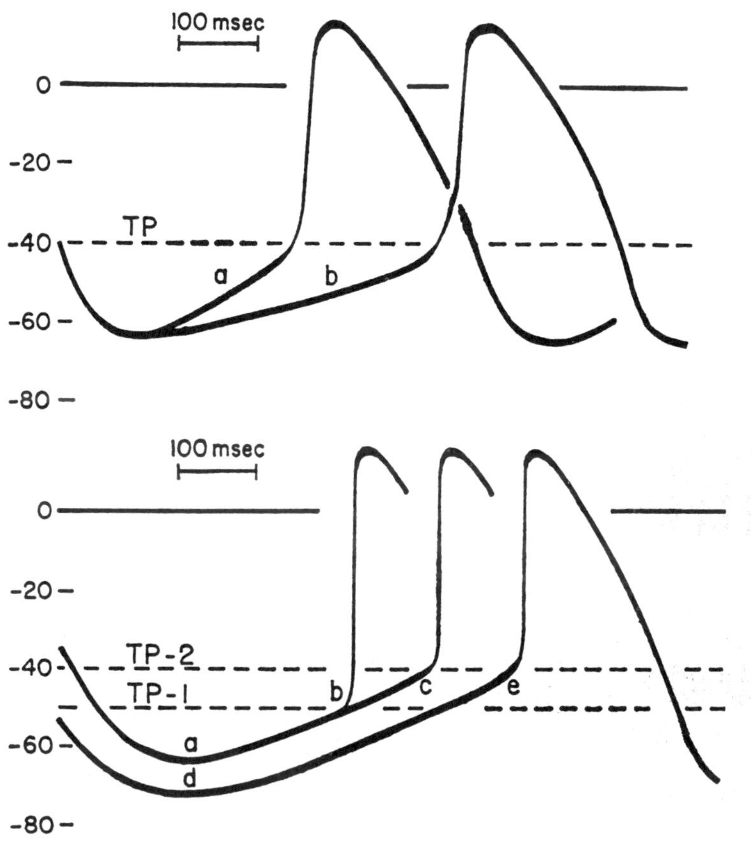


**Figure 1.** Diagram of transmembrane action potential recorded from sinus node fiber showing the mechanism responsible for impulse initiation and its change in frequency. In the upper diagram, the trace labelled *a* shows phase 4 depolarization (normal automaticity) that carries membrane potential to the threshold potential (TP), after which the action potential upstroke occurs. Trace *b* shows how a decrease in the slope or rate of phase 4 depolarization increases the time required for the transmembrane potential to reach threshold and thereby slow the rate. The diagram at the bottom shows how changes in maximum diastolic potential or threshold potential affect rate when the slope of phase 4 depolarization remains unchanged. Changing threshold potential from TP-1 to TP-2 increases the time required for phase 4 depolarization to bring membrane potential to the TP (trace *b–c*) and slows the rate. Increasing maximum diastolic potential from *a–d* has a similar effect. (Reproduced from Hoffman BF, Cranefield PF: *Electrophysiology of the Heart.* New York, McGraw-Hill Book Co., 1964, with the permission of the authors and the publisher.)

ic level to threshold and, thereby, alter the rate of impulse initiation. Such alterations in the rate of impulse initiation in the sinus node may lead to arrhythmias as will be discussed.

In addition to the sinus node, cells with pacemaking capability in the normal heart are located in some parts of the atria (plateau fibers along the crista terminalis and interatrial septum,[8] in the AV junctional region[9-11] and in the His Purkinje system.[7] The membrane currents causing spontaneous diastolic depolarization at ectopic sites have been studied most thoroughly in Purkinje fibers.[12,13] Many of the properties of the pacemaker current in Purkinje fibers appear to be similar to those of the sinus node. An inward current, carried primarily by Na ($i_f$)is initiated and increases slowly after repolarization, thereby depolarizing the membrane.[12,13] One additional important feature of this pacemaker current should be mentioned. The $i_f$ channels appear to have a gating mechanism controlling channel opening and closing that is dependent on the transmembrane voltage. At membrane potentials positive to about $-60$ mV, such as after the upstroke and during the early phases of repolarization, the channels are closed. However, in response to the potentials that occur after repolarization, negative to around $-50$ mV, the channels reopen, generating the inward current.[12,13] For this reason, when the steady state membrane potential of Purkinje fibers is reduced to $-50$ mV or less, as may sometimes occur in diseased regions of the heart, these normal pacemaker channels are not functional, and automaticity is not caused by the normal pacemaker mechanism (see discussion of abnormal automaticity later).

In the normal heart, the intrinsic rate of impulse initiation due to automaticity of cells in the sinus node is higher than that of the other potentially automatic cells and the latent pacemakers are excited by propagated impulses from the sinus node before they can depolarize spontaneously to threshold potential. Not only are latent pacemakers prevented from initiating an impulse because they are depolarized before they have a chance to fire but also the diastolic (phase 4) depolarization of the latent pacemaker cells actually is inhibited, because they are repeatedly depolarized by the impulses from the sinus node.[15,16] This inhibition can be demonstrated easily by suddenly stopping the sinus node, for example, by vagal stimulation. Impulses then usually arise from a subsidiary pacemaker, but that impulse initiation usually is preceded by a long period of quiescence.[17] Impulse initiation by the subsidiary pacemaker begins at a low rate and only gradually speeds up to a final steady rate, which is still slower, however, than the original sinus rhythm. The quiescent period following abolition of the sinus rhythm reflects the inhibitory influence exerted on the subsidiary pacemaker by the dominant sinus node pacemaker. This inhibition is called overdrive suppression. Overdrive suppression has been best characterized in microelectrode studies on isolated Purkinje fiber bundles exhibiting pacemaker activity[15] (Fig. 2); it results from driving a pacemaker cell faster than its intrinsic spontaneous rate and is mediated by an electrogenic current that results from enhanced activity of the $Na^+$-$K^+$ exchange pump.[18,19]

The sinus node, itself, also can be overdrive suppressed, if it is driven at a rate more rapid than its intrinsic rate.[20,21] Thus, there may be a quiescent period after termination of a rapid ectopic tachycardia before sinus rhythm resumes.[22] However, when overdrive suppression of the normal sinus node occurs, it is of lesser magnitude than that of subsidiary pacemakers overdriven at comparable rates.[20] The relative resistance of the normal sinus node to overdrive suppression may be important in enabling it to remain as the dominant pacemaker even when its rhythm is transiently

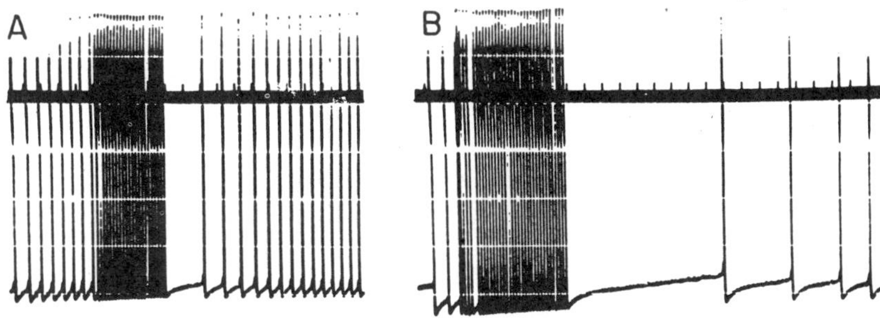

**Figure 2.** Overdrive suppression of normal automaticity in a Purkinje fiber. The first eight action potentials in panel A occurred sponaneously at the intrinsic firing rate of the Purkinje fiber. Note the phase 4 depolarization preceding the upstroke of the action potential. A period of rapid stimulation was then imposed for 25 sec (stimulus pulses are shown in the bottom trace). At the end of the period of stimulation, there was a short quiescent period followed by reappearance of the spontaneous rhythm that gradually increased to the control rate. In panel B, a longer period of overdrive (stimulus pulses shown in bottom trace) was followed by prolonged quiescence and a far slower return to the control rate. The time marks in the top trace occurred at 5 msec intervals. (Reproduced from Cranefield PF: *The Slow Response and Cardiac Arrhythmias*. Futura, Mt. Kisco, 1975, with the permission of the author and publisher.)

perturbed by external influences (such as transient shifts of the pacemaker to an ectopic site). The diseased sinus node, however, may be much more easily overdrive suppressable.[23]

Arrhythmias caused by the normal automaticity of cardiac fibers may occur for several different reasons. Such arrhythmias might result simply from an alteration in rate of impulse initiation by the normal sinus node pacemaker without a shift of impulse origin to an ectopic site; sinus bradycardia and tachycardia are such arrhythmias. The cellular mechanisms that can change the rate of sinus node impulse initiation have been described earlier.

A shift in the site of impulse initiation to one of the regions where subsidiary pacemakers are located is another factor that results in arrhythmias caused by a normal automatic mechanism. This would be expected to happen when any of the following occurs: (1) the rate at which the sinus node activates subsidiary pacemakers falls considerably below the intrinsic rate of the subsidiary pacemakers, or (2) impulse initiation in subsidiary pacemakers is enhanced.

The rate at which the sinus node activates subsidiary pacemakers may be decreased in a number of situations. Impulse initiation by the sinus node may be slowed or inhibited altogether by heightened activity in the parasympathetic nervous system[24] or as a result of sinus node disease.[25] Alternatively, there may be block of impulse conduction from the sinus node to the atria or block of conduction from the atria to the ventricles. Under any of these conditions there may be "escape" of a subsidiary pacemaker as a result of removal of overdrive suppression by the sinus pacemaker. Once overdrive suppression is removed the pacemaker with the fastest rate becomes the site of impulse origin after sinus node inhibition.[26]

Subsidiary pacemaker activity also may be enhanced, causing impulse initiation to shift to ectopic sites even when sinus node function is normal. Norepinephrine released locally from sympathetic nerves steepens the slope of diastolic depolarization of latent pacemaker cells[10,27] and diminishes the inhibitory effects of overdrive.[28] Localized effects may occur in the absence of sinus node stimulation.[29] Therefore, sympathetic stimulation may enable membrane potential of ectopic pacemakers to reach threshold before they are activated by an impulse from the sinus node, resulting in ectopic premature impulses or automatic rhythms.[30]

The flow of current between partially depolarized myocardium and normally polarized latent pacemaker cells also might enhance automaticity.[31] This mechanism has been proposed to be a cause of some of the ectopic beats that arise at the borders of ischemic areas in the ventricle.[32]

Inhibition of the electrogenic Na-K pump results in a net increase in inward current during diastole because such inhibition causes a decrease in the outward current normally generated by the pump.[18] Therefore, automaticity in subsidiary pacemakers may be increased. This might occur after ATP is depleted during prolonged hypoxia or ischemia or in the presence of toxic amounts of digitalis.[33] A decrease in the extracellular K level also enhances normal automaticity,[34] as does acute stretch.[35]

Working atrial and ventricular myocardial cells do not normally show spontaneous diastolic depolarization and do not initiate spontaneous impulses, even when they are not excited for long periods of time by propagating impulses. They do not have pacemaker membrane currents at their normal range of membrane potentials. However, when the resting potential of atrial or ventricular myocardial cells are experimentally reduced to less than about $-60$ V, spontaneous diastolic depolarization may occur and cause repetitive impulse initiation.[36,37] This is called *abnormal automaticity*. Likewise, cells such as those in the Purkinje system, which are normally automatic at high levels of membrane potential, also show abnormal automaticity when membrane potential is reduced [38,39] (Fig. 3). However, if a low level of membrane potential is employed as the only criterion for abnormal automaticity, the automaticity of the SA node would have to be considered abnormal. Therefore, an important distinction for abnormal automaticity is that the membrane potentials of fibers showing this type of activity are reduced markedly from their own normal level.[3]

At the low level of membrane potential at which abnormal automaticity occurs, it is likely that at least some of the ionic currents causing the automatic activity are not the same as those causing normal automatic activity. A likely cause of automaticity at membrane potentials of around $-50$ mV is deactivation of a $K^+$ current referred to as $ix_i$.[40] Under normal conditions, this current functions to repolarize the membrane after the upstroke of an action potential. In addition, the spontaneously occurring action potentials usually are slow responses (action potentials with upstrokes dependent on slow inward current[39]) because the fast inward $Na^+$ current is inactivated at the low levels of membrane potential.

Myocardial fibers with low resting potentials will not fire au-

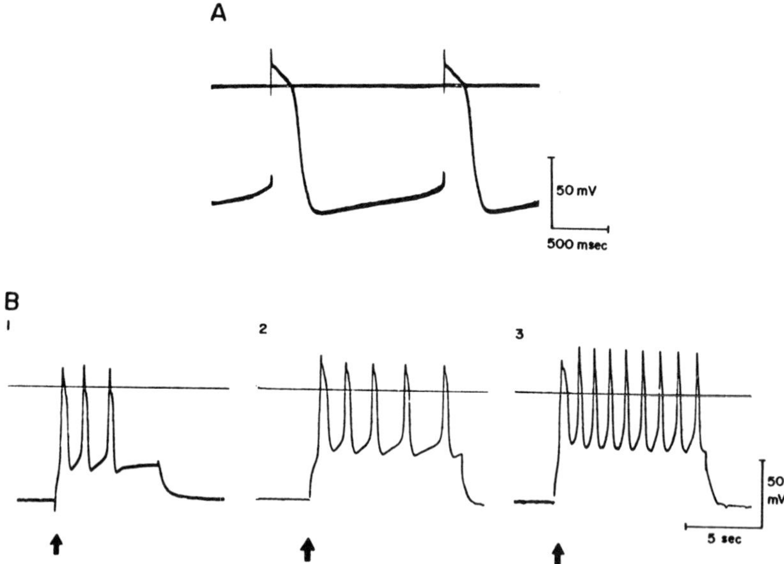


**Figure 3.** Normal and abnormal automaticity in a canine Purkinje fiber. Panel A shows automatic firing of a Purkinje fiber with a maximum diastolic potential of −85 mV. Panel B shows the abnormal automaticity that can occur when membrane potential is decreased. At the left (1), when the fiber was depolarized (at the arrow) to a membrane potential of −45 mV by injectng a long-lasting current pulse through a microelectrode, 3 automatic action potentials occurred. In the center (2), a larger amplitude current pulse at the arrow reduced membrane potential to −40 mV, resulting in more sustained automatic activity. At the right (3), a still larger current pulse (at the arrow) reduced membrane potential to −30 mV and automatic activity occurred at a still faster rate. Automaticity in atrial or ventricular muscle also occurred when the membrane potential was decreased in a similar way. (From Wit AL, Friedman PF: Bases for ventricular arrhythmias accompanying myocardial infarction. *Arch Int Med* 1975; 135:459, 1975, with permission of the publisher).

tomatically if the sinus node drives them faster than their intrinsic abnormal automatic rate. An abnormal automatic focus should manifest itself and cause an arrhythmia when the sinus rate decreases below the intrinsic rate of the focus or when the rate of the focus increases above that of the sinus node, as was discussed for latent pacemakers with normal automaticity. A similar interplay between maximum diastolic potential, threshold potential, and rate of phase 4 depolarization determines the rate of impulse initiation by the abnormal pacemaker. However, there is an important distinction between the effects of the dominant sinus pacemaker on the two kinds of foci; that is, abnormal automaticity is not over-drive suppressed to the same extent as the normal automaticity that occurs at high levels of membrane potential.[41] Moreover, the amount of suppression of spontaneous diastolic depolarization by overdrive is related directly to the level of membrane potential at which the automatic rhythm occurs.[41] For example, Purkinje fibers showing automaticity at membrane potentials of −60 to −70 mV still manifest some overdrive suppression, although less than those fibers with automaticity at −90 mV. Automaticity in Purkinje fibers with membrane potentials less than −60mV is hardly suppressed by short periods of overdrive. At normal sinus rates, there may be little overdrive suppression of pacemakers with abnormal automaticity. Because of the lack of overdrive suppression, even transient sinus pauses or occasional long sinus cycle lengths may permit the ectopic focus to capture the heart for one or more beats. On the other hand, an ectopic pacemaker with normal automaticity probably would be quiescent during relatively short, transient sinus pauses, because they are overdrive suppressed.

It is also possible that the depolarized level of membrane potential at which abnormal automaticity occurs might cause entrance block into the focus and prevent it from being overdriven by the sinus node.[42] This would lead to parasystole, an example of an arrhythmia caused by a combination of an abnormality of impulse conduction and initiation.

The firing rate of an abnormally automatic focus also might be enhanced above that of the sinus node leading to arrhythmias in the absence of sinus node suppression or conduction block between the focus and surrounding myocardium. The automatic rate is a direct function of the level of membrane potential—the greater the depolarization, the faster the rate.[36,37] Experimental studies have shown firing rates in muscle and Purkinje fibers of 150−200/min at membrane potentials less than −50 mV, and these rates appear to be sufficiently rapid to enable these pacemakers to control the heart. Catecholamines also increase abnormal automaticity.[43]

## Afterdepolarizations and Triggered Activity

Afterdepolarizations are oscillations in membrane potential that follow an action potential. These oscillations are divided into two subcategories: early afterdepolarizations precede full repolarization of the membrane; and delayed afterdepolarizations follow repolarization. Both of these types of afterdepolarizations, in turn, are capable of initiating the arrhythmias referred to as *triggered*. Triggered arrhythmias must be initiated by a conducted or stimulated action potential (the trigger) and cannot arise during a period of quiescence, such as that caused by sinus node inhibition. This contrasts with the characteristics of automaticity.

*Early Afterdepolarizations*

Early afterdepolarizations most frequently occur during repolarization of an action potential that has been initiated from a high level of membrane potential (usually between $-75$ and $-90$ mV). They may appear as oscillations at the plateau level of membrane potential or later, during phase 3 of repolarization. When the oscillation is large enough the decrease in membrane potential leads to an increase in inward (depolarizing) current, and a second action potential occurs prior to complete repolarization of the first. The second action potential occurring during repolarization is triggered in the sense that it is evoked by an early afterdepolarization that, in turn, is induced by the preceding action potential. Without the preceding action potential there would be no second upstroke. The second action potential also may be followed by other action potentials, all occurring at the low level of membrane potential characteristic of the plateau or phase 3 (Fig. 4). The sustained rhythmic activity that ensues may continue for a variable number of impulses and terminates when the increase in membrane potential associated with repolarization of the initiating action potential returns membrane potential to a high level. Triggered activity may occur again when the next action potential is initiated from the high level of membrane potential. Sometimes, repolarization to the high level of membrane potential may not occur, and membrane potential may remain at the plateau level or at a level intermediate between the plateau and the resting potential. The sustained rhythmic activity then may continue at the reduced level of membrane potential.

Little is known about the ionic mechanisms that cause early afterdepolarizations although they are likely to result from abnormalities in the repolarizing membrane currents. Normally, the net outward membrane current during the plateau shifts membrane potential progressively in a negative direction. An early afterdepolarization might occur if there is a shift in the current voltage relationship resulting in a region of net inward current during the plateau range of membrane potentials. This would retard or prevent repolarization[45] and might lead to a secondary depolarization

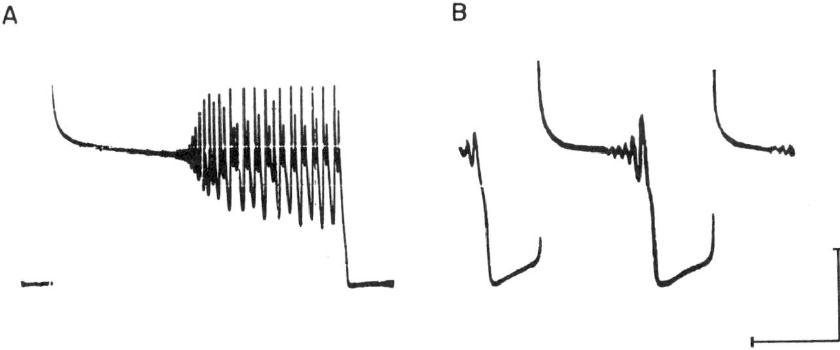

**Figure 4.** Panel A shows early afterdepolarizations and triggered activity in a Purkinje fiber from a monkey heart at the plateau level of the action potential. The triggered activity resulted because the time course for repolarization was markedly prolonged. Panel B shows action potentials recorded from another fiber, which had spontaneous diastolic depolarization at a high level of membrane potential. Small membrane oscillations were occurring during the plateau. (Reproduced from Wit AL, Wiggens R, Cranefield PF: Some effects of electrical stimulation on impulse initiation in cardiac fibers: Its relevance for the determination of the mechanism of clinical cardiac arrhythmias, in Wellens, HJJ, Janse M, Lie H (eds): *The Conduction System of the Heart.* Stenfert Kroesse Leiden, 1976, pp. 163–181.)

during the plateau or phase 3 if a regenerative inward current is activated. The second upstroke, and any subsequent action potentials that arise from the low levels of membrane potential during the plauteau, are slow responses (Fig. 4); that is, the inward current responsible for the upstroke flows through the slow channel because the fast channel is in the inactivated state.[39] Action potentials that arise during phase 3 (Fig. 5) might have upstrokes caused by current flowing through partially reactivated fast Na channels or a combination of slow and fast channels.

Conditions that increase the inward current components or decrease the outward current components during repolarization are expected to induce the shift in the current-voltage relationship that causes early afterdepolarizations. Early afterdepolarizations leading to triggered activity in isolated cardiac preparations may be caused by factors present in the heart in situ under some pathological conditions. Among these factors are hypoxia,[46] high $pCO_2$,[47] and high concentrations of catecholamines.[48] Data are not yet available to elucidate how they exert their effects. Since catecholamines, hypoxia, and elevated $pCO_2$ may be present in an ischemic or infarcted region of the ventricles, it is possible that

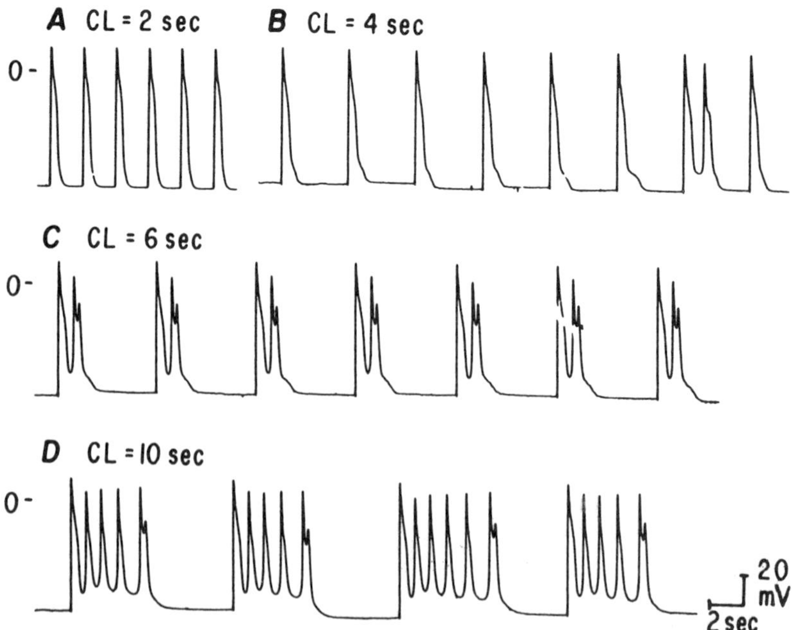


**Figure 5** Early afterdepolarizations in Purkinje fibers. Panel A shows the transmembrane potentials recorded from a Purkinje fiber stimulated at a cycle length of 2 sec (CL = 2 sec). Repolarization appears to be normal. When the stimulus cycle length was decreased to 4 sec (panel B) an early afterdepolarization appeared during phase 3 of repolarization. At the right, a second upstroke or triggered action potential arose from the early afterdepolarization. At a stimulus cycle length of 6 sec (panel C), a single triggered action potential occurred during phase 3 of each stimulated action potential. An early afterdepolarization also occurred during the plateau of the triggered action potential. At a stimulus cycle length of 10 sec (panel D), a burst of triggered action potentials occurred during phase 3 of each stimulated action potential (arrows point to stimulated action potentials). (Reproduced from Damiano BP, Rosen MR: Effects of pacing on triggered activity induced by early afterdepolarizations. *Circulation* 1984; 69:1013, with permission of the American Heart Association.)

early afterdepolarizations may cause some of the arrhythmias that occur soon after myocardial ischemia.

Some drugs used clinically that markedly prolong the time course for repolarization, such as the β receptor blocking drug sotalol[49] and the antiarrhythmic drug N-acetyl procainamide[50] also might cause early afterdepolarizations and triggered activity. These drugs in high concentrations have been shown to cause cardiac arrhythmias in experimental animals and in patients that may be triggered.[50,51]

Since the occurrence of early afterdepolarizations is facilitated by a decrease in net repolarizing current, a slowing of the rate at which the triggering action potentials are elicited also might favor the occurrence of the afterdepolarizations[52] (Fig. 5). As the drive rate slows, the action potential duration prolongs, reflecting a decrease in net outward current. It, therefore, seems likely that some tachycardias that occur after a period of bradycardia might be caused by early afterdepolarizations.[53,54] It also has been suggested that tachycardias in patients with the long QT interval syndrome (in which there may be a long ventricular action potential duration) are triggered.[54]

*Delayed Afterdepolarizations*

Delayed afterdepolarizations are oscillations in membrane potential that occur after repolarization of an action potential and are induced by that action potential (Fig. 6). One or more oscillations may occur after each action potential. Delayed afterdepolarizations may be subthreshold, but when they are large enough to bring the membrane potential to the threshold of a regenerative inward current a nondriven (triggered) impulse arises, which also may be followed by an afterdepolarization. The impulse is said to be triggered, since it would not have occurred without the preceding action potential.[39,44]

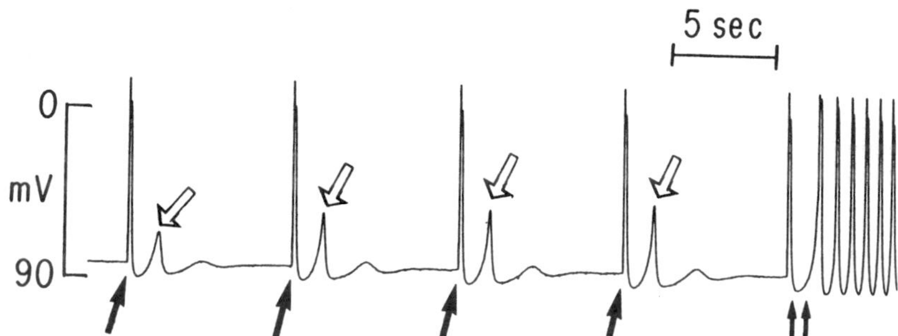



**Figure 6.** Delayed afterdepolarizations caused by catecholamines recorded from an atrial fiber in an isolated, superfused preparation of canine coronary sinus tissue. The black arrows point to the stimulated action potentials and the unfilled arrows to the large afterdepolarizations that follow each action potential. A second, smaller afterdepolarization follows the large one. The afterdepolarization amplitude is increasing with each stimulated impulse until it reaches threshold and causes triggered activity (double black arrow at the right).

Delayed afterdepolarizations occur under a number of conditions in which there is either a large increase in the intracellular Ca or an abnormality in the sequestration or release of calcium by the sarcoplasmic retriculum or a combination of the two. One of the causes most widely recognized is toxic amounts of cardiac glycosides, which cause an increase in $Ca_i$.[55,56] Cardiac glycosides inhibit the $Na^+$-$K^+$ pump, thereby leading to an increase in $Na_i$.[57] This in turn increases the intracellular $Ca^{++}$ through a $Na^+$-$Ca^{++}$ exchange mechanism.[58] Catecholamines can cause delayed afterdepolarizations,[10,59,60] possibly because they enhance Ca entry into cardiac fibers by increasing the slow inward current.[61]

Delayed afterdepolarizations also may occur in the absence of drugs or catecholamines. They have been identified in fibers in the upper pectinate muscles bordering the crista terminalis in the rabbit heart,[62] in hypertrophied ventricular myocardium,[63] in human atrial myocardium,[64] and in Purkinje fibers surviving on the subendocardial surface of canine infarcts.[65]

The mechanism by which elevated intracellular Ca causes delayed afterdepolarizations has been explored in studies utilizing voltage clamp techniques to control the depolarization of the membrane and to measure ionic currents.[66–69] Delayed afterdepolarizations result from a transient inward current activated by repolarization after a depolarizing voltage clamp pulse. The link between the depolarization (whether caused by a voltage clamp or by an action potential) and the subsequent transient inward current may involve release and reuptake of Ca from the sarcoplasmic reticulum. Normally, release is initiated by the depolarization phase of the action potential and reuptake is complete by the end of the action potential. However, if the sarcoplasmic reticulum is overloaded with Ca, it may not be able to take up all the Ca or there may be a secondary release of Ca after repolarization.[70] The increased level of intracellular Ca in the cytoplasm at this time (after the action potential) is proposed to alter sarcolemmal permeability, causing activation of a nonspecific membrane channel that allows an inward movement of a positive charge carried mainly by Na, and the delayed afterdepolarization occurs.[71] There are some dissenting opinions, however, concerning the mechanism for the inward current during the delayed afterdepolarization. It also has been proposed that this current results from electrogenic exchange of Ca for Na.[69,72] The exact mechanism, therefore, requires further clarification.

Delayed afterdepolarizations may not be large enough to reach threshold, in which case triggered activity does not occur. Triggering may result in fibers showing subthreshold afterdepolarizations, if the rate is increased at which the fiber is driven (Fig. 7). A decrease in the length of even a single drive cycle (i.e., a premature impulse) may increase the amplitude of the afterdepolarization of the action potential that follows the short cycle. As the premature impulse occurs earlier and earlier after the previous impulse, the amplitude of the afterdepolarizations that follow the premature impulse increases and may reach threshold, initiating triggered activity. The likelihood of a premature impulse initiating triggered activity is increased at more rapid basic drive rates. In cardiac Purkinje fibers made toxic by too much digitalis, at least two afterdepolarizations usually are present at relatively slow rates of drive. The first afterdepolarization is larger than the second. As the drive cycle length is decreased to around 500 msec, the amplitude of the first oscillation increases to its maximum and triggered activity may occur sometimes. If it does not occur and drive cycle length is decreased further, the amplitude of the second afterdepol-

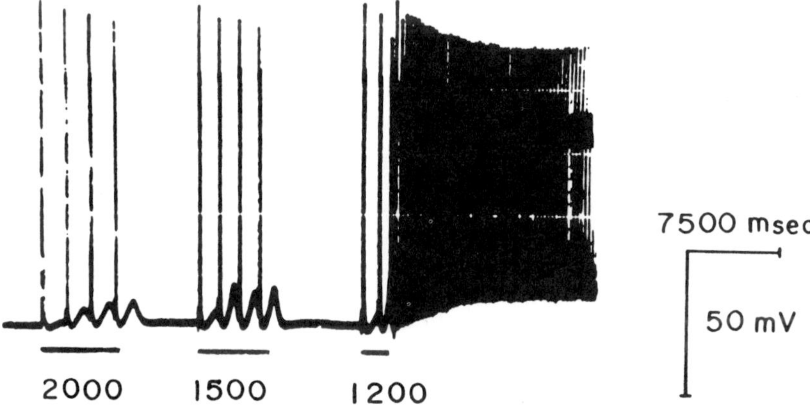


**Figure 7.** Effects of stimulus rate on afterdepolarization amplitude. The transmembrane potentials shown were recorded from an atrial fiber in the canine coronary sinus superfused with Tyrode's solution containing norepinephrine. The records at the left were recorded when the fiber was stimulated at a cycle length of 2000 msec for 4 impulses (underlined). The afterdepolarization following the last driven impulse had an amplitude of 10 mV. In the center, four impulses were stimulated at a cycle length of 1500 msec. The afterdepolarization following the last driven impulse had an amplitude of 17 mV. At the right, after two impulses were stimulated at a cycle length of 1200 msec (underlined) sustained rhythmic activity was triggered. The rate was too rapid for the individual upstrokes to be apparent. Maximum diastolic potential decreased during the initial period of triggered activity.

arization increases while the first declines, and triggered action potentials may arise from the second oscillation.[73]

There may be some differences in the characteristics of triggered activity resulting from delayed afterdepolarizations, depending upon the cause. The initial period of triggered activity in atrial fibers caused by catecholamines often is characterized by a gradual decrease in the cycle length, after which a relatively constant cycle length occurs.[10,74] This decrease in cycle length may be accompanied by a decrease in maximum diastolic potential, at least partly a result of accumulation of $K^+$ outside the cell during rapid activity due to restricted diffusion in the extracellular space.[75] The decrease in maximum diastolic potential contributes to the gradual acceleration in the rate of triggered activity, since the rate increases as membrane potential decreases in the same way as described for abnormal automaticity. Similar characteristics also have been shown for triggered activity caused by factors other than catecholamines in atrial, ventricular, and Purkinje fibers. On the other hand, during triggered activity in Purkinje fibers exposed to toxic amounts of digitalis, there usually is not a gradual increase in rate, but rather the maximum triggered rate is attained after a few impulses.[76]

Triggered activity often terminates spontaneously. When catecholamine induced triggered activity in atrial fibers of the coronary sinus terminates, the rate usually slows gradually before termination. This gradual slowing is accompanied by a progressive increase in the maximum diastolic potential. A delayed afterdepolarization usually follows the last triggered impulse.[10,74] The spontaneous termination of triggered activity in canine coronary sinus fibers (and probably in other types of cardiac fibers, as well) is caused, at least in part, by an increase in the rate of electrogenic sodium extrusion.[74] Triggered activity caused by digitalis toxicity probably stops by another mechanism. Termination of a triggered burst usually is not associated with gradual slowing and hyperpolarization but often by speeding of the rate, a decrease in action potential amplitude, and depolarization. Termination probably is not related to activity of the $Na^+$ pump, since the pump is inhibited by the digitalis.

## Abnormal Impulse Conduction and Reentry

The second major cause of arrhythmias is abnormal impulse conduction. One means whereby conduction abnormalities can cause arrhythmias has been discussed already; that is, the escape of subsidiary pacemakers that occurs when there is sinoatrial or atrioventricular block. Abnormal impulse conduction also causes reentrant excitation, a mechanism for arrhythmias that does not depend on pacemaker activity. During sinus rhythm, the conducting impulse usually dies out after sequential activation of the atria and ventricles, because it is surrounded by tissue that it recently excited and that, therefore, is refractory. A new impulse must arise in the sinus node for subsequent activation. Under special conditions, the propagating impulse may not die out after complete activation of the heart but may persist to reexcite (reenter) the atria or ventricles after the end of the refractory period.

For reentry to occur, a region of block must be present, at least transiently.[77] The block is necessary to provide the return pathway for the reentering impulse to the region it is to reexcite. Transient block causing reentry, can occur in the heart after premature excitation (discussed later). Reentry also may occur when there is permanent block, but the block then must be unidirectional. A unidirectional block often occurs in cardiac fibers in which excitability and conduction are depressed.

In addition, for reentry to occur, the impulse must always find excitable tissue in the direction in which it is propagating. This requires that the conduction time around the reentrant pathway be longer than the effective refractory period of the cardiac fibers that compose the pathway. If it is not, conduction of the reentering impulse would block. Normal heart muscle (excluding nodal fibers) has a refractory period that ranges from about 150 to 500 msec and a conduction velocity that ranges from about 0.5 to 2 m/sec. Therefore, the impulse conducting at a normal velocity of at least 0.5 m/sec in a reentrant pathway must conduct for at least 150 msec before it can return and reexcite a region it previously has excited. This means the conduction pathway must be at least 7.5 cm long for reentry to occur in cardiac fibers with normal properties of conduction and refractoriness. Such long reentrant pathways, functionally isolated from the rest of the heart, rarely exist. Clearly, the length of the pathway necessary for reentry can be shortened if the conduction velocity is slowed and/or the refractory period is reduced. For example, if conduction velocity is slowed to 0.05 m/sec (as can occur in diseased cardiac fibers or in the normal sinus or AV node), the reentrant circuit need be no more than 7.5 mm in length. Circuits of this size can readily exist in the heart. Therefore, slowed conduction in combination with unidirectional block are prerequisites that permit reentry to occur.

The "loop" of tissue that enables reentry to occur is called *the reentrant circuit*. It can be located almost anywhere in the heart and can assume a variety of sizes and shapes. The circuit may be an anatomical structure, such as a ring of cardiac fibers in the peripheral Purkinje system. The circuit also may be functional and its existence, size, and shape determined by electrophysiological properties of cardiac cells rather than anatomy. The size and location of an anatomically defined reentrant circuit obviously remains fixed and results in what may be termed *ordered reentry*. The size and location of reentrant circuits dependent on functional properties rather than anatomy also may be fixed, but they also may change with time, leading to *random* reentry. Random reentry probably is associated most often with atrial or ventricular fibrillation, whereas ordered reentry can cause most other types of arrhythmias.[3]

## Mechanisms for Slow Conduction

There can be a number of causes for the slowed conduction and block that predispose to the occurrence of reentry. The speed at which the impulse propagates in cardiac fibers is dependent on certain features of their transmembrane action potentials and passive electrical properties.[78] Alterations in either (by cardiac pathology) can result in reentrant arrhythmias. An important feature of the transmembrane potentials of working (atrial and ventricular) myocardial and Purkinje fibers that govern the speed of propagation is the magnitude of the inward Na current flowing through the fast Na channels in the sarcolemma during the upstroke and the rapidity with which this current reaches its maximum intensity. A reduction in this inward current, leading to a reduction in the rate and amplitude of depolarization, may decrease axial current flow, slow conduction, and lead to conduction block. Such a reduction may result from inactivation of Na channels caused by a reduction of the membrane potential.[79,80] Premature activation of the heart, therefore, can induce reentry, because premature impulses conduct slowly in regions of the heart where the cardiac fibers are not completely repolarized (where $Na^+$ channels are to some extent inactivated) and conduction of premature impulses may block in regions where cells have not yet repolarized to about $-60$ mV. Hence, the prerequisites for reentry—slow conduction and block—can be brought about by premature activation.

Reentry also might occur in cardiac cells with persistently low levels of resting potential, which may be between $-60$ and $-70$ mV, caused by disease. At these resting potentials, a significant fraction of the $Na^+$ channels is inactivated and, therefore, unavailable for activation by a depolarizing stimulus. The magnitude of the net inward current during phase 0 of the action potential is reduced and consequently both the speed and amplitude of the upstroke is diminished, decreasing axial current flow and slowing conduction significantly.

The slow inward current that causes the action potential plateau inactivates much more slowly than the fast Na current and gradually diminishes as the cell repolarizes.[81] Under special conditions, this slow inward current also may underlie the occurrence of the slow conduction that causes reentrant arrhythmias.[39] Although the fast Na channel may be largely inactivated at membrane potentials near $-50$ mV, the slow inward channel is not inactivated and still is available for activation.[39,80,81] Under certain conditions in cells with resting potentials less than $-60$ mV (such as when membrane conductance is very low or when catecholamines are present), this normally weak slow inward current may give rise to the regenerative depolarization characteristic of a propagated action potential. This propagated action potential dependent on slow inward current alone is *the slow response*.[39] Since this inward current is weak, conduction velocity is slow and both unidirectional and bidirectional conduction block may occur.[39] Slow reponse action potentials can occur in diseased cardiac fibers with low resting potentials, but they also occur in some normal tissues of the heart, such as cells of the sinoatrial and atrioventricular nodes where the maximum diastolic potential is normally less than about $-70$ mV.[39,82]

The slow conduction and block necessary for reentry also can be caused by factors other than the decrease in inward current accompanying a decrease in membrane potential. An increased resistance to axial current flow, which is expressed as *effective axial resistance* (resistance to current flow in the direction of propagation dependent on the intracellular and extracellular resistivities), may decrease conduction velocity.[83,84] Whether an increase in extracellular resistance to current flow sufficient enough to impair conduction and cause arrhythmias occurs during pathological states is not yet known. It is likely, however, that sufficient increases in intracellular resistance can occur. Although the intracellular resistance depends on both the resistance of the cytoplasm and the resistance at the intercalated discs that couple cells together, the changes in intracellular resistance causing slow conduction and arrhythmias probably result mainly from changes in resistance at the discs.

During conduction of the impulse, axial current flows from one myocardial cell to the adjacent cell through the gap junctions of the discs, which normally have a relatively low resistance,[78] and therefore, the resistance, extent, and distribution of these junctions have a profound influence on conduction. This influence can be seen even in the normal atrial or ventricular myocardium. In regions where the cardiac muscle fibers are packed closely together and arranged parallel to each other in a uniform manner, conduction in the direction parallel to the myocardial fiber orientation (along the long axis of the myocardial fibers) is much more rapid than in the direction perpendicular to the long axis.[83-85] Conduction perpendicular to the long axis of the fibers can be as slow as 0.1 m/sec even though resting and action potentials of the muscle fibers are normal. The slow conduction is caused by an effective axial resistivity, which is higher in the direction perpendicular to fiber orientation than parallel to fiber orientation. This higher axial resistivity results in part from fewer and shorter intercalated discs connecting myocardial fibers in a side-to-side direction than in the end-to-end direction. Conduction in the normal myocardium, therefore, might be slow enough to cause reentry.

Pathological alterations in anatomy also may cause slow conduction by increasing axial resistance through effects on coupling between cells. Fibrosis in the heart separates myocardial fibers, reducing the number of discs connections and decreasing the extent or area of connections that remain. An example is the effect of fibrosis resulting from the healing of an infarct on the myocardial fibers that survive in the infarcted region (Fig. 8). The broad, wide discs at the longitudinal ends of normal cells no longer are present because of the deformation of the cells by the connective tissue. Only short segments of intercalated discs remain in some regions. Conduction is very slow, despite the presence of normal resting potentials and normal action potentials, probably because there is a high resistance to current flow through the shortened discs[86,87] (Fig. 9). Similarly, fibrosis occurring in diseased or aged atrial myocardium may lead to slow conduction.[88]

In addition to structural changes, a rise in intracellular Ca might slow conduction by increasing resistance to current flow through gap junctions in the discs, since Ca levels profoundly affect the resistance of the gap junction.[89] This may occur during pro-

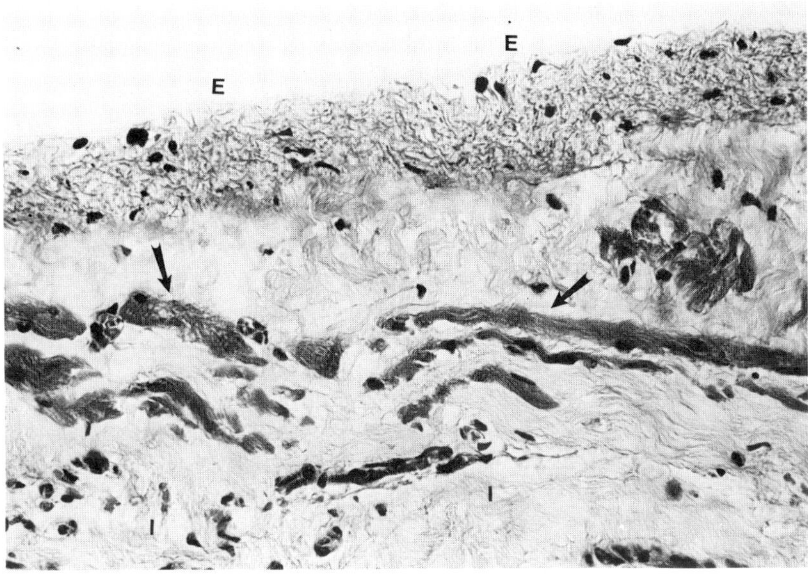


**Figure 8.** Surviving muscle fibers on the epicardial surface of the healed myocardial infarct in the canine heart. Beneath the epicardium (E), a few layers of viable muscle (arrows) remain 16 months after coronary occlusion. Directly beneath this muscle is the healed infarct (I). The entrapped muscle fibers are separated and distorted by connective tissue.

longed periods of ischemia.[90] Cardiac glycosides also increase resistance at the discs by increasing intracellular Ca.[91]

The effective axial resistivity also is dependent on the size and shape of the myocardial cells. Resistance to current flow may increase markedly and conduction may be slowed in regions where cells branch or where there are abrupt increases in cell size or number.[83,84,92,93]

## Reentrant Arrhythmias

Reentry can occur in different regions of the heart, utilizing either anatomical or functional pathways. Slow conduction and block may have a number of different cellular mechanisms. Conceivably, any of these mechanisms may occur in either an anatomical or functional reentrant pathway.

### Anatomical Pathways

Reentrant excitation caused by the slow conduction and block that accompany depression of the action potential upstroke (either

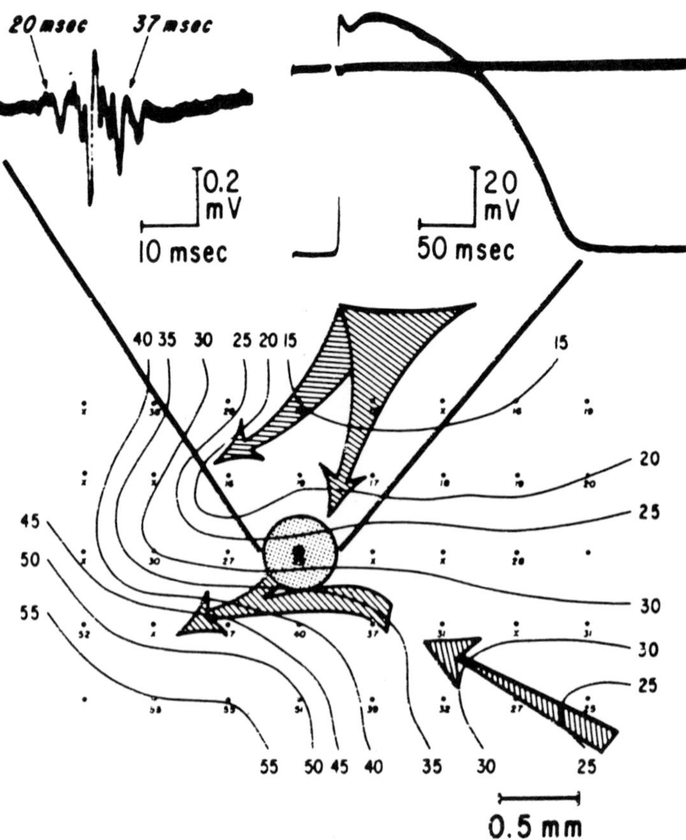



**Figure 9.**   Activation map of an epicardial region from a healed canine infarct (2 months old), superfused with Tyrode's solution in a tissue chamber. The points at which action potentials were recorded to construct this map are shown by the dots. A representative action potential is shown at the top right, and a fractionated electrogram recorded with a bipolar electrode (from region of the stippled circle on the map) is shown at the top left. A distance scale is at the bottom right. Activation is very slow despite the normal transmembrane potentials. (Reproduced from Gardner PI, Ursell PC, Fenoglio JJ Jr, et al: Electrophysiologic and anatomic basis for fractionated electrograms recorded from healed myocardial infarcts. *Circulation* 1985; 72:596−611; with permission of American Heart Association.)

because of premature excitation or because of a persistent reduction in the resting membrane potential) may occur in gross anatomically distinct circuits (around an anatomical obstacle). Reentrant excitation involving an anatomically distinct circuit and obstacle is exemplified by reentry in a loop of cardiac fiber bundles, such as a loop of Purkinje fiber bundles in the distal conduction system.[94] Anatomical circuits also might be formed by bundles of surviving muscle fibers in healed infarcts or in fibrotic regions of the atria or ventricles. The critically slow conduction and block may be caused by depressed transmembrane potentials, such as in the atria of hearts with cardiomyopathy[95] or by increased effective axial resistivity as in healed infarcts.[86] Gross anatomical circuits also are involved in reentry utilizing the bundle branches, which may cause ventricular tachycardia;[96] reentry utilizing an accessory AV connecting pathway, which may cause supraventricular tachycardia;[97] and reentry around the tricuspid ring, which may cause atrial flutter.[98]

*Functional Pathways*

Gross anatomical loops and anatomical obstacles are not a prerequisite for the occurrence of reentry. A kind of reentry termed *reflection* occurs in unbranched bundles of Purkinje fibers in which conduction is slow because the resting and action potentials are depressed.[39] During reflection, excitation occurs slowly in one direction along a bundle of fibers and is followed by excitation occurring in the opposite direction. The returning (reflected) impulse may be caused by reentry due to functional longitudinal dissociation of the bundles. Antzelevitch, Jalife, and Moe also have described another mechanism that may cause reflection and that is dependent on delayed activation of part of a bundle resulting from electrotonic excitation of a region distal to an inexcitable segment.[99,100]

Another mechanism that can cause reentry in functional pathways is the *leading circle* mechanism originally described by Allessie et al. in experiments on atrial muscle.[101–103] Reentry is initiated by precisely timed premature impulses in regions normally activated at regular rates of stimulation. Initiation of reentry is made possible by the different refractory periods of atrial fibers in close proximity to one another.[101] The premature impulse that initiates reentry blocks in fibers with long refractory periods and conducts in fibers with shorter refractory periods, eventually returning to the initial region of block after excitability recovers there. The impulse then may continue to circulate around a central area, which is kept refractory because it is bombarded constantly by impulses propagating toward it from all sides of the circuit. This central area provides a functional obstacle that prevents excitation from propagating across the fulcrum of the circuit.

Functional reentry also occurs in the epicardial border zone of infarcts in the canine heart.[104–106] This region is comprised of a thin sheet of ventricular muscle that survives on the epicardial surface of the infarcts.[86] During tachycardias induced by premature ventricular stimulation, circuitous excitation of the border zones occurs. The reentrant circuits may be in the form of a figure of eight[104]—two reentrant circuits joined by a common pathway (Fig. 10). Activation occurs around a central line of conduction delay or block (thick black line in Fig. 10). During sinus rhythm, the epicardial border zone is activated uniformly, sometimes without any evidence of conduction delay or block.

The anisotropic properties of atrial and ventricular myocardium also may predispose to functional reentrant circuits.[83,84] Conduction transverse to the long axis of myocardial cells may be slow enough to permit recovery of excitability and reexcitation of regions that have been excited previously.

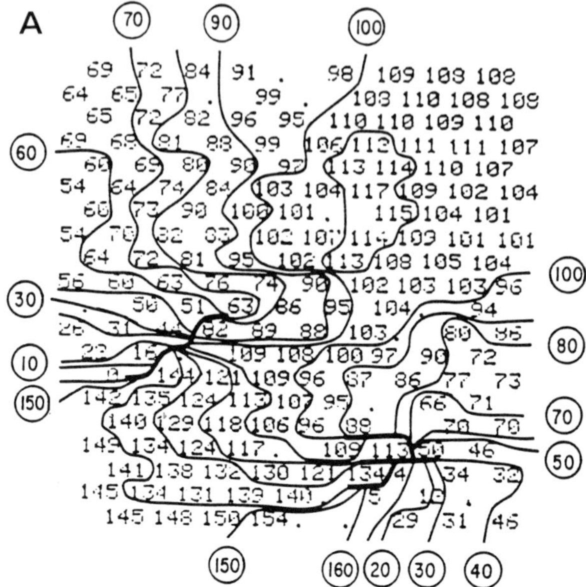

**Figure 10.**

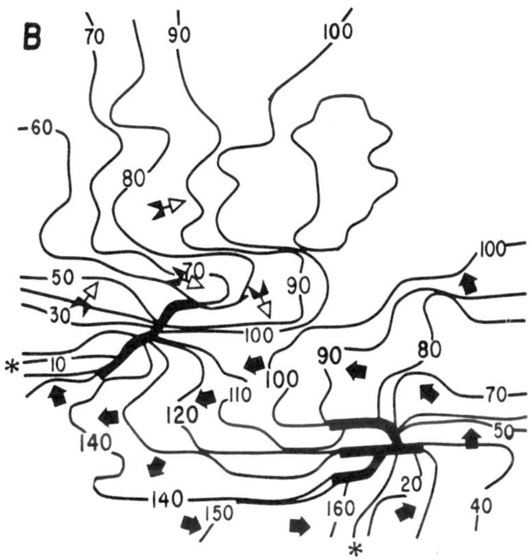


**Figure 10.** Activation map of the epicardial border zone of the canine infarct during ventricular tachycardia induced 3 days after occlusion of the left anterior descending coronary artery (LAD). In the top panel, the activation times are plotted from 192 bipolar electrodes on a map of the electrode array (LAD on the left margin, base at the top, apex at the bottom). Isochrones are drawn at 10 msec intervals. Panel B shows only the isochrones without the individual activation times used to calculate them. The arrows point out the sequence of isochrones that indicate the activation pattern. Two simultaneous reentrant circuits are present. One, beginning at the 10 msec isochrone is indicated by the asterisk at LAD margin and the other, beginning at the 10 msec isochrone on the lower (apical margin), also is indicated by the asterisk.

## Conclusions

Experimental studies on the electrophysiology of cardiac muscle and Purkinje fibers both in vivo and in vitro have led to the classification of mechanisms causing cardiac arrhythmias discussed in this chapter. Although there also is evidence from clinical electrophysiological investigation that these mechanisms cause certain clinical arrhythmias, it is not always possible to identify with certainty a cause-effect relationship between an electrophysiological mechanisms and a specific clinical arrhythmia. Ideally, this will come as a product of future research. But, why is this goal an important one? As more is learned about the cellular mechanism causing abnormal rhythm, the possibility for developing means to modify or abolish these mechanisms improves. Chemicals and drugs can be developed that would alter the function of membrane channels and thereby affect the action potential. An appropriate effect might abolish the generation of impulses causing an arrhythmia. In this symposium, emphasis is placed on the development of drugs to influence the membrane channels that participate in repolarization and prolong the time course of the action potential and refractoriness as a means to prevent reentrant excitation. Other drugs may be developed to influence membrane channels, causing automaticity or afterdepolarizations and prevent abnormal impulse initiation. Therefore, it may be possible eventually to determine precisely the cellular mechanism causing a clinical arrhythmia and use a drug specifically designed to abolish that mechanism as the therapeutic agent.

## References


1. Cranfield PF, Wit AL, Hoffman BF: Genesis of cardiac arrhythmias. *Circulation* 1973; 47:190–204.
2. Hoffman BF, Cranefield PF: The physiological basis of cardiac arrhythmias. *Am J Med* 1964; 37:670–684.
3. Hoffman BF, Rosen MR: Cellular mechanisms for cardiac arrhythmias. *Circ Res* 1981; 49:1–15.
4. DiFrancesco D, Ojeda C: Properties of the current $i_f$ in the sinoatrial node of the rabbit compared with those of $i_{K2}$ in Purkinje fibers. *J Physiol* 1980; 308:353–367.
5. Reuter H: Ion channels in cardiac cell membranes. *Ann Rev Physiol* 1984; 46:473–484.
6. Yanagihara K, Irisawa H: Potassium current during the pacemaker depolarization in rabbit sinoatrial node cell. *Pflueg Arch* 1980; 388:255–260.
7. Hoffman BF, Cranefield PF: *Electrophysiology of the Heart.* New York, McGraw-Hill, 1960.
8. Hogan PM, Davis LD: Evidence for specialized fibers in the canine atrium. *Circ Res* 1968; 23:387–396.
9. Kokubun S, Nishimura M, Noma A, et al: The spontaneous action potential of rabbit atrioventricular node cells. *Jap J Physiol* 1980; 30:529–540.
10. Wit AL, Cranefield PF: Triggered and automatic activity in the canine coronary sinus. *Circ Res* 1977; 41:435–445.
11. Wit AL, Fenoglio JJ Jr, Wagner BM, et al: Electrophysiological properties of cardiac muscle in the anterior mitral valve leaflet and the adjacent atrium in the dog: Possible implications for the genesis of atrial dysrhythmias. *Circ Res* 1973; 32:731–745.
12. DeFrancesco D: A new interpretation of the pacemaking current in calf Purkinje fibers. *J Physiol* 1981; 314:359–376.
13. DiFrancesco D: A study of the ionic nature of the pacemaker current in calf Purkinje fibers. *J Physiol* 1981; 314:377–393.

14. Kokubun S, Nishimura M, Noma A, et al: Membrane currents in rabbit atrioventricular node cell. *Pflueg Arch* 1982; 393:15−22.
15. Vassalle M: Electrogenic suppression of automaticity in sheep and dog Purkinje fibers. *Circ Res* 1970; 27:361−377.
16. Vassalle M: The relationship among cardiac pacemakers: Overdrive suppression. *Circ Res* 1977; 41:269−277.
17. Vassalle M, Caress DL, Slovin AJ, et al: On the cause of ventricular asystole during vagal stimulation. *Circ Res* 1967; 20:228−241.
18. Glitsch HG: Characteristics of active Na transport in intact cardiac cells. *Am J Physiol* 1979; 236:H189−199.
19. Gadsby DC, Cranefield PF: Direct measurement of changes in sodium pump current in canine cardiac Purkinje fibers. *Proc Natl Acad Sci USA* 1979; 76:1783−1787.
20. Jordan JL, Yamaguchi I, Mandel WJ, et al: Comparative effects of overdrive on sinus and subsidiary pacemaker function. *Am Heart J* 1977; 93:367−374.
21. Kodama I, Goto J, Ando S, et al: Effects of rapid stimulation on the transmembrane action potentials of rabbit sinus node pacemaker cells. *Circ Res* 1980; 46:90−99.
22. Gang ES, Reiffel JA: Sinus node recovery times following the spontaneous termination of supraventricular tachycardia and following overdrive pacing: A comparison. *Am Heart J* 1983; 105:210−215.
23. Breithardt G, Seipel L, Loogan F: Sinus node recovery time and calculated sinoatrial conduction time in normal subjects and patients with sinus node dysfunction. *Circulation* 1977; 56:43−49.
24. Toda N, West TC: Changes in sino-atrial node transmembrane potentials on vagal stimulation of the isolated rabbit atrium. *Nature* 1965: 205:808−809.
25. Ferrer MI: *The Sick Sinus Syndrome*. Mt. Kisco, N. Y., Futura, 1974.
26. Hope RR, Scherlag BJ, El-Sherif N, et al: Hierarchy of ventricular pacemakers. *Circ Res* 1976; 39:883−888.
27. Tsien RW: Effect of epinephrine on the pacemaker potassium current of cardiac Purkinje fibers. *J Gen Physiol* 1974; 64:293−319.
28. Pliam MB, Krellenstein DJ, Vassalle M, et al: The influence of norepinephrine, reserpine and propranolol on overdrive suppression. *J Electrocardiol* 1975; 8:17−24.
29. Armour JA, Hageman GR, Randall WC: Arrhythmias induced by local cardiac nerve stimulation. *J Physiol* 1972; 223:1068−1075.
30. Vassalle M, Levine MJ, Stuckey JH: On the sympathetic control of ventricular automaticity; the effects of stellate ganglion stimulation. *Circ Res* 1968; 23:249−258.
31. Katzung BG, Hondeghem LM, Grant AO: Cardiac ventricular automaticity induced by current of injury. *Pflueg Arch* 1975; 360:193−197.
32. Janse MJJ, van Capelle FJL: Electrotonic interactions across an inexcitable region as a cause of ectopic activity in acute regional myocardial ischemia. A study in intact porcine and canine hearts and computer models. *Circ Res* 1982; 50:527−537.
33. Rosen MR, Merker C, Gelband H, et al: Effects of ouabain on phase 4 of Purkinje fiber transmembrane potential. *Circulation* 1973; 47:681−689.

34. Vassalle M: Cardiac pacemaker potentials at different extra- and intracellular K concentrations. *Am J Physiol* 1965: 208:770–775.
35. Deck KA: Anderungen des Rhyepotentials und der Kabileigenschaften von Purkinje—faden bei der Dehnung. *Pflueg Arch* 1964; 280:131–140.
36. Katzung BG, Morgenstern JA: Effects of extracellular potassium on ventricular automaticity and evidence for a pacemaker current in mammalian ventricular myocardium. *Circ Res* 1977; 40:105–111.
37. Surawicz B, Imanishi S: Automatic activity in depolarized guinea pig ventricular myocardium: Characteristics and mechanisms. *Circ Res* 1976; 39:751–759.
38. Imanishi S: Calcium-sensitive discharges in canine Purkinje fibers. *Jap J Physiol* 1971; 21:443–463.
39. Cranefield PF: *The Slow Response and Cardiac Arrhythmias.* Mt. Kisco, N.Y., Futura, 1975.
40. Noble D, Tsien RW: The kinetics and rectifier properties of the slow potassium current in cardiac Purkinje fibers. *J Physiol (London)* 1968; 195:185–214.
41. Dangman KH, Hoffman BF: Studies on overdrive stimulation of canine cardiac Purkinje fibers: Maximum diastolic potential as a determinant of the response. *J Am College Cardiol* 1983; 2:1183–1188.
42. Ferrier GR, Rosenthal JE: Automaticity and entrance block induced by focal depolarization of mammalian ventricular tissues. *Circ Res* 1980; 47:238–248.
43. Hume J, Katzung BG: Physiological role of endogeneous amines in the modulation of ventricular automaticity in the guinea pig. *J Physiol* 1980; 309:275–286.
44. Cranefield PF: Action potentials, afterpotentials and arrhythmias. *Circ Res* 1977; 41:415–423.
45. Gadsby DC, Cranefield PF: Two levels of resting potential in cardiac Purkinje fibers. *J Gen Physiol* 1977; 70:725–746.
46. Trautwein W, Gottstein V, Dudel J: Der Aktionsstrom der Myokardfaser im Sauerstoffmangel. *Pflueg Arch* 1954; 260:40–60.
47. Coraboef E, Boistel J: L'action des taux eleves de gaz carbonique suur le tissu cardiaque etudiee a l'aide de microelectrodes intracellulaires. *Compt Rend Soc Biol (Paris)* 1953; 147:654–665.
48. Brooks C McC, Hoffman PF, Suckling EE, et al: *Excitability of the Heart.* New York, Grune and Stratton, 1955.
49. Strauss HC, Bigger JT Jr, Hoffman BF: Electrophysiological and beta-receptor blocking effects of MJ 1999 on dog and rabbit cardiac tissues. *Circ Res* 1970; 26:661–678.
50. Dangman KH, Hoffman BF: In vivo and in vitro antiarrhythmic and arrhythmogenic effects of N-acetyl procainamide. *J Pharmacol Exp Ther* 1981; 217:851–862.
51. Elonen E, Neuvonan PJ, Tarssnan L, et al: Sotalol intoxication with prolonged Q–T interval and severe tachyarrhythmias. *Br Med J* 1979; 1:1184.
52. Damiano BP, Rosen MR: Effects of pacing on triggered activity induced by early afterdepolarizations. *Circulation* 1984; 69:1013–1025.
53. Krikler DM, Curry PVL: Torsades de pointes: An atypical ventricular tachycardia. *Br Heart J* 1976: 38:117–120.

54. Brachmann J, Scherlag BJ, Rosentraukh LV, et al: Bradycardia-dependent triggered activity: relevance to drug-induced multiform ventricular tachycardia. *Circulation* 1983; 68:846–856.

55. Rosen MR, Gellard H, Hoffman BF: Correlation between effects of ouabain on the canine electrocardiogram and transmembrane potentials of isolated Purkinje fibers. *Circulation* 1973; 47:65–72.

56. Ferrier GR, Saunders JH, Mendez C: A cellular mechanism for the generation of ventricular arrhythmias by acetylstrophanthidin. *Circ Res* 1973; 32:600–609.

57. Akara T, Brody TM: The role of $Na^+$, $K^+$-ATPase in the inotropic action of digitalis. *Pharmacol Rev* 1977; 29:187–188.

58. Sheu SS, Fozzard HA: Transmembrane $Na^+$ and $Ca^{++}$ electrochemical gradients in cardiac muscle and their relationship to force development. *J Gen Physiol* 1982; 80:325–351.

59. Nathan D, Beeler GW: Electrophysiologic correlation of the inotropic effects of isoproteranol in canine myocardium. *J Mol Cell Cardiol* 1975; 7:1–15.

60. Dangman KH, Danilo P Jr, Hordof AJ, et al: Electrophysiologic characteristics of human ventricular and Purkinje fibers. *Circulation* 1982; 65:362–368.

61. Reuter H: Localization of beta adrenergic receptors and effects of noradrenaline and cyclic nucleotides on action potentials, ionic currents and tension in mamalian cardiac muscle. *J Physiol (London)* 1974; 242:429–451.

62. Saito T, Otaguro M, Matsubara T: Electrophysiological studies on the mechanism of electrically induced sustained rhythmic activity in the rabbit right atrium. *Circ Res* 1978; 42:199–206.

63. Aronson RS: Afterpotentials and triggered activity in hypertrophied myocardium from rats with renal hypertension. *Circ Res* 1981; 48:720–727.

64. Mary-Rabine L, Hordof AJ, Danilo P, et al: Mechanisms for impulse initiation in isolated human atrial fibers. *Circ Res* 1980; 47:267–277.

65. El-Sherif N, Gough WB, Zeiler RH, et al: Triggered ventricular rhythm in 1-day-old myocardial infarction in the dog. *Circ Res* 1983; 52:566–579.

66. Kass RS, Tsien RW, Weingart R: Ionic basis of transient inward current induced by strophanthidin in cardiac Purkinje fibers. *J Physiol (London)* 1978; 281:209–226.

67. Kass RS, Lederer WJ, Tsien RW, et al: Role of calcium ions in transient inward currents and aftercontractions induced by strophanthidin in cardiac Purkinje fibers. *J Physiol (London)* 1978; 281:187–208.

68. Vassalle M, Mugelli A: An oscillatory current in sheep cardiac Purkinje fibers. *Circ Res* 1980; 48:618–631.

69. Karaguezian HS, Katzung BG: Voltage-clamp studies of transient inward current and mechanical oscillation induced by ouabain in ferret papillary muscle. *J Physiol (London)* 1982; 327:255–268.

70. Tsien RW, Kass RS, Weingart R: Cellular and subcellular mechanisms of cardiac pacemaker oscillations. *J Exp Biol* 1979; 81:205–215.

71. Colquhoun D, Neher E, Reuter H, et al: Inward current channels

activated by intracellular calcium in cultured cardiac cells. *Nature* 1981; 294:752–754.

72. Arlock P, Katzung BG: Effects of sodium substitutes on transient inward current and tension in guinea-pig and ferret papillary muscle. *J Physiol* 1985; 360:105–120.

73. Rosen MR, Danilo Jr P: Digitalis induced delayed afterdepolarizations, in Zipes DP, Bailey JC, Elharrar V (Eds): *The Slow Inward Current and Cardiac Arrhythmias.* The Hague, Martinus Nijhoff, 1980, pp. 417–436.

74. Wit AL, Gadsby DC, Cranefield PF: Electrogenic sodium extrusion can stop triggered activity in the canine coronary sinus. *Circ Res* 1981; 49:1029–1042.

75. Kline RP, Siegal MS, Kupersmith J, et al: Effects of strophanthidan on changes in extracellular $K^+$ during triggered activity in the arrhythmic canine coronary sinus. *Circulation* 66 1982; Supp II–356.

76. Rosen MR, Reder RF: Does triggered activity have a role in the genesis of cardiac arrhythmias? *Ann Int Med* 1981; 94:794–801.

77. Wit AL, Cranefield PF: Reentrant excitation as a cause of cardiac arrhythmias. *Am J Physiol* 1978; 235:H1–17.

78. Fozzard HA: Conduction of the action potential, in Berne RM, Sperelakis, N, Geiger SR: *Handbook of Physiology,* Section 2, the Cardiovascular System, Volume I, *The Heart.* Baltimore, Williams and Wilkens Co., 1979, pp. 335–357.

79. Weidmann S: The effect of the cardiac membrane potential on the rapid availability of the sodium carrying system. *J Physiol (London)* 1955; 127:213–224.

80. Reuter H: Properties of two inward membrane currents in heart. *Ann Rev Physiol* 1979; 41:413–424.

81. Tsien RW: Calcium channels in excitable cell membranes. *Ann Rev Physiol* 1983; 45:341–358.

82. Zipes DP, Mendez C: Action of manganese ions and tetrodotoxin on atrioventricular nodal transmembrane potentials in isolated rabbit hearts. *Circ Res* 1973; 32:447–454.

83. Spach M, Miller WT, Geselowitz DB, et al: The discontinuous nature of propagation in normal canine cardiac muscle: Evidence for recurrent discontinuities of intracellular resistance that effect the membrane currents. *Circ Res* 1981; 48:39–54.

84. Spach MS, Muller WT, Dolber PC, et al: The functional role of structural complexities in the propagation of depolarization in the atrium of the dog: Cardiac conduction disturbances due to discontinuities of effective axial resistivity. *Circ Res* 1982; 50:175–191.

85. Clerc L: Directional differences of impulse spread in trabecular muscle from mammalian heart. *J Physiol (London)* 1976; 255:335–346.

86. Ursell PC, Gardner PI, Albala A, et al: Structural and electrophysiological changes in the epicardial border zone of canine infarcts during infarct healing. *Circ Res* 1985; 56:436–451.

87. Gardner PI, Ursell PC, Fenoglio JJ, Jr. et al: Electrophysiologic and anatomic basis for fractional electrograms recorded from healed myocardial infarcts. *Circulation* 1985; 72:596.

88. Spach MS, Dolber PC: Relating extracellular potentials and their de-

rivatives to anisotropic propagation at a microscopic level in human cardiac muscle: Evidence for uncoupling of side-to-side fiber connections with increasing age. *Circ Res* 1986; 58:356–371.

88. Spach MS, Dolber PC: Relating extracellular potentials and their derivatives to anisotropic propagation at a microscopic level in human cardiac muscle: Evidence for uncoupling of side-to-side fiber connections with increasing age. *Circ Res* 1986; 58:356–371.

89. Page P, Shibata Y: Permeable junctions between cardiac cells. *Ann Rev Physiol* 1981; 43:431–447.

90. Wojtezak J: Contractures and increase in internal longitudinal resistance of cow ventricular muscle induced by hypoxia. *Circ Res* 1979; 44:88–95.

91. Weingart R: The actions of ouabain on intercellular coupling and conduction velocity in mammalian ventricular muscle. *J Physiol (London)* 1977; 264:341–365.

92. Joyner RW: Effects of the discrete pattern of electrical coupling on propagation through an electrical syncytium. *Circ Res* 1982; 50:192–200.

93. Joyner RW, Veenstra R, Rawling D, et al: Propagation through electrically coupled cells. Effects of a resistive barrier. *Biophysical J* 1984; 45:1017–1025.

94. Wit AL, Cranefield PF, Hoffman BF: Slow conduction and reentry in the ventricular conducting system II. Singly and sustained circus movement in networks of canine and bovine Purkinje fibers. *Circ Res* 1972; 30:11–22.

95. Boyden PA, Tilley LP, Albala A, et al: Mechanisms for atrial arrhythmias associated with cardiomyopathy: A study of feline hearts with primary myocardial disease. *Circulation* 1984; 69:1036–1047.

96. Moe GK, Mendez C, Han J: Aberrant AV impulse propagation in the dog heart; a study of functional bundle branch block. *Circ Res* 1965; 16:261–286.

97. Gallagher JJ, Gilbert M, Sevenson RH, et al: Wolff-Parkinson-White syndrome: The problem, evaluation and surgical correction. *Circulation* 1975; 51:767–785.

98. Frame LH, Page RL, Hoffman BF: Atrial reentry around an anatomic barrier with a partially refractory exictable gap. A canine model of flutter. *Circ Res* 1986; 58:495–511.

99. Antzelevitch C, Jalife J, Moe GK: Characteristics of reflection as a mechanism of reentrant arrhythmias and its relationship to parasystole. *Circulation* 1980; 61:182–191.

100. Jalife J, Moe GK: Excitation, conduction and reflection of impulses in isolated bovine and canine cardiac Purkinje fibers. *Circ Res* 1981; 49:233–247.

101. Allessie MA, Bonke FIM, Schopman FJG: Circus movement in rabbit atrial muscle as a mechanism of tachycardia. II. Role of nonuniform recovery of excitabilty in the occurrence of unidirectional block, as studied with multiple microelectrodes. *Circ Res* 1976; 39:168–177.

102. Allessie MA, Bonke FIM, Schopman FJG: Circus movement in rabbit atrial muscle as a mechanism of tachycardia. *Circ Res* 1973; 33:54–62.

103. Allessie MA, Bonke FIM, Schopman FJG: Circus movement in rabbit atrial muscle as a mechanism of tachycardia. III. The "leading circle" concept: A new model of circus movement in cardiac tissue without the involvement of an anatomical obstacle. *Circ Res* 1977; 41:9–18.
104. El Sherif N, Smith A, Evans K: Canine ventricular arrhythmias in the late myocardial infarction period 8. Epicardial mapping of reentrant circuits. *Circ Res* 1981; 49:255–265.
105. Wit AL, Allessie MA, Bonke FIM, et al: Electrophysiological mapping to determine the mechanism of experimental ventricular tachycardia initiated by premature impulses. Experimental approach and initial results demonstrating reentrant excitation. *Am J Cardiol* 1982; 49:166–185.
106. Kramer JB, Saffitz JE, Witkkowski FX, et al: Intramural reentry as a mechanism of ventricular tachycardia during evolving canine MI. *Circ Res* 1985; 56:736.

# Chapter 2

# Genesis of Cardiac Arrhythmias: Relevance to Clinical Mechanisms

## Douglas P. Zipes and Robert F. Gilmour, Jr.

Normal cardiac rhythm occurs when spontaneous electrical impulses generated in the sinus node are transmitted via the specialized conducting pathways to working myocardium. This orderly progression of impulse formation and propagation ensures a synchronous sequence of contraction in atrial and ventricular myocardium. Many factors can disrupt cardiac rhythm by altering spontaneous activity in the sinus node and other potential pacemaker regions in the heart and by impairing impulse propagation. Significant abnormalities of automaticity or conduction can precipitate rhythm disturbances that compromise cardiac function, producing clinical symptoms or death.

The purpose of this chapter is to review present knowledge concerning clinical cardiac electrophysiological alterations that provoke cardiac arrhythmias.

## Abnormal Impulse Formation

Under appropriate circumstances, all types of cardiac cells can generate spontaneous activity. Normally, sinus and certain atrio-

*Supported in part by the Herman C. Krannert Fund; by Grants HL-06308 and HL-07182 from the National Heart, Lung, and Blood Institute of the National Institutes of Health, Bethesda, Maryland; and by the American Heart Association, Indiana Affiliate.*

From: *Control of Cardiac Arrhythmias by Lengthening Repolarization*, edited by Bramah N. Singh, MD, Futura Publishing Company Inc., Mount Kisco, NY, © 1988.

ventricular (AV) nodal cells and cells in the His-Purkinje system demonstrate diastolic or phase 4 depolarization that, if uninterrupted, brings the cell to threshold and initiates an action potential.[1] Phase 4 depolarization and automaticity may occur in tissues that are not normally automatic, such as atrial and ventricular muscle fibers. In addition, atrial and ventricular muscle, Purkinje fibers, and several other cardiac tissues can develop sustained rhythmic activity, distinct from automaticity, that is triggered by early or delayed afterdepolarizations. Abnormal impulse formation may be due to altered normal diastolic depolarization, abnormal automatic mechanisms, and triggered activity.

## Abnormal Impulse Conduction

Reentrant excitation occurs when an impulse excites a region of myocardium, conducts slowly around an area of inexcitable tissue, and returns to reexcite the original region. Unidirectional block in one limb of the circular pathway, prolonged conduction time in the other limb, and a relatively brief refractory period in the previously excited region are required to prevent the circulating wavefront from impinging on refractory tissue and extinguishing itself.

The classic description of reentrant excitation by Schmitt and Erlanger[2] requires an anatomical or electrophysiological obstacle around which a slowly conducting impulse circles (Fig. 1). However, experiments in atrial myocardium have demonstrated that the obstacle need not be fixed.[3] A premature stimulus can generate a propagating wavefront that establishes a vortex of conduction around a central area of electrotonically depolarized cells. These cells function as an inexcitable island, despite the fact that their electrophysiological properties are normal. The cycle length of this type of reentry is determined in large part by the refractory period of cells in the propagating wavefront. Shortening their refractory period shortens the tachycardia cycle length, until the leading edge of the propagating wavefront encounters the refractory tail of the previous wavefront and further propagation fails. A certain type of reentry, known as *reflection*, results from transmission of impulses back and forth along the same myocardial or Purkinje fiber, rather than around an obstacle.[4]

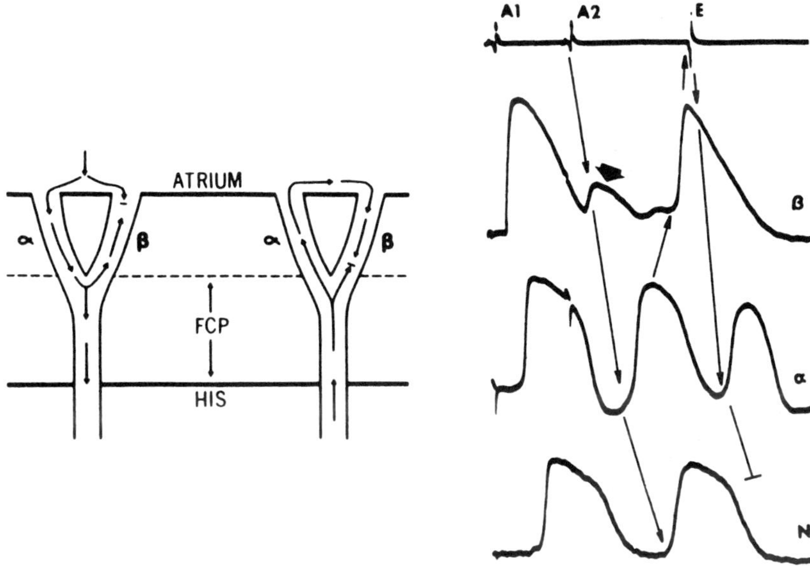


**Figure 1.** Atrial echoes. Left panel: Schematic representation of intra-nodal dissociation responsible for an atrial echo. A premature atrial response fails to penetrate the beta pathway, which exhibits unidirectional block, but propagates anterogradely through the alpha pathway. Once the final common pathway (FCP) is engaged, the impulse may return to the atrium via the now recovered beta pathway to produce an atrial echo. The neighboring diagram illustrates the pattern of propagation during generation of a ventricular echo. A premature response in the His bundle traverses the final common pathway, encounters a refractory beta pathway (unidirectional block), reaches the alpha pathway, and returns through a now recovered beta pathway to produce a ventricular echo.

Right panel: Recordings from the atrium (top tracing electrogram), cells impaled in the beta region (second tracing), alpha region (third tracing), and N portion of the AV node (bottom tracing) in an isolated rabbit preparation. The basic response to $A_1$ activated both alpha and beta pathways and the N cell (first tier of action potentials). The premature atrial response, $A_2$, caused only a local response in the beta cell (heavy arrow), was delayed in transmission to the alpha cell, and was further delayed in propagation to the N cell. Following the alpha response, a retrograde spontaneous response occurred in the beta cell and propagated to the atrium (E). This atrial response represents an atrial echo. The echo returned to stimulate the alpha cell but was not propagated to the N cell. (From Mendez C, Moe GK: Demonstration of a dual AV nodal conduction system in the isolated rabbit heart. *Circ Res* 19:378, 1966. By permission of the American Heart Association, Inc.)

## Interactions Between Abnormal Impulse Formation and Propagation

Since excitability, action potential amplitude, and maximum action potential upstroke velocity depend on the voltage at which activation occurs, impulse propagation into and out of spontaneously depolarizing regions may change significantly as diastolic depolarization proceeds.[5] Conversely, changes in conduction may affect the degree of entrance and exit block surrounding an automatic focus and alter the abiltiy of regenerative and subthreshold potentials to modulate pacemaker activity. Impulse conduction and automaticity also may interact due to the flow of injury current between regions of disparate electrophysiological properties.

An important clinical situation in which such interaction occurs is during parasystole. Automatic cells with the fastest rate of diastolic depolarizations usually suppress more slowly depolarizing foci, unless a block at some site between the dominant and latent pacemakers prevents resetting of the latent pacemaker. However, if entrance or exit block into or out of the automatic focus is incomplete, propagated impulses may induce subthreshold potentials distal to the site of block that predictably alter the discharge rate of a focus. Subthreshold depolarizing impulses that arrive in the focal area early in diastole delay the subsequent spontaneous discharge, whereas impulses that arrive later in diastole accelerate the subsequent discharge.[6]

## Electrophysiological Mechanisms Responsible for Clinically Occurring Arrhythmias

As stated earlier, the genesis of cardiac arrhythmias generally is divided into categories of disorders of impulse formation, disorders of impulse conduction, or combinations of both.[7] Present diagnostic tools do not permit unequivocal determination of the electrophysiological mechanisms responsible for most clinically occurring arrhythmias and usually do not allow convincing differentiation of the ionic mechanisms responsible for a particular arrhythmia. One can postulate only that a particular arrhythmia is "most consistent with" or "best explained by" one or the other electrophysiological mechanism. Furthermore, some tachyarrhythmias may be started by one mechanism and perpetuated by another. For example, premature ventricular depolarization due to abnormal automaticity may precipitate a ventricular tachycardia sustained by reentry. One tachyarrhythmia may give rise to another (Fig. 2). Given these comments, mechanisms demonstrated to cause abnormal electrical activity in a variety of clinical situations will be considered.

## Disorders of Impulse Formation

This category is defined as inappropriate discharge rate of the normal pacemaker, the sinus node (e.g., sinus rates too fast or too slow for the physiological needs of the patient), or discharge from an ectopic pacemaker that controls the atrial or ventricular rhythm for one complex or more. It is important to recall that such disorders of impulse formation can be due to a speeding or slowing of a *normal* pacemaker mechanism (e.g., phase 4 diastolic depolarization that is ionically normal for the sinus node or for an ectopic site such as a Purkinje fiber but inappropriately fast or slow) or due to an ionically *abnormal* pacemaker mechanism. The patient with persistent sinus tachycardia at rest or sinus bradycardia during exertion exhibits inappropriate sinus nodal discharge rates, but

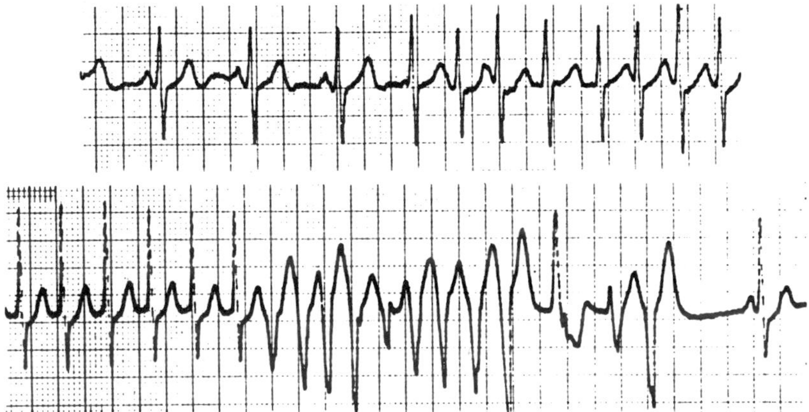

**Figure 2.** Supraventricular tachycardia inducing a ventricular tachycardia. In the top portion of this recording, a premature atrial complex (fourth P wave) initiates a sustained episode of supraventricular tachycardia, which initially demonstrates some alteration in cycle length. The supraventricular tachycardia becomes regular (bottom tracing) and initiates a short episode of a nonsustained ventricular tachycardia, which then results in termination of the supraventricular tachycardia.

the ionic mechanisms responsible for sinus nodal discharge still may be normal. Conversely, when a patient experiences ventricular tachycardia during an acute myocardial infarction, abnormal ionic mechanisms probably are operative to generate this tachycardia. Although pacemaker activity generally is not found in ordinary working myocardium, myocardial ischemia conceivably can bestow abnormal pacemaker properties on cells such as ventricular muscle fibers, permitting them to depolarize automatically. Rhythms due to automaticity may be slow atrial, junctional, and ventricular escape rhythms, certain types of atrial tachycardias (such as those produced by digitalis), accelerated junctional (nonparoxysmal junctional tachycardia) (Fig. 3), and idioventricular rhythms and parasystole.

Electrophysiological concepts about parasystole have been revised drastically in the last several years.[8,9] Classically, parasystole has been considered similar to a fixed-rate, asynchronously

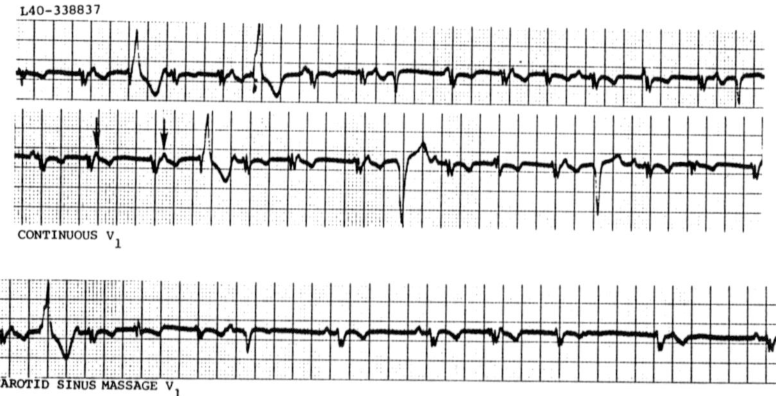


**Figure 3.**   Nonparoxysmal AV junctional tachycardia in a healthy young adult. This tachycardia occurs at a fairly regular interval. ("W-shaped" complexes) and is interrupted intermittently with atrial captures that produce functional right and left bundle branch block. Two P waves are indicated by arrows. The junctional discharge rate is approximately 120 beats/min (cycle length = 500 msec) and the rhythm irregular, sometimes shortened by atrial captures or delayed by concealed conduction that resets and displaces the junctional focus. In the bottom strip, carotid sinus massage slows the junctional as well as the sinus discharge rate. (From Zipes DP: Specific arrhythmias: Diagnosis and treatment. In E Braunwald (ed): *Heart Disease. A Textbook of Cardiovascular Medicine.* Philadelphia, WB Saunders, p 706, 1984. By permission.)

discharging pacemaker. As such its timing is not altered by the dominant rhythm, it produced depolarization when the myocardium was excitable, and the intervals between discharges were multiples of a basic interval. Complete entrance block, constant or intermittent, insulated and protected the parasystolic focus from surrounding electrical events and accounted for such activity. Occasionally, the focus exhibited exit block, during which it failed to depolarize excitable myocardium. As indicated earlier, data from recent experiments have shown that, in fact, the dominant cardiac rhythm may modulate parasystolic discharge to speed up or slow down its rate via electrotonic interactions with the dominant rhythm across an area of depressed excitability. Complex interactions of complete silence, concealed or manifest bigeminy, trigeminy, quadrigeminy, and periods of more complex group beating may occur owing to the entraining effects of the dominant rhythm on the ectopic focus. Clinical examples support these experimental observations.

## Disorders of Impulse Conduction

Reentry probably is the cause of most tachyarrhythmias, including various kinds of supraventricular and ventricular tachycardias, flutter and fibrillation (Figs. 4 and 5). It is important to remember, however, that initiation or termination of tachycardia by pacing stimuli, the demonstration of electrical activity bridging diastole, fixed coupling, and a variety of other clinically used techniques, although consistent with reentry, do not constitute proof of its existence.

## Atrial Flutter and Fibrillation

Mapping studies[10,11] in animals and mapping and stimulation studies in man provide some evidence to suggest that many forms of atrial flutter are due to reentry.

Much indirect evidence supports reentry as a cause of fibrillation, but this is difficult to prove beyond question. Several studies have established that a critical mass of myocardium is required to maintain fibrillation,[12] lending support to Moe's hypothesis that fibrillation is maintained by multiple wavelets of reentry, influenced by the mass of the tissue, refractory periods, and conduction velocity.[13] Demonstration of entrainment probably offers the most evidence of reentry.[14]

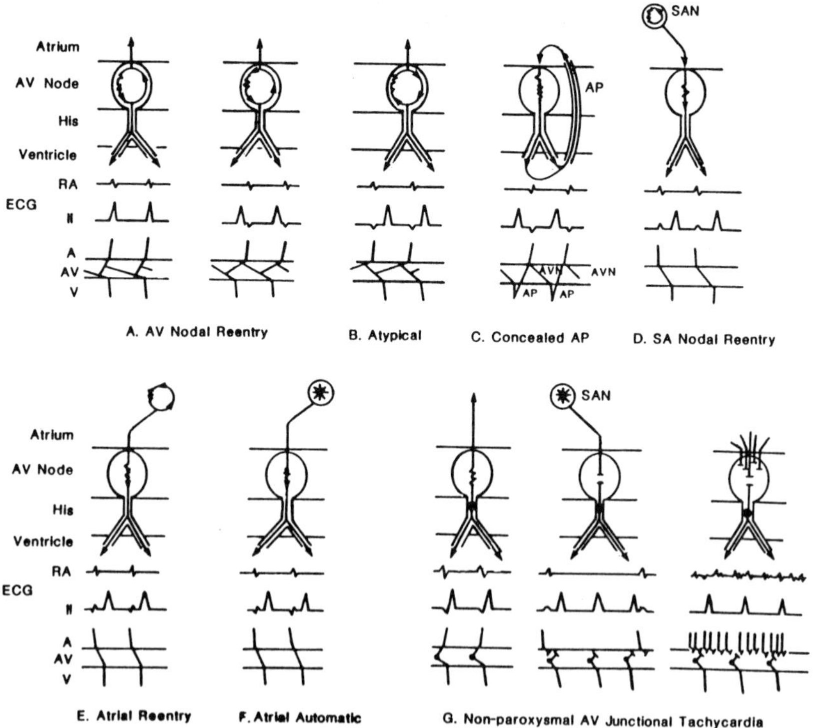


**Figure 4.** Diagrammatic representation of various tachycardias. In the top portion of each example is a schematic of the presumed anatomical pathways; in the bottom half, the ECG presentation and the explanatory ladder diagram are depicted. A: AV nodal reentry. In the left example, reentrant excitation is confined to the AV node, with retrograde atrial activity simultaneous to ventricular activity owing to anterograde conduction over the slow AV nodal pathway and retrograde conduction over the fast AV nodal pathway. In the right example, atrial activity occurs slightly later than ventricular activity, owing to retrograde conduction delay. B: Atypical AV nodal reentry due to anterograde conduction over a fast AV nodal pathway and retrograde conduction over a slow AV nodal pathway. C: Concealed accessory pathway. Reciprocating tachycardia is due to anterograde conduction over the AV node and retrograde conduction over the accessory pathway. Retrograde P waves occur after the QRS complex. D: Sinus nodal reentry. The tachycardia is due to reentry within the sinus node, which then conducts to the rest of the heart. E: Atrial reentry. Tachycardia is due to reentry within the atrium, which then conducts to the rest of the heart. F: Automatic atrial tachycardia. Tachycardia is due to automatic discharge in the atrium, which then conducts to the

## Sinus and Atrial Reentry

Reentry in parts of the atrium has been reported to occur in several experimental models as well as in humans. The sinus node shares with the AV node electrophysiological features such as the potential for dissociation of conduction, i.e., an impulse can be made to conduct in some nodal fibers but not in others. Evidence from a number of studies in humans and animal[14] supports the concept that sustained reentry in the sinus node can occur and cause supraventricular tachycardia (Fig. 6). Examples of supraventricular tachycardia purported to be due to atrial reentry have been cited,[15] but their relative infrequency in the published literature suggests that this is not a commonly recognized cause of supraventricular tachycardia in humans. Distinguishing atrial tachycardia due to automaticity from atrial tachycardia sustained by reentry over very small areas (i.e., microeentry) is very difficult, and therefore conclusions regarding clinical electrophysiological mechanisms of this supraventricular tachycardia based on currently available information must be accepted cautiously.

Microelectrode studies on isolated rabbit AV nodal preparations provide evidence to support longitudinal AV nodal dissociation and reentry.[16-18] Cells in the upper portion of the AV node can be dissociated during propagation of premature stimuli, so that one group of cells can discharge in response to a premature stimulus at a time when another group of cells fails to discharge. The impulse then can propagate to the mid and lower portions of the AV node and turn around without needing to activate the His bundle to produce an atrial echo (Fig. 1). Experiments using multiple simultaneous microelectrode recordings and episodes of sustained AV nodal tachycardia in isolated rabbit atria[19] largely confirmed these observations.

Reentry, initiated by a critical degree of AV nodal conduction delay[20] can be localized to the AV node, possibly occurring over functionally distinct dual AV nodal pathways.[21] The premature

---

rest of the heart; it is difficult to distinguish from atral reentry. G: Nonparoxysmal AV junctional tachycardia. Various presentations of this tachycardia are depicted with retrograde atrial capture. AV dissociation with the sinus node in control of the atria, and AV dissociation with atrial fibrillation (From Zipes DP: Specific arrhythmias: Diagnosis and treatment. In E Braunwald (ed): *Heart Disease. A Textbook of Cardiovascular Medicine.* Philadelphia, WB Saunders, p 695, 1984. By permission.)

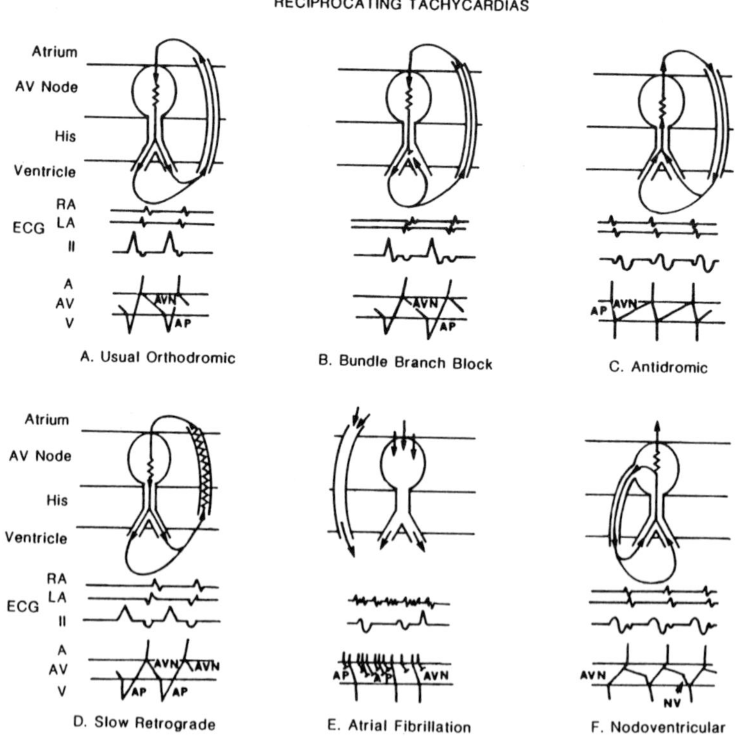



**Figure 5.** Schematic diagram of tachycardias associated with accessory pathways, format as in Figure 4. A: Orthodromic tachycardia with antegrade conduction over the AV node–His bundle route and retrograde conduction over the accessory pathway (left-sided for this example as depicted by LA activation preceding RA activation). B: Orthodromic tachycardia and ipsilateral functional bundle branch block. C: Antidromic tachycardia with anterograde conduction over the accessory pathway and retrograde conduction over the AV node–His bundle. D: Orthodromic tachycardia with a slowly conducting accessory pathway. E: Atrial fibrillation with the accessory pathway as a bystander. F: Anterograde conduction over a portion of the AV node and a nodoventricular pathway and retrograde conduction over the AV node. (From Zipes DP: Specific arrhythmias: Diagnosis and treatment. In E Braunwald (ed.): *Heart Disease. A Textbook of Cardiovascular Medicine.* Philadelphia, WB Saunders, p 716, 1984. By permission.)

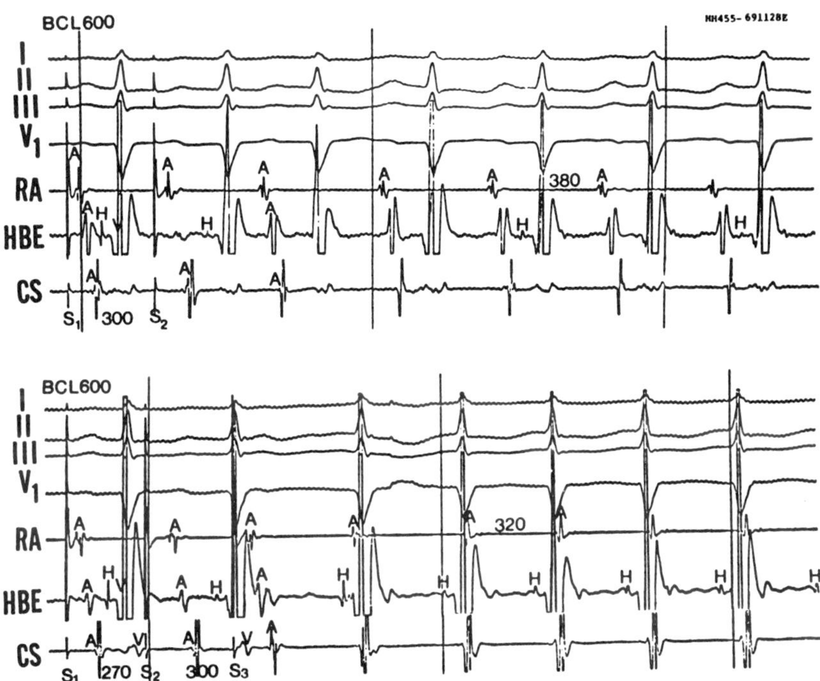


**Figure 6.** Sinoatrial nodal reentry. Premature stimulation of the high right atrium at an $S_1-S_2$ interval of 300 msec initiates an atrial tachycardia with an activation sequence similar to that occurring during high right atrial pacing. Activation in the His bundle is recorded inconsistently but, given the normal QRS complex, must occur prior to each ventricular depolarization. In the lower recording, premature atrial stimulation at an $S_1-S_3$ interval of 300 msec initiates an AV nodal reentry. Retrograde low right atrial activation recorded in the HBE lead occurs prior to ventricular activation and is followed by left atrial (CS) and high right atrial activation. Note the difference in atrial activation sequence in the top and lower panels, contrasting the presence of sinoatrial nodal reentry and AV nodal reentry in the same patient. I, II, III, $V_1$ indicate scalar recordings; RA, right atrial electrogram; HBE, His bundle electrogram; CS, coronary sinus electrogram.

atrial response can block anterogradely in one AV nodal pathway that conducts more rapidly (fast pathway, or beta pathway) but has a longer refractory period than a second pathway (slow pathway, or alpha pathway). The premature atrial response travels to the ventricle over the slow alpha pathway and back to the atrium over the fast beta pathway (Fig. 7). Less commonly, the premature atrial response can block in the slow pathway and travel in the fast pathway anterogradely, using the slow pathway retrogradely. A plot of the $A_1-A_2$ interval versus the $A_2-H_2$ or $H_1-H_2$ interval shows a "break" in the curve when the $A_2-H_2$ interval suddenly prolongs, presumably as conduction now travels over the slow pathway. Tachycardia usually begins at that point (Fig. 8).

## Preexcitation Syndrome

The accumulated anatomical and electrophysiological data support a reentrant mechanism to explain tachycardias related to an accessory pathway more than they support that mechanism for any other kind of tachycardia.[22-24] Electrophysiological studies have demonstrated that, in most pateints who have reciprocating tachycardia associated with the Wolff-Parkinson-White syndrome, the accessory pathway conducts more rapidly than does the normal AV node but takes a longer time to recover excitability; i.e., the anterograde refractory period of the accessory pathway exceeds that of the AV node.

Consequently, a premature atrial complex that occurs sufficiently early blocks anterogradely in the accessory pathway and continues to the ventricle over the normal AV node and His bundle. After the ventricles have been excited, the impulse is able to enter the accessory pathway retrogradely and return to the atrium. A continuous conduction loop of this kind establishes the circuit for the tachycardia. Although exceptions occur, the usual activation wave during such a reciprocating tachycardia in a patient with an accessory pathway occurs in this fashion: anterogradely over the normal AV node—His—Purkinje system and retrogradely over the accessory pathway resulting in a normal QRS complex (Figs. 9 and 10). In some patients, the accessory pathway may be capable only of retrograde conduction,[23,25] but the circuit and mechanism of tachycardia remain the same. Less commonly, the accessory pathway may conduct only anterogradely.[23,26]

In addition to the response of the reciprocating tachycardia to premature stimulation, one of the strongest lines of evidence supporting a reentrant mechanism is that interruption of the presumed reentrant loop at widely separated points (by surgically cutting the normal AV node—His bundle pathway or the accessory pathway) eliminates the ability to develop supraventricular tachycardia.

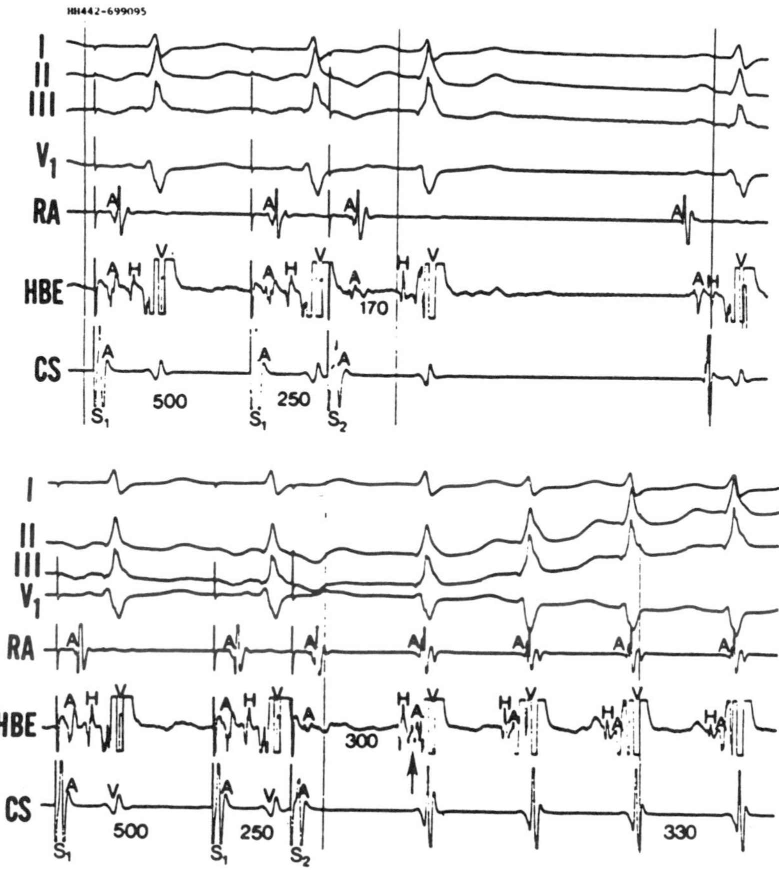

**Figure 7.** Initiation of AV nodal reentrant tachycardia in a patient with dual atrioventricular nodal pathways. Upper and lower panels show the last two paced beats of a train of stimuli delivered to the coronary sinus at a pacing cycle length of 500 msec. The results of premature atrial stimulation at an $S_1-S_2$ interval of 250 msec on two occasions are shown. In the upper panel, $S_2$ was conducted to the ventricle with an AH interval of 170 msec and then was followed by a sinus beat. In the lower panel, $S_2$ was conducted with an AH interval of 300 msec and initiated AV nodal reentry. Note that the retrograde atrial activity occurs (arrow) prior to the onset of ventricular septal depolarization and is superimposed on the QRS complex. Retrograde atrial activity begins first in the low right atrium (HBE lead) and then progresses to the high right atrium (RA) and coronary sinus (CS) recordings. (From Zipes DP: Specific arrhythmias: Diagnosis and treatment. In E Braunwald (ed): *Heart Disease. A Textbook of Cardiovascular Medicine.* Philadelphia, WB Saunders, p 707, 1984. By permission.)

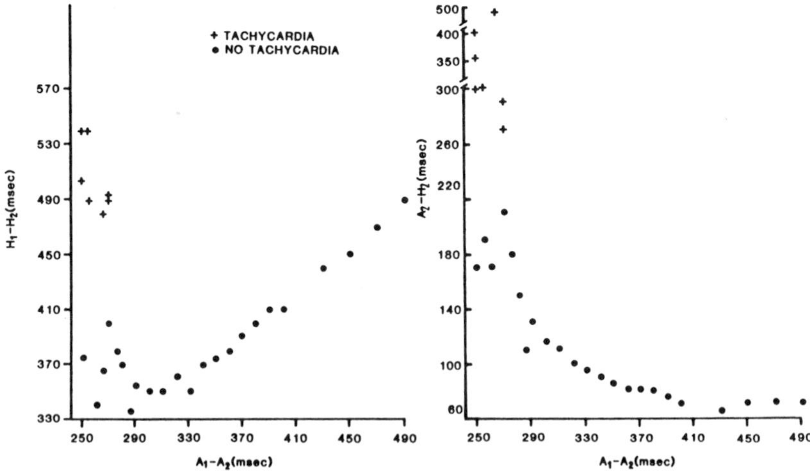


**Figure 8.**   $H_1-H_2$ intervals (left) and $A_2-H_2$ intervals (right) at various $A_1-A_2$ intervals showing discontinous AV nodal curves. At a critical $A_1-A_2$ interval, the $H_1-H_2$ interval and the $A_2-H_2$ interval increase markedly. At the break in the curves, AV nodal reentrant tachycardia is initiated. (From Zipes DP: Specific arrhythmias: Diagnosis and Treatment. In E Braunwald (ed): *Heart Disease. A Textbook of Cardiovascular Medicine*. Philadelphia, p 708, 1984. By permission.)

Other pathways may constitute the circuit for reciprocating tachycardias in patients who have some form of the Wolff-Parkinson-White syndrome. Conduction may proceed anterogradely over the accessory pathway and retrogradely over the AV node–His bundle, so-called antidromic tachycardia. Two accessory pathways may form the circuit. In the Lown-Ganong-Levine syndrome (short PR interval and normal QRS complex),[27] conduction over a James fiber[28] that connects the atrium to the distal portion of the AV node and His bundle, has been a postulated pathway although the presence of this entity as a distinct syndrome is unlikely.[29]

For some patients, electrophysiological findings may be consistent with communications between the AV node and the ventricle (nodoventricular) or the His bundle–bundle branches and the ventricle (fasciculoventricular).[30] Tachycardia in patients with nodoventricular fibers may be due to reentry using these fibers as the anterograde pathway and the His-Purkinje fibers and a portion of the AV node retrogradely. No direct relationship may exist between fasciculoventricular fibers and tachycardia.

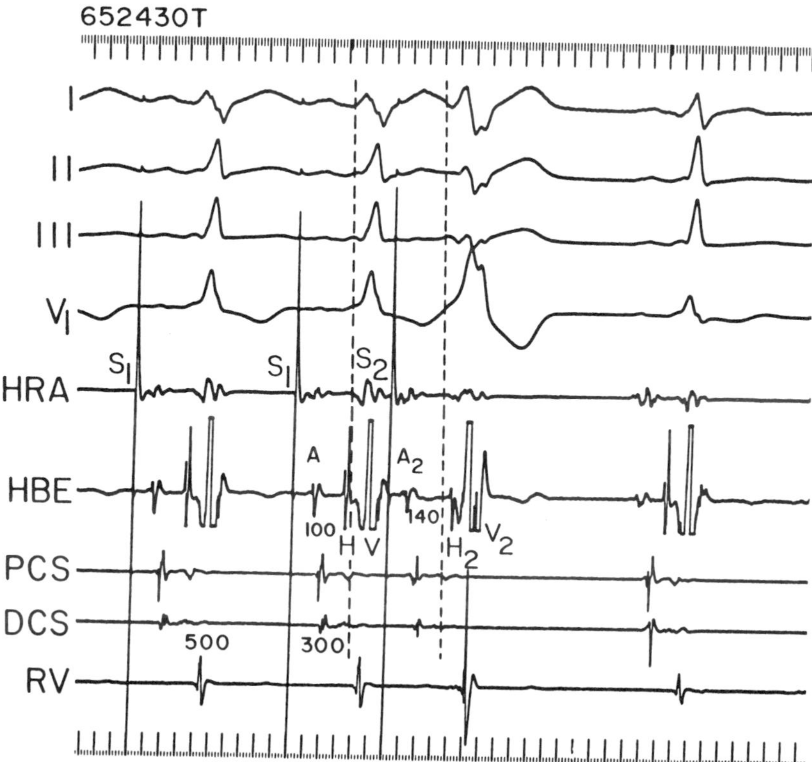



**Figure 9.** WPW tachycardia. Following high right atrial pacing at a cycle length of 500 msec ($S_1$–$S_1$), premature stimulation at a coupling interval of 300 msec ($S_1$–$S_2$) produces physiological delay in AV nodal conduction resulting in an increase in the AH interval from 100 to 140 msec but no delay in the AV interval. Consequently, activation of the His bundle occurs following activation of the QRS complex (second interrupted line) and the QRS complex becomes more anomalous in appearance due to increased ventricular activation over the accessory pathway. I, II, III, and $V_1$ are scalar leads I, II, III, and $V_1$ respectively; HRA, high right atrium; HBE, His bundle electrogram; PCS, proximal coronary sinus electrogram; DCS, distal coronary sinus electrogram; RV, right ventricular electrogram. Time lines are at 50 and 10 msec intervals. $S_1$ is stimulus of the drive train; $S_2$ premature stimulus. A, H, V indicate atrial His bundle and ventricular activation during the drive train; $A_2$, $H_2$, $V_2$, atrial, His, and ventricular activation during the premature stimulus. (From Zipes DP, Mahomed Y, King RD, et al: Wolff-Parkinson-White syndrome: Cryosurgical treatment. *Indiana Med* 79:433, 1986. By permission.)

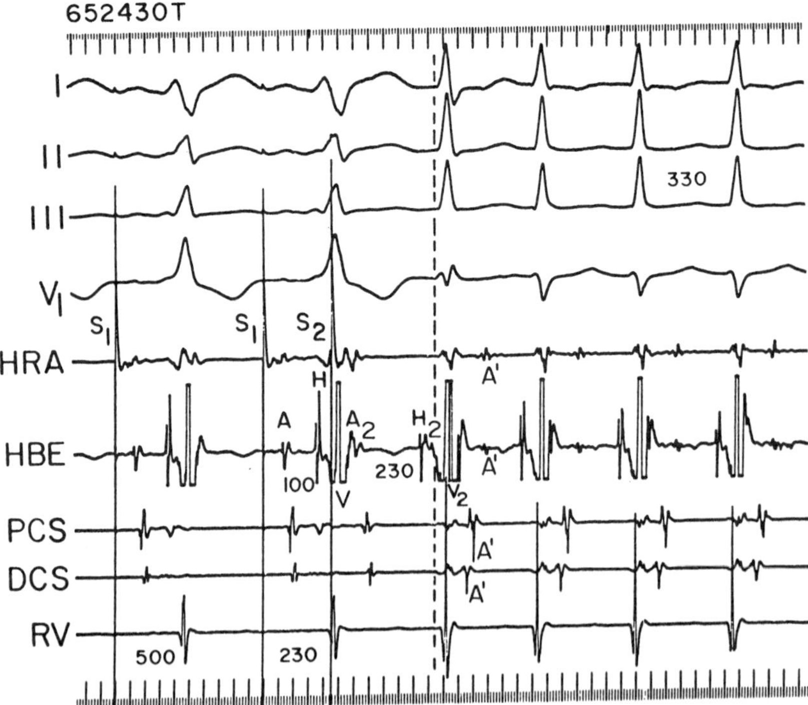

**Figure 10.** Precipitation of reciprocating atrioventricular tachycardia. Premature stimulation at a coupling interval of 230 msec prolongs the AH interval to 230 msec and results in anterograde block in the accessory pathway and normalization of the QRS complex (slight functional aberrancy in the nature of incomplete right bundle branch block occurs). Note that $H_2$ precedes the onset of the QRS complex (dashed line). Following $V_2$, the atria are excited retrogradely (A'), beginning in the distal coronary sinus then following by atrial activation in leads recording from the proximal coronary sinus, His bundle, and high right atrium. A supraventricular tachycardia is initiated at a cycle length of 330 msec. (Conventions in Fig. 9). (From Zipes DP, Mahomed Y, King RD, et al: Wolff-Parkinson-White syndrome: Cryosurgial treatment. *Indiana Med* 79:434, 1986. By permission.)

## Ventricular Reentry

Reentry within ventricular muscle, with or without participation of Purkinje fibers, probably is responsible for many ventricular tachycardias. In addition, reentry has been demonstrated to occur over the bundle branches in the in situ dog heart[31] (Fig. 11)

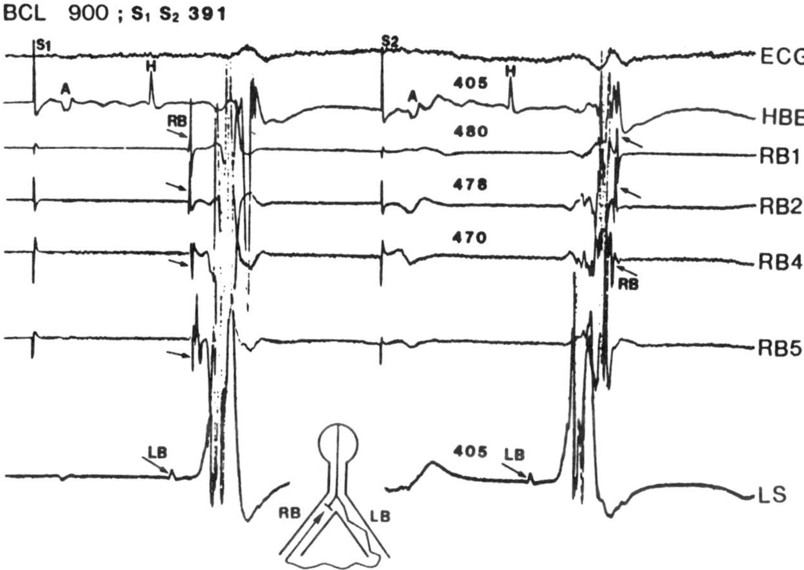


**Figure 11.** Reentry in the bundle branches of the dog heart. Recordings have been made with an electrode in the His bundle area (HBE), a multipolar plaque electrode sewn on the right bundle branch portraying activation from base to apex direction in electrograms $RB_1$ to $RB_5$ and from the left bundle branch (LB) in the left septal lead (LS). During the last basic cycle, $S_1$ applied to the atrium causes conduction to proceed from the His bundle through the left and right bundle branches to the ventricle. Note the orderly progression of conduction from $RB_1$ to $RB_5$. At a premature right atrial interval of 391 msec, conduction is blocked distal to His, travels to the ventricle over the left bundle branch without any delay between left bundle branch deflections, and then activates the right bundle branch retrogradely from $RB_4$ to $RB_2$ to $RB_1$. Retrograde right bundle branch deflection in $RB_5$ cannot be seen. Insert shows activation sequence in bundle branches following $S_2$. (From Glassman RD, Zipes DP: Site of anterograde and retrograde functional right bundle branch block in the intact canine heart. *Circulation* 64:1277, 1981. By permission of the American Heart Association.)

and probably in humans as well[32,33] However, bundle branch reentry does not appear to be a common cause of sustained ventricular tachycardia in the dog or in humans.[34] Reentry within ventricular muscle is difficult to prove because the large muscle mass makes complete mapping of the reentrant loop and interruption of the pathway difficult. In general, experimental studies provide supportive evidence of reentry.

Ischemia, both acute and chronic, has been a favorite model to investigate because it generates fragmented, delayed activation that may be conducive to the generation of reentrant excitation.[35–38] However, even the demonstration of continuous electrical activity spanning diastole, linked temporally and perhaps causally to the generation of sustained ventricular arrhythmia, constitutes only circumstantial proof. For example, such continuous electrical activity could be produced by oscillatory pacemaker activity conducting with delay to the surrounding myocardium and could be unrelated to reentry. Several recent animal studies using an extensive array of extracellular electrodes have provided important information concerning the sequence of activation during ventricular tachyarrhythmias, strongly suggesting in some of the studies that reentry is the responsible mechanism.

## Summary

As new mechanisms for the development of cardiac arrhythmias are identified, the tests used to identify previously described mechanisms may need to be revised. For example, initiation and termination of a presumed reentrant tachycardia by a single premature stimulus does not exclude triggered activity or initiation and annihilation of pacemaker activity as possible mechanisms. Therefore, it still is not possible, given present discriminating techniques, to be unequivocally certain about the mechanisms responsible for most clinically occurring cardiac arrhythmias. Nevertheless, much information has accumulated that has provided for better understanding of the mechanisms responsible for clinically occurring arrhythmias.

## References


1. Vassalle M: Cardiac automaticity and its control. In ML Levy and M Vassalle (eds.): *Excitation and Neural Control of the Heart*, Washington, DC, American Physiological Society, 1982, p. 59.
2. Schmitt FO, Erlanger J: Directional differences in the conduction of the impulse through heart muscle and their possible relation to extrasystolic and fibrillatory contractions. *Am J Physiol* 87:326, 1928.
3. Allessie MA, Bonke FIM, Schopman FJG: Circus movement in rabbit atrial muscle as a mechanisms of tachycardia. III. The "leading circle" concept: A new model of circus movement in cardiac tissue without the involvement of an anatomical obstacle. *Circ Res* 41:9, 1977.

4. Antzelevitch C, Jalife J, Moe GK: Characteristics of reflection as a mechanism of reentrant arrhythmias and its relationship to parasystole. *Circulation* 61:182, 1980.
5. Gilmour RF, Salata JJ, Zipes DP: Rate-related suppression and facilitation of conduction in isolated canine cardiac Purkinje fibers. *Circ Res* 57:35, 1985.
6. Jalife J, Moe GK: Effect of electrotonic potentials on pacemaker activity of canine Purkinje fibers in relation to parasystole. *Circ Res* 39:801, 1976.
7. Zipes DP: Genesis of cardiac arrhythmias: Electrophysiologic considerations. In E Braunwald (ed.): *Heart Diseases: A Textbook of Cardiovascular Medicine ed. 3*. Philadelphia, W. B. Saunders, p. 605, 1988.
8. Jalife J, Antzelevitch C, Moe GK: Models of parasystole and reflection. In MB Rosenbaum and MV Elizari (eds.): *Frontiers of Cardiac Electrophysiology*. The Hague, Martinus Nijhoff, p. 217, 1983.
9. Nau GJ, Aldariz AE, Acunzo RS, et al: Modulation of parasystolic activity by nonparasystolic beats. *Circulation* 66:462, 1982.
10. Boineau JP, Mooney CR, Hudson RD, et al: Observations on reentrant excitation pathways and the refractory period distributions in spontaneous and experimental atrial flutter in the dog. In HE Kulbertus (ed.) *Reentrant Arrhythmias*. Baltimore, University Park Press, p. 72, 1977.
11. Pastelin G, Mendez C, Moe GK: Participation of atrial specialized conduction pathways in atrial flutter. *Circ Res* 42:386, 1978.
12. Zipes DP: Electrophysiological mechanisms involved in ventricular fibrillation. *Circulation* 51−52 (Suppl III):120, 1975.
13. Moe GK, Abildskov JA: Atrial fbrillation as a self-sustaining arrhythmia independent of focal discharge. *Am Heart J* 58:59, 1969.
14. Waldo AL, Plumb VJ, Henthorn RW: Observations on the mechanism of atrial flutter. In Surawicz B, Reddy CP, Prystowsky EN (eds): *Tachycardia*. The Hague, Martinus Nighoff, p. 213, 1984.
15. Allessie MA, Bonke FIM: Direct demonstration of sinus nodal reentry in the rabbit heart. *Circ Res* 44:557, 1979.
16. Watanabe Y, Dreifus LS: Inhomogeneous conduction in the AV node: A model for reentry. *Am Heart J* 70:505, 1965.
17. Mendez C, Moe GK: Demonstration of dual AV conduction system in the isolated rabbit heart. *Circ Res* 19:378, 1966.
18. Janse MJ, VanCapelle FJL, Freud GE, et al: Circus movement within the AV node as a basis for supraventricular tachycardia as shown by multiple microelectrode recording in the isolated rabbit heart. *Circ Res* 28:403, 1971.
19. Wit AL, Goldreyer BN, Damato AN: An *in vitro* model of paroxysmal supraventricular tachycardia. *Circulation* 43:862, 1971.
20. Bigger JT, Goldreyer BN: The mechanism of supraventricular tachycardia. *Circulation* 42:673, 1970.
21. Denes P, Wu D, Dhingra C, et al: Demonstration of dual AV nodal pathways in patients with paroxysmal supraventricular tachycardia. *Circulation* 48:549, 1973.
22. Durrer D, Schoo L, Schuilenburg RM, et al: The role of premature beats in the initiation and the termination of supraventricular tachy-

cardia in the Wolff-Parkinson-White syndrome. *Circulation* 36:644, 1967.
23. Zipes DP, DeJoseph RL, Rothbaum DA: Unusual properties of accessory pathways. *Circulation* 49:1200, 1974.
24. Gallagher JJ: The pre-excitation syndromes. *Prog Cardiovasc Dis* 20:285, 1978.
25. Coumel P, Attuel P: Reciprocating tachycardia in overt and latent pre-excitation: Influence of functional bundle branch block on the rate of the tachycardia. *Eur J Cardiol* 1:423, 1974.
26. Hammill SC, Pritchett LC, Klien GJ, et al: Accessory atrioventricular pathways that conduct only in the antegrade direction. *Circulation* 62:1335, 1980.
27. Lown B, Ganong WF, Levine SA: The syndrome of short PR interval, normal QRS complex and paroxysmal rapid heart action. *Circulation* 5:693, 1952.
28. James TN: The Wolff-Parkinson-White syndrome. Evolving concepts of its pathogenesis. *Prog Cardiovasc Dis* 13:159, 1970.
29. Jackman WM, Prystowsky EN, Naccarelli GV, et al: Reevaluation of enhanced atrioventricular nodal conduction: Evidence to suggest a continuum of normal atrioventricular nodal physiology. *Circulation* 67:441, 1983.
30. Gallagher JJ, Smith WM, Kasell JH, et al: Role of Mahaim fibers in cardiac arrhythmias in man. *Circulation* 64:176, 1981.
31. Glassman RD, Zipes DP: Site of antegrade and retrograde functional right bundle branch block in the intact canine heart. *Circulation* 64:1277, 1981.
32. Akhtar M, Gilbert C, Wolfe FG, et al: Reentry within the His–Purkinje system: Elucidation of reentrant circuit using right bundle branch and His bundle recordings. *Circulation* 58:295, 1978.
33. Lloyd EA, Zipes DP, Heger JJ, et al: Sustained ventricular tachycardia due to bundle branch block reentry. *Am Heart J* 104:1095, 1982.
34. Josephson ME, Horowitz LN, Farshidi A, et al: Recurrent sustained ventricular tachycardia. I. Mechanisms. *Circulation* 57:431, 1978.
35. Boineau JP, Cox JL: Slow ventricular activation in acute myocardial infarction: A source of reentrant premature ventricular contractions. *Circulation* 48:703, 1973.
36. Waldo AL, Kaiser GA: Study of ventricular arrhythmias associated with acute myocardial infarction in the canine heart. *Circulation* 47:1222, 1973.
37. El-Sherif N, Scherlag BJ, Lazzara R, et al: Reentrant ventricular arrhythmias in the late myocardial infarction period. I. Conduction characteristics in the infarction zone. *Circulation* 55:686, 1977.
38. Wit Al, Allessie MA, Bonke FIM, et al: Electrophysiologic mapping to determine the mechanism of experimental ventricular tachycardia initiated by premature impulses: Experimental approaches and initial results demonstrating reentrant excitation. *Am J Cardiol* 49:166, 1982.

# Chapter 3

# Comparative Mechanisms of Action of Antiarrhythmic Agents: Significance of Lengthening Repolarization

Bramah N. Singh

The exact manner in which various antiarrhythmic agents act in controlling disorders of cardiac rhythm still is poorly defined. However, in recent years, there has been considerable growth in knowledge, especially with the increasing application of the intracellular microelectrode, voltage-clamp, and "patch-clamp" techniques to isolated heart muscle.[1-4] Initially, the focus was on the interpretation of pharmacodynamic effects from the gross parameters of the transmembrane potentials from various parts of the heart. Attention has been directed at alterations in conduction velocity, refractoriness, and threshold of excitability of the myocardial cell relative to changes in the rate of depolarization and repolarization during a complete cycle.[5-8] More recently, attention has shifted to the delineation of the effects of drugs on specific ionic conductances[9,10] and on the recovery kinetics of the ionic channels[11-15] in response to abrupt changes in stimulation frequency. The precise relevance of these newer findings in controlling cardiac dysrhythmias still remains to be established. Nevertheless, the data indicate that the differences between the overall

*Supported by grants from the Medical Research Service of the Veterans Administration and the American Heart Association, the Greater Los Angeles Affiliate, Los Angeles, California.*

From: *Control of Cardiac Arrhythmias by Lengthening Repolarization,* edited by Bramah N. Singh, MD, Futura Publishing Company Inc., Mount Kisco, NY, © 1988.

electrophysiologic actions of antiarrhythmic compounds may be considerably greater than hitherto appreciated. The purpose of this chapter is to discuss the effects of antiarrhythmic agents on action potentials generated in various cardiac fibers. The description of these effects is preceded by a discussion of the current but simple ideas of the genesis of the cardiac action potential in relation to changes in myocardial refractoriness, conduction, and threshold of excitability.

## Cardiac Electrophysiology

In excitable tissues, such as skeletal muscle and nerve, the electrical activity is uniform and mediated by similar ionic mechanisms. In contrast, the electrical activity in different types of cardiac fibers is represented by action potentials of varying configurations. These are associated with varying functions and are characterized by quantitatively different electrophysiologic parameters, such as refractory periods, conduction velocity, and the duration of repolarization.

In the heart the electrical activity begins spontaneously in a rhythmic fashion in the sinoatrial (SA) node (designated as *pacemaker*) and spreads sequentially throughout the atria and is transmitted over internodal pathways to the atrioventricular (AV) node. The properties of the internodal pathways resemble those of ventricular Purkinje fibers in terms of conduction velocity and refractory periods. The conduction velocity in the AV node is slowed markedly, accounting for the normal delay of the impulse here during its transmission to the His–Purkinje fibers and the ventricular myocardium, in which the conduction velocity once again accelerates considerably. The differences in conduction velocity and other electrophysiologic properties among different types of cardiac fibers appear to be related to the differences in the ionic basis for the depolarization and repolarization phases of the action potentials. There are further differences in these tissues in different animal species.

The electrical impulses in cardiac tissue are generated by a sequential alteration in the relative permeability of the myocardial membrane to different ions. A knowledge of the sequence of such ionic changes mediating rapid depolarization, repolarization, and spontaneous diastolic depolarization during the inscription of the action potential (AP) in pacemaking and nonpacemaking tissues is essential to the understanding of the origin of arrhythmias and how antiarrhythmic drugs exert their salutary effects. Ions are transferred across the myocardial membranes through channels that can discriminate among different charge carriers, the channel selectivity being reflected in the equilibrium potential for individual ions involved in the generation of the cardiac action potential.[16,17] The current flow through the ion-specific channels is regulated by voltage- and time-dependent activation and inactivation gates.[18]

## Ionic Basis of Various Types of Cardiac Action Potentials

Based on the maximal rate of depolarization and the membrane potential from which the upstroke is initiated, two types of cardiac action potentials may be distinguished. The first type (e.g., in atrial, ventricular, and His–Purkinje fibers) has a fast upstroke velocity arising from markedly negative membrane potentials. The second type (e.g., in SA and AV nodes) has a much slower rate of rise and a much more positive activation voltage. These differences may reflect two distinct types of excitatory inward currents, one carried by sodium ions and the other predominantly (but not exclusively) by calcium ions.

*Sodium Current*

The cardiac action potential is a phasic electrical activity separable into five phases, particularly well delineated in the case of action potentials dependent on sodium ions for depolarization. The surface and ionic correlates of a transmembrane action potential in a fast-channel dependent cardiac muscle are shown in Figure 1. Phase 0, representing the sudden depolarization when the membrane potential (MP) is brought to threshold, is mediated by a kinetically fast current ("fast response") and a kinetically slow current ("slow response"). The fast response is mediated by a change in sodium ion conductance.[19] The change is sudden and brief, lasting only a few milliseconds, and its intensity, as determined by the upstroke velocity of phase 0 ($V_{max}$), is a function of the membrane potential from which the action potential is generated (Fig. 2). $V_{max}$ has been used as a valid index of sodium channel availability, although recent evidence has questioned its linearity in this regard.[20] However, the parameter continues to be used for measuring the effects of physiologic and pharmacologic interventions on sodium channel function.[6] The measurements of single-Na channel

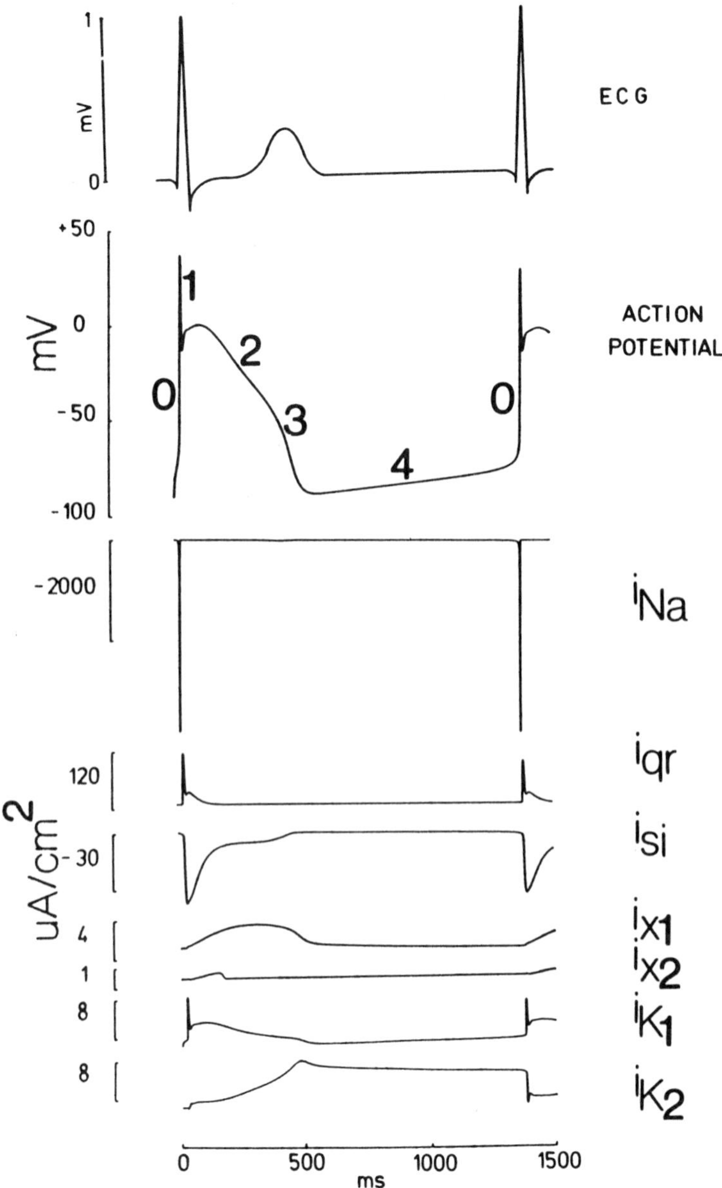


**Figure 1.** Ionic and surface electrocardiographic correlates of the idealized cardiac action potential (phases 0 to 4 denote the various phases of action potential during one complete cardiac cycle). Inward currents are indicated by negative deflections and outward currents by positive deflections.

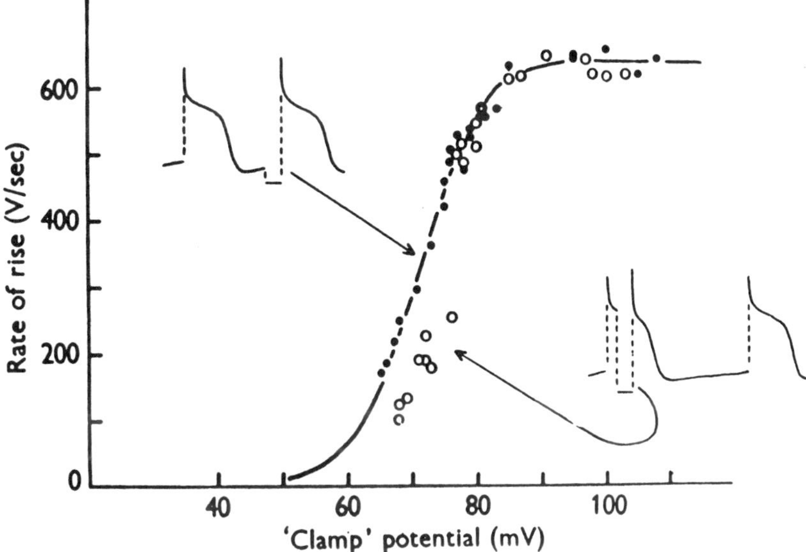


**Figure 2.**   Relationship between membrane potential ("clamp" potential) and the rate of rise of the elicited action potential. Note the sigmoidal relationship; also note that at about -50 mV the fiber is inexcitable (completely refractory) to an applied stimulus. (From Weidmann S: The effect of the cardiac membrane potential on the rapid availability of the sodium carrier system. *J Physiol* 127:213, 1955. By permission of the author and the journal.)

currents have provided the basis for the understanding of Na current kinetics that appear identical both in cultured cells and in isolated cardiac muscle.[9,21,22] In nerve, sodium current has been interpreted in terms of a closed resting state, an open activated state, and a closed inactivated state. In cardiac muscle, this has provided the basis for defining the differences in the binding and reactivation kinetics of different local anesthetic types of antiarrhythmic compounds.[15] It also should be emphasized that the level of membrane potential affects the fraction of sodium channels that remain open and are available for impulse transmission. For example, in the plateau range of potentials, many are inactivated (i.e., closed). Thus, the time course of recovery from inactivation at diastolic potentials determines the availability of the sodium channels for impulse conduction and the period over which the cells remain inexcitable (refractory) to an applied stimulus. The sodium channel is inhibited specifically by tetrodotoxin (TTx), which, however, does not affect the kinetics of the channel.

In mammalian Purkinje fibers, the maximum diastolic potential (MDP) is between -80 and -90 mV with an upstroke velocity often exceeding 500 V/sec and the associated conduction velocity is about 5 meters/sec. The threshold potential for the activation of the action potential is about -65 mV. Purkinje fibers may exhibit spontaneous pacemaker activity but the activation voltage, unlike that in the sinus node, is considerably more negative. Atrial and ventricular myocardium also demonstrate action potentials that are dependent on the fast-channel for depolarization. Thus, they also have the maximum diastolic potential (MDP), usually exceeding -80mV but, unlike the Purkinje fibers, these tissues do not normally show pacemaker activity. Neither atrial nor ventricular muscle fibers demonstrate a marked early "notch" preceding the plateau phase of the action potential, but the upstroke velocity of phase 0 is rapid, as is the associated conduction velocity.

*Calcium current*

In contrast, the second (slow) inward current is carried essentially by calcium ions, with a small component of sodium ions, and the threshold for the activation of the slow channel is about -35 mV.[17] Thus, normally, it is activated as the fast channel depolarizes the cell. The slow channel in ventricular muscle begins to inactivate at about 500 msec from the onset of depolarization so that the slow current only starts to attenuate near the end of the plateau phase of the action potential. In magnitude, the slow current is about 100 times less than the peak sodium current. Physiologically, it mediates conduction in nodal tissues,[17,23] is responsible for excitation-contraction coupling in cardiac muscle, and is crucial to the generation of the plateau phase of the atrial, ventricular, and the specialized conducting tissues of the heart.[17,24]

Voltage-clamp studies have shown that the slow current is sensitive to alterations in calcium concentrations; it is enhanced by catecholamines[25] and depressed by acetylcholine[26] and certain metallic ions, such as manganese, lanthanum, cobalt, and nickel as well as organic molecules (verapamil, nifedipine, nisoldipine, and diltiazem, among others), which now have been designated as calcium antagonists (to be discussed later). However, recent observations have suggested that whereas numerous agents block the slow channel, there are differences in their specificities and modes of action.[24] The slow channel is not inhibited by TTx and its voltage dependence and kinetics of its gating mechanism differ from those of the fast sodium channel. Reuter and Scholz[27] have shown that the slow channel is not completely selective for calcium ions. It was found that Na and K ions also may move through the slow channel, but they have over 100 times less the permeability of calcium.

Slow response action potentials are normally found in the sinoatrial and atrioventricular nodes and in pathological situations in which the fast response has been inactivated. Experimentally, slow-channel potentials may be induced in atria, ventricles, or Purkinje fibers by inactivating the fast channel by high concentrations of potassium in a medium also containing catecholamines.[17] In the case of the SA node the MDP is about -65 mV and the maximum rate of depolarization is about 10 V/sec, reflecting the magnitude of the inward current responsible for the voltage change. The electrical activity of the AV node resembles that of the SA node but there is less of a proclivity for pacemaker activity. The MDP is about -60 mV and the rate of rise of the action potential about 10 V/sec.

## Outward or Repolarizing Currents in the Myocardium

These are best established in Purkinje fibers and in ventricular muscle (see Fig. 1). Here, the plateau phase is maintained by a fine balance between the inward and outward current flow, with a small net transfer of charge. Repolarization occurs when the net outward transfer of charge increases due to a stepwise increase in the inactivation of the slow current and the slow activation of a number of time- and voltage-dependent currents, carried largely but not exclusively by potassium. It is also known that a component of the fast Na channel is inactivated slowly and extends into the plateau range of action potentials, particularly in the Purkinje fibers[28] The existence of this is inferred from the effects of tetrodotoxin, which tends to accelerate the early phases of repolarization in Purkinje fibers. Unlike the case with the depolarizing currents, the nature of the repolarizing currents is less well understood. Agents that might selectively block individual outward currents have not been described.

### Delayed Rectification

Noble and Tsien[29] described a time-dependent outward current (designated as $I_x$) that could be activated in the plateau range of the action potentials with a fast ($I_{x1}$) and slow ($I_{x2}$) time constants of inactivation. This current is called the *delayed rectifier* in relation to the repolarizing currents in skeletal muscle and nerve. Such a current also has been described in the SA node and in atrial and ventricular tissues. The second potassium current ($i_{k1}$), which is voltage dependent only, also appears to contribute to repolarization. Its kinetics are poorly defined.

### Transient Outward Current

This current, sometimes alled $I_{qr}$, or *dynamic chloride current,* was found in early voltage clamp studies[30] during the early phase repolarization, particular in Purkinje fibers. Recent studies have suggested that the most likely charge carrier for this current is potassium ions.[31] This transient outward current is now designated as $I_{to}$ and has been found to have two components: one sensitive to calcium, the other not. It appears to be responsible for the "notch" in the early part of repolarization phase of the action potential in Purkinje fibers and to a lesser extent in the ventricular muscle. The physiologic significance of the $I_{to}$ is unknown.

### Pacemaker Current

The ionic basis of the pacemaker current was first investigated in Purkinje fibers using the voltage clamp studies.[32] It is likely that the pacemaker phenomenon is due to one of three possible mechanisms: (1) slow increase in sodium permeability, (2) slow diminution of potassium permeability, and (3) a slow decline in the outward current carried by the sodium pump. The characteristics of the pacemaker current, designated as $i_{k2}$, was investigated by Noble and Tsien,[32] whose data supported the second possibility. Whether this is the mechanism for the spontaneous diastolic depolarization in the natural pacemaker however is less clear. Recent experimental studies[33–36] on the nature of the pacemaker current have suggested that the mechanism of pacemaking is more complicated than previously thought. It appears that $i_{k2}$ may be due, in part, to a time-dependent inward current carried by sodium with an outward component carried by potassium.

As far as the pacemaker current in the sinus node is concerned, it is important to emphasize that whatever ionic mechanisms for its origins are postulated, they must take cognizance of the fact that acetycholine decreases spontaneous diastolic depolarization and adrenaline accelerates it. Acetylcholine increases passive potassium conductance and both epinephrine and acetycholine affect gated channels in the heart. Tsien[37] showed that epinephrine affected $i_{k2}$ kinetics in such a way that its decay was accelerated in the diastolic potential range. This may account for the steepness of the slope of diastolic depolarization in the SA node. However, an augmentation of the slow calcium current induced by catecholamines in the SA node would result in faster pacing in the pacemaker cells. This emphasizes the potential significance of the slow calcium inward current in the genesis of the pacemaker current in the SA node.

## Threshold, Excitability, and Refractoriness in Cardiac Muscle

Myocardial fibers exhibit the property of *excitability*: The membrane of these cells can be stimulated to produce an electrophysiologic response, an action potential. Excitability may be quantified by the amount of current needed to depolarize an area of the membrane to threshold potential so that an action potential is generated. The minimum current required to elicit such a response is termed the *threshold*. The excitability of the myocardial cell varies with time during the cardiac cycle, and it is related intimately to the property of refractoriness. The voltage dependence of refractory period in cardiac muscle was clearly established by Weidmann,[19,38] and the salient features, as applicable to fast and slow channel fibers, are illustrated in Figure 3.

The study of the relationship between membrane potential and $V_{max}$, commonly known as *membrane responsiveness*, has shown that, until the membrane is repolarized to -55 mV or so in fibers that are dependent on fast sodium channel activity for depolarization, it cannot be reactivated, irrespective of the stimulus strength. This level of repolarization thus defines the end of the *absolute refractory period* (ARP), a parameter that is voltage dependent and varies in length with the action potential duration (Fig. 2). Thus, any intervention that lengthens the APD (e.g., bradycardia, hypocalcemia, hypothyroidism) prolongs the ARP; conversely, those that shorten the APD (e.g., halothane, anoxia, tachycardia) tend to abbreviate the ARP. The ARP of cardiac muscle needs to be distinguished from the *effective refractory period* (ERP), which is the main determinant of the number of *propagated* impulses that the heart is able to generate per unit time. It thus is longer in duration than the ARP and, since the generation of a propagated impulse is critically dependent on the recovery of excitability, the ERP, under certain circumstances, may outlast the entire duration of cardiac repolarization. The recovery of excitability in this context is related to the recovery of the sodium-carrier mechanism to a finite

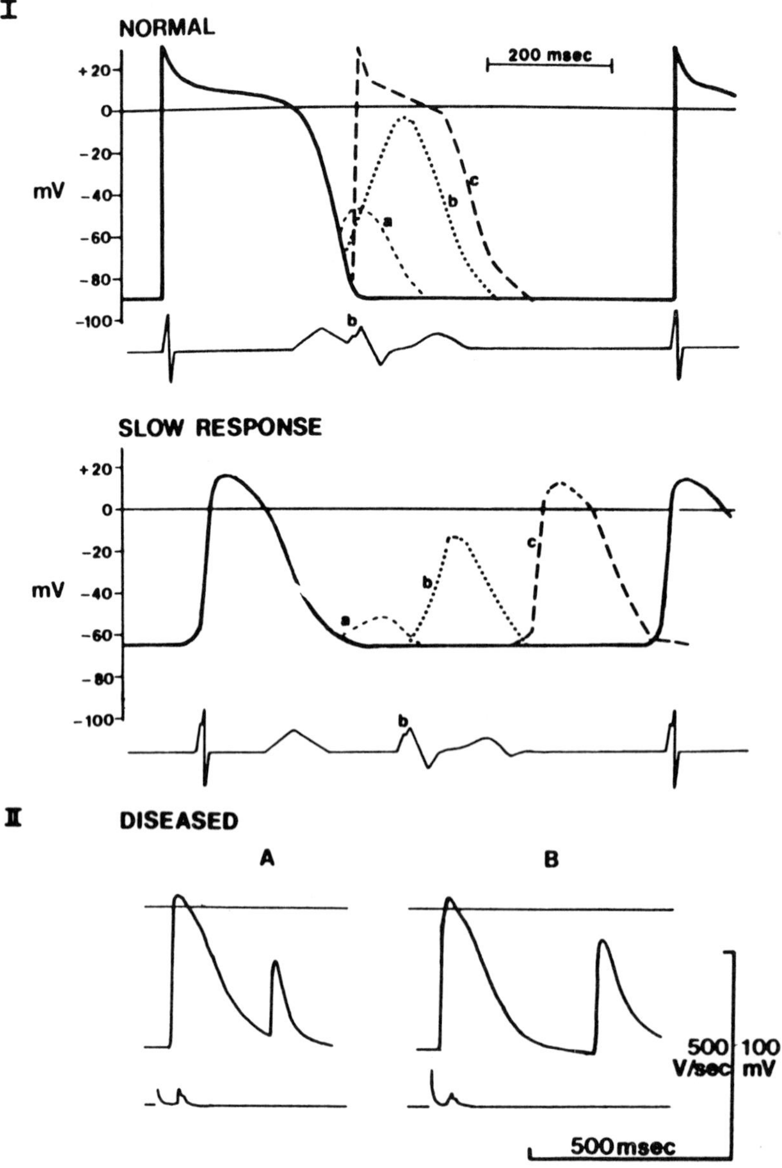


**Figure 3.** Characteristics of fast response and slow response (I), and action potentials from diseased myocardium (II) in relation to the surface electrogram. Note the differences between the fast response and slow response fibers to an applied extrastimulus. In the former a conducted action potential is elicitable before repolarization is completed. In the latter, the effective refractory period outlasts the entire duration of the action potential. In the diseased fibers, the action potentials shown represent attenuated fast responses. (From Singer DH, Baumgarten CM, Ten Eick RE: Cellular electrophysiology of ventricular and other dysrhythmias: Studies on diseased and ischemic hearts. In, Sonnenblick EH, Lesch M (eds): *Sudden Cardiac Death*, New York, Grune and Stratton, p 13, 1981. By permission of the authors and publishers.)

degree; the inhibition of the fast response, as might be produced by local anesthetic drugs, may lengthen markedly the ERP with a trivial or no change in the overall action potential duration (and hence, the ARP). It therefore is apparent that the lengthening of the refractory period in cardiac muscle may arise on the basis of selective or isolated lengthening of the time course of repolarization because of the voltage dependence of the refractory period, and it would be associated with no change in conduction velocity. The effective refractory period also may be prolonged by a delay in the reactivation of the sodium channel following the passage of an impulse. Since this would occur independent of the time course of repolarization, it may be termed a *time-dependent change* in the effective refractory period. The concept of time- and voltage-dependent refractoriness in cardiac muscle with respect to the fast and slow channel potentials is illustrated in Figure 3.[39]

## Cardiac Action Potentials and the Autonomic Nervous System

Directly or indirectly, many cardioactive compounds affect the autonomic nervous system. For example, quinidine, disopyramide, and to a lesser extent procainamide exert anticholinergic effects. On the other hand, verapamil, diltiazem, and amiodarone noncompetitively block adrenergic excitation. Therefore, it is necessary to differentiate those changes in the cardiac action potential produced by a particular agent as a result of its effect on the autonomic nervous system and those that are the intrinsic effects of the compound itself.

The most striking effects of autonomic transmitters, adrenergic and cholinergic, are on the SA and AV nodal potentials. Adrenergic agonists increase the slope of phase 4 depolarization in the SA nodal cells and exert a tendency for the maximum diastolic potential to become more negative and for the amplitude of the action potential to increase. The effects of acetylcholine and vagal stimulation appear to be the converse of sympathomimetic amines. Cholinergic agents decrease the slope of phase 4 depolarization by decreasing the rate of diastolic depolarization and hyperpolarize the membrane by effects on potassium and, possibly, calcium conductance.[40]

The net effect of catecholamines is to augment the amplitude and the rate of rise of the action potentials in the AN and N regions of the AV node with an effect on the resting membrane potential. These changes are accompanied by an enhancement of conduction and a shortening of the effective and the functional refractory periods. The cells in the N$-$H region are affected little by catecholamines but, in those that exhibit phase 4 depolarization, the rate of firing is accelerated by an increase in the rate of depolarization. These overall in vitro changes provide the basis for delineating the effects of sympathetic excitation and blockade in vivo and in the AV node.

Again, the effects of acetylcholine, vagal stimulation, and cholinergic agents are the converse to those found with adrenergic stimulation. Vagomimetic agents reduce the upstroke velocity and the action potential amplitude and delay conduction velocity in the AV node with a prolongation of the refractory period. A concentration-dependent failure of conduction may occur, principally at the level of cells in the AN and N regions of the AV node with those in the NH region being relatively unaffected.

The effects of adrenergic and cholinergic agents on the action potential parameters in fast-channel dependent tissues such as atria, Purkinje fibers, and ventricular myocardium are complex. Little is known about the sympathetic regulation of the His$-$Purkinje system in vivo. However, when the Purkinje fibers are paced at a rate sufficient to overdrive spontaneous activity, beta-receptor agonists tend to modestly decrease the action potential duration in these fibers. The effects of acetylcholine in Purkinje fibers is variable and often species-dependent. Very high concentrations are necessary to demonstrate a measurable effect on the action potential duration and refractoriness.[40,41]

In the case of atrial and ventricular fibers, the adrenergic effects on the action potential are qualitatively similar: There is only a minor effect on the action potential from fibers that normally are polarized despite a marked increase in contractile force.[41] Under the action of sympathetic amines, the action potential tends to be more positive in the plateau range of potentials for a slightly longer period of time compared to controls. However, the precise nature of the ionic changes that underlie these changes has not been clearly defined. In the case of partially depolarized fibers, especially following high concentrations of external potassium, catecholamines may augment markedly the upstroke velocity of the resulting slow response potentials, increasing their amplitude and markedly prolonging their duration of repolarization.

The effects of cholinergic agents in the atria are striking, being characterized by a marked acceleration of the time course of repolarization and hyperpolarization of the membrane compared to the maximum diastolic potential during control.[41] These effects are related to an increase in potassium conductance. Such a change is accompanied by a markedly negative inotropic effect. The effects of cholinergic influences on the ventricular myocardium are complex but, in general, much less significant than those on the atria. The effects are minimal in the normal ventricular myocardium, in which the negative inotropic effect evident in atrial tissue largely is absent. In markedly depolarized fibers, acetylcholine may inhibit the slow inward current augmented by adrenergic stimulation.

The remainder of this chapter discusses the effects of various electrophysiolgic classes of antiarrhythmic agents[7,8] on the action potentials from different types of myocardial fibers. The major focus will be on data derived from studies using the standard microelectrode techniques. However, wherever information on the ionic correlates of such changes are available, these are discussed. The overall in vitro effects are related to the effects established in vivo either by the use of recordings of the monophasic action potential by suction electrodes[42] or intracavitary electrodes as well as those obtained by surface electrocardiography.

## Effects of Antiarrhythmic Agents on Cardiac Action Potentials

Over the years numerous attempts have been made to interpret the fundamental mode of actions of antiarrhythmic agents from their effects on the cardiac action potentials.[7,8] Initially, the experimental data dealt almost exclusively with isolated healthy mammalian myocardium and thus the effects of pharmacologic agents were interpreted from the changes that occurred in the normal action potentials in the sinus node, atria, AV node, ventricles, and the His-Purkinje fibers. Subsequently, there has been an increasing appreciation that such data may not be extrapolated readily to the diseased myocardium, which usually forms the substrate for the genesis of the clinically occurring cardiac dysrhythmias.[39] Thus, newer in vitro and in vivo experimental models need to be developed to allow for these deficiencies in the acquisiton of data for the interpretation of the mode of action of antiarrhythmic agents in the clinical setting. Of particular interest has been the characterization of abnormally occurring action potentials, such as attentuated fast-channel potentials (e.g., in ischemic myocardium), slow-channel potentials (e.g., in diseased atria, ventricular aneurysm), and on afterdepolarizations.[43] Two types of afterdepolarizations already have been described (see Chapters 1 and 2). The early afterdepolarizations occur as oscillations that interrupt phase 2 or phase 3 of the repolarization phase of the action potential. Such oscillations lead to a repetitive rhythm that has been termed *triggered.*[44] The charge carriers for these action potentials have not been elucidated completely but they have been shown to be blocked by local anesthetic agents, such as lidocaine and procainamide, or in calcium channel blockers, such as verapamil. Delayed afterdepolarizations are oscillations in the membrane potential that follow complete repolarization and often are preceded by transient hyperpolarization. When these oscillations reach threshold, they produce triggered rhythms that exhibit the phenomenon of overdrive acceleration. Again, the precise ionic basis of afterdepolarizations is unclear, but they are induced by digitalis intoxication and are depressed by fast channel blockers, calcium channel blockers, but by beta blockers only if they are induced by a combination of catecholamines and digitalis. Triggered automaticity is now considered a disturbance of impulse formation and, along with enhanced automaticity, a mechanism of certain cardiac arrhythmias in addition to that which produces a dysrhythmia due to reentry.[45] Thus, in the elucidation of the mode of action of antiarrhythmic agents, it is no longer sufficient to define the action of these agents in normal and abnormal action potentials but it also is necessary to define their effects on action potentials that mediate the genesis of abnormal cardiac rhythms (see Chapter 1).

It now is clear that the recognition of those features of a compound that may be associated with a particular antiarrhythmic effect may serve a useful purpose; for example, to allow screening for an antiarrhythmic effect in the development of newer agents. The correlation of the structure of the compound with a particular antiarrhythmic and electrophysiologic effect also may be of value in this regard. Furthermore, the summated effects of one or more discrete mechanisms may form the basis of testing the hypothesis that combination therapy may be additive or even synergistic. It should be emphasized that no definitive answers to these issues as yet are available. However, it appears of value to characterize major antiarrhythmic mechanisms on the basis of (1) the fast channel blockade, (2) the blockade of the electrophysiologic effects of sympathetic excitation to the heart, (3) the inhibition of cardiac repolarization currents, and (4) the inhibition of the slow myocar-

Table 1
Major Electrophysiologic Classes of Antiarrhythmic Compounds

| I. Fast Sodium Channel Blockers | II. Sympathetic Blockers | III. Inhibitors of Repolarization | IV. Calcium Antagonists |
|---|---|---|---|
| a. Quinidine | Propranolol | Sotalol | Verapamil |
| Procainamide | Timolol | Amiodarone | Tiapamil |
| Disopyramide | Oxprenolol | N-acetylprocainamide | Nifedipine |
| | Alprenolol | Bretylium | Gallopamil |
| b. Lidocaine | Nadolol | Melperone | Bepridil |
| Mexiletine | Atenolol | | Perhexiline |
| Tocainide | Acebutolol | | |
| Phenytoin Sodium | Sotalol | | |
| Ethmozine | Metoprolol | | |
| Aprindine | Labetolol | | |
| | (plus others) | | |
| c. Flecainide | | | |
| Encainide | | | |
| Lorcainide | | | |
| Propafenone | | | |
| Indecainide | | | |
| Recainam | | | |

*Also, other dihydropyridines. Lidoflazine is not included as a calcium antagonist because it has no significant effect on the myocardial slow channel.

dial inward current.[7,8,46–50] These effects, in different ways, lead to an increase in the threshold of excitability (including fibrillation threshold) and in the refractory period in different types of cardiac muscles. How different antiarrhythmic agents (Table 1), conventional ones and those under investigation, might alter these parameters will be discussed briefly in the remainder of this chapter.

## Fast Channel Blockers and the Cardiac Action Potential

There are numerous chemically heterogeneous compounds that exert antiarrhythmic actions and their major electrophysiologic effects are mediated through the inhibition of the fast sodium channel in the myocardium. These agents are potent local anesthetics in nerve with a comparable depressant effect on conduction velocity in cardiac tissues, although the actions evident in the myocardium are of very much lower concentrations than those in nerve.[7,8,46–51]

The dominant electrophysiologic property of fast channel blockers is their ability to reduce the $V_{max}$, a property associated with an increase in the threshold of excitability, a depression in conduction velocity, and a marked prolongation in the time-dependent effective refractory period in cardiac muscle.[46-51] Another way of expressing the effects of fast channel blockers is to relate the alterations in the maximal rate of rise of the action potential to the membrane potential (discussed earlier (i.e., on "membrane responsiveness"). Fast channel blockers shift this relationship in the hyperpolarizing direction.[38] These changes occur without a significant alteration in the resting membrane potential (except in toxic concentrations) but are invariably associated with the inhibition of the spontaneous diastolic depolarization in automatic fibers. These effects on the so-called pacemaker cells usually are apparent at lower concentrations than those on conduction or the threshold of excitability. Thus, it will be evident that fast channel blockers, as a group, are likely to be effective in controlling arrhythmias not only by depressing conduction and prolonging refractoriness but also by depressing automaticity—a broad spectrum antiarrhythmic action. However, it must be recognized that many fast channel blockers have additional properties, which may influence their overall action in the myocardium. For example, in the cases of *quinidine, disopyramide, and procainamide*, there is the feature of the prolongation of action potential duration. This possibly confers on these compounds an additional antiarrhythmic activity while the QT lengthening may lead to torsade de pointes.[52] In a subclassification of antiarrhythmic agents,[50,51] these agents (see Table 2) therefore have been designated as 1a. In contrast, agents such as *lidocaine, mexiletine, tocainide, aprindine, phenytoin sodium, pirmenolol, and ethmozin*, which block the fast channel but either shorten the action potential duration or have no effect, have been subcategorized as 1b. Finally, those fast channel blockers that have a markedly depressant effect on conduction velocity in cardiac muscle but that exert a differential effect on the duration of the action potential in Purkinje fibers and ventricular muscle (shortening the former and either having no effect or lengthening somewhat in the latter) have been designated as 1c. This subgroup includes *flecainide, encainide (and its metabolites), propafenone, indecainide, recainam, lorcainide, and possibly cibenzoline*. Thus, it is important to distinguish those parameters of various fast channel blockers that may be attributed to sodium channel blockade and those unrelated to it. In vivo, fast channel

**Table 2**
**Electrophysiologic Subclassification of Fast Sodium Channel Blockers in Cardiac Muscle**

| Subclasses | Ia | Ib | Ic |
| --- | --- | --- | --- |
| 1. $V_{max}$ at normal or low stimulation rates | Depress | Little effect | Depress markedly |
| 2. $APD_{90}$ | Increase modestly | Either no change or shorten | Differential effect: increase in ventricular muscle (or no change) and markedly shorten in Purkinje fibers |
| 3. QRS and HV | Increase modestly | Little effect (except in diseased tissues) | Increase markedly |
| 4. ERP | Increase significantly | Little or no increase (except in diseased or depolarized fibers) | Increase modestly |
| 5. Onset-offset kinetics of rate-dependent block of sodium channel | Intermediate in rapidity | Fast | Slow |
| 6. Major examples | Quinidine<br>Procainamide<br>Disopyramide | Lidocaine<br>Tocainide<br>Mexiletine | Encainide<br>Flecainide<br>Lorcainide |

inhibition is associated with the prolongation of the QRS duration on the surface electrocardiogram and the lengthening of infranodal conduction (i.e., HV interval on His bundle electrocardiography). There also is lengthening of the effective refractory period in ventricular myocardium, bypass tracts, and in the His–Purkinje system with a lesser effect in the atria and variable effects in the AV node.

Other features of blocking the inward sodium current should be recognized. First, since $V_{max}$ is dependent on the level of membrane potential from which the action potential takes off, it is clear that interventions that affect the level of the resting membrane potential will, of necessity, influence membrane responsiveness. For example, hypokalemia, which hyperpolarizes the membrane, will attenuate the overall effects of those agents that exert a depressant action on $V_{max}$; the converse will occur in hyperkalemia.[48] Similarly, in myocardial ischemia, a situation in which fibers are markedly depolarized, the effects of fast channel blockers on membrane responsiveness and conduction velocity will be accentuated. The same may hold for the clinical contexts in which the membrane potential is depressed because of disease. Second, there is clear evidence that the blockade of the fast sodium channel is frequency- or use-dependent[11–15] i.e., the reduction in the $V_{max}$ increases as a function of stimulus frequency and the magnitude of its decrease is significantly greater at the end of a train of impulses than at the beginning. Thus, the steady-state effect on $V_{max}$ increases with the increasing stimulus frequencies. Moreover, it been established that during diastole, the use-dependent depression of the $V_{max}$ recovers much more slowly at more positive than at negative membrane potentials.

These observations, which also hold true for calcium channel blockers (discussed later), recently have formed the basis for the application of the so-called receptor modulated hypothesis developed in studies on nerve[53,54] to cardiac muscle to account for actions of fast channel blockers as antiarrhythmic agents.[51] Central to the receptor modulated hypothesis is the postulate that the interaction of certain antiarrhythmic agents with the myocardial sodium channel are time and voltage dependent.[15] It was suggested that these agents bind to the receptor site or very close to the ionic channel and that the binding affinity of the drug to the channel is modulated by the state of the channel. Thus, in terms of this hypothesis, the kinetics of fast channel blockers may vary in accordance with their affinity for binding with the rested, activated, or inactivated channel states.[15] It also was suggested that the drug-associated channels differed from drug-free channels in so far as they transmitted impulses more slowly or not at all and their voltage dependence was shifted in the hyperpolarizing direction. This hypothesis has drawn a great deal of interest recently since the concept of differential binding of a drug in relation to the state of the channel suggests a potential explanation for the differences in the effects of various fast channel blockers with respect to their effects on the reactivation kinetics of the fast sodium channel. For example, it has been found that the so-called Class 1b agents (e.g., lidocaine, mexiletine, and tocainide) have very fast kinetics of onset and offset of rate or use-dependent block of the fast channel, whereas Class 1c agents (e.g., flecainide and encainide) are extremely slow and Class 1a (e.g., quinidine, procainamide, and disopyramide) have an intermediate potency in this regard. It also recently has been suggested that these differences are of potential clinical significance.[14,55]

# Effects of Quinidine, Procainamide, and Disopyramide on Cardiac Action Potential

Although structurally disparate, these agents share certain common electrophysiologic properties, apart from their effects on the fast sodium channel. For example, all three compounds exert a modest effect in lengthening the cardiac action potential and their rate-dependent fast channel blocking effect is associated with a similar kinetics of inactivation and reactivation.[14,51]

## Quinidine

The net effects of quinidine on the cardiac action potential is due to an interplay of its direct effect on depolarization and repolarization in cardiac muscle and the indirect effects due to its anticholinergic and its noncompetitive alpha- and beta-receptor blocking actions.[56] The interaction with the autonomic transmitters varies considerably with different types of myocardial fibers relative to adrenergic and cholinergic innervation of the heart.[40,41]

The most striking electrophysiologic effect of quinidine in cardiac muscle is as a depressant on the fast sodium channel. Weidmann[38] showed that in goat Purkinje fibers, quinidine shifted the membrane responsiveness curve to more negative membrane potentials. Subsequent studies[57-66] have revealed a number of other features of quinidine action. It was found that the maximal rate of rise in the action potential in atria, ventricular muscle, and Purkinje fibers[56-60] was reduced as a function of drug concentration; this effect was associated with an increase in the threshold of excitability and an increase in the effective but not the absolute refractory period of cardiac muscle. Except at extremely high concentrations, the membrane potential was not affected. In part, the effect on the effective refractory period is due to the modest lengthening of the action potential duration, but it should be emphasized that the depressant effects of the drug on depolarization and conduction velocity overshadow its effects on the lengthening of repolarization. Thus, the drug has the propensity to prolong the effective refractory period both by the voltage and the time-dependent mechanisms.

It also should be stressed that the effects of quinidine on depolarization is more pronounced in tissues subjected to ischemia,[67] hypoxia,[62] high levels of potassium,[68] and above all, when such tissues are stimulated at high frequencies.[57] Thus, it is evident that quinidine has the propensity to selectively depress conduction velocity and excitability in depolarized tissues. In terms of the receptor-modulated theory, the rested and inactivated states of the sodium channels have a low affinity for quinidine whereas the open and activated states have a high affinity for the drug.[56,62] The time constant of recovery of $V_{max}$ after a train of impulses is about 5 to 6 seconds, accentuated by acidosis and shortened by alkalosis.

Although the ionic basis of the effect is not clear, quinidine, at relatively low drug concentrations, markedly reduces phase 4 depolarization, best demonstrated in isolated tissues. However, because the anticholinergic effect of the drug appears to exceed its antiadrenergic actions, in vivo this rarely is translated into a decrease in the spontaneous firing frequency of the sinus node nor into a depressant effect on conduction (AH interval) or refractoriness in the AV node.[69,70] A depressant effect on both the sinus node and the AV node however is likely in the event of autonomic insufficiency due to pharmacologic blockade or disease. In contrast, there is lengthening of the infranodal conduction (HV interval) and widening of the QRS interval consistent with the drug's effect on the fast sodium channel. The ionic currents that mediate the lengthening of cardiac repolarization under the influence of quinidine remain to be identified, but on surface electrocardiograms, there invariably is a prolongation of the QT interval associated with the lengthening of the effective refractory period in atria, ventricle, His-Purkinje system, and the accessory tracts in the heart. These effects, in part accountable in terms of the drug's effect on the fast channel and its kinetics and in part to delayed repolarization, likely form the basis of the known antiarrhythmic actions of quinidine, reflecting the combined influence of direct and autonomically mediated actions. Quinidine does not appear to exert a significant effect on the slow myocardial channel. Whether it has an effect on early or late afterdepolarizations giving rise to triggered rhythms is uncertain.

*Procainamide*

The overall effects of procainamide on cellular electrophysiology is very similar to those of quinidine in terms of actions on phase 4 depolarization and upstroke velocity of phase 0, including the onset-offset kinetics of rate-dependent block of the sodium channel, although procainamide has not been studied as widely as has quinidine.[56] The effects of quinidine and procainamide on phases 2 and 3 of the cardiac action potential in the so-called therapeutically meaningful concentrations are comparable.[59] In these concentrations, procainamide has no effect on the maximum diastolic potential, but as in the case of other agents with local anesthetic properties,[60,67] it reduces the $V_{max}$ and the action potential amplitude in atrial, ventricular, and His-Purkinje fibers. Procainamide also shifts the threshold potential to more negative potentials, so that more current is needed to initiate an action potential. The drug decreases conduction velocity.

The most consistent effects of procainamide are to delay repolarization and to prolong the effective refractory period in atria, ventricle, and the His-Purkinje fibers.[71-75] It is noteworthy that the increase in the effective refractory period produced by procainamide is greater than the lengthening of the action potential, indicating that the change in refractoriness is due additionally to the delay in the reactivation of the sodium channel following inactivation. Again, as in the case of quinidine, the ionic mechanisms mediating the delay in repolarization induced by procainamide are not known. However, it is known that the delay in repolarization and the prolongation of the effective refractory period in Purkinje fibers are greater in regions in which they are shorter initially than in those in which they are longer.[71] Such an effect, reported for a number of antiarrhythmic agents including lidocaine,[76] may reduce the existing heterogeneity in myocardial refractoriness and excitability. It may constitute an antiarrhythmic mechanism.[76]

Procainamide exerts no significant effect on slow channel potentials but it decreases the slope of phase 4 depolarization in spontaneously firing Purkinje fibers.[73] This also is associated with an elevation of the threshold potential. In a study of sheep Purkinje fibers, unlike liodcaine or quinidine, procainamide had no significant effect on the so-called pacemaker current.[77] Thus, it is likely that the effect of procainamide on automatic activity in the sinus node or in Purkinje fibers is mediated through the drug's effect on the fast sodium channel. However, little is known about the drug's effect on abnormal automaticity or on early or late afterdepolarizations. It nevertheless is possible that the lengthening of the action potential duration, especially in the setting of hypokalemia, may lead to low voltage oscillations in the plateau range of potentials and produce torsades de pointes.

The in vivo electrophysiologic effects of procainamide are concordant with its known in vitro actions. Unlike quinidine, the direct effects of procainamide are modified little, if at all, by autonomic interactions, and except in the setting of disease, SA and AV nodal conduction times are affected minimally. The antegrade effective or the functional refractory periods of the AV node are not influenced by procainamide. The AH and PR intervals remain unchanged. The dominant effect is the lengthening of the QRS duration and the HV interval. These effects, in therapeutically relevant concentrations, are associated with a significant lengthening of the effective refractory periods of the atria, ventricles, His-Purkinje system, and of the bypass tracts.[78] The effect on the refractory period is a composite one. In part, it is due to delayed repolarization as reflected in the prolongation of the QT interval; and in part, due to the delayed reactivation of the fast sodium channel.[14]


*Disopyramide*

Disopyramide (4-diisopropylamino 2 phenyl-2-[2-pyridyl] butyramide phosphate) was synthesized and characterized as an antiarrhythmic agent over 20 years ago.[79] Although structurally it resembles neither quinidine nor procainamide, its electrophysiologic effects on cardiac muscle are very similar to those of these compounds. For example, in isolated rabbit atria, Sekiya and Vaughan Williams (60) found that quinidine and disopyramide had comparable depressant effects on $V_{max}$ of the action potential while delaying the terminal phases of repolarization to a modest extent. Similar results also were obtained subsequently in other isolated atrial, ventricular, and Purkinje fiber preparations in which disopyramide was found to reduce spontaneous activity, to prolong the effective refractory period, and to increase atrioventricular conduction time.[80-84] However, there was no effect on the slow response,[84] although this effect is not excluded completely at higher concentrations, since one explanation of the drug's negative inotropic effect may be related to the inhibition of the slow inward current. As in the case of quinidine and other local anesthetic type of antiarrhythmic agents,[15,48] alterations in the levels of external potassium in the perfusion media over a 2−6 mM range profoundly altered the electrophysiologic effects of disopyramide in isolated Purkinje fibers, again emphasizing the essential similarities between the overall actions of the drug and those of other fast channel blockers. It should also be emphasized that as in the case of quinidine, the effects of disopyramide on the fast channel is frequency-dependent[14] with the onset-offset kinetics of rate-dependent block being very much slower than those for the newer potent fast channel blockers such as flecainide or encainide. The time constant of reactivation of disopyramide-induced block has been reported to be about 13 seconds, compared to 16–17 seconds for flecainide.

The effects of disopyramide, have been reported in ischemic or infarcting myocardium with partially depolarized fibers. For instance, in canine Purkinje fibers surviving experimental infarcts induced by coronary artery ligation, disopyramide slowed conduction to a greater extent in areas of infarction than in those normally perfused.[85] It is conceivable that this may be a significant mechanism whereby the drug alters unidirectional block to a bidirectional one in aborting reentrant ventricular tachyarrhythmias in acute ischemia. It is recognized that the electrophysiologic and hemodynamic effects of disopyramide in isolated tissue preparations as well as intact animals and humans may be influenced significantly by the drug's associated anticholinergic properties.[82,86,87] For example, whereas sinus node automaticity is consistently depressed by the drug in in vitro preparations, in vivo the net effect on sinus frequency is variable and often the anticholinergic actions of disopyramide nullifies or even reverses the expected bradycardic response.[82,84] Similarly, AV conduction is affected little or may even be facilitated by the drug in patients with normal AV transmission. A predominantly depressant effect, however, may occur in situations in which the conduction through the AV node is compromised by disease. These considerations are in line with the somewhat variable electrophysiologic effects of disopyramide reported in patients studied by His bundle electrocardiography.[87,88] The interaction with anticholinergic and adrenergic effects and direct effects of disopyramide are not confined to nodal tissues. For example, Mirro et al.[89] showed that in Purkinje fibers disopyramide lengthened the action potential duration but when the compound was superfused during the simultaneous activation of beta-adrenergic and cholinergic receptors, the action potential duration was shortened because of the anticholinergic effects of disopyramide.

These observations therefore indicate that the net drug's in vivo electrophysiologic effect in experimental animals and in humans arises on the basis of the drug's direct myocardial effects and those due to its anticholinergic properties. The effect on the sinus cycle length is variable; the PR and AH intervals shorten but the HV interval and the QRS duration lengthen. The AV nodal refractory period is not influenced by the drug but following cholinergic blockade with atropine, both sinus node function and AV nodal conduction and refractoriness are depressed by disopyramide. From the standpoint of the antiarrhythmic actions of the drug, it is noteworthy that the effective refractory period in the atria, ventricles, His-Purkinje system and the bypass tracts (in the retrograde and the anterograde directions) is consistently prolonged during intravenous as well as oral administration of disopyramide. However, it is not clear to what extent such an effect on refractoriness is due to action potential lengthening and to what extent it might be due to the delay in the reactivation of the inactivated sodium channel under the influence of the compound.

## Fast Channel Blockers with Fast Onset-Offset Kinetics of Rate-Dependent Sodium Channel Block

This subcategory of fast channel blockers includes a chemically heterogeneous group of compounds: lidocaine and its congeners (mexiletine and tocainide), aprindine, phenytoin sodium, and the newer agent ethmozine. Both in terms of the gross parameters of the action potential and the kinetics of the rate-dependent block of the fast sodium channel, these agents share common properties. First, in normally polarized myocardial fibers, these agents have little effect on the maximum rate of depolarization of the action potential at low rates of stimulation and they either shorten the action potential duration or have no effect.[15,84] Second, as in the case of all fast channel blockers, their depressant effect on $V_{max}$ is not only frequency-dependent but the kinetics of the onset and offset of the rate-dependent block to a steady state is extremely rapid. These newer findings of their effects on the action potential appear to be of direct clinical relevance.[13]

### Lidocaine

This local anesthetic agent, first synthesized in 1946, is now used widely for the short-term management of life-threatening ventricular arrhythmias. Structurally, it is a tertiary amine that has an amide linkage to an aromatic residue. Although there have been discrepancies in reports on the electrophysiologic effects of lidocaine on cardiac muscle,[7,48,90-93] recent observations have established clearly that the compound exerts its fundamental action by inhibiting the fast sodium channel.[994-99] However, it has been demonstrated that such an action is influenced a great deal by stimulation frequency,[14] membrane voltage,[96,97] levels of extracellular potassium,[48] and pH.[98]

In concentrations that are found in the serum of successfully treated patients, lidocaine exerts no significant effects on the resting membrane potential in atria, ventricles, and His–Purkinje system; it has only a modest depressant effect on $V_{max}$ of phase 0 of the action potential, not sufficient to retard conduction velocity at concentrations between 1.5–6 µg.ml. However, these effects become increasingly greater as a function of drug concentration and rate of stimulation of the fiber. The rate-dependent block induced by lidocaine is of particular interest. At stimulation frequencies less than 1 Hz lidocaine has little effect on $V_{max}$; as the ferquency is decreased, there is a very rapid decline with a new steady-state effect being achieved over 2–4 beats. There is an equally rapid recovery from inactivation after a period of rest. It appears that lidocaine has the greatest affinity for open sodium channels but tends to dissociate rapidly from them in the resting state at the time the membrane potential has returned to the maximum diastolic value. Therefore, the compound has a weak blocking effect on sodium conductance at rest and when the rate of fiber stimulation is low.

For these reasons, it will be evident that lidocaine will exert a markedly depressant effect on $V_{max}$ in fibers with attenuated fast response potentials as in myocardial ischemia, especially in the setting of high external levels of potassium and low pH.

Lidocaine shortens the action potential duration in atrial, ventricular, and Purkinje fibers that are normally polarized; the extent of shortening is the greatest in the Purkinje fibers in which the duration of repolarization is the longest. It has been suggested in the past that such a shortening may result from an effect on K conductance,[74] but the most recent data suggests that it is probably due to an effect on the TTx-sensitive inactivated sodium channels persisting into the plateau range of the action potentials.[63,77] The abbreviation of the action potential is accompanied by a corresponding *shortening* of the effective refractory period (ERP), but this is somewhat less than the shortening of the action potential duration (APD). Thus, the ERP/APD ratio is increased. However, as might be expected, lidocaine *increases* the effective refractory period in partially depolarized ventricular muscle or Purkinje fibers. Under these circumstances, the duration of the effective refractory period outlasts the duration of the action potential under the influence of lidocaine, the increase in the refractory period being due to the fact that the drug dissociates more promptly from Na channels in the rested state than in the inactivated state.

Except in very high concentrations, lidocaine has no effect on the slow response potentials. However, in normally polarized fibers lidocaine (1–10 µg/ml) depresses the slope of phase 4 depolarization in Purkinje fibers with no effect on the sinus node in the same drug concentrations.[90,93] There is evidence that the drug may abolish early afterdepolarizations in Purkinje fibers by accelerating repolarization[75] but in the human atria no effect on afterdepolarization was found.[99] Nevertheless, the drug does depress late afterdepolarizations induced by digitalis in Purkinje fibers.[100]

The in vivo electrophysiologic effects[101–103] of lidocaine appear to be due largely to its direct myocardial effects, as there is no significant interaction with the autonomic nervous system. Sinus node function is not altered by the drug in the absence of conduction system disease; however, sinus arrest and bradycardia may result in diseased nodes. In humans, there is no effect on the PR, AH, HV, and QRS intervals in therapeutic serum concentrations consistent with the in vitro observations that the drug has no slow channel inhibitory effect and low affinity for the sodium channels in the rested state and at low stimulus frequency. The atrial refractory period is shortened with a variable effect on AV nodal refractoriness. Even in toxic concentrations, lidocaine does not affect the ventricular effective refractory period but it consistently shortens the ERP in the His–Purkinje system, resulting from the shortening of the action potential duration in this tissue. It must be emphasized that, consonant with the observation that the drug depresses $V_{max}$ in partially depolarized tissues, lidocaine produces infranodal block in diseased conduction system and lengthens the ERP in the ischemic myocardium. It also may increase the ventricular fibrillation threshold of the ischemic myocardium. Electrophysiologic studies have shown that the drug has a minimal effect on the anterograde or retrograde conduction and refractoriness in the bypass tracts in the WPW syndrome in man. The overall electrophysiologic data are in accord with the clinical observation that the drug is effective only in the control of ventricular arrhythmias with little or no effect in those of supraventricular origin.

*Mexiletine* is a relatively new local anesthetic antiarrhythmic agent whose chemical structure and electrophysiologic properties closely resemble those of lidocaine[27] but differs significantly in its anticonvulsant and pharmacokinetic properties. In recent years the drug has emerged as a significant agent for the chronic prophylactic therapy of ventricular arrhythmias.

The mode of antiarrhythmic action of mexiletine has been elucidated in a variety of in vitro and in vivo experimental models as well as in man. The overall data are consisent with the data that the drug has cardiac effects very similar to those of lidocaine,[104] depressing the fast response of the cardiac action potential in a manner characteristic of Class I antiarrhythmic agents.[15]

When tested in the frog sciatic nerve, mexiletine was found to be a strong local anesthetic having a potency comparable to that of lidocaine.[104,105] In isolated atrial or ventricular muscle as well as Purkinje fibers, the drug exerts its major effects in a manner very similar to those of lidocaine. For example, in concentrations between 1 and 5 μg/ml, mexiletine reduces the maximal rate of depolarization of the action potential, thus enhancing the threshold of excitability, decreasing conduction velocity, and prolonging the ERP while having little effect on the resting membrane potential or on sinus node automaticity.[104–108] Of particular interest has been the observation that, as in the case of lidocaine, mexiletine produces a concentration-dependent abbreviation of the action potential duration in Purkinje fibers associated with modest shortening in the length of the ERP.[106] The effect on repolarization in ventricular muscle is minimal as in the effect on ERP at normal or low stimulus frequency. However, the abbreviation in the duration of the action potential found in the Purkinje fibers appears to be always of a greater magnitude than that in the effective refractory period. Thus, ERP/APD ratio increases under the action of the drug. Nevertheless, in toxic concentrations mexiletine, as in the case of lidocaine, may lengthen the ERP but it does so even in therapeutically relevant concentrations in ischemic tissues,[109] an effect that is in line with the drug's affinity for binding with sodium channels in partially depolarized fibers. Overall, in terms of the receptor modulated hypothesis, mexiletine closely resembles lidocaine in exhibiting a steep relationship between $V_{max}$ and stimulus frequency (or heart rate) and a rapid onset and offset kinetics of rate-dependent block of sodium channels.[110] As indicated by Campbell,[13,14] such an effect is in accord with the clinical observation that lidocaine and its congeners (mexiletine and tocainide) selectively depress early diastolic extrasystoles whereas Class Ia fast channel blockers (e.g., dispyramide) suppress extrasystoles at all coupling intervals. The fact that mexiletine has little or no effect on normal beats is in line with the observation that the drug essentially is without effect on the QRS and HV intervals at heart rates within the normal range. Mexiletine has not been shown to have a significant effect on the calcium-mediated slow response.

Mexiletine has no effect on the autonomic nervous system nor does it interfere with the function of biogenic amines. It has neither antihistaminic activity nor alpha- or beta-adrenergic blocking properties.

The data from clinical observations with mexiletine are in general agreement with those from experimental studies. However, marked differences in the action of the drug in patients with normal conduction compared to those with conduction disturbances have emerged.

In patients with normal sinus node function, mexiletine has been found to exert little effect on spontaneous frequency or recovery time following overdrive suppression.[111-113] In contrast, severe bradycardia and abnormal prolongation of the sinus node recovery time have been found in patients with sick sinus disease.[114] Mexiletine has been found to have little effect on atrial refractoriness consistent with the knowledge that the drug is ineffective in atrial fibrillation or flutter. The effects of mexiletine on AV nodal function also are somewhat inconsistent. For example, using concentrations of the drug in the therapeutic range, McComish et al.[112] reported shortening of the effective refractory of the AV node in nine patients, from a mean value of $437 \pm 11$ to $398 \pm 8$ msec. They found no significant effects on AV or His-Purkinje conduction times. In direct conflict with these are the findings of Roos et al.,[111,113] who demonstrated that the drug increased AV nodal conduction time at paced atrial rates and shifted the Wenckebach point to a lower atrial rate. In their study, the effective refractory period of the AV node was not altered consistently, while the functional refractory period increased in most patients. The HV interval representing distal or infra-Hisian conduction, was increased in about 30 percent of the patients while the effective refractory period of the His-Purkinje system also was prolonged by the drug. The depressant effect of the drug was more pronounced in patients with preexisting impairment of impulse generation and conduction. This is consistent with the effects of the drug in partially depolarized fibers.

*Tocainide* (2-amino-2'-6' propionoxylidide hydrochloride) is a primary analog of lidocaine and has striking similarities to mexiletine in its overall properties as an antiarrhythmic agent.[114,115] As with mexiletine, the major therapeutic interest in this new compound relates to the fact that it is orally active; it differs from lidocaine in lacking two ethyl groups, which protects the compound from first-pass hepatic elimination after oral ingestion.

There is a paucity of data on the in vitro and in vivo pharmacologic effects of tocainide on cardiac muscle, but the available information suggests that the spectrum of the drug's antiarrhythmic action is virtually identical to that of mexiletine and lidocaine.[114,115] In isolated superfused Purkinje fibers, tocainide decreased the action potential duration at 50 percent repolarization, but more significantly, it depressed the maximal rate of rise of phase 0 ($dV/dt_{max}$) of the action potential.[7,116] As in the case of lidocaine, the relationship relating the stimulus frequency and the depression of $V_{max}$ is steep and the onset and offset kinetics of the rate-dependent block fast. Tocainide has an affinity for partially depolarized fibers but it appears to have no effect on slow channel potentials but it depresses the normal automatic activity in Purkinje fibers.

Electrophysiologic studies in patients with relatively normal conduction have revealed no significant effects on AV conduction time or the HV interval[117] at mean plasma concentrations between 7.4 and 10.6 μg/ml. Small but consistent decreases in the right ventricular as well as His-Purkinje effective refractory period also were apparent with tocainide, but these results need to be interpreted in relation to those with mexiletine in which marked differences were demonstrated in the effects of the drug on various electrophysiologic parameters in patients with and without preexisting conduction abnormalities.

As might be expected, tocainide has little effect on the $Q-T_c$ interval in most patients, although in a few, some decrease, not reaching statistical significance, may be noted.[117] Similarly, at normal heart rates, tocainide does not alter the QRS duration or the HV interval with minimal effects on the effective refractory period in the atria, ventricles, His-Purkinje system, or the bypass tracts. Again, as in the case of mexiletine, these effects are consistent with the in vitro electrophysiologic actions of the compound and they provide the basis for the interpretation of the antiarrhythmic effects of tocainide.

*Aprindine*

Aprindine [N, N-diethyl-N'-(2-indanyl)-N'-phenyl-1,3-propanediamine] is a powerful Class I antiarrhythmic agent against a variety of ventricular and supraventricular arrhythmias.[7,115]

The major effect of aprindine in therapeutically meaningful concentrations is depression of the upstroke velocity of phase 0 of the action potential in atrial, ventricular, and Purkinje fibers;[118-120] the effects of the drug in Purkinje fibers is evident at lower concentrations than those in atrial and ventricular fibers. In addition, aprindine shortens the action potential duration (APD) and the ERP in Purkinje fibers but tends to increase the ratio of the ERP–APD. The shortening of the action potential duration in atrial, ventricular, or Purkinje fibers is not due to effects on $K^+$ conductance or outward potassium currents. Rather, it might result from a decrease in the TTx-sensitive inward sodium current during the plateau phase of the action potential.[77] The maximal rate of depolarization is reduced more at high stimulation frequencies, at high potassium levels, and to a much greater extent than with comparable concentrations of lidocaine. However, the kinetics of the rate-dependent block of the fast sodium channel in the case of aprindine has not been determined critically but appears to be of the same order of magnitude as that for lidocaine, mexiletine, and tocainide.

Diastolic depolarization and spontaneous activity in Purkinje fibers as well as those induced by stretch and hypoxia are uniformly depressed or abolished by aprindine but there appears to be no direct effect on slow channel activity;[120] transient afterdepolarizations induced by acetylstrophanthidin also are suppressed by the drug, findings that have relevance to the effects of the drug in arrhythmias due to triggered automaticity.

Electrophysiologic observations with aprindine in intact animals and humans are in general agreement with the in vitro data. For example, when the drug was injected directly into the sinus nodal arterty in the dog, spontaneous sinus frequency was decreased; when injected into the AV nodal artery, the functional refractory period and the conduction time of the AV node were lengthened greatly.[120] Similarly, intravenous doses of the drug prolonged the AH and HV intervals as well as the ventricular effective refractory period in the dog.[120] The effect on the intranodal conduction is not explained but may result either from a vagal effect or one that is mediated through the selective blockade of the slow channel in the AV node. Such a negative dromotropic effect of the drug also is found in studies in humans, in whom aprindine increased the AH and HV intervals and QRS duration while lengthening the effective refractory period of the atria and ventricle as well as the AV node.[52,121-124] In agreement with the general action of Class I agents, aprindine blocked conduction in the accessory pathway of patients with the Wolff-Parkinson-White syndrome more often and more consistently in the anterograde than in the retrograde direction.[52,121] On the basis of these overall electrophysiologic observations, one might expect the drug to exhibit a wide spectrum of antiarrhythmic efficacy against supraventricular and ventricular dysrhythmias in the experimental and clinical context.

*Phenytoin Sodium*

Although primarily an anticonvulsive agent and one that shares structural similarities to baributurates, the antiarrhythmic action of phenytoin has been recognized for over two decades. The effects of phenytoin on the cardiac action potential resembles those of lidocaine and its congeners and it does exhibit local anesthetic properties in nerve as well as the cardiac membrane.[48] The overall effects of the compound are influenced greatly by its significant anticholinergic actions especially on the AV node, by its interaction with electrolyte (especially potassium) concentrations,[48,125,126] and also by the state of the fiber (i.e., whether normally polarized or partially depolarized).[127]

In low concentrations (1−5 μg/ml) and in the presence of low potassium (3 mM or lower), the membrane may be hyperpolarized, $V_{max}$ either is not affected or may be increased with a concomitant augmentation in conduction velocity[128,129] especially in atrial fibers. The increase in conduction velocity may occur particularly in the presence of high concentrations of cardiac glycosides. Higher concentrations of the drug especially in the presence of normal or higher concentrations lead to a decrease in $V_{max}$ with a shift of the membrane responsiveness curve in the hyperpolarizing direction.[48] However, in equimolar concentrations such an effect is not as great as with procainamide or quinidine.

Therapeutically relevant concentrations of phenytoin shorten the action potential duration of Purkinje fibers with somewhat less shortening of the ERP.[48] The effect on APD and ERP is less striking in the case of ventricular and atrial fibers. Phenytoin sodium depresses the spontaneous phase 4 depolarization in Purkinje fibers both in normally polarized fibers and in those with more positive maximum diastolic potential than normal.[130] This effect leads to the slowing of the automatic firing in such fibers. The slope of spontaneous diastolic depolarization augmented by catecholamines is depressed by the drug. In high concentrations, phenytoin sodium has the propensity to slow the sinus automaticity in the rabbit heart,[129] while the drug suppresses the delayed afterdepolarizations induced by toxic levels of cardiac glycosides[127] in Purkinje fibers but there appears to be no data on the effects of the compound on early afterdepolarization.

The in vivo electrophysiologic effects of phenytoin[131] are somewhat similar to those of mexiletine or tocainide, namely a minimally depressant effect unless cardiac disease is present. The effect on the sinus automaticity is variable, reflecting a balance between the drug's direct and indirect effects; a direct depressant effect may predominate in the of case of sinus node dysfunction. The ERP in the atria, ventricles, and His-Purkinje system or the bypass tracts are affected minimally at normal heart rates. Variable effects also have been reported in the case of conduction and refractoriness at the level of the AV node. For example, the drug may sometimes shorten AV nodal conduction time and decrease the ERP. Whether this is a direct effect or it indicates a significant anticholinergic effect of the drug is unclear. There have been reported studies on the action of phenytoin sodium on the transmembrane action potentials recorded from the AV nodal cells. When the drug is given orally for protracted periods of time, no increases in the PR interval have been noticed. Nor has there been reports of increases in the QRS duration or the $QT_c$ interval. The effects of the drug on the ERP of the atria, ventricle, or the His-Purkinje system in humans are poorly defined, but small decreases have been reported. This is consistent with the shortening of the action potential duration noted in in vitro studies. It is possible however that at fast stimulation frequencies an increase in the time-dependent ERP as well as a prolongation of infranodal conduction time may result from the effects of the drug on $V_{max}$ in ventricular fibers and in the His-Purkinje system.

*Ethmozine*

This is an investigational antiarrhythmic agent that is a phenothiazine derivative that appears to have a spectrum of antiarrhythmic activity that encompasses both ventricular and supraventricular tachyarrhythmias.[132,133] The effects of the drug on all facets of the cardiac action potential in various types of myocardial fibers are poorly defined. However, the available data indicate that the drug exerts its major actions by inhibiting the fast sodium channel in the heart.

In canine Purkinje fibers, the drug has been found to depress $V_{max}$, reduce the amplitude of the action potential, and shift the membrane responsiveness curve in the negative direction on the voltage axis.[133,134] This effect was found to be related to drug concentration. Ethmozine has no significant effect on slow channel dependent potentials. As in the case of many Class Ib agents, ethmozine shortens the action potential duration in Purkinje fibers, but the effect of the drug in atria and ventricles is not clearly defined. Further studies are needed to define the nature of the rate-dependent block that the compound may produce in relation to the changes in the ERP as a function of frequency of stimulation, level of membrane potential, and electrolyte and pH changes.

Somewhat surprisingly, the drug does not appear to affect the slope of phase 4 depolarization in spontaneously firing Purkinje fibers, but it slows the firing rate by elevating the threshold potential[137] to more positive potentials. It is noteworthy that the drug has a strikingly depressant effect on abnormal automaticity in stretched Purkinje fibers, in those superfused with barium chloride, or those removed from areas of one-day old infarcts in the canine model of experimental coronary occlusion. In these situations, the compound depresses the slope of spontaneous diastolic depolarization and decreases the firing rate with sometimes a complete suppression of spontaneous activity.[137] From the standpoint of effects on automaticity, it is of interest that ethmozine also decreases the amplitude of delayed afterdepolarizations in Purkinje fibers removed from one-day old infarcts and in fibers superfused with large concentrations of cardiac glycosides.[137]

In vivo, ethmozine does not appear to influence the sinus cycle length; orally administered ethmozine minimally lengthens the PR interval and the QRS duration but exerts no significant effect on the $QT_c$ interval.


## Fast Channel Blockers with Slow Onset-Offset Kinetics of Rate-Dependent Block of $V_{max}$

As indicated, numerous agents recently have been introduced that are potent fast-channel blockers but with a slow-onset and offset kinetics of rate-dependent block. As a subclass, these agents markedly depress conduction under resting conditions but exert little effect on refractoriness of cardiac muscle. They exert a paradoxical effect on repolarization in ventricular muscle and in Purkinje fibers junction, shortening it markedly in the latter and either having no effect or lengthening it somewhat in the former.[136] The best studied are flecainide, encainide (and its metabolites), and propafenone; newer and still poorly studied ones include cibenzoline, lorcainide, indecainide, and recainam, which are characterized insufficiently and will not be discussed further in this chapter.

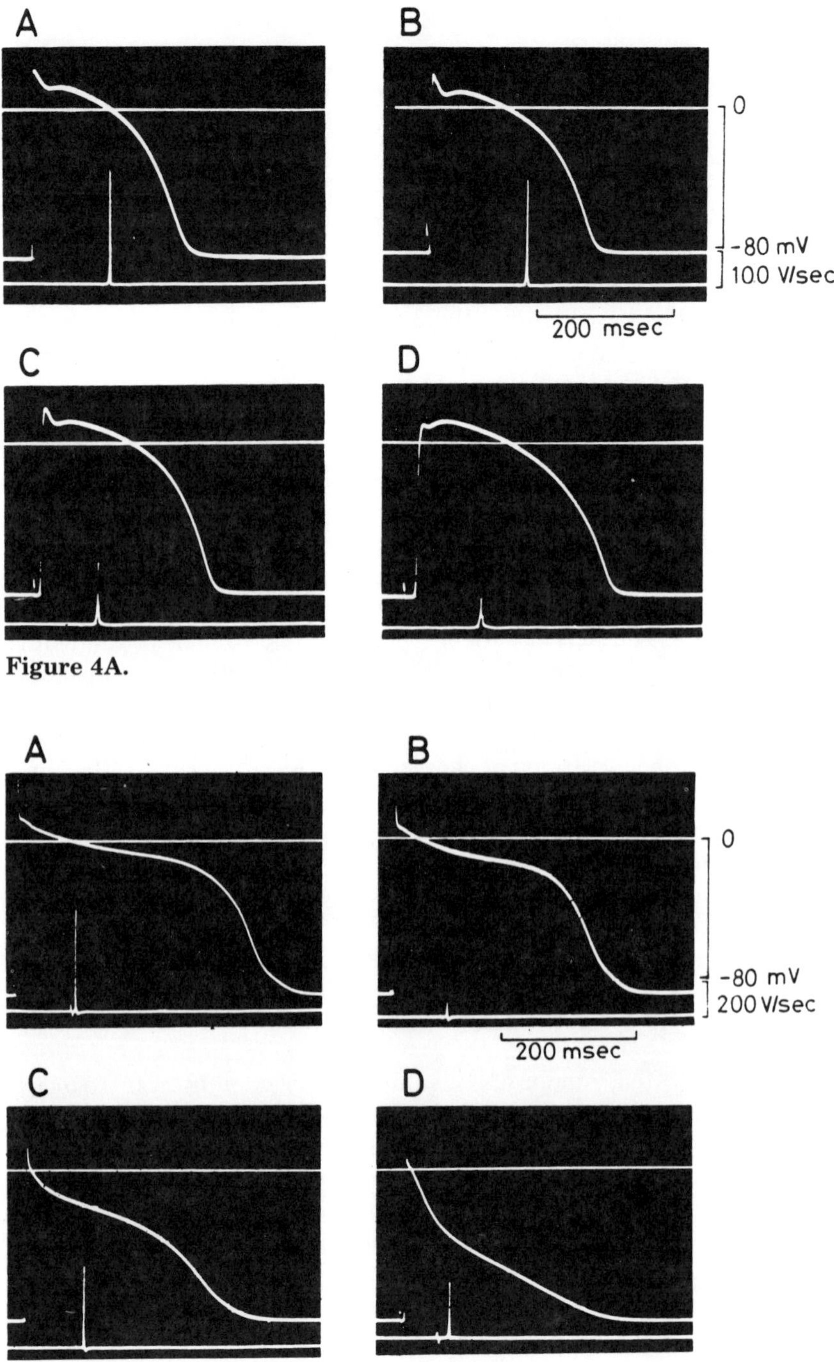


Figure 4A.

Figure 4B.

*Flecainide*

Flecainide produces a concentration-dependent decrease in $V_{max}$, action potential amplitude, overshoot potential with an increase in the ERP in atria, ventricles, and Purkinje fibers.[136] A characteristic feature of the compound is the fact that the action potential duration was lengthened by flecainide in ventricular muscle and shortened in Purkinje fibers (Fig. 4). At high concentrations (10 μg/ml), flecainide depresses slow channel dependent fibers. Purkinje fiber automaticity induced by isoproterenol was slowed by flecainide by the elevation of threshold potential.

The dominant effects of flecainide in various isolated cardiac tissues demonstrated by numerous investigators are consistent with a potent inhibitory action on the fast sodium current as indicated by the decrease in $V_{max}$ and the shift of the membrane responsiveness curve in the hyperpolarizing direction.[135-137] The data of Borchard and Boisten[137] and of Campbell[12] emphasize the use-dependent nature of the inhibitory effect of flecainide on sodium channels demonstrated over a wide range of stimulus frequencies. The onset and offset kinetics of flecainide with respect to its effect on the rate-dependent block of $V_{max}$ was analyzed by Campbell[12,14] and found to be among the slowest for fast sodium channel blockers.

From the standpoint of the overall antiarrhythmic actions of flecainide, the drug's effect on myocardial refractoriness is perhaps of the greatest significance. However, the importance of the disparate effects of the drug on the ERP of the Purkinje fibers and of ventricle muscle is uncertain. The ERP in Purkinje fibers is shortened significantly at all effective drug concentrations despite comparable decreases in $V_{max}$; thus it appears that the decreases in the voltage-dependent ERP due to the marked abbreviation of the $APD_{90}$ exceeded the lengthening of time-dependent Na-mediated ERP in this tissue. At 10 μg/ml drug concentration, the two appar-

---

**Figure 4.**   Differential effects of flecainide on the action potential duration in canine ventricular muscle (Figure 4a) and in Purkinje fibers (Figure 4b). For each of the two series, A = control, B = after 0.1 μg/ml flecainide, C = 1.0 μg/ml flecainide, and D = on 10.0 μg/ml flecainide. Note that whereas flecainide shortens the APD in Purkinje fibers, it lengthens it in ventricular muscle. This overall effect appears to be characteristic of the so-called Class 1c fast sodium channel blockers. (From Ikeda N, Singh BN, Davis LD, et al: Effects of flecainide on the electrophysiologic properties of isolated canine and rabbit myocardial fibers. *J Am Coll Cardiol* 5:303, 1985. By permission of the authors and the Journal.)

ently competing effects are however "balanced" so that no significant net effect on the ERP was found.

It is conceivable however that such a "balance" in the disparate changes induced by flecainide in ventricular muscle and Purkinje fiber repolarization may not always be achieved. This may lead to exaggerated heterogeneity in the recovery of excitability with a tendency for focal reexcitation. It is possible that this is the basis for the observed arrhythmogenicity of flecainide[138] and other so-called Class 1c compounds, such as encainide and its metabolites (discussed later), which also exert a similar differential electrophysiologic effect on Purkinje fibers and ventricular muscle (discussed later). It is noteworthy that antiarrhythmic drugs such as diphenylhydantoin and lidocaine,[24,25] which act primarily by inhibiting Na-channels, also accelerate repolarization and may shorten the ERP over certain drug concentrations, but they do this in Purkinje fibers as well as in ventricular muscle. It has been suggested that the shortening of the $APD_{90}$ by lidocaine was due to an increase in time-dependent K conductance (discussed later). Recently, however, voltage clamp studies have suggested that the shortening of the $APD_{90}$ by lidocaine is caused by the suppression of tetrodotoxin (TTx) sensitive steady-state Na current.[77] The TTx-sensitive steady-state Na current apparently contributes more to the Purkinje fiber plateau than to that of the ventricular muscle fibers, since tetrodotoxin was found to abolish the difference that exists between the APD of Purkinje fibers and ventricular fibers.[77] Thus, it is possible that, as in the case of lidocaine, flecainide exerts an inhibitory action on the TTx-sensitive steady-state Na current accounting for the observed shortening of the $APD_{90}$ and $APD_{50}$ in Purkinje fibers due to the drug. The shortening of the APD also is antagonized partially by elevating $Ca^{++})^{\circ}$ and, at least in high concentrations, flecainide inhibits the slow channel;[135] this suggests that slow channel inhibition also may contribute to the observed shortening of the APD.

The clinical electrophysiologic effects of flecainide are consistent with overall in vitro data.[139–143] For example, Hellestrand et al.[143] showed that intravenous flecainide lengthened the QRS duration, prolonged the HV interval, and increased the effective refractory period in the atria, ventricle, and the accessory tracts with a minimal lengthening of the $QT_c$ interval. Similar findings have been demonstrated from the recordings of the right ventricular monophasic action potentials given flecainide intravenously.[139] As in the case of the in vitro studies, the magnitude of the increase in the action potential duration was small and did not influence the $QT_c$ interval of the surface electrocardiogram, suggesting that the modest increases in the ventricular ERP observed in the same study in humans were due essentially to a time-dependent inhibition of the sodium channel.

*Encainide*

Structurally, encainide resembles procainamide, but its effect on the cardiac action potential shows striking differences. Although the compound has not been studied as extensively as flecainide, the overall effects of these two compounds on the cardiac action potential as well as their antiarrhythmic actions resemble each other closely. The electrophysiologic effects of the two active metabolites of encainide are qualitatively similar to those of the parent compound[147] and will not be discussed further.

Encainide has no effect on the resting membrane potential, but it depresses $V_{max}$ in Purkinje fibers, atria, ventricles, and the His-Purkinje fibers and shifts the membrane responsiveness curve in the hyperpolarizing direction.[144,146] As in the case of flecainide, such a change is accompanied by a modest lengthening of the ERP with a marked depressant effect on conduction velocity. The rate-dependent block of the fast sodium channel block induced by encainide is associated with slow onset and offset kinetics; the block is accentuated in partially depolarized fibers. The drug exerts no significant effect on the slow channel potentials.

Encainide shortens the action potential duration markedly in the Purkinje fibers with a lesser shortening of the ERP[144] but the compound has no significant effect in ventricular muscle at normal heart rates. At high concentrations, encainide reduces the slope of phase 4 depolarization and decreases the spontaneous firing frequency of Purkinje fibers that are partially depolarized or have maximum diastolic potentials.[145] At present, there is little data on the effects of encainide on triggered automaticity.

There are differences between the effects of the intravenous and oral encainide in vivo.[146–149] For example, following the intravenous administration of the drug, intranodal conductin is not affected but the QRS duration is widened; the QT interval is lengthened but due essentially to the prolongation of the JT interval rather than due to ST segment. Intravenous encainide has no effect on the ERP in the atria, ventricle, or the AV node.[146] In contrast, following oral therapy for over 3 days, AV nodal conduction is slowed and atrial and ventricular ERP are prolonged, as is the ERP in the accessory tracts of the heart.[146] It is surmised that these differences are due to the activity of the drug's metabolites.

The similarity in the electrophysiologic profile of encainide and flecainide indicate that the antiarrhythmic and arrhythmogenic potential of the two compounds is likely to be similar.

*Propafenone*

Developed in West Germany, this compound recently has been widely studied elsewhere for its potential to control ventricular and supraventricular tachyarrhythmias. The effects of the compound on the cardiac action potential has been determined in numerous mammalian species.[150–153] Propafenone exhibits a complex aggregate of electrophysiologic effects due to intrinsic effects on depolarization and repolarization phases of the fast channel potentials in the heart modified somewhat by its propensity to block beta-adrenergic receptors[152] on the one hand and the slow myocardial channels[152] especially at high drug concentrations on the other.

Numerous studies[150–153] have confirmed that the major effects of the drug is to block the fast $Na^+$-dependent potentials in the atria, ventricles, and His-Purkinje fibers in a concentration-dependent manner. In these fibers, in concentrations that are clinically relevant, the drug had no effect on the resting membrane potential but increased the excitability threshold and prolonged the ERP, although not to the same extent as it slowed conduction velocity. As is characteristic of this subclass of antiarrhythmic agents, propafenone exhibits a strong resting or tonic block and a potent phasic block of its effect on $Na^+$ channel.[152,153] This is consistent with a relatively slow dissociation rate constant for its binding to the sodium channel in contrast to lidocaine or mexiletine, which have high dissociation rate constants and the property to suppress extrasystoles closely coupled to the antecedent beats or short-cycle length tachycardias. In contrast, propafenone is expected to influence cardiac excitability and refractoriness at all cycle lengths even at normal heart rates.

There have been some discrepancies in the reported data on the effects of propafenone on the action potential duration. For example, whereas Duke and Vaughan Williams[152] found that in the rabbit the drug modestly prolonged the APD in all cardiac tissues, Kohlhardt[153] and Ledda et al.[151] found a significant shortening of the APD, at least in the Purkinje fibers. Again, as in the case of flecainide and encainide, propafenone has a less striking effect on the ERP than on conduction at low stimulus frequencies. In the case of the effects of the drug on sinus node automaticity, it depresses the slope of phase 4 depolarization and reduces the amplitude of the action potential. The latter effect is likely to be due to the blockade of the slow channel, whereas the effect on the slope of diastolic depolarization may be attributed to the drug's antiadrenergic and calcium antagonistic effects, as well as its fast channel blocking actions. At present, there is a paucity of data on the effects of propafenone on triggered automaticity.

The in vivo effects of propafenone on the electrocardiographic intervals and on conduction intervals and refractoriness in various tissues[154–156] is predictable on the basis of the in vitro findings. For example, the drug has been shown to have little effect on the sinus cycle length but to exert a depressant effect on intranodal (AV) conduction. Thus, the PR interval increases, as does the QRS duration, but with no change in the $QT_c$ interval.[156] During His bundle electrocardiography, propafenone was found to increase the HV interval and AV nodal Wenkebach during right atrial pacing; during programmed electrical stimulation of the heart, in one study, the right ventricular ERP was found to be increased 24 msec following the intravenous injection of the drug. In another study, the antegrade ERP of the accessory tracts of the heart was increased significantly by propafenone. It must be emphasized that although there is a broad correlation between the in vitro and in vivo effects of propafenone, further work needs to be undertaken to define the role of beta-blocking and apparent calcium antagonistic effects in determining the overall electrophysiologic profile of propafenone as an antiarrhythmic compound.

## Sympathetic Antagonists and Cardiac Action Potential

For many decades, numerous observations have suggested a convincing rationale for the role of sympathetic antagonists in the control of disorders of cardiac rhythm, since augmented adrenergic activity has been implicated in the genesis of a variety of ventricular and supraventricular dysrhythmias (see Singh & Venkatesh)[157]. For example, it long has been known that ablation of the sources of sympathetic transmitters to the heart, whether presynaptic or competitive or noncompetitive receptor blockade, reduced the tendency to cardiac arrhythmias.[158] In the case of the congenital long QT interval syndrome,[159,160] a disorder in which there is a marked tendency for spontaneous onset of ventricular tachycardia and fibrillation presumably due to sympathetic imbalance in the heart (see Chapter 4), beta-blockade and left stellate ganglionectomy have been shown to correct the arrhythmogenic tendency in a large number of patients.[158] Furthermore, the relationship between potentially lethal arrhythmias and sympathetic activity recently has come into sharp focus because of the numerous clinical trials that have shown that prophylactic beta-adrenergic blockade in the survivors of acute myocardial infarction reduces the incidence of sudden death by 18−35 percent.[157] It now is clear that sympathetic antagonism by whatever means is likely to be a significant and discrete antiarrhythmic mechanism. For this reason, it is of practical and theoretical importance to relate, if possible, the observed salutary antiarrhythmic effects of sympathetic inhibitors to their electrophysiologic actions. The discussion that follows however will focus essentially on the electrophysiologic properties of competitive beta-adrenergic antagonists. The autonomic interactions with the cardiac action potential has been discussed earlier. It provides the background to the discussion that ensues.

## Beta-Adrenergic Blockade and Cardiac Action Potentials

In discussing the antiarrhythmic actions of beta blockers, the thesis will be developed that these agents exert their major effects by antagonizing the well-known electrophysiologic effects of catecholamines.[161,162] The additional actions that some of the agents (e.g., sotalol with respect to repolarization and propranolol in the case of depolarization at high drug concentrations) exhibit will be considered as arising independently of adrenergic blockade. The issue about the potential differences between the effects on the action potential of acute beta-blockade and those following chronic drug administration also will be discussed briefly. For the purposes of this discussion, it is assumed that the property of cardioselectivity present in certain beta blockers is of little electrophysiologic consequence.[157]

In concentrations that produce substantial beta blockade, none of the plethora of beta-antagonists now available exerts an effect on the resting membrane potential, action potential amplitude, or the maximal rate of rise of the action potential. Thus, these agents do not affect conduction velocity or membrane responsiveness in fast sodium channel−dependent fibers. Similarly, there is no influence on the effective or the functional refractory periods.

It is known, however, that some of the beta blockers (e.g., propranolol, oxprenolol, acebutalol, alprenolol) in high drug concentrations exert local anesthetic effects on nerve, and on the cardiac membrane they reduce sodium conductance,[162] an effect that is particularly evident in partially depolarized fibers as might be found in the ischemic myocardium. In these circumstances, beta blockers may depress conduction velocity, shift the membrane responsiveness curve in the hyperpolarizing direction and prolong the effective refractory period. Such effects also may be noted in relatively normal myocardium in the presence of high levels of catecholamines in the superfusion medium. The effect of propranolol has been the most extensively studied in this regard. It has been shown that in high concentrations, the drug's membrane-depressant effect leads to a decrease in the effective refractory period with a somewhat greater shortening of the action potential; these actions may be related to the propensity of the drug to inhibit sodium conductance which is particularly marked in Purkinje fibers, being less striking in atrial and ventricular fibers.

The most consistent and easily demonstrable effect of beta blockade is on the enhanced rate of spontaneous diastolic depolarization induced by catecholamines in the sinus pacemaker and in automatically firing Purkinje fibers.[163] The slope of spontaneous diastolic depolarization in this setting is depressed without an effect on the threshold potential or the amplitude of the action potential. The overall effect is on the rate of firing in the fiber. The effect of beta blockade is not as well studied in the spontaneously firing fibers in the middle region of the AV node. However, from the known effects of sympathetic blockade on intranodal conduction and AV nodal refractoriness, it may be inferred that beta-blockers must exert a depressant effect on phase 4 depolarization in this structure.

At present, there is a paucity of data on the effects of beta-blockers on triggered automaticity. However, propranolol has been shown to decrease the amplitude of delayed afterdepolarizations and to stop triggering in atrial muscle or Purkinje fibers exposed to high concentrations of catecholamines or cardiac glycosides,[164] findings clearly of clinical significance.

In a series of studies, an interesting observation has been reported by Raine and Vaughan Williams[165] on the changes in the cardiac action potentials in the rabbit myocardium from animals treated chronically with a variety of beta blockers. They found that agents such as propranolol and acebutolol produced a modest but significant lengthening of the action potential duration[165] but without effect on the upstroke velocity of phase 0. It was postulated that such a change represented a physiologic adaptation to chronic sympathetic blockade. The clinical counterparts of these studies have been conflicting. Studies with the monophasic action potential measurements using suction electrodes have both confirmed and failed to document the prolongation of repolarization,[166,167] whereas the measurement of the $QT_c$ intervals in humans following chronic beta blockade have shown that repolarization following propranolol may shorten, prolong, or not change[167,168] in duration. In any event, the overall data are consistent with the knowledge that if beta blockade does prolong the cardiac action potential duration, the overall change is very much less than that produced by drugs such as amiodarone, sotalol, n-acetylprocainamide (discussed later), or even quinidine, procainamide or disopyramide (discussed later). For this reason, it is unlikely that the effects of beta blockade on cardiac repolarization is of crucial significance in mediating the antidysrhythmic actions of this class of antiarrhythmic agents.

The in vivo electrophysiologic effects of beta blockade are in accord with their in vitro effects and vary with the autonomic tone. The dominant effect is on the SA and AV nodes: Beta blockade increases the sinus node recovery time, increases AH interval, but has no effect on the HV interval. On the surface electrocardiogram, there is lengthening of the PR interval, no effect on the QRS duration, and generally no effect on the $QT_c$ interval, although a slight shortening may be found[168] especially in the case of propranolol. There is only a minor increase in the atrial ERP with no significant effect on ERP in the ventricle, His-Purkinje system, or the accessory tracts of the heart.[169] These effects relate solely to beta blockade and, in the case of agents that exert additional actions such as membrane-depressant properties (e.g., propranolol and acebutolol in high concentrations) or the prolongation of cardiac repolarization (e.g., sotalol), time- and voltage-dependent refractoriness may be lengthened. Whether the ERP in ventricular or atrial muscle increases as a function of chronic beta blockade independent of these additional properties is unknown at present but merits further investigation.

## Antiarrhythmic Agents that Act Principally by Lengthening Cardiac Repolarization

It has long been recognized that delayed repolarization in cardiac muscle may be associated with an increased tendency for serious ventricular arrhythmia.[159,160] The fact that the converse also might hold however has been appreciated as well,[46] although a number of clinical observations long have suggested that lengthening the cardiac action potential might be antiarrhythmic.[170] For example, it is known that in cases of extreme hypocalcemia, there is a marked prolongation of cardiac repolarization, but the occurrence of arrhythmias is rare.[50] Similarly, in hypothyroidism, a situation in which there is uniform prolongation of repolarization,[171,172] arrhythmias of all kinds are extremely uncommon. In contrast, in thyrotoxicosis, in which atrial action potentials are markedly abbreviated,[171] a high incidence of atrial fibrillation is well documented. These clinical and experimental observations therefore are consistent with the possibility that the lengthening of cardiac repolarization per se may be associated with a corresponding increase in the voltage-dependent ERP and may constitute a discrete antiarrhythmic mechanism.[46] Historically, it is of interest that quinidine, the archetype of antiarrhythmic agent, has been known to inhibit depolarization and to lengthen repolarization. Thus, its overall antiarrhythmic action may result from a summate effect of changes in these parameters. Recent focus is on the development of compounds that have a selectivity of action in lengthening the refractory period by prolonging repolarization. Although there does not appear to be many compounds that are completely selective in their propensity to lengthen cardiac repolarization, a number recently have been recognized as having the property to control arrhythmias mainly by inhibiting the repolarization currents in cardiac muscle. The major agents are bretylium, sotalol, N-acetylprocainamide, and amiodarone, which has been studied experimentally and clinically the most extensively.

*Bretylium*

The antiarrhythmic effects of bretylium were first recognized in 1965,[173] although the drug was initially introduced as an antihypertensive agent in 1959.[174] It then was recognized that bretylium markedly reduced the vulnerability of the heart to ventricular fibrillation[175] and was particularly effective in suppressing ventricular dysrhythmias complicating acute infarction in dogs as well as in humans.[176,177]

The mode of action of bretylium always has been the subject of much controversy, the main points at issue being whether the drug exerts its observed antiarrhythmic effects by impairment of neuronal release of catecholamines or by its direct electrophysiologic actions on cardiac muscle. It is known that a low concentration of bretylium during the early phases of the drug's effect on heart muscle is associated with catecholamine release.[178] This accounts for the fact that in rabbit atrial muscle an initial increase in conduction velocity, spontaneous sinus rate, and a decrease in the effective refractory period as well as the threshold of excitability are usually found.[176] Higher concentrations and prolonged contact with the drug result in predominantly depressant effects, but in atrial muscle, no change in the action potential duration is found.[179] Moreover, in partially depolarized myocardial fibers, the action potential duration is shortened and the membrane is hyperpolarized, effects that also are accountable in terms of catecholamine release, since they are not apparent in animals pretreated with reserpine.[180] In contrast, in normal myocardial and Purkinje fbers, bretylium consistently *lengthens* the action potential duration as well as the effective refractory period[181,182] in a homogeneous fashion, akin to that produced by the chronic administration of amiodarone. It thus is possible that the major mechanism of antiarrhythmic action of bretylium may stem from its ability to homogeneously prolong the action potential duration. The fact that this does not occur in atrial muscle is consistent with the knowledge that supraventricular arrhythmias are poorly responsive to bretylium. It also is noteworthy that the drug is particularly effective in refractory ventricular arrhythmias occurring in the context of acute myocardial infarction. The results of the electrophysiologic effects of bretylium on subendocardial Purkinje fibers from infarcted canine fibers reported by Cardinal and Sasyniuk[183] therefore are relevant. The drug produced the greatest increases in the action potential duration in cells in the proximal parts of the free-running anterior bundle in the region free of infarction and the least in those cells within the infarcted region, where the action potential duration already had lengthened (as a result of ischemia) before bretylium was superfused. These differential effects resulted in a reduction of the disparity in action potential durations (and in refractory periods) between the normal and infarcted regions. Such an action may be of crucial significance for the antifibrillatory effect of bretylium in myocardial ischemia.

*N-acetylprocainamide (NAPA)*

Over ten years ago, it was found that in numerous animal species as well as in humans, the para-amino group of procainamide was metabolized to N-acetylprocainamide and during chronic therapy with the parent compound the concentrations of the metabolite often approached or exceeded those of procainamide.[184] The electrophysiologic properties of NAPA are discussed in detail in Chapter 10. Only the salient features are presented here for completeness.

There are significant differences in the effects of procainamide and NAPA,[185-188] most clearly defined in isolated heart muscle by Dangman and Hoffman.[189] They reported that NAPA (10–40 μg/ml), unlike procainamide, had no effect on the $V_{max}$ in Purkinje fiber action potentials and had no effect on the resting membrane potential or action potential amplitude. By inference, therefore, the drug had no effect on the fast sodium current in fast channel–dependent fibers consistent with a lack of effective membrane responsiveness. The main effect was the significant lengthening of the action potential duration and the effective refractory period as a function of drug concentration. The latter property is similar to that of procainamide. In tissues other than the Purkinje fibers dependent on fast channel depolarization (e.g., ventricles), NAPA (20–40 μg/ml) consistently lengthened the action potential duration and the effective refractory period as a function of drug concentration. The effects on atrial fibers were similar to those from the ventricle.

The effects of NAPA on normal or abnormal automaticity also differed from those of the parent compound.[189] For example, the drug exerted no significant effect on spontaneous activity in Purkinje fibers nor did it alter phase 4 depolarization engendered by the superfusion of Purkinje fibers in varying concentrations of barium ions. Similarly, NAPA had no measurable effects on "slow response" potentials with automatic characteristics. The fact that NAPA had little effect on normal automaticity in canine Purkinje fibers also was supported by Dangman and Hoffman's observations[189] that the compound had no effect on the junctional pacemaker in dogs with complete atrioventricular block. In contrast, lidocaine and procainamide had a depressant effect. However, the lack of a depressant effect of NAPA on Purkinje fiber automaticity in the study by Dangman and Hoffman[189] is in conflict with those of Bagwell et al.,[194] who reported that NAPA (10–20 μg/ml) reduced the automatic rate in Purkinje fibers.

In regard to the potential arrhythmogenic effects of NAPA the toxic concentrations of the metabolite were found to induce slight depolarization with accelerated automaticity in some fibers and to produce early afterdepolarization in others. However, neither features could be induced predictably. Whether these effects in the setting of prolonged repolarization in ventricular muscle form the basis for the development of torsade des pointes in humans remains conjectural at present.

The differences between the electrophysiologic effects of NAPA and procainamide also have been found in intact animals and in humans.[191-194] Jaillon and Winkle[191] gave a successive sequence of bolus injections followed by a 45-minute of constant intravenous infusion in chloralose-anesthetized dogs prior to intracardiac electrocardiography and programmed electrical stimulation. Both procainamide and NAPA increased the atrial and ventricular refractory periods and the $QT_c$ interval, whereas increases in the QRS duration and in the HV interval (a measure of infranodal atrioventricular conduction) occurred only after procainamide. These data are consistent with the in vitro findings. They emphasize that the electrophysiologic effects of NAPA are accountable on the basis of the drug's propensity to lengthen cardiac repolarization.

The clinical electrophysiologic effects of NAPA are concordant with those established in isolated cardiac muscle and in intact animal preparations.[192,193] The data before and after the intravenous injection of NAPA in patients undergoing electrophysiologic studies from the study (see Chapter 12) reported by Sung et al.[192] showed that NAPA had no effect on sinus cycle length, sinus node recovery time, conduction intervals (such as the AH, HV, PR, or the QRS), AV nodal functional or effective refractory periods, or the AV nodal Wenckebach cycle length. However, when the drug was infused to plasma concentrations of $12-30$ µg/ml, the atrial and ventricular refractory periods were lengthened significantly, as was the $QT_c$ interval of the surface electrocardiogram. Again, as in the case of experimental studies, these effects differ from those of the parent compound, which increases the HV interval and prolongs the QRS duration as a result of a depressant effect on the fast sodium channel. The effects of NAPA on the accessory tracts of the heart have not been defined but the known electrophysiologic effects of the drug suggest that the effective refractory period of the accessory tract is likely to be prolonged by the compound via prolongation of repolarization.

*Sotalol*

From the standpoint of effect on the cardiac action potential, sotalol is unique among beta-adrenoceptor antagonists.[46,195] Its net electrophysiologic action stems from the combined effects of blocking beta receptors and lengthening cardiac repolarization.[46]

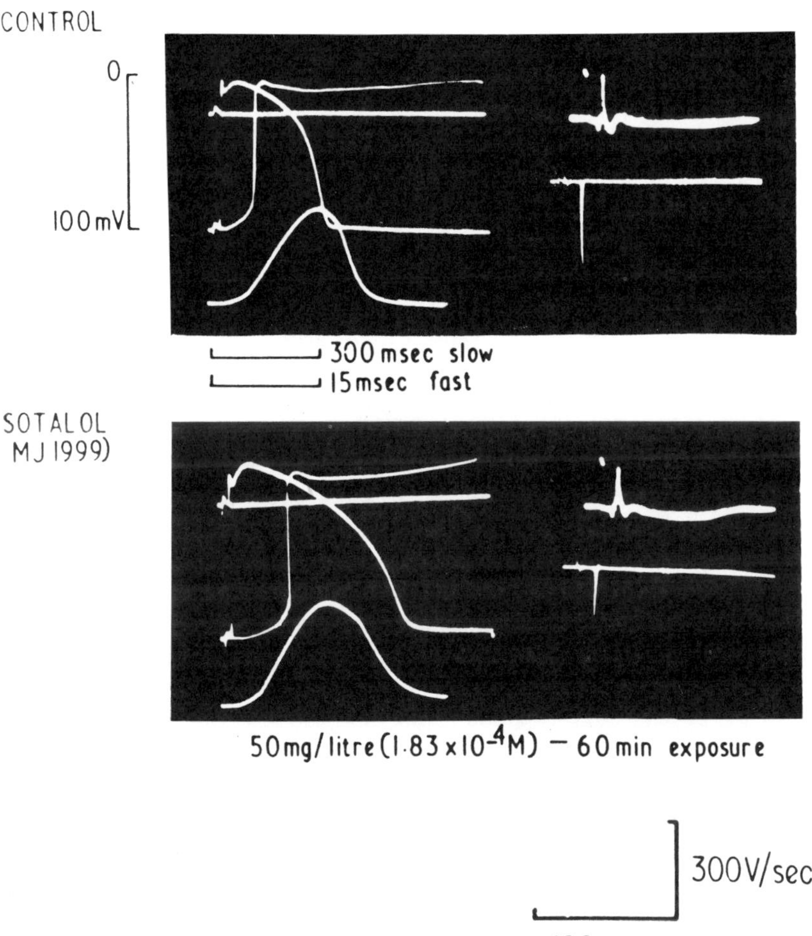


**Figure 5.**  The effect of sotalol (MJ1999) on the transmembrane action potentials recorded from cat papillary muscle. The horizontal line on the left at the top of each panel represents zero potential; the middle trace represents the action potential at slow and fast sweep speeds; the bottom trace represents isometric tension. The upper trace on the right represents surface potential and the lower, the differential signal for the maximal rate of rise of the action potential. Note that sotalol has little or no effect on the upstroke velocity (maximal rate of rise) of phase 0 or on isometric tension. The dominant effect is the lengthening of the action potential duration and hence, by inference, the effective refractory period, a Class III action. (From Singh BN: A study of the pharmacological actions of certain drugs and hormones with a particular reference to cardiac muscle. D. Phil. thesis, England, University of Oxford.)

Representative findings illustrating the effects of dl-sotalol in cat papillary muscles are shown in Figure 5. The major effects of the compound in the concentrations used is to lengthen the APD without affecting the maximal rate of rise of the action potential in atria, ventricles, Purkinje fibers, and in the sinoatrial node, in which the compound depresses the slope of phase 4 depolarization.[46,196] The prolongation of the APD is accompanied by a corresponding increase in the absolute and effective refractory period.

Recent data[197] utilizing the effects of the levo (l-) and the dextro (d-) isomers of the compound have provided reasonably conclusive evidence that the lengthening of the action potential duration is unrelated to the beta-blocking effect of the compound. For example, in the studies of Kato et al.[197] at a concentration ($10^{-5}$ M) at which d-sotalol had negligible beta-blocking activity, there were no statistically significant differences between the effects of d- and l-sotalol on the $APD_{90}$ either in Purkinje fibers (15 percent versus 19 percent) or in ventricular (Fig. 6) muscle (14 percent versus 20 percent). Similarly, at this drug concentration, the changes in the ERP in the Purkinje fibers (16 percent versus 19 percent) and in ventricular muscle (14 percent versus 21 percent) did not differ significantly. In the case of the atria, although the changes induced were less striking, the electrophysiologic effects of the two compounds also were quantitatively similar including those on phase 4 depolarization in the sinus pacemaker cells. Furthermore, in the Purkinje fibers and in ventricular muscle the overall effects of d- and l-sotalol were nearly identical to those of the racemic compound. Thus, the data of Kato et al.[197] further confirm that, unlike most other beta-adrenoceptor blocking drugs,[198] dl-sotalol lengthens the effective refractory period of cardiac muscle by prolonging the action potential duration with little or no effect on the maximal rate of rise of the action potential. These findings are in accord with earlier reports from different laboratories.[46,195,196]

The overall actions of the stereoisomers reported by Kato et al.[197] confirm and extend the observations of Carmeliet.[199] At concentrations equal to or below $10^{-4}$ M, he found that the main electrophysiologic effect of sotalol and its isomers was to prolong the action potential duration. At higher concentrations, there was shortening of the action potential duration (Fig. 7) and a significant reduction in $V_{max}$ due to the inhibition of the tetrodotoxin-sensitive ("window") inward sodium current. Thus, the observed lengthening of the action potential duration effected by sotalol is

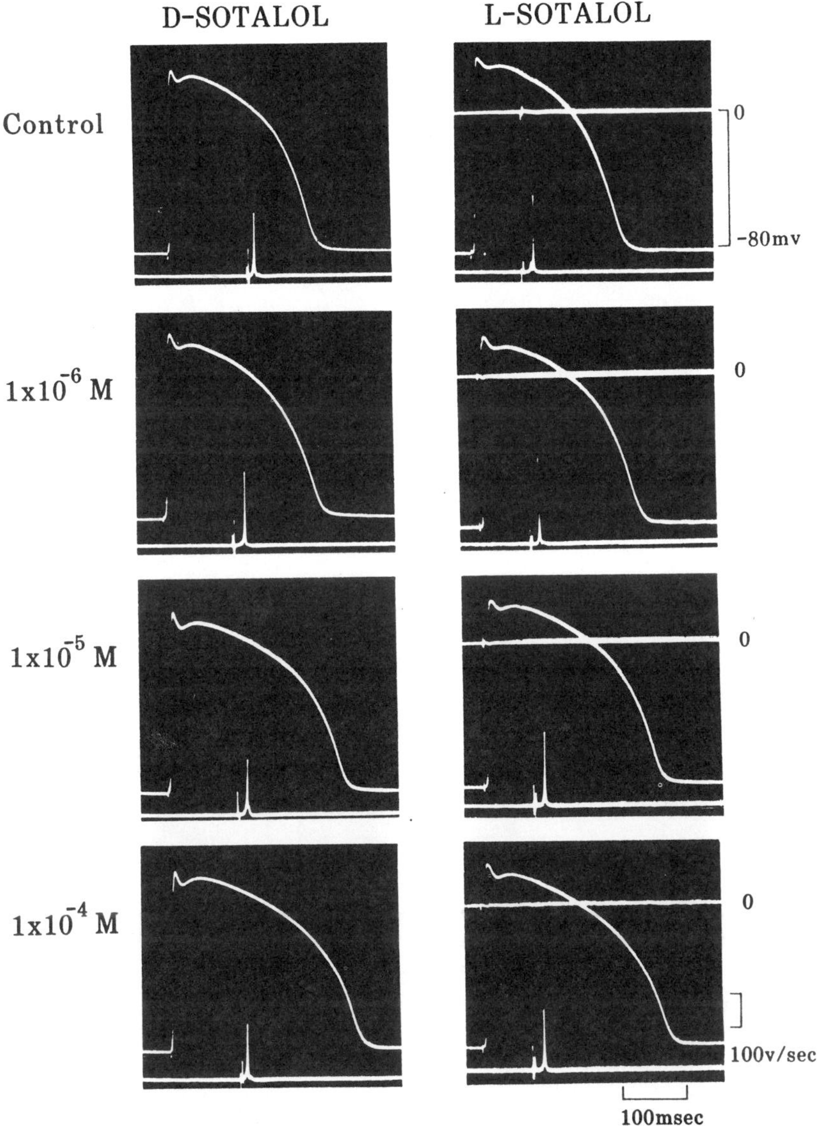


**Figure 6.**    Effects of d-sotalol and l-sotalol on the action potential parameters in canine ventricular muscle. Note the concentration-dependent lengthening of the action potential duration of a similar magnitude induced by the two isomers of sotalol. At the highest concentration (1 x $10^{-4}$M), $V_{max}$ is reduced. (From Kato R, Yabek S, Ikeda N, et al: Electrophysiologic effects of dextro- and levo-isomers of sotalol in isolated cardiac muscle. *J Am Coll Cardiol* 7:116, 1986. By permission of the authors and of the American College of Cardiology.)

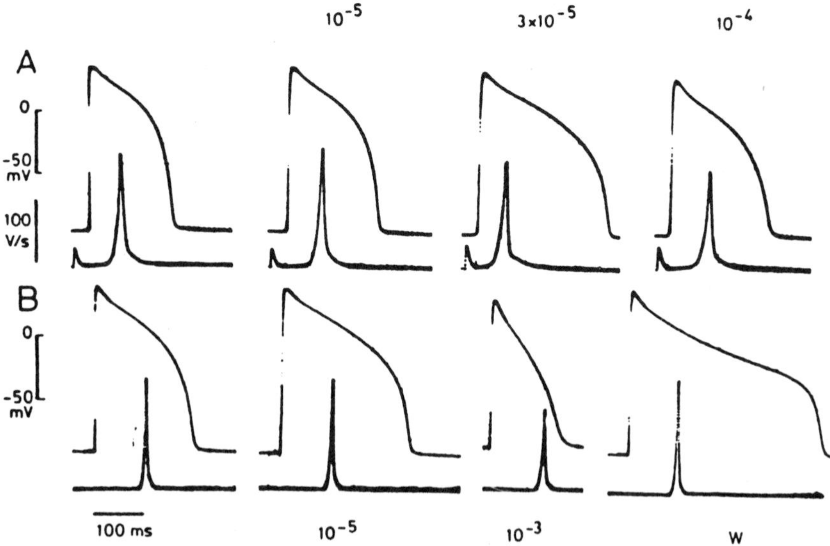


**Figure 7.** The effects of varying concentrations of dl-sotalol on ventricular action potentials. The upper traces show transmembrane potentials, the lower the differentiated rate of rise of the upstroke. The drug concentrations shown are in moles; W = after superfusion with a control solution. Note the marked reduction in the rate of rise of the action potential induced by $10^{-3}$ M sotalol with an associated abbreviation in the action potential duration (APD). At lower concentrations APD increases, which is pronounced during the washout (W) phase. (From Carmeliet E: Electrophysiologic and voltage clamp analysis of sotalol effects in cardiac muscle and Purkinje fibers, *J Exp Pharmacol Ther* 232:817, 1985. By permission of the author and of the journal.)

mediated through adrenergic antagonism since the dextro-isomer, devoid of beta-blocking activity, was equipotent with the levo-isomer in lengthening repolarization and refractoriness. These changes therefore must represent the intrinsinc property of sotalol with respect to outward repolarization currents. The voltage clamp studies of Carmeliet[199] have indicated that the lengthening of the action potential duration by sotalol may be due to a substantial reduction in the plateau outward K current in association with a small decrease in the background current. These electrophysiologic effects raise two theoretical possibilities. First, the lengthening of repolarization will delay the inactivation of the slow calcium channel, which will tend to augment myocardial contractility. This is consonant with the findings of Kaumann and Olson,[195] who indeed have reported a positive inotropic effect due to sotalol in the cat papillary muscle in association with markedly lengthened action potential duration. In the case of the dextro-isomer of sotalol, such an effect is likely to be more pronounced, since it will not be attenuated by the associated beta-receptor blockade. Second, the inhibition of the outward K currents by sotalol and its isomers will lengthen the refractory period. Our data,[197] indicating that d-sotalol lengthens the ERP to the same extent as the l-isomer or the racemic compound, constitutes a valid assumption that the compound is likely to be a potent antiarrhythmic agent.

In vivo studies in experimental animals and in humans have provided further confirmation of the fact that the dominant action of sotalol is to prolong repolarization in all cardiac tissues.[200-205] In humans, intravenously administered sotalol has been found to increase the $QT_c$ interval of the electrocardiogram and to increase the effective refractory period of the atria, ventricles, AV node, His-Purkinje system, and the accessory tracts in the heart.[200-205] Furthermore, intravenous sotalol has also been shown to prolong the duration of the monophasic action potentials recorded by suction electrodes.[206-208] Intravenously or orally administered sotalol has no significant effect on the HV interval or the QRS duration but, as might be expected for a beta antagonist, there is lengthening of intranodal conduction (AH interval).

*Amiodarone*

Amiodarone hydrochloride has attracted considerable experimental and clinical interest in recent years.[211-232] Its extreme potency in the prophylactic control of most supraventricular and ventricular arrhythmias is now well established.[211-215] However, the fundamental mechanism whereby amiodarone induces its salutary effects remains uncertain, because the effects of the drug on the cardiac action potential are of much theoretical as well as practical importance. The details form the subject of Chapter 14 and the interrelationships with thyroid hormone metabolism are examined in Chapter 15; for completeness, the major features are presented here in brief.

As in the case of numerous antiarrhythmic agents, the overall effects of amiodarone on the cardiac action potentials may result from its direct as well indirect actions. When the action of amiodarone on cardiac muscle is considered, several features of its pharmacology appear of importance. First, the drug is not soluble in the usual physiologic media, and thus, superfusion studies in isolated cardiac tissues can be undertaken only in homologous plasma or blood or in an especially modified extracellular environment.[217,218] Studied in this way, the data show that the drug has a modest effect in lengthening the action potential duration in most cardiac tissues (except in Purkinje fibers where it shortens it), a substantial depressant effect on sinus-node potential, and a rate-dependent depression of fast sodium channel function in atria, ventricles, and Purkinje fibers at high concentrations and especially in the setting of inactivated sodium channels. Although the data are not complete, the effects of the metabolite appear to be similar. Second, when the drug is given intravenously in experimental animals and in humans, the electrophysiologic effects are much less striking than those noted after the chronic administration at a constant dose over long periods of time.[217,219] Third, the elimination half-life of amiodarone is extremely long (see Chapter 6) and variable[209,220] and the steady-state effect of the compound cannot be predicted on the basis of the plasma and tissue drug levels of the parent compound or its active metabolite, desethylamiodarone.[221] For these reasons, the acute and the chronic effects of amiodarone and its metabolite need to be differentiated. In part, the acute effects may result from the drug's propensity to antagonize adrenergic receptors and to block the slow channel.

The most striking and consistent electrophysiologic effects of amiodarone occur when the drug is administered chronically.[217] The electrophysiologic changes induced by amiodarone following chronic drug administration closely resemble those (see Chapter 14) produced by thyroid gland ablation.[172,173] Such an effect is not due to the iodine contained in the amiodarone molecule, since the administration of iodine alone in doses equivalent to those contained in the effective dose of amiodarone had no significant effect on the APD of atrial action potentials.[217] On the other hand, the concomitant administration of amiodarone and thyroid hormone prevented the development of repolarization changes evident after admiodarone alone.[217] These observations raise the possibility that the fundamental electrophysiologic effect of amiodarone at least in part may be mediated by the selective blockade of $T_3$ action on cardiac muscle. For the present, this remains a tenable hypothesis that requires experimental verification (see Chapter 14).


## Slow Calcium Channel Blockers and Cardiac Action Potentials

Under voltage clamp conditions, and in concentrations of drugs that are therapeutically relevant, all calcium antagonists inhibit the slow inward current in a dose-dependent manner.[233–235] The effect is apparent in concentrations at which the fast sodium current is unaffected,[236,237] indicating the selectivity of the inhibitory action of this class of drugs on the myocardial slow channel. However, it should be emphasized that such channel selectivity is not absolute[238] and differences exist in the sensitivities of different agents in this regard. For example, extremely low concentrations of nifedipine ($10^{-7}$ to $10^{-5}$ M) depressed the slow current in a dose-dependent manner[39,239] with no effect on the sodium channel. In contrast, verapamil and $D_{600}$ in high concentrations may depress the fast sodium channel; the effect is particularly noticeable in the case of the dextroisomers[240–242] but most of the studies have been undertaken with racemic mixtures.[7,15,243] Differences also have been found between nifedipine and verapamil with respect to their effects on the kinetic parameters of the slow inward current. Nifedipine has been shown[244] to have no effect on the rate of activation and inactivation of the slow current, nor was it found to delay the recovery from the inactivation (i.e., refractoriness). Thus, the action of nifedipine on the slow channel resembles that of textrodotoxin on the fast sodium channel in so far as it inhibits the slow inward current without altering the gating mechanisms of the channel. It also is of interest that the electrophysiologic actions of nifedipine were not frequency-dependent, and stimulus frequencies between 5 to 60/min produced similar effects. However, a recent study[245] has demonstrated a modest frequency-dependent depressant effect of nifedipine on $V_{max}$ in slow channel potentials. In marked contrast, verapamil, especially its levo-isomer, was shown to block the slow inward current in a frequency-dependent manner[233,239,240] and both verapamil and $D_{600}$ altered the kinetics of the slow current. There agents slowed the activation of the slow current while producing a striking delay in the recovery from inactivation,[233,236,246] a property that may be particularly significant in the AV node, in which a marked change in refractoriness has been reported.

Numerous compounds with a great deal of heterogeneity in chemical structure have been found to block the slow myocardial channel in the heart.[243,247] On a molar basis, their potencies to block the slow channel in isolated tissues also may differ significantly. Because of the structural diversity of these compounds, it is not surprising that many have additional electrophysiologic effects on the myocardium and their fundamental effects on the slow channel–mediated actions (e.g., in the SA and AV nodes) may be altered markedly. For example, nifedipine and the other dihydro-pyridines[247] are potent slow channel inhibitors in vitro without other associated electrophysiologic effects. They have a strikingly depressant effect on slow channel function in isolated tissues, but such effects in the AV and SA nodes are nearly completely nullified in vivo because of their reflex actions impinging upon these structures. In contrast, the effects of verapamil and its congeners (gallopamil and tiapamil) and diltiazem on the AV node and SA nodes are associated with significant depression in vitro and in vivo.[243,247] It also is of interest that *perhexiline* is a compound that blocks the slow and the fast channel in approximately the same drug concentrations;[8] *bepridil hydrochloride* blocks the slow channel in low concentrations and at higher concentrations it depresses the fast sodium channel and prolongs cardiac repolarization in all tissues except in Purkinje fibers, in which it shortens repolarization.[248] Thus, it has a complex aggregate of electrophysiologic effects in vitro and in vivo. The effects of verapamil, diltiazem, nifedipine, and bepridil will be discussed somewhat further in the remainder of this chapter.

In contrast to the voltage clamp data, the results obtained with the effects of the various calcium antagonists using standard microelectrode techniques in normal fast response fibers (atria, ventricles, and Purkinje fibers) are reasonably uniform. None of the compounds in low concentrations has an effect on the upstroke velocity of phase 0; "membrane responsiveness" is unaltered, as is conduction velocity or the resting membrane potential;[249,250] and the overall effects, as initially shown by Kolhardt[236] resemble that obtained when using extracellular media devoid of calcium. As might be expected, the effective refractory period is not affected significantly by verapamil as other calcium antagonists in atrial, myocardial, or Purkinje fibers.[251,252] A typical example of the type of effect caused by a calcium antagonist in a fast response fiber is shown in Figure 8. The major effect is on isometric contraction, which is markedly attenuated with no effect on the maximal rate of depolarization and with a slight but consistent acceleration of the plateau phase of the action potential. Such an effect of repolarization, noted with nifedipine, verapamil, $D_{600}$ (gallopamil), and diltiazem[233,239,253-256] may be attributed to the inhibition of the slow current with a secondary effect on potassium conductance.[257] However, an independent action by these compounds on the outward potassium current is not excluded. Figure 8 shows that the depression of the contractile response by calcium antago-

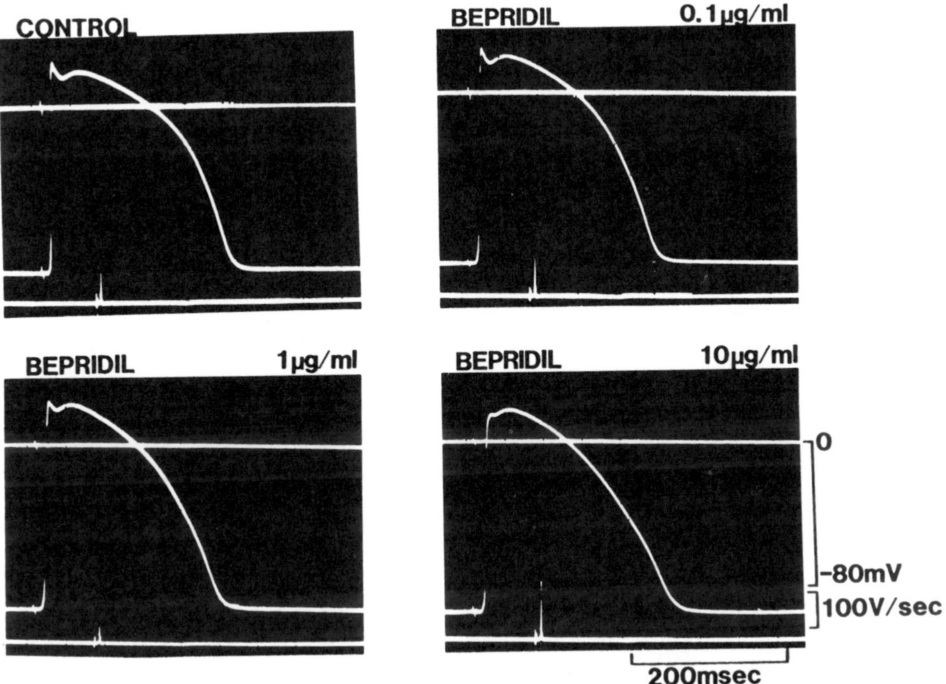


**Figure 8.**   Effects of various concentrations of bepridil on the canine ventricular myocardial action potentials. Note the dose-related reduction in $V_{max}$ and greater lengthening of $APD_{90}$. (From Kato R, Singh BN: Effect of bepridil on the electrophysiologic properties of isolated canine and rabbit myocardial fibers. *Am Heart J* 11:271, 1986. By permission of the authors and of the American Heart Association.)

nists may be reversed by ouabain as well as epinephrine, but only the latter restores the electrophysiologic changes induced as a consequence of slow channel inhibition.

The most striking effects of slow-channel inhibition by calcium antagonists in healthy tissues are found predictably in those structures normally slow channel–dependent for their excitation, namely the sinoatrial and atrioventricular nodes.[251,258–260] In isolated preparations, the sinus node frequency is markedly slowed[47,261] due to the depression in the rate of spontaneous diastolic depolarization, but there is no effect on threshold potential. Similar dose-dependent effects are found in the isolated AV node (Fig. 9) especially in the upper and middle portions, in which the slow response fibers are depressed but the resting membrane potential is not altered. Both in the SA and AV nodes, the rate of rise

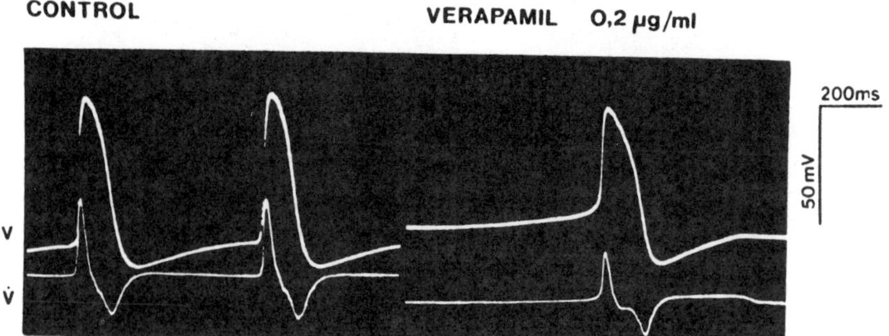


**Figure 9.** Effects of verapamil superfusion on slow response potentials in the AV node. Note the depression of the slope of phase 4 depolarization and elevation of threshold potential. (From Tritthart HA: Pharmacology and electropharmacology of calcium ion antagonists. *J Clin Invest Med* 3:1, 1980. By permission of the author and of the journal.)

and overshoot of the action potentials are lowered and conduction velocity is decreased. Excitability and impulse conduction tend to become extremely rate-dependent in these tissues under the action of these drugs, with a marked lengthening of the effective refractory period[260] particularly in the AV node. As alluded to earlier, however, nifedipine has less effect on AV nodal conduction, but a recent dose-response relationship for this compound[262] in isolated rabbit AV node has confirmed its in vitro depressant effect on intranodal conduction time. Perhaps, it also should be mentioned that slow response fibers in parts of the heart independent of the SA and AV nodes also are sensitive to the action of calcium antagonists,[243] but the precise physiologic or clinical significance of these observations is unknown (discussed later).

Cranefield, Aronson, and Wit[263] demonstrated that Purkinje fibers that were spontaneously active in a media containing high potassium, low sodium, and 4.0 mM Ca were markedly depressed in rate and amplitude on superfusion with low concentrations of verapamil; similarly, fibers exposed to low concentrations of Na and developing repetitive activity following bursts of long depolarizing impulses could be inhibited by verapamil.[263] Cardiac fibers in the mitral leaflets having slow response characteristic under normal conditions tend to develop repetitive activity when exposed to catecholamines;[249] such fibers also may develop after depolarizations due to a slow inward current. Verapamil, in concentrations with no effect on atrial potentials, abolishes such delayed depolarization either spontaneously or after catecholamines in mitral valve fibers.[249] Delayed afterdepolarizations induced by cardiac glycosides[249,251] also are abolished by verapamil, an electrophysiologic effect that may account for the drug's efficacy in the control of certain digitalis-induced dysrhythmias.[264]

Abnormally occurring slow responses sensitive to the depressant actions of calcium antagonists also have been reported in tissues removed from atria[265] and ventricles[266] during open heart surgery. Such studies have shown the presence of typical slow response fibers with low resting membrane potentials with spontaneous activity as well as low conduction velocity. Although such action potentials are promptly abolished in vitro by calcium antagonists such as verapamil, their role in the genesis of clinically occurring atrial and ventricular tachyarrhythmias remains obscure. Slow response potentials also are known to develop in the context of acute myocardial infarction when, in the experimental animal, a coronary artery is abruptly occluded.[267] Such an abnormality develops both during the early and late phases following coronary artery occlusion. The significance of the slow response in this context is unclear.

*Bepridil*

Bepridil hydrochloride is a relatively new calcium antagonist that appears to have a complex pharmacologic profile.[248,268–273] Kato and Singh[274] have shown that the drug exerts a complex aggregate of electrophysiologic effects not only with a varying selectivity of action in terms of drug concentrations but also with respect to the quantitatively and qualitatively variable actions in different myocardial fibers. For example, at the lowest concentration of the drug, the sole measurable effect was a depressant one in slow channel–dependent potentials and in the sinus node. At higher concentrations, there were concentration-dependent decreases in the upstroke velocity of phase 0 or membrane responsiveness in fast-channel dependent potentials accompanied by increases in the effective refractory period (Fig. 10). These changes were the least striking in the case of ventricular tissue when compared to the atria or the Purkinje fibers. Similarly, at high concentrations, there were increases in the action potential duration in the atrial and ventricular fibers, whereas the converse occurred in Purkinje fibers. Here, a concentration-dependent acceleration of repolarization occurred. In the case of changes in the effective refractory period, the effects of bepridil were most marked in the case of rabbit atria, raising the possibility of a correspondingly greater po-

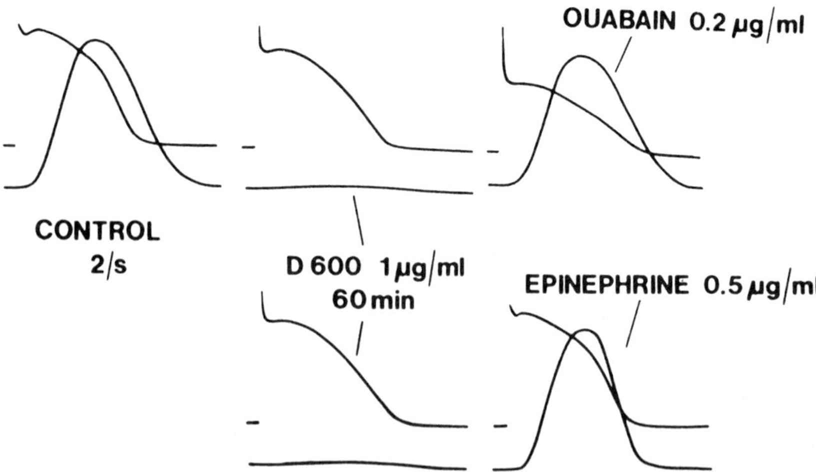


**Figure 10.** Effects of a calcium antagonist ($D_{600}$) on ventricular myocardial action potential contraction. Note that the drug nearly abolishes isometric contraction and accelerates the plateau phase of the action potential. The mechanical effects are reversed by ouabain and epinephrine. (From Tritthart HA: Pharmacology and electropharmacology of calcium ion antagonists. *Clin Invest Med* 3:1, 1980. By permission of the author and of the journal.)

tency in atrial rather than ventricular tachyarrhythmias. Thus, depending on drug concentration and on the myocardial tissue, bepridil has the potential to exert a complex array of electrophysiologic effects in the heart. In vivo, such actions may be modulated by the reflex effects engendered by the drug's vasodilator propensity,[274] due to its calcium channel blocking action in vascular smooth muscle interacting with its intrinsic noncompetitive adrenergic inhibitory properties.[248]

The data of Kato and Singh[274] in the dog and the rabbit confirm and extend previous observations in myocardial tissues from a variety of animals[268–273] and provide new information on the concentration and tissue dependencies of the electrophysiologic actions of bepridil. The fact that the compound depressed phase 4 depolarization and reduced the amplitude of pacemaker potentials in the sinoatrial node and reduced and finally abolished slow channel potentials in Purkinje fibers is consistent with a calcium antagonistic effect. This is further supported by the observation that the effect was reversed in a competitive fashion by increasing extracellular calcium ion concentration. The data of Kato and Singh[274] on the automaticity of the rabbit sinus node as those of

Goto and Sperelakis[273] are consistent with a bradycardic effect in experimental animals[269] and in humans.[248,275,276] These effects as well as the depressant ones in the AV node with the associated lengthening of the effective refractory period reported by Vogel et al.[271] are likely to be explained by the drug's known effects on the myocardial calcium-dependent slow channels.

The results of clinical electrophysiologic studies with be-pridil[248,275–277] are in accord with the experimental findings. For example, when bepridil was administered intravenously, it decreased sinus cycle length, increased intranodal conduction time (AH), and prolonged the effective and the functional refractory periods of the AV node. These effects are similar to those of verapamil or diltiazem. However, unlike these conventional calcium antagonists, intravenous bepridil increased the effective refractory periods of atria and ventricle and prolonged the QRS duration as well as the infranodal conduction time (HV interval). Such effects are in line with the drug's propensity to block the fast sodium channels in the heart. Finally, unlike other calcium antagonists, intravenously administered bepridil lengthens the $QT_c$ interval of the surface electrocardiogram,[248,275] again consistent with the increases in the action potential duration in ventricular fibers contributing to the observed increases in the effective refractory period in the myocardium.

## Conclusions

There now is a plethora of antiarrhythmic compounds of varied structural diversity and complex electropharmacologic profiles. How precisely they control experimentally induced and clinically occurring cardiac arrhythmias still is poorly understood. However, valuable insights into the origin of arrhythmias and the ways antiarrhythmic agents work may be provided by studies of their electrophysiologic effects, as defined by the microelectrode, voltage-clamp, and patch-clamp techniques in isolated cardiac muscle preparations and cells, when correlated with those obtained by suction electrodes and electrode catheter recordings in whole animals and in humans. Such data have been examined. It is suggested that further refinements of this approach may provide a rational basis for the pharmacologic control of cardiac arrhythmias. Attention is drawn to the fact that "isolated" or selective lengthening of the action potential duration appears to constitute a distinct antiarrhythmic mechanism. Under which circumstances and in the presence of which additional features this may constitute the ideal approach to control disorders of cardiac arrhythmias remains essentially unclear. However, lengthening of repolarization is known to increase the tachycardia cycle length and to prevent the degeneration of the tachycardia into fibrillation. Such an antifibrillatory property clearly is an integral prerequisite in a pharmacologic agent for patients with life-threatening arrhythmias, since the terminal event in this setting is ventricular fibrillation. It is suggested that the most promising pharmacologic approach to the control of arrhythmic deaths is a homogeneous prolongation of repolarization and refractoriness in ventricular myocardium.

# References


1. Fozzard HA: Cardiac muscle: Excitability and passive electrical properties. *Prog Cardiovasc Dis* 19:343, 1977.
2. Hauswirth O, Singh BN: Ionic mechanisms in heart muscle in relation to the genesis and the pharmacologic control of cardiac arrhythmias. *Pharmacol Rev* 30:5, 1978.
3. Neher E, Saksmann B: Single channel currents recorded from membrane of denervated frog muscle fibers. *Nature* 260:799, 1976.
4. Hamill OP, Marty A, Neher E, et al: Improved patch-clamp technique for high-resolution current recordings from cells and cell-free membrane patches. Pflueg Arch 391:85, 1981.
5. Vaughan Williams EM: Classification of antidysrhythmic drugs. *Pharmacol Ther* 12:115, 1975
6. Hondeghem LM: Validity of $V_{max}$ as a measure of the sodium current in cardiac and nervous tissue. *Biophysical J* 23:147, 1978
7. Singh BN, Collett JT, Chew CYC: New perspectives in the pharmacologic therapy of cardiac arrhythmias. *Prog Cardiovasc Dis* 22:243, 1980
8. Vaughan Williams EM: *Antiarrhythmic Action and the Puzzle of Perhexiline*. London, Academic Press, 1980.
9. Lee KS, Hume JR, Giles W, et al: Sodium current depression by lidocaine and quinidine in isolated ventricular cells. *Nature* 291:325, 1981.
10. Cohen CJ, Bean BP, Tsien TW: Maximum upstroke velocity ($V_{max}$) as an index of available sodium conductance: Comparison of $V_{max}$ and voltage clamp measurements of $I_{Na}$ in rabbit Purkinje fibers. *Circ Res* 54:636, 1984.
11. Hondeghem LM, Katzung B: Time- and voltage-dependent interactions of antiarrhythmic drugs with cardiac sodium channels. *Biochem Biophys Acta* 472:373, 1977.
12. Campbell TJ, Vaughan Williams EM: Voltage and time-dependent depression of maximum rate of depolarization of guinea-pig ventricular action potentials by two new antiarrhythmic drugs, flecainide and lorcainide. *Cardiovasc Res* 17:251, 1983.

13. Campbell TJ: Resting and rate-dependent depression of maximum rate of depolarization ($V_{max}$) in guinea-pig ventricular action potentials by mexiletine, disopyramide and encainide. *J Cardiovasc Pharmacol* 5:291, 1983.

14. Campbell TJ: Kinetics of onset of rate-dependent effects of Class I antiarrhythmic drugs are important in determining their effects on refractoriness in guinea-pig ventricle and provide a theoretical basis for their subclassification. *Cardiovasc Res* 17:344, 1983.

15. Hondeghem LM, Katzung BG: Antiarrhythmic agents: The modulated receptor mechanism of action of sodium and calcium channel-blocking drugs. *Ann Rev Pharmacol Toxicol* 24:387, 1984.

16. Reuter H: Ion channels in cardiac cell membranes. *Ann Rev Physiol* 46:473, 1984.

17. Tsien RW: Calcium channels in excitable cell membranes. *Ann Rev Physiol* 45:341, 1983.

18. Trautwein W: Membrane currents in cardiac muscle fibers. *Physiol Rev* 53:793, 1973.

19. Weidmann S: The effect of the cardiac membrane potential on the rapid availability of the sodium carrier system. *J Physiol* 127:213, 1955.

20. Buchanan JW, Saito T, Gettes LS: The effects of antiarrhythmic drugs, stimulation frequency, and potassium-induced resting membrane potential changes on conduction velocity and $dV/dt_{max}$ in guinea pig myocardium. *Circ Res* 56:696, 1985.

21. Cachelin AB, De Peyer JE, Kokubun S: Sodium channels in cultured cardiac cells. *J Physiol* 340:389, 1983.

22. Colatsky TJ: Voltage clamp measurements of sodium channel properties in rabbit cardiac Purkinje fibers. *J Physiol* 305:215, 1980.

23. Fleckenstein A: Specific pharmacology of calcium antagonists in myocardium, cardiac pacemakers and vascular smooth muscle. *Ann Rev Pharmacol Toxicol* 17:149, 1977.

24. Kass RS, Tsien RW: Multiple effects of calcium antagonists on plateau currents in cardiac Purkinje fibers. *J Gen Physiol* 66:169, 1975.

25. Kass RS, Wiegers SE: Ionic basis of concentration-related effects of noradrenaline on the action potentials of cardiac Purkinje fibers. *J Physiol* 322:541, 1982.

26. Giles W, Noble SJ: Changes in membrane currents in bullfrog atrium produced by acetylcholine. *J Physiol* 261:103, 1976.

27. Reuter H, Scholz A: A study of ion selectivity and the kinetic properties of the calcium-dependent slow inward current in the mammalian cardiac muscle. *J Physiol* 264:17, 1977.

28. Coroboeuf E, Deroubaix E, Coulombe A: Effect of tetrodotoxin on action potentials of the conducting system in the dog heart. *Amer J Physiol* 236:H561, 1979.

29. Noble D, Tsien RW: Outward membrane currents activated in the plateau range of potentials of Purkinje fibers. *J Physiol* 200:255, 1969.

30. Fozzard HA, Hiraoka M: The positive dynamic current and its inactivation properties in cardiac Purkinje fibers. *J Physiol* (London) 234:569, 1973.

31. Kenyon JL, Gibbons WR: 4-aminopyridine and the early outward

current of sheep cardiac Purkinje fibers. *J Gen Physiol* (London) 73:139, 1979.

32. Noble D, Tsien RW: The kinetics and the rectifier properties of the slow potassium current in cardiac Purkinje fibers. *J Physiol* 195:185, 1968.

33. Kass RS: The ionic basis of electrical activity of the heart. In N Sperelakis (ed.): *Physiology and Pathophysiology of the Heart*. Boston, Martinus Nijhoff Publishers, p 83, 1984.

34. Baumgarten CM, Isenberg G: Depletion and accumulation in the extracellular clefts of cardiac Purkinje fibers. *Pflueg Arch* 368:19, 1977.

35. Maylie JM, Morad M, Weiss J: A study of pacemaker potential in rabbit sino-atrial node measurement of potassium activity under voltage clamp conditions. *J Physiol* 311:161, 1981.

36. Di Francesco D: A new interpretation of the pacemaker current $i_{k2}$ in Purkinjie fibers. *J Physiol* 314:359, 1981.

37. Tsien RW: Effects of epinephrine on the pacemaker potassium current of cardiac Purkinje fibers. *J Gen Physiol* 64:293, 1977.

38. Weidmann S: Effect of calcium ions and local anesthetics on the electrical properties of Purkinje fibers. *J Physiol* 129:568, 1955.

39. Singer DH, Baumgarten CM, Ten Eick RE: Cellular electrophysiology of ventricular and other arrhythmias: Studies on diseased and ischemic hearts. In EH Sonnenblick, M Lesch (eds): *Sudden Cardiac Death*. New York, Grune and Stratton, p 13, 1981.

40. Watanabe AM, Bailey JC: The role of the autonomic central nervous system in mediating and modifying the action of cardiac antiarrhythmic drugs. *Ann NY Acad Sci* 432:90, 1984.

41. Levy MN: Neural control of cardiac rhythm and contraction. In MR Rosen, BF Hoffman (ed.): *Cardiac Therapy*. Boston, Martinus Nijhoff Publishers, p 73, 1983.

42. Olsson B, Varnauskas E, Korsgren M: Further improved method for measuring action potentials of the intact heart. *J Electrocardiol* 4:19, 1971.

43. Wit AL: Cellular electrophysiologic mechanisms of cardiac arrhythmias. *Ann NY Acad Sci* 432:1, 1984.

44. Cranefield PF: Action potentials, afterpotentials and arrhythmias. *Circ Res* 41:415, 1977.

45. Rosen MR, Reder RF: Does triggered activity have a role in the genesis of cardiac arrhythmias? *Ann Int Med* 94:794, 1981.

46. Singh BN, Vaughan Williams EM: A third class of antiarrhythmic action. Effects on atrial and ventricular intracellular potentials and other pharmacologic actions on cardiac muscle of MJ1999 and AH3474. *Br J Pharmacol* 39:675, 1970.

47. Singh BN: A study of the pharmacological actions of certain drugs and hormones with a particular reference to cardiac muscle. D. Phil. thesis, England, University of Oxford, 1971.

48. Singh BN, Vaughan Williams EM: Effect of altering potassium concentration on the action of lidocaine and diphenylhydantoin on rabbit atrial and ventricular muscle. *Circ Res* 29:286, 1971.

49. Singh BN, Vaughan Williams EM: A fourth class of antiarrhythmic action? Effect of verapamil on ouabain toxicity, on atrial and ventric-

ular intracellular potentials and on other features of cardiac function. *Cardiovasc Res* 6:109, 1972.

50. Singh BN, Hauswirth O: Comparative mechanisms of action of antiarrhythmic drugs. *Am Heart J* 87:367, 1974.

51. Vaughan Williams EM: A classification of antiarrhythmic actions reassessed after a decade of new drugs. *J Clin Pharmacol* 24:129, 1984.

52. Singh BN: Rational basis of antiarrhythmic therapy: Clinical pharmacology of commonly used antiarrhythmic drugs. *Angiology* 29:206, 1978.

53. Hille B: Local anesthetics: Hydrophilic and hydrophobic pathways for the drug-receptor interaction. *J Gen Physiol* 69:497, 1977

54. Courtney KR: Mechanism of frequency-dependent inhibition of sodium currents in myelinated nerve by the quaternary lidocaine derivative GEA 968. *J Pharmacol Exper Ther* 195:225, 1975.

55. Harrison DC: Antiarrhythmic drug classification: New science and practical applications. *Amer J Cardiol* 56:185, 1985.

56. Mason JW, Hondeghem LM: Quinidine. *Ann NY Acad Sci* 432:162, 1984.

57. Johnson EA, McKinnon JM: The differential effects of quinidine and pyrilamine on the myocardial action potential at various rates of stimulation. *J Pharmacol Exp Ther* 120:460, 1957.

58. Vaughan Williams EM: The mode of action of quinidine on isolated rabbit atria interpreted from intracellular records. *Br J Pharmacol* 13:276, 1958.

59. Hoffman BF: The action of quinidine and procainamide on single fibers of dog ventricle in specialized conduction system. *Ann Acad Bras Circ* 29:365, 1958.

60. Sekiya A, Vaughan Williams EM: A comparison of the antifibrillatory actions and effects on intracellular cardiac potentials of pronethalol, disopyramide and quinidine. *Br J Pharmacol* 21:473, 1963.

61. Chen C-M, Gettes LS, Katzung BG: Effect of lidocaine and quinidine on steady-state characteristics and recovery kinetics of $dV/dt_{max}$ in guinea pig ventricular myocardium. *Circ Res* 37:20, 1975.

62. Hondeghem LM, Grant AD, Jensen RA: Antiarrhythmic drug action: Selective depression of hypoxic cardiac cells. *Am Heart J* 87:602, 1974.

63. Colatsky TJ: Mechanism of action of lidocaine and quinidine on action potential duration in rabbit cardiac Purkinje fibers. *Circ Res* 50:17, 1982.

64. Grant AO, Trantham JL, Brown KK, et al: pH-dependent effects of quinidine on the kinetics of $dV/dt_{max}$ in guinea pig ventricular myocardium. *Circ Res* 50:210, 1982.

65. Weld FM, Coromilas J, Rottman JN, et al: Mechanisms of quinidine-induced depression of the maximum upstroke velocity in ovine cardiac Purkinje fibers. *Circ Res* 50:369, 1982.

66. Nattell S, Elharrar V, Zipes DP, et al: pH-dependent electrophysiologic effects of quinidine and lidocaine in canine Purkinje fibers. *Circ Res* 48:55, 1981.

67. Hondeghem LM: Effects of lidocaine, phenytoin and quinidine on the ischemic canine myocardium. *J Electrocardiol* 9:203, 1976.

68. Watanabe Y, Dreifus LS, Likoff W: Electrophysiologic antagonism and synergism of potassium and antiarrhythmic agents. *Amer J Cardiol* 12:702, 1963.

69. Josephson ME, Seides SF, Batsford WP, et al: The electrophysiologic effects of intramuscular quinidine on atrio-ventricular conducting system in man. *Am Heart J* 87:55, 1974.

70. Mason JW, Winkle RA, Rider AK, et al: The electrophysiologic effects of quinidine in the transplanted human heart. *J Clin Invest* 59:481, 1977.

71. Rosen MR, Gelband H, Merker C, et al: Effects of procainamide on the electrophysiologic properties of the canine ventricular conducting system. *J Pharmacol Exp Ther* 185:438, 1973.

72. Hoffman BF, Rosen MR, Wit AL: Electrophysiology and pharmacology of arrhythmias. VII Cardiac effects of quinidine and procainamide. *Am Heart J* 90:117, 1975.

73. Rosen MR, Gelband H, Hoffman BF: Canine electrocardiographic and electrophysiologic changes induced by procainamide. *Circulation* 46:528, 1972.

74. Arnsdorf M, Bigger JT: The effects of procainamide on components of excitability in long mammalian cardiac Purkinje fibers. *Circ Res* 38:115, 1976.

75. Arsndorf M: The effects of antiarrhythmic drugs on triggered sustained activity in cardiac Purkinje fibers. *J Pharmacol Exp Ther* 201:689, 1977.

76. Wittig J, Harrison LA, Wallace AG: Electrophysiologic effects of lidocaine on distal Purkinje fibers of the canine heart. *Am Heart J* 86:69,1973.

77. Carmeliet E, Saikawa T: Shortening of the action potential and reduction of pacemaker activity by lidocaine, quinidine, and procainamide in sheep cardiac Purkinje fibers: An effect on Na K currents? *Circ Res* 50:257, 1982.

78. Josephson ME, Caracta AR, Riccuitti MA, et al: Electrophysiologic properties of procainamide in man. *Am J Cardiol* 33:596, 1974.

79. Mokler CM, Van Arman CG: Pharmacology of a new antiarrhythmic agent -di-isopropyl-amino- -phenyl-2 (2-pyridyl) butyramide (SC-7031). *J Pharmacol Exp Ther* 136:114, 1962.

80. Dreifus LS, Zbigniew F, Sexton DM: Electrophysiological and clinical effects of a new antiarrhythmic agent: Disopyramide. *Am J Cardiol* 31:129, 1973.

81. Kus T, Sasyniuk BI: Electrophysiological actions of disopyramide phosphate on canine ventricular muscle and Purkinje fibers. *Circ Res* 37:844, 1975.

82. Danilo P, Rosen MR: Cardiac effects of disopyramide. *Am Heart J* 92:532, 1976.

83. Danilo P, Hordof AJ, Rosen MR: Effects of disopyramide on electrophysiologic properties of canine cardiac Purkinje fibres. *J Pharmacol Exp Ther* 201:701, 1977.

84. Vaughan Williams EM: Disopyramide. *Ann NY Acad Sci* 432:189, 1984.

85. Sasyniuk BI, Kus T: Electrophysiologic actions induced by disopyr-

amide phosphate in normal and infarcted hearts. *J Int Med Res*4(Suppl 1):20, 1978.

86. Levites R, Anderson G: Differential electrophysiologic effects of disopyramide phosphate in canine myocardial ischemia. *Am J Cardiol* 39:292, 1977.

87. Befeler B, Castellanos A, Wells DE: Electrophysiologic effects of the antiarrhythmic agent disopyramide phosphate. *Am J Cardiol* 35:282, 1975.

88. Spurrell RAJ, Thorburn CW, Camm J: Effects of disopyramide on electrophysiological properties of specialised conduction system in man and an accessory atrioventricular pathway in Wolff-Parkinson-White syndrome. *Br Heart J* 37:870, 1975.

89. Mirro MJ, Manalan AS, Bailey JC, et al: Anticholinergic effects of disopyramide and quinidine on guinea pig myocardium: Mediation by direct muscarinic receptor blockade. *Circ Res* 47:855, 1980.

90. Bigger JT, Mandel WJ: Effect of lidocaine on transmembrane potentials of ventricular muscle and Purkinje fibers *J Clin Invest* 49:63, 1970.

91. Mandel WJ, Bigger JT: Effect of lidocaine on isolated canine and rabbit atrial tissues. *J Pharmacol Exp Ther* 178:81, 1971.

92. Bigger JT, Mandel WJ: Effect of lidocaine on conduction in canine Purkinje fibers and at the ventricular muscle Purkinje fiber junction. *J Pharmacol Exp Ther* 174:487, 1970

93. Davis LD, Temte JV: Electrophysiologic actions of lidocaine on canine ventricular muscle and Purkinje fibers. *Circ Res* 24:639, 1969.

94. Colatsky TJ: Mechanism of action of lidocaine and quinidine on action potential duration in rabbit cardiac Purkinje fibers: An effect on steady state sodium currents. *Circ Res* 50:17, 1982.

95. Rosen MR, Merker C, Pippenger CE: The effects of lidocaine on ECG and electrophysiologic properties of Purkinje fibers. *Am Heart J* 91:191, 1976.

96. Brennan FJ, Cranefield PF, Wit AL: Effects of lidocaine on slow response and depressed fast response action potentials of canine cardiac Purkinje fibers. *J Pharmacol Exp Ther* 204:312, 1978.

97. Lazzara R, Hope RR, El-Sherif N, Scherlag BJ: Effects of lidocaine on hypoxia and ischemic cardiac cells. *Am J Cardiol* 41:872, 1978.

98. Grant AO, Strauss LJ, Wallace AG, et al: The influence of pH on the electrophysiologic effects of lidocaine in guinea pig ventricular myocardium. *Circ Res* 47:542, 1980.

99. Mary-Rabine L, Hordof AJ, Danilo P, et al: Mechanism for impulse initiation in isolated human atrial fibers. *Circ Res* 47:267, 1980.

100. Rosen MR, Danilo P: Effects of tetrodotoxin, lidocaine, verapamil, and AHR-2666 on ouabain-induced delayed afterdepolarization in canine Purkinje fibers. *Circ Res* 46:117, 1980.

101. Barrett PA, Laks MM, Mandel WJ, et al: The electrophysiologic effects of intravenous lidocaine in the WPW syndrome. *Am Heart J* 100:22, 1980.

102. Rosen KM, Lau SH, Weiss MB, et al: The effect of lidocaine on atrioventricular and intraventricular conduction in man. *Am J Cardiol* 25:1, 1970.

103. Jospehson ME, Caracta AR, Lau SH, et al: Effects of lidocaine on refractory periods in man. *Am Heart J* 84:778, 1972.
104. Singh BN, Vaughan Williams EM: Investigations of the mode of action of a new antidysrhythmic drug. Ko 1173. *Br J Pharmacol* 44:1, 1972.
105. Vaughan Williams EM: Mexiletine in isolated tissue models. *Postgrad Med J* 53(Suppl I):30, 1977.
106. Yamaguchi I, Singh BN, Mandel WJ: Electrophysiological actions of mexiletine on isolated rabbit atria and canine ventricular muscle and Purkinje fibers. *Cardiovasc Res* 13:288, 1979.
107. Weld FM, Bigger JT, Swistel D, et al: Electrophysiological effects of mexiletine (Ko 1173) on ovine cardiac Purkinje fibers. *J Pharmacol Exp Ther* 210:222, 1979.
108. Arita M, Goto M, Nagomoto Y, et al: Electrophysiologic actions of mexiletine (Ko 1173) on canine Purkinje fibers and ventricular muscle. *Br J Pharmacol* 67:143, 1979.
109. Burke GH, Berman ND: Differential electrophysiologic effects of mexiletine on normal and hypoxic canine Purkinje fibers. *J Cardiovasc Pharmacol* 7:1096, 1985.
110. Hohnloser S, Weirich J, Antoni H: Effects of mexiletine on steady-state characteristics and recovery kinetics of $V_{max}$ and conduction velocity in the guinea pig myocardium. *J Cardiovasc Pharmacol* 4:232, 1982.
111. Roos JC, Paalman ACA, Dunning AJ: Electrophysiological effects of mexiletine in man *Br Heart J* 38:1262, 1976.
112. McComish M, Robinson C, Kitson D, et al: Clinical electrophysiological effect of mexiletine. *Postgrad Med J* 53(Suppl I):85, 1977.
113. Roos JC, Paalman DCA, Dunning AJ: Electrophysiological effects of mexiletine in man. *Postgrad Med J* 53(Suppl I):92, 1977.
114. Coltart DJ, Berndt TB, Kernoff R: Antiarrhythmic and circulatory effects of Astra W36095, a new lidocaine-like agent. *Am J Cardiol* 34:35, 1974.
115. Zipes DP, Troup PJ: New antiarrhythmic drugs. *Am J Cardiol* 41:1005, 1978.
116. Oshita S, Sada H, Kojima M, et al: Effects of tocainaide and lidocaine on the transmembrane action potentials as related to the external potassium and calcium concentrations in guinea pig papillary muscles. *Naunyn Schmiedebergs Arch Pharmacol* 314:62, 1980.
117. Anderson JL, Mason JW, Winkle RA: Clinical electrophysiological effects of tocainide. *Circulation* 57:685, 1978.
118. Verdonck F, Vereecke J, Vlengels A: Electrophysiological effects of aprindine on isolated heart preparations. *Eur J Pharmacol* 26:338, 1974.
119. Steinberg MI, Greenspan K: Intracellular electrophysiological alterations in canine cardiac conducting tissue induced by aprindine and lidocaine. *Cardiovasc Res* 10:236, 1976.
120. Elharrar V, Foster PR, Zipes DP: Effects of aprindine HC1 on cardiac tissues. *J Pharmacol Exp Ther* 195:201, 1975.
121. Zipes DP, Gavin WE, Foster PR: Aprindine for treatment of supraventricular tachycardias with particular application to Wolff-Parkinson-White syndrome. *Am J Cardiol* 40:586, 1977.

122. Seipel L, Both B, Breithardt G: Action of antiarrhythmic drugs in His bundle electrogram and sinus node function. *Acta Cardiol* (Brussels) 18(Suppl):251, 1974.

123. Schlepper M, Neuss H: Changes of refractory periods in the AV conduction system induced by antiarrhythmic drugs. A study using His bundle recordings. *Acta Cardiol* (Brussels) 18(Suppl):269, 1974.

124. Knoll DA, Lucchessi BR: Antiarrhythmic and antifibrillatory properties of aprindine. *J Pharmacol Exp Ther* 194:427, 1975.

125. Jensen RA, Katzung BG: Electrophysiologic properties of diphenylhydantoin in rabbit atria. *Circ Res* 26:17, 1970.

126. Katzung BG, Jensen RA: Depressant action of diphenylhydantoin on the electrical and the mechanial properties of isolated rabbit and dog atria: Dependence on sodium and potassium. *Am Heart J* 80:80, 1970.

127. Rosen MR, Danilo P, Alonso MB, et al: Effects of therapeutic concentrations of diphenylhydantoin on the transmembrane potentials of normal and depressed Purkinje fibers. *J Pharmacol Exp Ther* 197:594, 1974.

128. Bigger JT, Strauss HC, Bassett AL, et al: Actions of diphenylhydantoin on the electrophysiologic properties of canine Purkinje fibers. *Circ Res* 22:221, 1968.

129. Strauss HC, Bigger JT, Bassett AL, et al: Actions of diphenylhydantoin on the electrical properties of isolated canine and rabbit atria. *Circ Res* 22:463, 1968.

130. Bigger JT, Weinberg DI, Kovalik ATW, et al: Effect of diphenylhydantoin on automaticity and excitability of the canine heart. *Circ Res* 21:757, 1967.

131. Dhatt MS, Gomes JAC, Reddy CP, et al: Effects of phenytoin on refractoriness and conduction in the human heart. *J Cardiol Pharmacol* 1:3, 1979.

132. Podrid PJ, Lyakishev A, Lown B, et al: Ethmozine, a new antiarrhythmic drug for suppressing premature ventricular complexes. *Circulation* 61:450, 1980.

133. Danilo P, Langan WB, Rosen MR, et al: Effects of the phenothiazine analog EN313 on ventricular arrhythmias in the dog. *Eur J Pharmacol* 45:127, 1977.

134. Rosen MR, Wit AL: Electropharmacology of antiarrhythmic drugs. *Am Heart J* 106:829, 1983.

135. Ikeda N, Singh BN, Davis LD, et al: Effects of flecainide on the electrophysiologic properties of isolated canine and rabbit myocardial fibers. *J Am Coll Cardiol* 5:303, 1985.

136. Cowan JC, Vaugan Williams EM: Characterization of a new oral antiarrhythmic drug, flecainide R-818. *Eur J Pharmacol* 73:333, 1981

137. Borchard U, Boisten M: Effect of flecainide on action potentials and alternating current-induced arrhythmias in mammalian myocardium. *J Cardiovasc Pharmacol* 4:205, 1982

138. Muhiddin K, Nathan AW, Hellestrand KJ, et al: Ventricular tachycardia associated with flecainide. *Lancet* 2:1220, 1983

139. Olsson SB, Edvardsson N: Clinical electrophysiologic study of antiarrhythmic properties of flecainide: Acute intraventricular delayed

conduction and prolonged repolarization in regular paced and premature beats using intracardiac monophasic action potentials with programmed stimulation. *Am Heart J* 102:864, 1981.

140. Hodess AB, Follansbee WP, Spear JF, et al: Electrophysiological effects of a new antiarrhythmic agent, flecainide, on the intact canine heart. *J Cardiovasc Pharmacol* 1:427, 1979.

141. Seipel L, Abendroth RR, Breithard TG: Electrophysiological effects of flecainide (R-818) in man. *Circulation* 62(Part III):153, 1980.

142. Nathan A, Hellestrand K, Bexton R, et al: The proarrhythmic effects of the new "antiarrhythmic" drug flecainide acetate. *J Am Coll Cardiol* 1:709, 1983.

143. Hellestrand KJ, Bexton RS, Nathan AV, et al: Acute electrophysiological effects of flecainide acelate on cardiac conduction and refractoriness in man. *Br Heart J* 48:140, 1982.

144. Elharrar V, Zipes DP: Effects of encainide and metabolites (MJ14030 and MJ19444) on canine Purkinje fibers and ventricular fibers. *J Pharmacol Exp Ther* 220:440, 1982.

145. Carmeliet E: Electrophysiological effects of encainide on isolated cardiac muscle and Purkinje fibers and on the Langendorff perfused guinea pig heart. *Eur J Pharmacol* 61:247, 1980.

146. Jackman WM, Zipes DP, Nacarelli GV, et al: Electrophysiology of oral encainide. *Am J Cardiol* 49:1270, 1982.

147. Winkle RA, Peters F, Kates RE, et al: Clinical pharmacology and antiarrhythmic efficacy of encainide in patients with ventricular arrhythmias. *Circulation* 64:290, 1981.

148. Sami M, Mason JW, Peters F, et al: Clinical electrophysiologic effects of encainide, a newly developed antiarrhythmic agent. *Am J Cardiol* 44:526, 1979.

149. Carey EL, Duff HJ, Roden DM, et al: Relative electrocardiographic and antiarrhythmic effects of encainide and its metabolite in man. *Circulation* 64:IV-264, 1981.

150. Kohlhardt M, Seifert C: Inhibition of $V_{max}$ of the action potential by propafenone and its voltage-time and pH-dependence in mammalian ventricular myocardium. *Naunyn Schmiedebergs Arch Pharmacol* 315:55, 1980

151. Ledda F, Mantelli L, Manzini S, et al: Electrophysiologic and antiarrhythmic properties of propafenone in isolated cardiac preprarations. *J Cardiovasc Pharmacol* 3:1162, 1981.

152. Duke IS, Vaughan Williams EM: The multiple modes of action of propafenone. *Eur Heart J* 5:115, 1984.

153. Kohlhardt M: Block of sodium currents by antiarrhythmic agents: Analysis of the electrophysiologic effects of propafenone in heart muscle. *Am J Cardiol* 54:13D, 1984.

154. Seipel L, Breithardt G, Both A, et al: Effects of propafenone on the sinus nodes and intracardiac conduction in man. *Drug Dev Eval* 1:45, 1977.

155. Prystowsky EN, Heger JJ, Chilson DA, et al: Antiarrhythmic and electrophysiologic effects of propafenone. *Am J Cardiol* 54:26D, 1984.

156. Breithardt G, Borgreffe M, Wiebringhaus E, et al: Effects of propafenone in the Wolff-Parkinson-White syndrome: Electrophysiologic findings and long-term follow-up. *Am J Cardiol* 54:29D, 1984.

157. Singh BN, Venkatesh N: Prevention of myocardial reinfarction and of sudden death in survivors of acute myocardial infarction: Role of prophylactic beta-adrenoceptor blockade. *Am Heart J* 107:189, 1984.
158. Schwartz PH: Idiopathic long QT syndrome: Progress and questions. *Am Heart J* 109:399, 1985.
159. Surawicz B, Knoebel S: Long QT: Good, bad or indifferent? *J Am Coll Cardiol* 4:498, 1984.
160. Jervell A, Lange-Nielsen F: Congenital deaf-mutism, functional heart disease with prolongation of the QT interval and sudden death. *Am Heart J* 54:59, 1957.
161. Wit Al, Hoffman BF, Rosen MR: Electrophysiology and pharmacology of cardiac arrhythmias. IX. Cardiac electrophysiologic effects of beta adrenergic receptor stimulation and blockade. *Am Heart J* 90:795, 1975.
162. Davis LD, Temte JV: Effects of propranolol on the transmembrane potentials of ventricular muscle and Purkinje fibers of the dog. *Circ Res* 22:661, 1968
163. Rosen MR, Hordof AJ, Ilvento JP, et al: Effects of adrenergic amines on electrophysiologic properties and automaticity of neonatal and adult canine Purkinje fibers. *Circ Res* 40:390, 1977.
164. Hewett K, Rosen MR: Beta-adrenergic modulation of the digitalis-induced delayed afterdepolarization and triggered activity. *Am J Cardiol* 49:913, 1982.
165. Raine AEG, Vaughan Williams EM: Adaptation to prolonged beta-blockade on rabbit atrial, Purkinje and ventricular potentials and papillary muscle contractions. *Circ Res* 48:804, 1981.
166. Edvaardsson N, Olsson B: Effects of acute and chronic beta-blockade on ventriocular repolarization in man. *Br Heart J,* 45:626, 1981.
167. Duff H, Roden DM, Brorson L, et al: Electrophysiologic actions of high plasma concentrations of propranolol in human subjects. *J Am Coll Cardiol* 2:1134, 1983.
168. Stern S, Eisenberg S: The effect of propranolol on the electrocardiogram of normal subjects. *Br Heart J* 77:192, 1969.
169. Rosen KM, Barwolf C, Ehsani A, et al: Effects of lidocaine and propranolol on the normal and anomalous pathways in patients with pre-excitation. *Am J Cardiol* 30:801, 1972.
170. Singh BN, Nademanee K: Control of cardiac arrhythmias by selective lengthening of repolarization: Theoretic considerations and clinical observations. *Am Heart J* 109:421, 1985.
171. Freedberg AS, Papp JG, Vaughan Williams EM: The effect of altered thyroid state on atrial intracellular potentials. *J Physiol* 207:357, 1970.
172. Johnson PN, Freedberg AS, Marshall JM: Action of thyroid hormone on the transmembrane potentials from sino-atrial node cells and atrial cells in isolated atria of rabbits. *Cardiology* 58:273, 1973.
173. Leveque PE: Antiarrhythmic action of bretylium. *Nature* 207:203, 1965.
174. Boura ALA, Green AF: The action of bretylium: Adrenergic neurone blocking and other effects. *Br J Pharmacol* 14:536, 1959.
175. Bacaner MB: Bretylium tosylate for suppression of induced ventricular fibrillation. *Am J Cardiol* 17:528, 1966.

176. Terry G, Vellani CW, Higgins MR, et al: Bretylium tosylate in treating refractory ventricular arrhythmias complicating myocardial infarction. *Br Heart J* 32:21, 1970.
177. Day HW, Bacaneer M: Use of bretylium tosylate in management of acute myocardial infarction. *Am J Cardiol* 27:177, 1971.
178. Gillis RA, Clancy MM, Anderson RJ: The deleterious effects of bretylium in cats with digitalis-induced ventricular tachycardia. *Circulation* 47:976, 1973.
179. Papp JG, Vaughan Williams EM: The effect on intracellular atrial potentials of bretylium in relation to its local anesthetic potency. *Br J Pharmacol* 35:352, 1969.
180. Watanabe Y, Josipovic V, Dreifus LS: Electrophysiologic mechanisms of bretylium tosylate. *Circulation* 38(Suppl VI):202, 1968.
181. Bigger JT, Jaffe CC: The effect of bretylium tosylate on the electrophysiologic properties of ventricular muscle and Purkinje fibers. *Am J Cardiol* 27:82, 1971.
182. Wit Al, Steiner C, Damato AN: Electrophysiologic effects of bretylium tosylate on single fibers of the canine specialized conducting system and ventricle. *J Pharmacol Exp Ther* 173:344, 1970.
183. Cardinal R, Sasyniuk BI: Electrophysiological effects of bretylium tosylate in subendocardial Purkinje fibers from infarcted canine hearts. *J Pharmacol Exp Ther* 204:159, 1978.
184. Drayer DF, Reidenberg MM, Levy RW: N-acetylprocainamide: An active metabolite of procainamide. *Proc Soc Exp Biol Med* 146:358, 1974.
185. Refsum H, Frislid K, Lunde PKM et al: Effects of N-acethylprocainamide as compared with procainamide in isolated rat atria. *Eur J Pharmacol* 33:47, 1975.
186. Minchin RF, Ilett KF, Paterson JW: Antiarrhythmic potency of procainamide and N-acetylprocainamide in rabbits. *Eur J Pharmacol* 47:51, 1978.
187. Amlie JP, Nesje OA, Frislid K, et al: Serum levels and electrophysiological effects of N-acetylprocainamide as compared with procainamide in the dog heart in situ. *Acta Pharmacol Toxicol* 42:280–286, 1978.
188. Reynolds RD, Kamath BL: N-acetylprocainamide and ischemia-induced ventricular fibrillation in the dog. *Eur J Pharmacol* 59:115, 1979.
189. Dangman KHP, Hoffman BF: In vivo and in vitro antiarrhythmic and arrhythmogenic effects of N-acetylprocainamide. *J Pharmacol Exp Ther* 217:851, 1981.
190. Bagwell EE, Walle T, Drayer DE, et al: Correlation of the electrophysiological and antiarrhythmic properties of N-acetylmetabolite of procainamide with plasma and tissue drug concentrations in the dog. *J Pharmacol Exp Ther* 197:38, 1976.
191. Jaillon P, Winkle RA: Electrophysiologic comparative study of procainamide and N-acetylprocainamide in anesthetized dogs: Concentration-response relationships. *Circulation* 60:1385, 1979.
192. Sung RJ, Zulfikar J, Saxena S: Electrophysiologic properties and antiarrhythmic mechanisms of intravenous N-acetylprocainamide in patients with ventricualr dysrhythmias. *Am Heart J* 105:811, 1983.

193. Jaillon P, Rubenson D, Peters F, et al: Electrophysiologic effects of N-acetylprocainamide in human beings. *Am J Cardiol* 47:1136, 1981.

194. Roden DM, Reele SB, Higgins SB, et al: Antiarrhythmic efficacy, pharmacokinetics and safety of N-acetylprocainamide in human subjects: Comparison with procainamide. *Am J Cardiol* 46:483, 1980.

195. Kaumann AJ, Olson CB: Temporal relationship between long-lasting aftercontractions and action potentials in cat papillary muscles. *Science* 163:293, 1968.

196. Strauss HC, Bigger JT, Hoffman BF: Electrophysiological and beta-receptor blocking effects of MJ 1999 on dog and rabbit cardiac tissue. *Circ Res* 26:661, 1970

197. Kato R, Yabek S, Ikeda N, et al: Electrophysiologic effects of dextro- and levo-isomers of sotalol in insolated cardiac muscle. *J Am Coll Cardiol* 7:116, 1986.

198. Jewitt DE, Singh BN: The role of beta-adrenergic blockade in myocardial infarction. *Prog Cardiovasc Dis* 16:421, 1974.

199. Carmeliet E: Electrophysiologic and voltage clamp analysis of sotalol effects in cardiac muscle and Purkinje fibers. *J Exp Pharmacol Ther* 232:817, 1985.

200. Ward DE, Camm AJ, Spurrell RAJ: The acute cardiac electrophysiological effects of intravenous sotalol hydrochloride. *Clin Cardiol* 2:185, 1979.

201. Nathan W, Hellestrand KJ, Bextan RS, et al: Electrophysiological effects of sotalol--Just another beta-blocker? *Br Heart J* 47:515, 1982.

202. Toubol P, Atullah G, Kirkonian G, et al: Clinical electrophysiology of intravenous sotalol, a beta-blocking drug with Class III antiarrhythmic properties. *Am Heart J* 107:888, 1984.

203. Cobbe SM, Hoffman E, Ritzenhoff A, et al: Action of sotalol on potential re-entrant pathways and ventricular tachyarrhythmias in conscious dogs in the late postmyocardial infarction phase. *Circulation* 68:865, 1983.

204. Senges J, Lengfelder W, Jauernig R, et al: Electrophysiologic testing of therapy with sotalol for sustained ventricular tachycardia. *Circulation* 69:577, 1984.

205. Nademanee K, Feld GK, Hendrickson JA, et al: Electrophysiologic and antiarrhythmic effects of sotalol in patients with life-threatening ventricular tachyarrhythmias. *Circulation* 72:555, 1985.

206. Edvardsson N, Hirsch I, Emanuelson H, et al: Sotalol-induced delayed ventricular repolarization in man. *Eur Heart J* 1:335, 1980.

207. Edvardsson N, Olsson SB: Effects of acute and chronic beta-receptor blockade on ventricular repolarisation in man. *Br Heart J* 45:628, 1981.

208. Echt DS, Bert LE, Clusin WT, et al: Prolongation of the human cardiac monophasic action potential by sotalol. *Am J Cardiol* 50:1082, 1982.

209. Singh BN: Amiodarone: Historical development and pharmacologic profile. *Am Heart J* 106:788, 1983.

210. Rosenbaum MB, Chiale PA, Halpern MS, et al: Clinical efficacy of amiodarone as an antiarrhythmic agent. *Am J Cardiol* 38:934, 1976.

211. Nademanee K, Hendrickson J, Kannan R, et al: Antiarrhythmic effi-

cacy and electrophysiologic actions of amiodarone in patients with life-threatening arrhythmias. *Am Heart J* 103:950, 1982.

212. Gomes JAC, Kang PS, Hariman RJ, et al: Electrophysiologic effects and mechanisms of termination of supraventricular tachycardia by intravenous amiodarone. *Am Heart J* 107:214, 1984.

213. Heger JJ, Prystowky EN, Jackman WN, et al: Amiodarone: Clinical efficacy and electrophysiology during long term therapy for recurrent ventricular tachycardia or ventricular fibrillation. *N Eng J Med* 305:539, 1981.

214. Graboys TB, Podrid PJ, Lown B: Efficacy of amiodarone for refractory supraventricular tachyarrhythmias *Am Heart J* 106:870, 1983.

215. Rosenbaum MB, Chiale PA, Haedo A, et al: Ten years of experience with amiodarone. *Am Heart J* 106:957, 1983.

216. Polster P, Broekhuysen J: The adrenergic antagonism of amiodarone. *Biochem Pharmacol* 25:131, 1976.

217. Singh BN, Vaughn Williams EM: The effect of amiodarone, a new anti-anginal drug, on cardiac muscle. *Br J Pharmacol* 39:657, 1970.

218. Yabek S, Kato R, Singh BN: Acute electrophysiologic effects of amiodarone and desethylamiodarone in isolated cardiac muscle. *J Cardiovasc Pharmacol* (in press).

219. Wellens HJJ, Brugada P, Abdollah H, et al: A comparison of the electrophysiologic effects of intravenous and oral amiodarone in the same patient. *Circulation* 69:120, 1984.

220. Holt DW, Tucker GT, Jackson PR, et al: Amiodarone pharmacokinetics. *Am Heart J* 106:840, 1983.

221. Kato R, Venkatesh N, Yabek S, et al: The comparative electrophysiologic effects of desethylamiodarone and amiodarone after chronic dosing in rabbits. Submitted for publication, 1986.

222. Mason JW, Hondeghem LM, Katzung BG: Amiodarone blocks inactivated cardiac sodium channels. *Pflueg Arch* 396:79, 1983.

223. Mason JW, Hondeghem LM, Katzung BG: Block of inactivated sodium channels and of depolarization-induced automaticity in guinea-pig papillary muscle by amiodarone. *Circ Res* 55:277, 1984.

224. Aomine M, McCullough J, Mayuga R, et al: Cellular electrophysiologic effects of acute exposure to admiodarone on guinea pig heart. *Fed Proc* 43:961, 1984.

225. Venkatesh N, Padbury J, Singh BN: Effects of amiodarone and desthylamiodarone on rabbit myocardial beta-adrenoceptors and serum thyroid hormones--Absence of relationship to serum and myocardial drug concentrations. *J Cardiovasc Pharmacol* 8:989, 1986.

226. Gloor HO, Urthaler F, James TN: Acute Effects of amiodarone upon the canine sinus node and atrioventricular junctional region. *J Clin Invest* 71:1457, 1983.

227. Goupil N, Lenfant J: The effects of amiodarone on the sinus node activity of the rabbit heart. *Eur J Pharm* 39:23, 1976.

228. Olsson B, Brorson L, Varnauskas E: Antiarrhythmic action in man: Observations from monophasic action potential recordings and amiodarone treatment. *Br Heart J* 35:1255, 1973.

229. Wellens HJJ, Brugada P, Abdalla AH: Effect of amiodarone in paroxysmal supraventricular tachycardia with or without Wolff-Parkinson-White syndrome. *Am Heart J* 106:876, 1983.

230. Zipes DP, Prystowsky EN, Heger JJ: Amiodarone: Electrophysiologic actions pharmacokinetics and clinical effects *J Am Coll Cardiol* 3:1059, 1984.
231. Finerman WB Jr, Hamer A, Peter T: Electrophysiologic effects of chronic amiodarone therapy in patients with ventricular arrhythmias. *Am Heart J* 104:987, 1982.
232. Waxman HL, Groh WC, Marchlinski FE, et al: Amiodarone for control of sustained ventricular tachyarrhythmias: Clinical and electrophysiological effects in 51 patients. *Am J Cardiol* 50:1066, 1982.
233. Ehara T, Kaufmann R: The voltage and time dependent effects of (-)verapamil on the slow inward current in isolated cat ventricular myocardium. *J Pharmacol Exp Ther* 207:49, 1978.
234. Nawrath H, Ten Eick RE, McDonald TF: On the mechanism underlying the action of D600 in slow inward current and tension in mammalian myocardium. *Circ Res* 40:408, 1977.
235. Tritthart HA, Volkmann R, Weiss R: Calcium mediated action potentials in mammalian myocardium: Alterations of membrane response induced by changes of Ca or by promoters and inhibitors of transmembrane Ca inflow. *Naunyn Schmiedebergs Arch Pharmacol* 280:239, 1973.
236. Kohlhardt M, Bauer B, Krause H, et al: New selective inhibitors of the transmembrane Ca conductivity in mammalian myocardial fibers. Studies with the voltage clamp technique. *Experiments* 28:288, 1972.
237. Tritthart HA: Pharmacology and electropharmacology of calcium ion antagonists. *Clin Invest Med* 3:1, 1980.
238. Shigenobu K, Schneider JA, Sperelakis N: Verapamil blockade of slow $Na^+$ and $Ca^{++}$ responses in myocardial cells. *J Pharmacol Exp Ther* 190:280, 1974.
239. Bayer R, Rodenkirchen R, Kaufman R: The effects of nifedipine on contraction and monophonic action potentials of isolated cat ventricular myocardium. *Naunyn Schmiedebergs Arch Pharmacol* 301:29, 1977.
240. Bayer R, Kalusche D, Kaufmann R: Inotropic and electrophysiological actions of verapamil and D600 in mammalian myocardium. III. Effects of the optical isomers on transmembrane action potentials. *Naunyn Schmiedebergs Arch Pharmacol* 290:81, 1976.
241. Raschack M: Relationship of antiarrhythmic to inotropic activity and antiarrhythmic qualities of the optical isomers of verapamil. *Naunyn Schmiedebergs Arch Pharmacol* 294:285, 1976.
242. Kaumann AJ, Uchibel OD: Reversible inhibition of potassium contractures by optical isomers of verapamil and D600 on slow muscle fibers of the frog, *Naunyn Schmiedebergs Arch Pharmacol* 292:21, 1976.
243. Singh BN, Hecht HS, Nademanee K, et al: Electrophysiologic and hemodynamic effects of slow-channel blocking drugs. *Prog Cardiovasc Dis* 25:103, 1982.
244. Kohlhardt M, Fleckenstein A: Inhibition of the slow current by nifedipine in mammalian ventricular myocardium. *Naunyn Schmiedebergs Arch Pharmacol* 298:267, 1977.

245. Woods JP, West TC: Frequency-dependence of $V_{max}$ in K-depolarized guinea-pig ventricle: Effects of nifedipine and verapamil. *J Cardiovasc Pharmacol* 7:197, 1985.
246. Kohlhardt M, Krause H, Kubler M, et al: Kinetics of inactivation and recovery of the slow inward current in the mammalian ventricular myocardium. *Pfluegs Arch* 355:1, 1975.
247. Singh BN, Baky S, Nademanee N: Second-generation calcium antagonists: Search for greater selectivity and versatility. *Amer J Cardiol* 55:214B, 1985.
248. Singh BN, Nademanee K, Feld G, et al: Comparative electrophysiologic profiles of calcium antagonists with particular reference to bepridil hydrochloride. *Amer J Cardiol* 55:14C, 1985.
249. Cranefield PF, Aronson RS, Wit AL: Effect of verapamil on the normal action potential and on a calcium-dependent slow response of canine cardiac Purkinje fibers. *Circ Res* 34:204, 1974.
250. Rosen MR, Wit AL, Hoffman BF: Appraisal and reappraisal of cardiac therapy. Electrophysiology and pharmacology of cardiac arrhythmias. VI. Cardiac effects of verapmil. VI. Cardiac effects of verapamil. *Am Heart J* 89:665, 1975.
251. Okada R: Effect of verapamil on electrical activities of SA node, ventricular muscle, and Purkinje fibers in isolated rabbit hearts. *Japan Circ J* 40:329, 1976.
252. Rosen MR, Ilvento JP, Relband H, et al: Effects of verapamil on electrophysiological properties of canine cardiac Purkinje fibers. *J Pharmacol Exp Ther* 189:414, 1974.
253. Refsum H: The effect of a calcium antagonistic drug, nifedipine, on the rat atrial action potential at different calcium levels. *Acta Pharmacol Toxicol* 37:32, 1975.
254. Saikawa R, Nagamoto Y, Artia M: Electrophysiologic effects of diltiazem, a new slow-channel inhibitor, on canine fibers. *Japan Heart J* 18:235, 1977.
255. Nabata H: Effects of calcium antagonistic coronary vasodilators on myocardial contractility and membrane potentials. *Japan J Pharmacol* 27:239, 1977.
256. Nakajima H, Hoshiyama M, Yamashita K: Effect of diltiazem on electrical and mechanical activity of isolated cardiac muscle of guinea pig. *Japan J Pharmacol* 25:383, 1975.
257. Isenberg G: Cardiac Purkinje fibers ($Ca^{2+}$), controls steady state potassium conductance. *Pflueg Arch* 37:71, 1977.
258. Zipes DP, Fischer JC: Effects of agents which inhibit the slow-channel on sinus node automaticity and atrioventricular conduction in the dog. *Circ Res* 34:184, 1974.
259. Wit Al, Cranefield P: Effect of verapamil on the sinoatrial and atrioventricular nodes of the rabbit and the mechanism by which it arrests re-entrant atrioventricular nodal tachycardia. *Circ Res* 35:4123, 1974.
260. Strauss HC, Prystowsky EN, Scheinmn MM: Sinoatrial and atrial electrogenesis. *Prog Cardiovasc Dis* 19:385, 1977.
261. Refsum H, Landmark K: The effect of Ca antagonist drug, nifedipine, on the mechanical and electrical activity of the isolated rat atrium. *Acta Pharmacol Toxicol* 37:369, 1975.

262. Kawai C, Konishi T, Matsuyama E, et al: Comparative effects of three calcium antagonists, diltiazem, verapamil and nifedipine, on the sinoatrial and atrioventricular nodes. Experimental and clinical studies. *Circulation* 63:1035, 1981.

263. Cranefield PF, Aronson RS, Wit AL: Effect of verapamil on the normal action potential and on a calcium dependent slow response of canine cardiac Purkinje fibers. *Circ Res* 34:204, 1974.

264. Storstein O, Landmark KH: Verapamil in the treatment of atrial tachycardia with block. *Acta Med Scan* 198:482, 1975.

265. Hordof AJ, Edie R, Malm JR, et al: electrophysiologic properties and response to pharmacologic agents of fibers from diseased human atria. *Circulation* 54:774, 1976.

266. Spear JF, Horowitz LN, Hodess AB, et al: Cellular electrophysiology of human myocardial infarction: Abnormalities of cellular activation. *Circulation* 59:247, 1979.

267. Elarrar V, Zipes DP: Cardiac electrophysiologic alterations during myocardial ischemia. *Am J Physiol* 233:H329, 1977.

268. Labrid C, Grosset A, Dureng G, et al: Some membrane interactions with bepridil, a new antianginal agent. *J Pharmacol Exp Ther* 211:546, 1979

269. Kane KA, Winslow E: Antiarrhythmic and electrophysiological effects of a new antianginal agent, bepridil. *J Cardiovasc Pharmacol* 2:193, 1980.

270. Beaughard M, Ferrier M, Labrid C, et al: Studies on the bradycardia induced by bepridil on rabbit isolated hearts. *Br J Pharmacol* 75:293, 1982.

271. Vogel S, Cramptom R, Sperelakis N: Blockade of myocardial slow-channels by bepridil, a new antianginal. *J Pharmacol Exp Ther* 210:378, 1979.

272. Anno T, Furuta T, Itoh M, et al: Effects of bepridil on the electrophysiologic properties of guinea-pig ventricular muscles. *Br J Pharmacol* 81:589, 1984

273. Goto J, Sperelakis N: Depression of automaticity of the rabbit SA node by bepridil and nifedipine. *Eur J Pharmacol* 99:227, 1984.

274. Kato R, Singh BN: Effect of bepridil on the electrophysiologic properties of isolated canine and rabbit myocardial fibers. *Am Heart J* 111:271, 1986.

275. Rowland E, McKenna W, Krikler D: Electrophysiological and antiarrhythmic effects of bepridil in re-entry AV tachycardia--comparison with verapamil and ajamaline. *Circulation* 68:311, 1983.

276. Desoutar P, Haiat R: Modifications electrocardiographiques induite par le bepridil. *Arch Mal Coeur* 73:1237, 1980.

277. Duchenne-Marallaz P, Kantelip JP, Tyrolese JF: Effects of bepridil, a new antianginal agent, on ambulatory electrocardiography in human volunteers. *J Cardiovasc Pharmacol* 5:506, 1983.

# Chapter 4

# QT Interval Lengthening and Cardiac Arrhythmias

Peter J. Schwartz and Emanuela Locati

It seems such a long time ago when, in a well-known textbook of electrocardiography, one could read the following sentence: "The measurement of the QT interval has little usefulness."[1]

Several reviews have discussed the relationship between QT prolongation and sudden death[2-4] and have indicated that prolongation of the QT interval often is associated with enhanced risk for malignant arrhythmias. The electrophysiologic bases for interpreting QT prolongation as a proarrhythmic or as a protective condition also have been discussed in detail.[5-8] The unproven assumption, shared nonetheless by most investigators, is that when QT prolongation results from an homogeneous lengthening of action potential duration it may be associated with decreased risk for reentrant arrhythmias, whereas when it depends on the presence of nonhomogeneous areas with different recovery times it increases the risk for life-threatening arrhythmias. The present chapter will not enter into this controversy; rather, it will illustrate three clinical conditions where there is evidence that QT prolongation is associated with increased risk for sudden death. Besides the idiopathic long QT syndrome (LQTS), we will discuss the significance of a prolonged QT interval in patients with a prior myocardial infarction (MI) and in healthy newborns in relation to the propensity to sudden death.

From: *Control of Cardiac Arrhythmias by Lengthening Repolarization*, edited by Bramah N. Singh, MD, Futura Publishing Company Inc., Mount Kisco, NY, © 1988.

## QT Prolongations in Post-MI Patients

In 1976, Schwartz and Wolf for the first time reported on the association between a prolonged QT interval and an increased risk for subsequent sudden death among post-MI patients.[9,10]

During the following decade, a large number of related studies has appeared, mostly confirming the original report. These studies had different designs, periods of follow-up, number of patients, number of EKG tracings obtained in a single patient, exclusion criteria, and therapy. An overview of this topic has to take into a critical account the different methodologies employed: therefore, the original study by Schwartz and Wolf will be the first to be reviewed in detail.

That study[10] included 55 patients with recent myocardial infraction (MI) and 55 healthy controls matched for age, sex, race, weight, height, education, and occupation. The study group was drawn from a consecutive series of patients seen at the University of Oklahoma between 1962 and 1965. EKG tracings were recorded at 2-month intervals on both patients and controls over a 7-year period. At the end of 7 years of observation and after 3 additional years of follow-up, 27 of the 55 patients were still alive: 28 had died, all of them suddenly (within 24 hours after the beginning of symptoms); among the 55 controls only one had died, and he died suddenly.

The $QT_c$ was measured in post-MI patients and in controls from five nonconsecutive beats on each EKG tracing and the mean $QT_c$ value $\pm$ standard deviation (SD) was calculated. The mean $QT_c$ among controls was $418 \pm 15$ msec (mean $\pm$ SD), whereas among the patients it was significantly longer, $436 \pm 25$ msec. More important, a mean $QT_c$ interval greater than 440 msec was present in 57 percent of the deceased in contrast to 18 percent of the survivors; values greater than 450 msec were found in 36 percent of the deceased and in only 8 percent of the survivors. The mean $QT_c$ was significantly longer among the deceased ($443 \pm 27$ msec) than among the surviving patients ($429 \pm 20$ msec, $p > 0.05$) (Fig. 1). Of the 21 patients who had a mean $QT_c > 440$ msec, 16 (77 percent) died suddenly, and mortality was even higher (83 percent) among those having $QT_c > 450$ msec (Fig. 2); by contrast, of the 34 patients who had a mean $QT_c < 440$ msec, 12 (35 percent) died. The calculated risk for sudden death for patients with a previous MI and prolonged QT interval was respectively 2.16 and 2.36 times greater than for those with normal QT interval (Fig. 3).

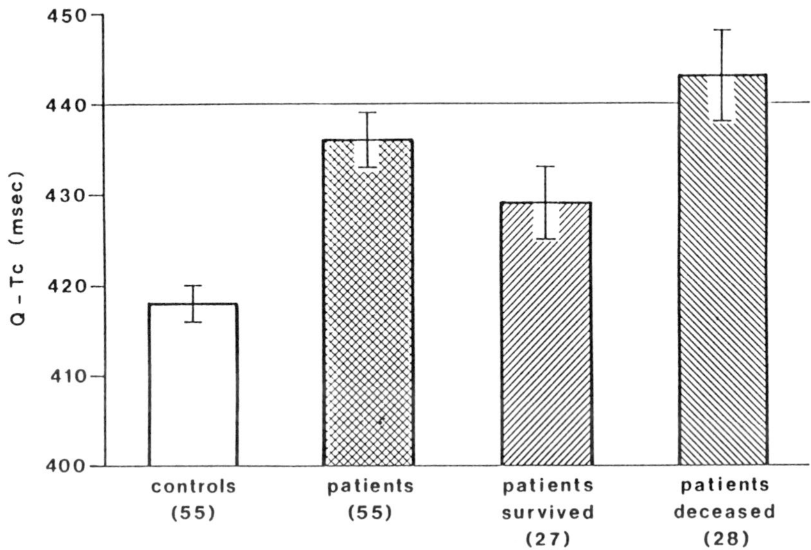

**Figure 1.** Comparison of mean QTc values among the group studied (Ref. 10. Reprinted with permission.).

The variability of $QT_c$ from month to month and from year to year, as determined by the mean differences in measurement $\pm$ standard error (SE), was greatest in the deceased patients (survivors $QT_c$ 20 $\pm$ 2msec, deceased $QT_c$ 28 $\pm$ 2; p < 0.025). Also, the heart rate (HR) was almost identical in post-MI patients (survivors and deceased) and in controls, those who died had a greater day-to-day variability of their HR values than the survivors, who did not differ from the controls in this sense. The finding of a greater variability in $QT_c$ and HR in the patients who died suddenly may suggest that they were more exposed to shifts in autonomic nervous activity.

Also the presence of frequent VPBs (more than 10 beats per minute) increased the risk of sudden death after MI by a factor of 2.19. A prolonged $QT_c$ with VPBs carried a risk of sudden death between five and six times higher than a normal $QT_c$ without VPBs (Table 1).[11] It is important to note that the post MI group did not include patients treated with quinidine or drugs that might have affected either the QT interval or survival. Of course, in the early 1960s, post-MI patients were not receiving beta-adrenergic blocking agents, or the many antiarrhythmic drugs currently in use.

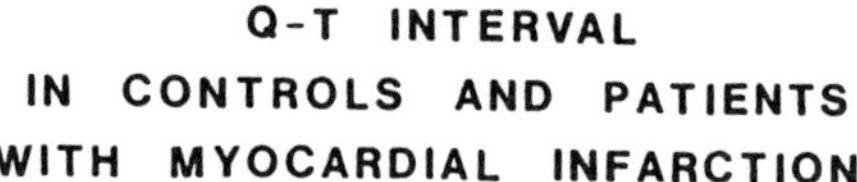



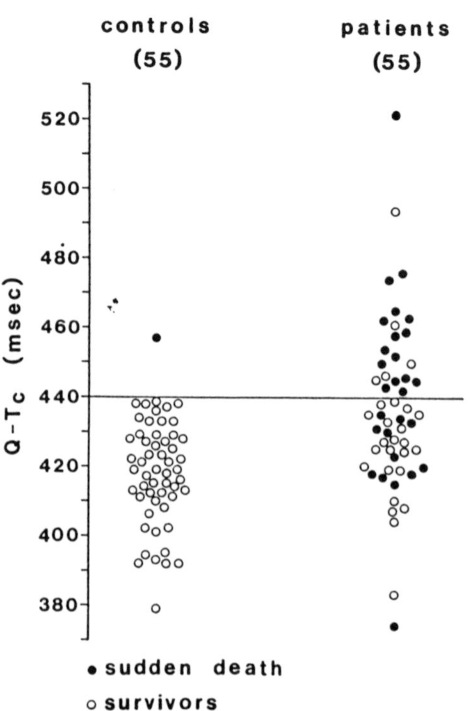



**Figure 2.** Distribution of QTc values among patients and controls (Ref. 10. Reprinted with permission.).

Thus, this study indicated that in patients with a myocardial infarction the presence of a prolonged QT interval could be used as a marker of an increased risk for sudden cardiac death. What caused the QT interval prolongation and how this is related to an increased risk for malignant arrhythmias is still controversial. It is possible that QT prolongation simply reflects the gross extent of myocardial damage, although it is interesting to note that it may instead reflect a nonhomogeneous distribution of cardiac sympathetic nerves involving more fibers originating from the right than the left stellate ganglion. This might give rise to the prolongation of the QT interval on the surface EKG tracing[12,13] and would create the arrhythmogenic sympathetic imbalance associated with left dominance[14] therefore favoring the onset of malignant arrhyth-

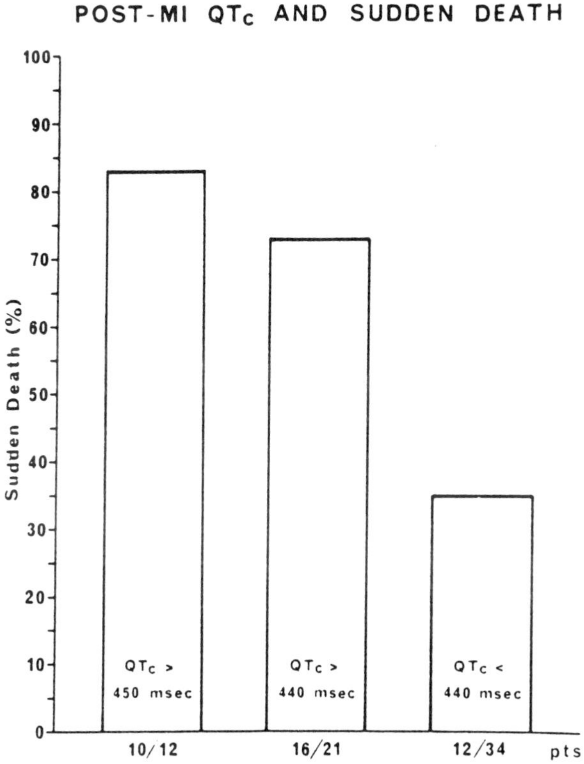

POST-MI QT$_C$ AND SUDDEN DEATH



**Figure 3.** Risk of sudden death in patients with prolonged QT interval (Ref. 24. Reprinted with permission.).

mias. Whatever the cause, this study indicated that the prolongation of the QT interval after myocardial infarction could be considered an important marker of increased myocardial electrical instability. Some of the numerous studies that deal with this general topic will be described briefly together with some general comments.

Haynes et al.[15] analyzed the QT$_c$ in a unique group of patients with coronary artery disease who had been resuscitated from out-of-hospital ventricular fibrillation (VF): 37 percent of those patients had a prolonged QT$_c$, compared to 18 percent of patients with a myocardial infarction not complicated by VF (p < 0.005).

A significant contribution to this subject came from the various studies performed by Anhve et al.[16,17] In 1980,[16] they studied 160 consecutive survivors of acute myocardial infarction under 66 years of age. Calculations of the QT interval duration were made during the first 2 days in the Coronary Care Unit (CCU), on the

**Table 1**
Interaction Between Prolonged $QT_c$* and PVCs in
Post-Myocardial Infarction Patients

|  | Mortality | Calculated Risk |
|---|---|---|
| $QT_c > 440$ | 76% | 5.33 |
| PVCs | 74% | 5.18 |
| $QT_c > 440$ and PVCs | 79% | 5.50 |
| $QT_c > 440$, no PVCs | 71% | 5.00 |
| $QT_c < 440$ and PVCs | 69% | 4.81 |
| $QT_c < 440$, no PVCs | 14% | — |

*in milliseconds

first post-CCU day, at discharge, and at 1–3, 6, and 12 months after discharge. Sixteen patients died during the first follow-up year. Twenty patients suffered reinfarction, five of whom died. Those patients who had major cardiac events during follow-up (reinfarction or death, particularly sudden death) had significantly longer $QT_c$ values ($434 \pm 35$ msec versus $417 \pm 42$ msec, $p > 0.001$) (Fig. 4). Also, a multivariate analysis of risk factors revealed that the $QT_c$ at discharge had significant independent value for predicting major cardiac events after discharge from the hospital.

In a subsequent multicenter study performed in 1984 by the same group,[17] a population of 257 patients (mean age $61 \pm 12.5$ years), with a clear-cut diagnosis of myocardial infarction and without therapy that could influence the QT interval, was followed prospectively after MI. Among them, a group of 214 patients was followed for 12 months: 201 survived and 13 died, with a mean age of $58 \pm 13$ and $67 \pm 10$ years respectively ($p < 0.05$). Of those 214 patients, 43 (20 percent) had a QT interval exceeding 440 msec and of these 43 patients, 10 (23 percent) died, 5 suddenly. By comparison, of the 171 patients without a prolonged $QT_c$ only 3 (1.8 percent) died ($p < 0.001$). As 10 out of 13 deceased patients had a $QT_c$ interval exceeding 440 msec, this yielded a sensitivity of 77 percent. Of the 201 survivors, 168 had a $QT_c$ less than 440 msec, which gave a specificity of 84 percent. This recent and large study clearly confirms the predictive value of QT prolongation in post-MI patients.

The BHAT experience[18] concluded that in a large group of about 4000 patients, a prolonged QTc indentified a high risk subset of post-myocardial infarction patients: the mortality being significantly higher in the patients with $QT_c > 440$ msec (6.6 versus

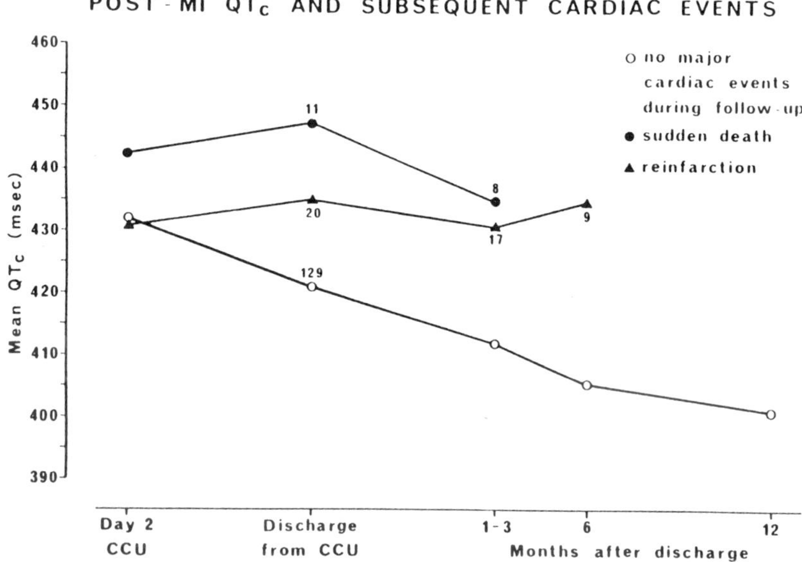


**Figure 4.** Mean QTc values in patients with reinfarction, sudden death, or no major cardiac events post myocardial infarction (Ref. 16. Reprinted with permission.).

3.7 percent, p < 0.01). The prognostic value of a prolonged QT interval was present in both the placebo and the propranolol treated groups. Also, in a study by Juul-Moller,[19] the patients with $QT_c$ at rest > 480 msec had 50 percent mortality after 1 year, compared with 9 percent in the patients with $QT_c$ at rest < 480 msec (p = 0.0002).

A Finnish study stated that $QT_c$ is not a useful prognostic tool in identifying patients at higher risk of dying after myocardial infarction.[20] However, when $QT_c$ = 440 was used as a cut-off point, despite their own conclusion, a significant difference was observed: in fact, the patients with normal QT interval ($QT_c$ < 440 msec) had a better survival throughout the follow-up period (78 percent versus 69 percent at 4 years, p < 0.05).

Two studies have showed that a prolonged QT interval is associated with other known coronary risk factors. Kramer et al.[21] showed that the prolongation of the QT interval significantly correlated with definite risk factors for sudden death; i.e., impaired left ventricular function and severe coronary artery disease. Also, the data reported by the MILIS study[22] showed that a prolonged

$QT_c$ was associated with other known predictors of sudden death, as frequent premature complexes and left ventricular dysfunction, although a prolonged $QT_c$ in this study was not an independent risk factor for sudden death.

In contrast with these two studies, Puddu and Bourassa,[23] showed that QT prolongation was not related to other known coronary risk factors, such as mean ejection fraction and number of diseased vessels. Nonetheless, the patients who died of sudden death had a significantly higher prevalence of QT prolongation during follow-up compared to survivors.

The prognostic significance of QT prolongation in the early phase post-MI is more controversial.[24] Although most of these studies in the early phase of myocardial infarction suggest a relationship between a prolonged $QT_c$ and subsequent events (mostly, life-threatening arrhythmias), conclusions from the results of these studies should be guarded. The early phase of a myocardial infarction is associated with several factors that may affect ventricular repolarization, like the administration of several cardioactive drugs, the direct effects of ischemia and necrosis, the outpouring of catecholamines possibly related to the psychologic stress. These factors may obscure changes of the QT interval; therefore, it is safer to measure the QT interval for prognostic purposes only once the acute phase is over and the patient is in more stable condition.

Although most reports have confirmed the observations of Schwartz and Wolf, they also presented some methodological limitations that will be discussed presently. A critical point of the original study, not well appreciated by most subsequent investigators, was the fact that what was prognostically important was the average QT interval as measured on several occasions. A single measurement of QT interval may be misleading, as shown by the fact that the high risk patients who had, on average, a prolonged QT interval occasionally could have normal values; the opposite was true as well. In other words, the occasional finding of a prolonged QT interval in a post-myocardial infarction patient should suggest only the need for repeated observations. If the finding is confirmed, then it would be correct to view this patient as being at higher risk than normal.

The use of cardioactive drugs constitutes a major problem. Some of these drugs affect the repolarization process; more important, others may protect from malignant arrhythmias some patients otherwise destined to sudden death. This fact interferes with the evaluation of any potential prognostic marker. Accordingly, studies on effectively treated patients can provide information on risk factors relative to mechanisms not affected by the administered drugs. Most of the recent studies on the predictive value of QT prolongation in post-MI patients have not taken into account the confounding role of therapy.

The measurement of the QT interval constitutes another significant problem (see Chapter 24), discussed repeatedly in the literature.[25-29] Because of the unavoidable degree of subjectivity in the determination of the "precise" point where the T wave ends, a high degree of internal consistency is necessary. For this reason, studies where a single experienced investigator made all the measurements of the QT interval seem more reliable than those in which several investigators have been responsible for measurements. Accordingly, it may be important for studies on the QT interval in post-MI patients to also have data on a "control" population, so that the "normal" values for given laboratory or investigators would become apparent.

Given these considerations, most evidence from the data available in the literature strongly supports the following conclusions: Among the post-myocardial infarction patients, a prolonged QT interval represents a marker of increased risk for subsequent mortality, particularly sudden cardiac death. Also, in some patients QT prolongation is associated with other traditional risk factors that may or may not add to the final prognosis. Finally, when a QT prolongation is identified occasionally, it still may indicate an augmented risk, but it is certainly safer to base a prognostic judgement on repeated measurements of the QT interval in several successive EKG tracings. Finally, the original suggestion[9,10] that among post-MI patients the analysis of the QT interval may contribute to a better identification of the individuals at higher risk still remains valid and useful.

## Idiopathic Long QT Syndrome

The clinical features of the idiopathic long QT syndrome (LQTS) are now well known.[30] In patients with a prolonged QT interval on the electrocardiogram, major cardiac events, as syncopal episodes and cardiac arrest, are precipitated by stressful situations and ultimately may determine sudden cardiac death. Also, alternation of the T wave often can be observed under the same conditions that provoke syncopal episodes and may precede the occurrence of torsades de pointes[30,31] (Fig. 5). The experimental reproduction of this phenomenon by the unilateral manipulation

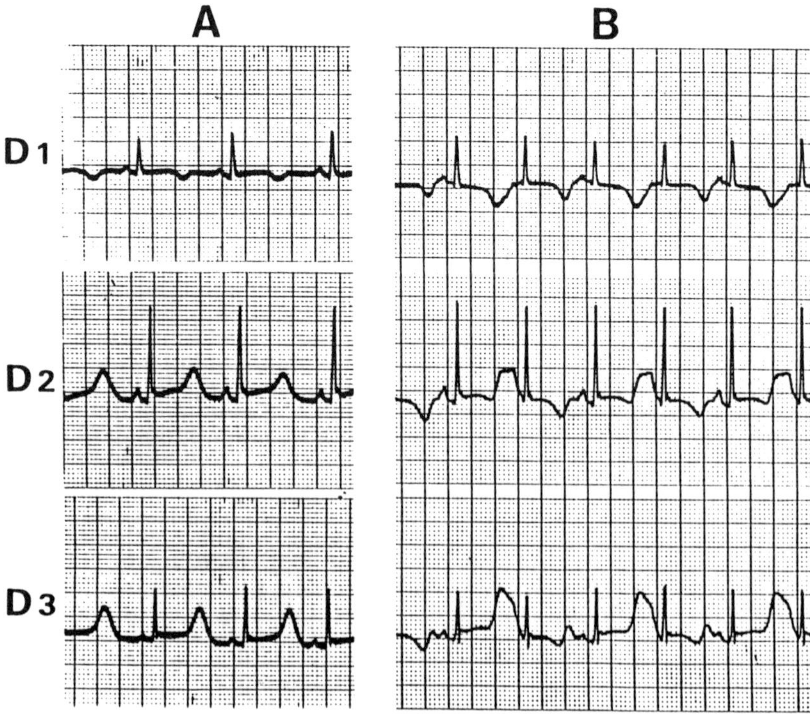


**Figure 5A. B.**   9 years of age, was affected by LQTS. A, ECG at rest. B, alternation of the T wave appeared during unintentionally induced fear. Note in D2 and in D3 the bizarre configuration of the T wave with the P wave, which in alternate beats begins during the ventricular repolarization (Ref. 31. Reprinted with permission.).

of the cardiac sympathetic innervation (Fig. 6) has played an important role in the development of the "sympathetic imbalance" theory.[32] These experimental observations subsequently were reproduced in patients with LQTS,[33] providing a significant and unusual bridge between experimental and clinical cardiology. The sympathetic imbalance theory harmonizes with the known facts regarding LQTS and may indeed represent the true pathogenetic mechanism of LQTS, although at this time it still requires definitive confirmation.

The appreciation of the critical role of the sympathetic nervous system in the genesis of the malignant arrhythmias typical of the LQTS and the better understanding of its pathogenetic mechanisms suggested a rational therapeutic approach based on the prevention of the effects of increases in sympathetic activity. Indeed, the selective antiadrenergic procedures (both pharmacological with

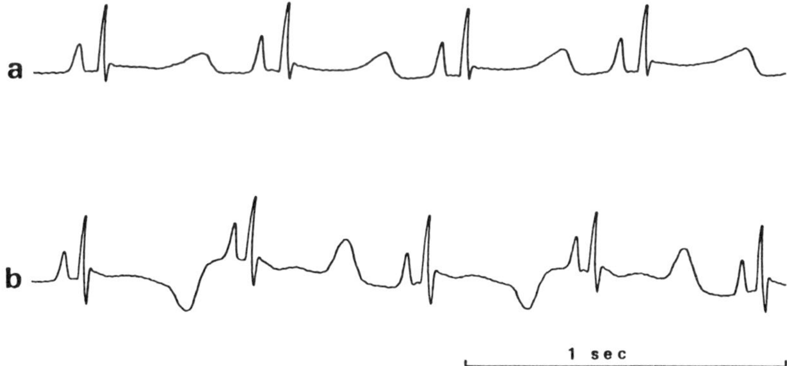


**Figure 6.** EKG of an anesthetized cat (D2). **a.** Control; **b.** 5 seconds after the cessation of a 30-second electrical stimulation of both stellate ganglia (left ganglion: 20 V, 2 msec, and 20 Hz; right ganglion: 10 V, 2 msec, and 20 Hz). Alternation in polarity of the T wave is evident (Ref. 32. Reprinted with permission.).

beta-adrenergic blocking agents and surgical with high thoracic left sympathectomy) have changed dramatically the long-term prognosis of this lethal disease.

## Pathogenetic Mechanisms

The strong association observed between the syncopal episodes and physical or emotional stress has pointed to a critical role of the sympathetic nervous system in the genesis of the malignant arrhythmias typical of LQTS. Experimentally, the QT interval was prolonged by either right stellectomy or left stellate ganglion stimulation.[12] Subsequently, it was possible to reproduce experimentally the typical alternation of the T wave by an analogous manipulation of the cardiac sympathetic activity.[32] Clinically, this rate phenomenon was observed in several patients with LQTS under the same circumstances that trigger the syncopal episodes.[32] These observations suggested that the patients with LQTS may have a congenital imbalance between right and left cardiac sympathetic innervation, with a left dominance. This would result in a prolongation of the QT interval at rest and particularly under stresssful conditions, when the sympathetic activity increases, often giving rise to episodes of alternation of the T wave.

The suggestion that a lower than normal right cardiac sympathetic activity might be the basic defect of LQTS, rather than a primary increase in left sympathetic activity, stemmed from the notion that sympathetic control of heart rate almost exclusively is exerted through the right-sided nerves,[34] together with the observation that most patients with LQTS have an unusually low resting heart rate and that many of them show an impaired heart rate response to exercise.[30,35] Actually, this concept was further confirmed by the fact that an experimentally induced sympathetic imbalance of this type, achieved by surgical removal of the right stellate ganglion in otherwise normal animals, produced changes consistent with the long QT syndrome.[30-36]

Recently, another indirect confirmation of the "sympathetic imbalance" theory came from two studies with body surface mapping:[36,37] both suggested the presence in patients with the LQTS of prolonged repolarization in the anterior ventricular wall, which is innervated primarily by right-sided sympathetic fibers. These data are entirely consistent with deficient right cardiac sympathetic tone in the patients affected by LQTS.

Also, it was shown in experimental and later in clinical conditions that a lower-than-normal right cardiac sympathetic activity might enhance the occurrence of ventricular arrhythmias; these studies have been reported in detail elsewhere.[30,35,38] Briefly, using different animal models and different techniques, it was possible to demonstrate that the sympathetic imbalance resulting from the ablation of the right stellate ganglion is quite arrhythmogenic. An opposite effect was observed with left stellate ganglion ablation: the protective effect of left stellectomy had therapeutic implications that extended beyond the problem of the LQTS.[39]

Despite the fact that the "sympathetic imbalance" theory fits with all the known characteristics of the syndrome, the interpretation of these data could be less unequivocal: the particularly high arrhythmogenic potential of the left-sided nerves also accounts for the possibility that the basic defect may be an unknown intracardiac abnormality that decreases electrical stability and sensitizes the myocardium to the effect of neutrally mediated catecholamine release.[30,40] In this case the left stellate ganglion would represent only the trigger for ventricular tachyarrhythmias. The unknown intracardiac abnormality in LQTS may be a primary abnormality in myocardial repolarization as a result of a genetic alteration in the voltage-dependent protein that regulates outward potassium current during phase 3 of the action potential.[41] Activation of the cardiac sympathetic nerves would trigger ventricular tachyarrhythmias by modifying potassium conductance[42] in an electrically unstable heart with delayed repolarization.

All in all, the information originating from the clinical and experimental observations support the hypothesis that the basic defect is a congenital imbalance in the cardiac sympathetic innervation with a dominance of the arrhythmogenic left-sided nerves that is likely to be secondary to a lower-than-normal right cardiac sympathetic activity. The syncopal episodes would be precipitated by sudden increases in sympathetic activity mostly mediated through the left stellate ganglion. The possibility of an unknown intracardiac abnormality sensitizing the myocardium to sudden sympathetic discharge still needs further supporting evidence.

## Clinical Aspects

The characteristic clinical features of the LQTS are syncopal spells associated with abnormally prolonged QT intervals on EKG tracing; also, some other abnormalities often are described. Frequently, low resting heart rate is observed, particularly striking in young children, as well as reduced capability to increase heart rate during exercise, and sudden pauses in sinus rhythm exceeding 1.2 seconds. In most patients, the T wave is abnormal not only for the duration but also for the peculiar morphologic abnormalities, such as biphasic, bifid, or notched configuraiton, suggestive of different repolarization time courses in different ventricular areas[30,38] (Fig. 7).

The realization that the spectrum of this disease may be broader than previously suspected[35] and may include some patients with a normal QT interval has important clinical implications. Indeed, several patients with normal QT intervals in whom ventricular fibrillation is triggered by emotional or physical stress have been reported repeatedly.[30,35] Whether these patients, or some of them, represent a variety of the spectrum of this disease or a slightly different abnormality still needs clarification.

The existence of patients with LQTS but without familial involvement, or even worse, without a clear-cut prolongation of the QT interval, makes the diagnosis more complex. The borderline cases are more difficult to diagnose, and yet the high risk of sudden death for untreated patients requires a correct diagnosis so that proper and effective treatment can be instituted. To obviate these problems, diagnostic criteria have been proposed:[30] the diagnosis of LQTS should be made in the presence of two major criteria or one major and two minor criteria (Table 2). The potential additional diagnostic values of the Valsalva maneuver, exercise stress

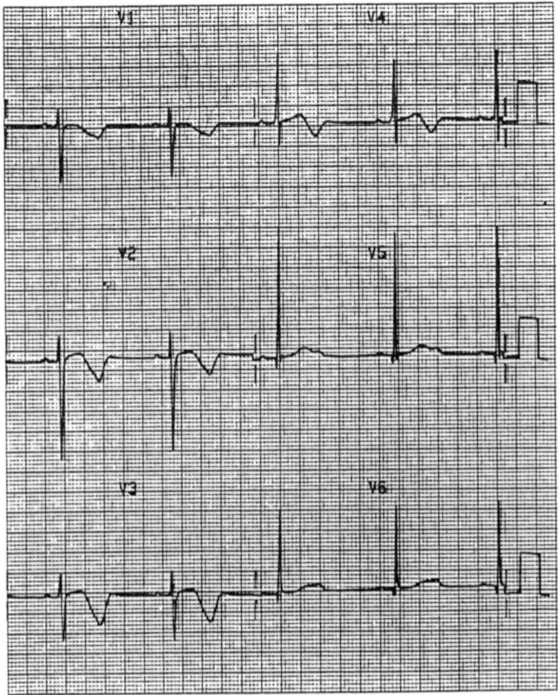


**Figure 7.** EKG of a patient affected by the idiopathic LQTS. Note the deep negative T wave in the right precordial leads (V1 to V3); the diphasic T wave in V4; the camel hump in the left precordial leads (V5 and V6); and the low heart rate (50 beats/min) for a young patient (Ref. 30. Reprinted with permission.).

test, monophasic action potential recording, and body surface mapping remain to be determined. At this time it is possible to state that programmed electrophysiologic stimulation is of no help in the management of patients with LQTS, particularly in children.[43] Basically, the diagnosis of LQTS usually can be achieved through a carefully collected clinical history and some selected noninvasive observations.

## Epidemiology

Several epidemiological aspects of the disease still require further clarification. Initially, LQTS was considered an hereditary disorder and two distinct clinical and genetic syndromes with prolongation of the QT interval were recognized: the Jervell

---

**Table 2**
**Diagnostic Criteria**

---

*MAJOR*
— Prolonged QT interval (QTc > 440) msec)
— Stress-induced syncope
— Family members with LQTS

*MINOR*
— Congenital deafness
— Episodes of T wave alternans
— Low heart rate
— Abnormal ventricular repolarization

---

and Lange-Nielsen syndrome with congenital deafness and recessive pattern of inheritance,[44] and the Romano-Ward syndrome with normal hearing and autosomal-dominant pattern of inheritance.[45,46] Actually, at present, the reported number of sporadic cases without familial involvement has greatly increased. Since the cardiac defect seems the same, regardless of the hereditary transmission, both familial and sporadic cases were grouped under the definition of "idiopathic" long QT syndrome.[35]

A recent report suggests a probable close linkage between the locus for the Romano-Ward type and the HLA locus.[47] In this single Japanese family, all 10 affected individuals had the same HLA haplotype (A9-BW54), whereas 0 of the 6 unaffected individuals had this haplotype. The identification of a genetic marker for LQTS may provide important insight into this disease, but this finding requires further confirmation.

At present, several general questions on the epidemiology of the LQTS have no definite answers. Specifically, it is not known what the risk is for an asymptomatic patient with idiopathic QT interval prolongation to become symptomatic. Also, is it possible to identify subgroups at higher or lower risk? What are the long-term effects of the various treatments employed? Answers to these questions necessarily have to come from comprehensive information gathered through a large prospective study of this uncommon disease. For this reason, in 1979 an international prospective registry was instituted to enroll cases of LQTS diagnosed worldwide.[48] At present, approximately 950 patients have been enrolled: 196 probands (first individual to be identified as affected within a family) and their family members. In the first report on the initial group of about 200 LQTS patients,[41] multivariate analysis identified as independent risk factors for post-enrollment major cardiac events (syncope or sudden death), congenital deafness, previous history of syncope, and female sex. Two types of treatment (left stellate ganglionectomy and beta-blocker therapy) were associated with a significant reduction in the occurrence of cardiac events during follow-up.

Some comments are necessary as regards the mortality in the LQTS. In a previous review of 203 cases of LQTS,[31] the mortality was approximately 5 percent per year, during an estimated average follow-up of about 5 years. This represented an early survey of a large group of high risk patients (high proportion of congenital deafness and symptomatic patients, mostly not treated). Among the patients enrolled in the prospective study, the mortality was 1.3 percent per year, a value still remarkably high considering that the mean age in this population was 24 years. At present, the extensive use of effective therapies has modified significantly the natural history of LQTS, as it only could be observed many years ago, when most patients were not treated. Therefore, these data confirm the high degree of lethality in untreated patients with symptomatic LQTS and the necessity to use therapy with proven efficacy in the management of the disease.

## Therapy

Due to the high mortality rate of this disease in untreated patients, therapeutic procedures with proven efficacy should be started immediately after the diagnosis of the disease is confirmed in symptomatic patients.

At present, data on more than 750 patients collected and updated through the cooperation of physicians worldwide provided extensive observations on the mortality figures, that substantially were stable over the years[40] (Table 3). The mortality in untreated

**Table 3**
**Treatment and Mortality in the Long QT Syndrome**

|  | Patients | Mortality |
|---|---|---|
| Asymptomatics | 196 | – |
| Treatment unknown | 93 | – |
| No treatment | 157 | 71% |
| Miscellaneous treatment | 50 | 35% |
| Beta-blockers | 214 | 6% |
| Left sympathectomy | 53 | 7% |
| TOTAL LQTS PATIENTS | 763 | – |

symptomatic patients is extremely high (70 percent) and remains high (35 percent) when nonantiadrenergic therapies are used. The mortality falls to 6 percent among the more than 200 patients treated with beta blockers. Actually, the protective effect of beta blockade, although unquestionable, was probably overestimated; indeed, approximately 20 percent of the patients treated with beta blockers were not protected as they continued to have syncope and required high thoracic left sympathectomy.[49] It seems very likely that many of these patients, who continued to have syncopal episodes, would have encountered sudden death if they had not been operated.

The dramatic impact on survival of antiadrenergic interventions (beta-adrenergic blockade and high thoracic left sympathectomy) compared to no therapy or miscellaneous treatment also was determined in a study of a group of 233 patients for whom we had detailed information[38] (Fig. 8).

At present, 53 patients who were resistant to full-dose beta blockade (as indicated by the continuation of the syncopal episodes) have been treated with high thoractic left sympathectomy. In this subgroup at extremely high risk, only four late deaths (7.5 percent) have occurred, and the long-term survival was very good (96 percent after one year and 90 percent after 7 years)[50] (Fig. 9).

High thoracic left sympathectomy (HTLS) usually, but improperly, is referred to as *left stellectomy*. The extent of denervation is important. Actually, whereas in most animals the ablation of the stellate ganglion produces a major ipsilateral sympathetic denervation; in order to achieve a similar result in humans it is necessary to ablate the first 4–5 thoracic ganglia. Still, there is no need to remove the cephalic portion of the left stellate ganglion; in this way the Horner's syndrome is not produced.

After HTLS, some patients may still require treatment with beta blockers, usually at a dosage lower than that which was not effective in preventing syncope before surgery. Actually, our prospective study indicates that both antiadrenergic interventions, beta-blocking agents, and left stellectomy carry an independent and additive protective effect[43] and in most patients in whom neither therapy alone is sufficient, this combined therapy may be lifesaving.

The efficacy of high thoracic left sympathectomy may be determined only by the clinical follow-up of the patient, as it is independent of the presence or absence of EKG changes; most patients with LQTS have little or no change in the QT interval after left sympathectomy, despite total abolition of the syncopal episodes in

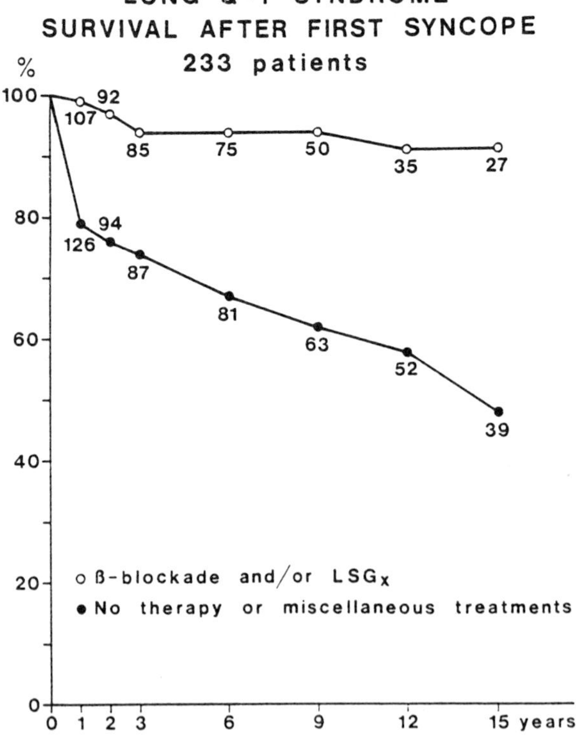


**Figure 8.** Effect of therapy on the survival, after the first syncopal episode, of 233 patients affected by the idiopathic LQTS. The protective effect of beta-adrenergic blockade and of left stellectomy (LSGx) is dramatically evident. For example, the mortality 3 years after the first syncope is 6% in the group treated with antiadrenergic interventions, and it is 26% in the group treated differently or not treated. Fifteen years after the first syncope, the respective mortality rates are 9% and 53% (Ref. 35. Reprinted with permission.).

the long-term follow-up. Therefore, the only criterion of therapeutic efficacy is survival associated with abolition of the syncopal episodes.

The ablation of the left-sided sympathetic nerves is the logical consequence of the understanding of the pathogenetic mechanisms of LQTS, and is to be used for those patients not protected by the higher tolerated dosage of beta-blocking agents.[40,50] Other therapies should be used only for those patients who continue to have syncope despite combined beta blockade and high thoracic left sympathectomy. Among them, verapamil may be of particular interest

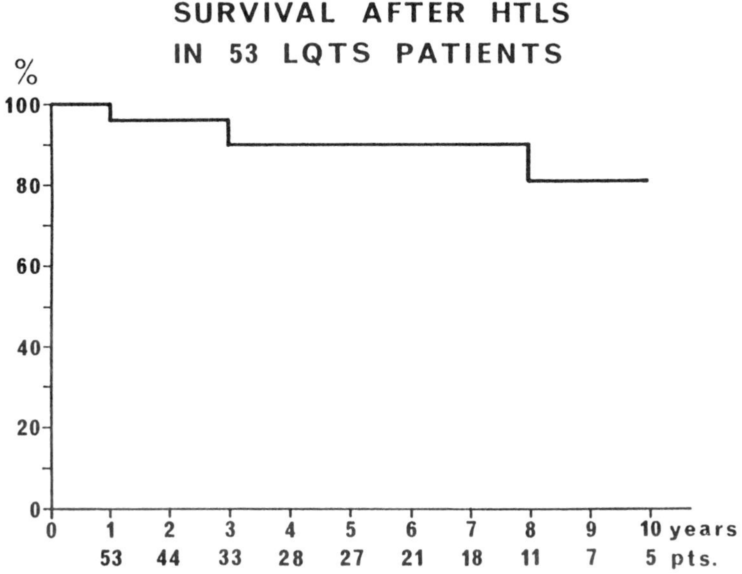


**Figure 9.** Effect of high thoracic left sympathectomy on survival (Ref. 52. Reprinted with permission.).

for the possible role of afterdepolarizations in LQTS.[51,52] However, the effectiveness of long-term oral treatment with calcium entry blockers is unknown and requires careful confirmation.

In conclusion, the use of antiadrenergic therapies has modified radically the prognosis for patients with LQTS. The prospective studies will further define the long-term effectiveness of this protection and whether a treated patient with LQTS has a near-normal life expectancy. When a patient with symptomatic LQTS is identified, treatment with beta blockers should be started immediately. If the syncopal episodes continue despite full-dose beta-blockade, high thoracic left sympathectomy should be performed without hesitation. Any other treatment has to be considered "experimental" and reserved for those patients who continue to have syncopal episodes despite high thoracic left sympathectomy and beta blockade.

## Sudden Infant Death Syndrome

The leading cause of mortality during the first year of life, after the neonatal period, is the Sudden Infant Death Syndrome (SIDS), also known as *cot* or *crib death*.[53] Its incidence is close to 2 per 1000 live births in most countries, even if in some (e.g., the Scandinavian countries), it is markedly lower. It is usually defined as "the sudden death of any infant or young child, which is unexpected by history, and in which a thorough postmortem examination fails to demonstrate an adequate cause for death."

Because of the high incidence, the catastrophic impact on the affected families, the mystery still surrounding these deaths, and the unsolved scientific problem, SIDS represents a major challenge for contemporary medicine.

Prevention of a given event, sudden death in this case, requires an adequate understanding of the mechanisms involved. As far as SIDS is concerned, these mechanisms seem still elusive.

There is almost a consensus that SIDS depends on a respiratory defect; nonetheless, the possibility of a primary cardiac death in SIDS was proposed in 1968[54] and is logically tenable.[55] The cardiac theory proposed that at least some cases of SIDS might depend on sudden sympathetic discharges taking place through an asymmetrically developed cardiac sympathetic innervation with left dominance,[56] similar to that congenitally present in the idiopathic long QT syndrome. This developmental imbalance would manifest itself with a temporary prolongation of the QT interval, evident either at birth or during the first few months of life, thus allowing early identification of the "at risk" babies.

A prospective study specifically designed to test this hypothesis, usually referred to as the *QT hypothesis*, currently is ongoing and has already provided interesting information.[57,58]

Beginning at the end of 1975, electrocardiograms were performed in unselected newborns on the fourth day of life, and the second, fourth, and sixth month. As of October 1986, 13,278 infants have been enrolled, and the 1 year survival data are available for 8000 infants. There have been 9 SIDS victims and 4 non-SIDS deaths. Two significant findings are already available.

The QT interval corrected for heart rate ($QT_c$) increases from $397 \pm 18$ (mean $\pm$ SD) to $409 \pm 15$ at the second month ($p < 0.0001$) and declines progressively with time, so that by the sixth month it is back to the same values present at birth.[22] Although all the 4 non-SIDS victims had a $QT_c$ well within the normal limits, 6 out of 9 of the SIDS victims had a markedly prolonged $QT_c$ (i.e., exceeding the mean by over 2 SD). Four SIDS infants actually had a $QT_c$ exceeding the mean by more than 3 SD.[58]

What inference can be drawn from this ongoing study? The difference in the $QT_c$ between the fourth day and second month of life is important not because of the absolute values, but because it indicates a trend within which a number of individuals (3.6 percent) have marked $QT_c$ prolongation (i.e., > 440 msec). This study demonstrates conclusively that the QT interval lengthens physiologically and temporarily during the first few months of life. Thus, there is a tendency—that in some infants $QT_c$ may become excessive—toward a reduction in cardiac electrical stability at the same time there is a peak incidence of SIDS. While more data on SIDS victims are needed, these results suggest that an unknown percentage (probably not less than 25 percent) of infants who subsequently become SIDS victims can be expected to have, on the fourth day of life, a prolonged QT interval.

Given the number of infants with a markedly prolonged $QT_c$ (18/1000) our data suggest that the risk of SIDS for these infants would be approximately 40/10,000 live births. If confirmed, this would become the single most important risk factor for SIDS.[59]

Thus, also among healthy infants, a prolongation of the QT interval may be a harbinger of life-threatening arrhythmias or sudden death.


## Conclusions

It was the theme of the present book that cardiac arrhythmias might be controlled by lengthening repolarization. Indeed, there is a conceptual background suggesting that, when action potential is increased homogeneously by drug administration, the susceptibility to reentrant arrhythmias is decreased. This concept needs to be reconciled with the observations that drug-induced torsades-de-pointes ventricular tachycardia is nearly always associated with prolongation of QT interval. This iatrogenic phenomenon is infrequent and well may represent abnormal individual responses that should not be generalized; on the other hand, it cannot be dismissed easily. Also, in patients with impaired coronary circulation the drug distribution may not be uniform, so that the lengthening of repolarization could be unequal, thus negating the potential benefits.

We have presented the evidence indicating that in several conditions, ranging from post-myocardial infarction patients to healthy infants, a prolongation of the QT interval is associated with a higher risk for sudden cardiac death. An understanding of the precise mechanisms linking the prolonged cardiac repolarization and the development of life-threatening ventricular arrhythmias may be crucial to the prevention of sudden arrhythmic deaths.

## References


1. Grant RP: *Clinical Electrocardiography.* New York, McGraw-Hill, p 63, 1957.
2. Surawicz B, Knoebel S: Long QT: Good, bad or indifferent? *J Am Coll Cardiol* 4:498, 1984.
3. James TN: QT prolongation and sudden death. *Mod Concepts Cardiovasc Dis* 38:35, 1969.
4. Somberg JC, Singh BN (eds): QT prolongation: Antiarrhythmic and arrhythmogenic effects. *Am Heart J* 109:395, 1985.
5. Han J, Goel BG: Electrophysiologic precursor of ventricular tachyarrhythmias. *Arch Int Med* 129:749, 1972.
6. Vaughan Williams EM: QT and action potential duration. *Br Heart J* 47:513, 1982.
7. Kuo CS, Munakata K, Reddy CP, et al: Characteristics and possible mechanisms of ventricular arrhythmias dependent on the dispersion of action potential duration. *Circulation* 67:1356, 1983.
8. Moss AJ, Schwartz PJ: Delayed repolarization (QT or QTU prolongation) and malignant ventricular arrhythmias. *Mod Concepts Cardiovasc Dis* 51:85, 1982.
9. Schwartz PJ, Wolf S: QT prolongation as predictor of sudden death in patients with myocardial infarction. *Proc 7th Eur Congr Cardiol* (Amsterdam) 1:53, 1986.
10. Schwartz PJ, Wolf S: QT prolongation as predictor of sudden death in patients with myocardial infarction. *Circulation* 57:1075, 1978.
11. Schwartz PJ: Prolonged QT interval to predict sudden death. *Circulation* 59:1079, 1979.
12. Yanowitz R, Preston JB, Abildskov JA: Functional distribution of right and left stellate innervation to the ventricles: Production of neurogenic electrocardiographic changes by unilateral alternation of sympathetic tone. *Circ Res* 18:416, 1966.
13. Abildskov JA: Adrenergic effects on the QT interval of the electrocardiogram. *Am Heart J* 92:210, 1966.
14. Schwartz PJ: Sympathetic imbalance and cardiac arrhythmias. In Randall WC (ed): *Nervous Control of Cardiovascular Function.* New York, Oxford University Press, p 225, 1984.
15. Haynes RE, Hallstrom AP, Cobb LA: Repolarization abnormalities in survivors of out-of-hospital ventricular fibrillation. *Circulation* 57:654, 1978.
16. Ahnve S, Helmers C, Lundman T: QTc intervals at discharge after acute myocardial infarction and long-term prognosis. *Acta Med Scand* 208:55, 1980.
17. Ahnve S, Gilpin E, Madsen EB, et al: Prognostic importance of QTc interval at discharge after acute myocardial infarction: A multicenter study of 865 patients. *Am Heart J* 108:395, 1984.
18. Peters RW, Barker A, Byington R, for the BHAT Study Group: Prognostic value of QTc prolongation: The BHAT experience. *Circulation* 70 (II):24, 1984.
19. Juul-Moller S: Corrected QT-Interval during one year follow-up after an acute myocardial infarction. *Eur Heart J* 7:299, 1986.
20. Pohjola-Sintonen S, Siltanen P, Haapakoski J: Usefulness of QTc in-

terval on the discharge electrocardiogram for predicting survival after acute myocardial infarction. *Am J Cardiol* 57:1066, 1986.

21. Kramer B, Brill M, Bruhn A, et al: Relation between the degree of coronary artery disease and of left ventricular function and the duration of the QT-interval in ECG. *Eur Heart J* 7:14, 1986.
22. Wheelan K, Mukharji J, Rude RE, et al for the MILIS Study Group: Sudden death and its relation to QT-interval prolongation after acute myocardial infarction: Two year follow-up. *Am J Cardiol* 57:745, 1986.
23. Puddu PE, Bourassae MG: Prediction of sudden death from QTc interval prolongation in patients with chronic ischemic heart disease. *J Electrocardiol* 19:203, 1986.
24. Locati E, Schwartz PJ: Prognostic value of QT interval prolongation in post myocardial infarction patients. *Eur Heart J* 8 (Suppl A): 121, 1978.
25. Lepeschkin E, Surawicz B: The measurement of the QT interval in the electrocardiogram. *Circulation* 6:378, 1952.
26. Browne KF, Zipes DP, Heger JJ, et al: Influence of the autonomic nervous system on the QT interval in man. *Am J Cardiol* 50:1099, 1982.
27. Ahnve S: Correction of the QT interval for heart rate: Review of different formulas and the use of Basett's formula in myocardial infarction. *Am Heart J* 109:568, 1985.
28. Ahnve S: Errors in the visual determination of corrected QT (QTc) interval during acute myocardial infarction. *J Am Coll Cardiol* 5:699, 1985.
29. Campbell RWF, Gardiner P, Amos A, et al: Measurement of the QT interval. *Eur Heart J* 6:81, 1985.
30. Schwartz PJ: Idiopathic long QT syndrome: Progress and questions. *Am Heart J* 2:399, 1985.
31. Schwartz PJ, Periti M, Malliani A: The long QT syndrome. *Am Heart J* 89:378, 1975.
32. Schwartz PJ, Malliani A: Electrical alternation of the T-wave: Clinical and experimental evidence of its relationship with the sympathetic nervous system and with the long QT syndrome. *Am Heart J* 89:45, 1975.
33. Crampton RS: Pre-eminence of left stellate ganglion in the long QT syndrome. *Circulation* 59:769, 1979.
34. Randall WC, Rohse WG: The augmentor action of the sympathetic cardiac nerves. *Circ Res* 4:470, 1956.
35. Schwartz PJ: The long QT syndrome. In HE Kulbertus, HJJ Wellens (eds): *Sudden Death*. The Hague, Martinus Nijhoff Publishers, p 358, 1980.
36. Schwartz PJ: Experimental reproduction of the long QT syndrome. *Am J Cardiol* 41:374, 1978.
37. Abildskov JA, Vincent GM, Evan AK, et al: Distribution of body surface potentials in familial Q–T interval prolongation. *Am J Cardiol* 47:480, 1981.
38. Schwartz PJ, Locati E: The idiopathic long QT syndrome. Pathogenetic mechanisms and therapy. *Eur Heart J* 6 (Suppl D): 103, 1985.
39. Schwartz PJ: The rationale and the role of left stellectomy for the prevention of malignant arrhythmias. *Ann NY Acad Sci* 427:199, 1985.
40. Schwartz PJ: Prevention of the arrhythmas in the long QT syndrome.

In HE Kulbertus (ed): *Medical Management of Cardiac Arrhythmias*. Edinburgh, Churchill Livingstone, p 152, 1984.
41. Moss AJ, Schwartz PJ, Crampton RS, et al: Hereditable malignant arrhythmias: A prospective study of the long QT syndrome. *Circulation* 71:17, 1985.
42. Kass RS, Wiegers SE: The ionic basis of concentration-related effect of noradrenaline on the action potential of calf cardiac Purkinje fibers. *J Physiol* 322:541, 1982.
43. Bhandari AK, Shapiro WA, Morady F, et al: Electrophysiologic testing in patients with the long QT syndrome. *Circulation* 71:63, 1985.
44. Jervell A, Lange-Nielsen F: Congenital deaf-mutism, functional heart disease with prolongation of the QT interval and sudden death. *Am Heart J* 54:59, 1957.
45. Romano C, Gemme G, Pongiglione R: Aritmie cardiache rare in eta' pediatrica. *Clin Pediatr* 45:656, 1963.
46. Ward OC: New familial cardiac syndrome in children. *J Irish Med Ass* 54:103, 1964.
47. Itoh S, Munemura S, Satoh H: A study of the inheritance pattern of Romano-Ward syndrome. *Clin Pediatr* 21:20, 1982.
48. Schwartz PJ: The idiopathic long QT syndrome: The need of a prospective study. *Eur Heart J* 4:529, 1983.
49. Moss AJ, McDonald J: Unilateral cervicothoracic sympathetic ganglionectomy for the treatment of long QT interval syndrome. *N Eng J Med* 285:903, 1970.
50. Locati E, Schwartz PJ, Moss AJ, et al: Long-term survival after cervico-thoracic sympathectomy in high risk long QT syndrome patients with refractory ventricular arrhythmias. *J Am Coll Cardiol* 7:235A, 1986.
51. Schechter E, Freeman CC, Lazzara R: Afterdepolarizaiton as a mechanism for the long QT syndrome: Electrophysiologic studies of a case. *J Am Coll Cardiol* 3:1556, 1984.
52. Schwartz PJ, Priori SG: Adrenergic arrhythmogenesis and long QT syndrome. In Vaughn Williams EM, Campbell TJ (eds): *Handbook of Experimental Pharmacology*. Basil, Switzerland, Springer Verlag, 1988.
53. Schwartz PJ: The sudden infant death syndrome. In EM Scarpelli, EV Cosmi (eds): *Reviews in Perinatal Medicine*. New York, Raven Press, p 475, 1981.
54. James TN: Sudden death in babies. *Am J Cardiol* 22:479, 1978.
55. Froggatt P, James TN: Sudden unexpected death in infants. Evidence on a lethal cardiac arrhythmia. *Ulster Med J* 52:136, 1973.
56. Schwartz PJ: Cardiac sympathetic innervation and the sudden infant death syndrome. A possible pathogenetic link. *Am J Med* 60:167, 1976.
57. Schwartz PJ, Montemerlo M, Facchini M, et al: The QT interval throughout the first six months of life: A prospective study. *Circulation* 66:496, 1982.
58. Segantini A, Varisco T, Monza E, et al: QT interval and the sudden infant death syndrome. A prospective study. *J Am Coll Cardiol* 7:1118A, 1986.
59. Schwartz PJ: The quest for the mechanism of the sudden infant death syndrome. Doubt and progress. *Circulation* (in press).

# Chapter 5

# Hemodynamic Effects of Class III Antiarrhythmic Agents

Martin A. Josephson and
Bramah N. Singh

In recent years there has been an increasing appreciation that cardiac arrhythmias, especially of ventricular origin, are associated with adverse prognosis and related a great deal to the degree of impairment of ventricular function. For example, it has been shown that premature ventricular contractions, simple or complex, occurring in subjects with normal hearts have no prognostic significance.[1] In contrast, complex ventricular ectopy associated with severely reduced myocardial function is a significant marker for sudden arrhythmic death.[2] Moreover, most cases of recurrent life-threatening ventricular arrhythmias tend to occur in patients with significantly reduced ventricular ejection fraction. For these reasons, the hemodynamic effects of agents used to suppress such arrhythmias are of practical importance. The issue was brought into sharp focus with the introduction of disopyramide for the treatment of ventricular arrhythmias, since a significant number of patients with a previous history of cardiac failure had an exacerbation when the drug was administered.[3]

The purpose of this chapter is to discuss critically the inotropic and hemodynamic effects of agents that appear to control cardiac arrhythmias by selectively lengthening repolarization. There are theoretical considerations that suggest that these agents, as a class, might exert fewer negatively inotropic actions than other classes of antiarrhythmic agents. The salient data in support of this contention are discussed briefly.

From: *Control of Cardiac Arrhythmias by Lengthening Repolarization*, edited by Bramah N. Singh, MD, Futura Publishing Company Inc., Mount Kisco, NY, © 1988.

## Prolongation of Repolarization and Myocardial Contractility

In 1959, Kavaler[4] provided evidence for augmented tension development as a function of sustained depolarization in isolated cardiac muscle. He devised a method whereby it was possible to depolarize a short strip of mammalian ventricular muscle by applying an external voltage. From the same segment of muscle, he recorded simultaneously myocardial tension by a force transducer and the time course of the transmembrane potential by the standard microelectrode technique. By this approach, he found that it was possible to increase the duration of the action potential from 50 msec to 2000 msec. This caused the tension to remain at near-peak levels over the period of 2 seconds, relaxation occurring only when the fibers were allowed to repolarize. That an augmentation of tension development does indeed occur as a function of prolonged repolarization was subsequently confirmed by Morad and Trautwein.[5]

The "discovery" of the slow calcium channel and the delineation of its kinetics[6] have provided a theoretical basis to account for the initial observations of Kavaler.[4] As mentioned elsewhere in this volume (see Chapter 3), the slow calcium channel is responsible for excitation-contraction coupling in working cardiac fibers. Its time constant of inactivation is long (about 500 msec in ventricular muscle) and is voltage dependent. Thus, any intervention that interferes with the normal processes of repolarization and produces a prolongation of the action potential duration in the setting of normal extracellular calcium ion concentration is likely to enhance the net transfer of calcium ion per excitation across the cardiac membrane and produce an increase in contractile force. If these theoretical considerations are tenable, one might expect agents that produce a significant lengthening of the action potential duration to exert a positive inotropic effect. It should be emphasized however that rarely does a pharmacologic agent exhibit a "pure" effect in vitro and particularly in vivo where the net effect often is a balance between direct cardiac and indirect extracardiac actions of a particular compound. Nevertheless, within this limitation, it appears that the concept of augmented myocardial contractility as a function of lengthened repolarization is valid and has clinical relevance in the case of certain antiarrhythmic compounds.

In 1968, Kaumann and Olson[6] duplicated the observations made by Kavaler.[4] They described a pharmacologic method for varying electrical and mechanical events in kitten papillary muscles. It was found that high concentrations of sotalol (27 µg/ml) led to a marked prolongation of the action potential duration associated with a significant increase in peak tension often accompanied by the development of aftercontractions, which could be correlated with the lengthening of repolarization. An example of the simultaneous recordings of the action potential and of isometric tension is shown in Figure 1. Recently, a positive inotropic effect associated with the prolongation of the action potential duration also has been demonstrated in the case of melperone (also see Chapter 14). Increasing concentrations of the drug produced a stepwise increase in contractile force (Fig. 2) pari passu with the lengthening of the action potential duration in isolated cardiac muscle.[7] Thus, the data with sotalol and melperone are consistent with the hypothesis that sustained depolarization increases tension development in cardiac muscle. It must be emphasized that, while this is demonstrated readily in cardiac muscle, the effect in vivo may not necessarily be translated into an augmented cardiac performance. The net in vivo effect will be determined by the associated pharmaco-

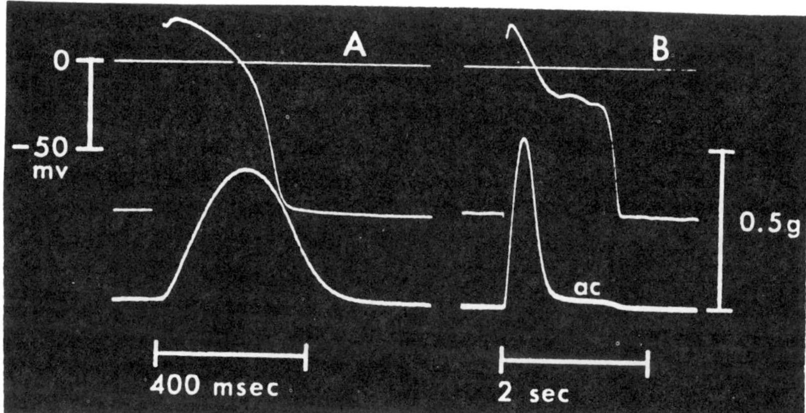



**Figure 1.** Effects of sotalol (27 µg/ml) on the action potential and isometric tension in papillary muscle from the kitten heart. The upper trace of each panel (A and B) shows zero potential; middle trace, transmembrane action potential; and lower trace isometric tension. Vertical calibration: membrane potential (left) and isometric tension (right). Horizontal calibration: time. A: Shows recordings under control conditions; B: Shows the effects of sotalol superfusion. Note that the drug augments peak isometric tension pari passu with the lengthening of the action potential. An aftercontraction (ac) develops during the lengthened phase 2 of the action potential. (From Kaumann AJ, Olson CB: Temporal relations between long-lasting aftercontractions and action potentials in cat papillary muscles. *Science* 161:293, 1968. By the permission of the authors and the journal.)

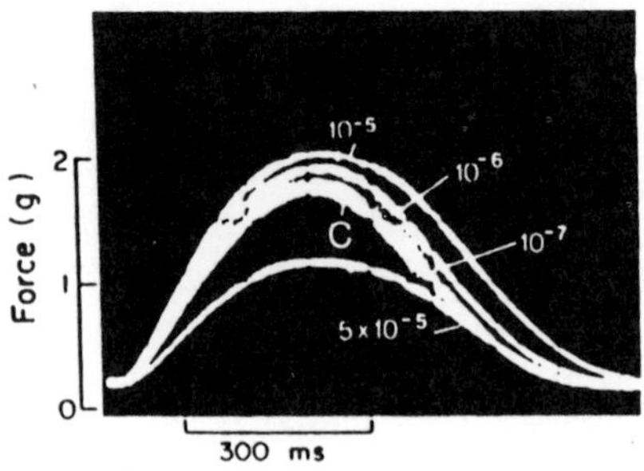

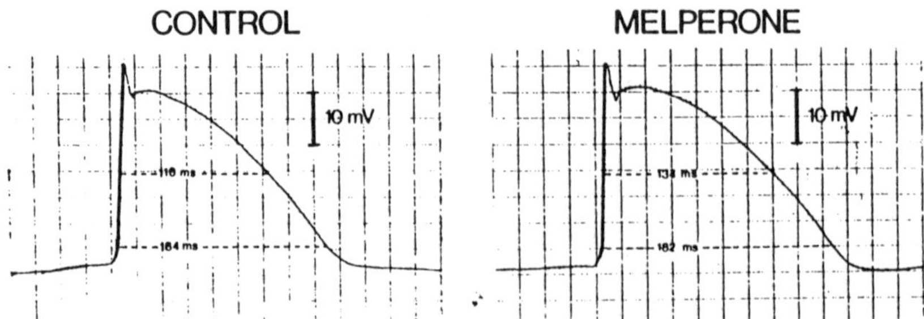



**Figure 2.** Effects of melperone on isometric tensions (upper panel) and on transmembrane potential (lower panel) in canine ventricular muscle. Note the stepwise increase in peak tension as a function of molar concentration of melperone ($10^{-7}$ to $10^{-5}$ M) compared to control; at the highest concentration ($5 \times 10^{-5}$), there is reduction in contractile force. The increases in contractile force were associated with a prolongation of the action potential duration (lower panel). (From Platou ES: Class III antarrhythmic action. Doctoral thesis, Norway, University of Tromsø. By the permission of the author.)

logic properties of individual compounds (e.g., beta blockade in the case of sotalol and noncompetitive sympatholytic effect in the case of amiodarone). These considerations clearly are of importance in delineating the hemodynamic effects of individual Class III antiarrhythmic compounds. The remainder of this chapter deals with the inotropic and hemodynamic effects of sotalol, amiodarone, and N-acetylprocainamide. The hemodynamic effects of bretylium are discussed in Chapter 13 and those of melperone in Chapter 14.

## Inotropic and Hemodynamic Effects of Sotalol

The hemodynamic effects of sotalol and its dose-relationships in patients with varying levels of ventricular function have not been fully evaluated. The net hemodynamic effects of the drug are likely to be a balance between the depressant actions of the drug due to the blockade of beta receptors and those tending to increase contractility by prolongation of the time course of calcium influx due to the lengthening of the action potential duration.

Numerous studies have indicated that unlike other beta-adrenergic blocking drugs devoid of intrinsic sympathomimetic actions, sotalol exerts either no depressant effect on myocardial contractility or may even increase it somewhat. As indicated elsewhere,[8] it appears that lengthening of the action potential duration induced by the drug may augment contractility, a phenomenon that has been demonstrated in isolated cardiac muscle[9–12] and seen with other beta-blockers such as propranolol (Fig. 3).

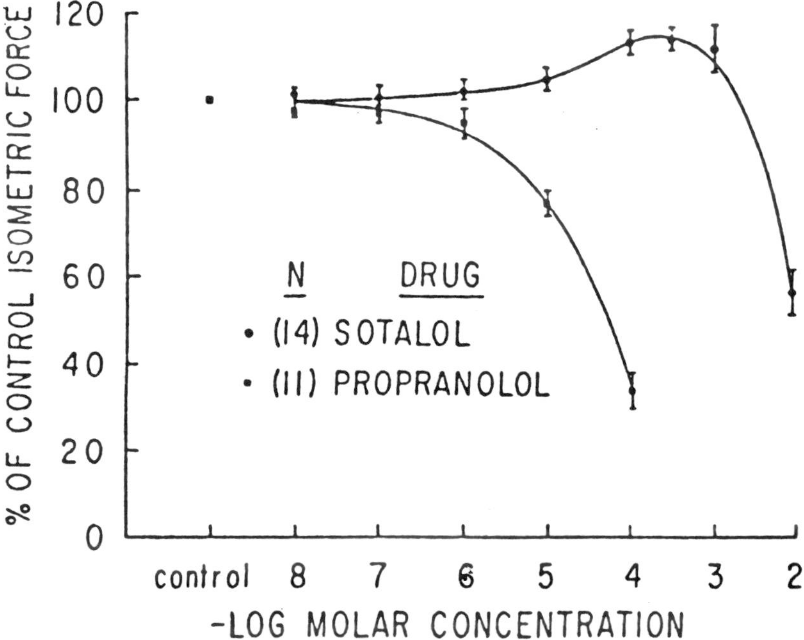


**Figure 3.** Changes in isometric force in isolated cat papillary muscle induced by sotalol (upper curve) and propranolol (lower curve). In sotalol the response is biphasic: there is an increase in isometric force over the lower range of drug concentrations before the depressant effect becomes evident. In contrast, with propranolol, there is a decrease in isometic contraction over the entire range of drug concentrations. (From Parmley WW, Rabinowitz B, Chuck L, et al: Comparative effects of sotalol and propranalol on contractility of papillary muscles and adenyl cyclase of myocardial extract of cat. *J Clin Pharmacol* 12:127, 1972. By permission of the authors and the journal.)

Increases in contractility up to 13–15 percent in isolated cardiac muscle have been reported,[13] an effect that is unrelated to an adrenergic mechanism, as it occurs in reserpinized preparations. Thus, it appears to be related to the property of the sotalol molecule, although no studies on the structure–activity relationship of such an action has been reported. However, such an effect, in part, may offset the depressant effect of beta blockade in a patient with cardiac decompensation. This feature distinguishes sotalol from conventional beta-blocking drugs; the available in vivo experimental data and clinical experience are in agreement with these postulates.

## Hemodynamic Effects of Sotalol in Animals

In anesthetized animals, numerous studies have indicated that the myocardial depressant effects of sotalol are significantly less than those of propranolol and other conventional beta-adrenergic blocking drugs. For example, when equipotent beta-blocking doses of propranolol and sotalol were given to anesthetized open-chest dogs and cardiac contractility was measured by Walton-Brodie strain-gauge arches sewn over the anterior wall of the left ventricle, sotalol reduced contractility only 20 percent whereas a reduction of 50 percent was effected by propranolol.[14] Similarly, in a canine aortic bypass preparation, propranolol produced a greater reduction in contractile force of the right ventricle and left ventricular $dp/dt_{max}$ and a greater increase in the left ventricular end diastolic pressure than equimolar doses of sotalol.[12] The differences in the effects of the two blocking agents were not accountable in terms of adrenergic actions as a similar pattern of responses was found in reserpinized animal preparations. Similar differences in the actions of sotalol and other beta-blockers have been reported by other investigators.[9,15] Of particular interest were the findings of Puri and Bing;[16] in closed-chest anesthetized dogs, they reported that sotalol decreased heart rate and rate-dependent hemodynamic functions but exerted no significant effects on stroke volume, stroke work index, or the tension time index per heart beat. The drug did not increase the left ventricular end diastolic pressure, a pattern of effect strikingly different from that induced by propranolol. These overall findings are consistent with those of Rogers et al.[17] in the conscious baboon, in which orally administered sotalol reduced cardiac output but only as a function of heart rate, since no change in stroke volume was noted, again emphasizing the differences in the hemodynamic effects of sotalol from those of propranolol. These data also are consistent with the findings of Brooks et al.[18] in open-chest anesthetized dogs, in which the authors determined force velocity curves from the isovolumic left ventricular pressure recordings in reserpinized and nonreserpinized animals before and after 1–6 mg/kg of intravenous sotalol. The data were acquired during right atrial pacing at a fixed rate so that the effects due to rate changes could be excluded. In none of the studies was there a shift in the force-velocity relationship, even at doses far exceeding the beta-blocking dose. Thus, the data indicated that sotalol produced no basic change in the contractile state of the intact heart at controlled heart rates.

## Hemodynamic Effects in Humans

There is a striking concordance between the actions of sotalol in experimental animals and those in man. Again, the pattern of hemodynamic changes induced by intravenous sotalol differs from that described for conventional beta blockers such as propranolol. In general, the net effects of the drug are characterized by a reduction in heart rate, increase in systemic vascular resistance, cardiac output (without a change in stroke volume), and little or no increases in the filling of the left ventricle or in pressures in the right heart.[18–23]

The studies of Brooks et al.[18] are of particular interest as they were performed in patients with cardiac failure. The dose of sotalol used was 0.2–0.6 mg/kg and the studies were carried out under resting conditions. Whether the left ventricular end diastolic pressure was elevated or not, the drug produced a consistent and proportionate reduction in heart rate and cardiac output without a change in stroke volume or in left ventricular end-diastolic pressure (Fig. 4), in contrast to what is consistently observed with conventional beta blockers such as propranolol or timolol. The findings of Brooks et al.[18] are supported by the observations of Thumala et al;[22] who found a similar reduction in cardiac output and heart rate, again without a fall in stroke volume at rest or during exercise. These authors also found small changes in the left ventricular end-diastolic pressure, both at rest and during exercise after sotalol and a reduction in the velocity of left ventricular contraction. It is noteworthy that Hutton et al.[23] reported a decrease in the $LVdp/dt_{max}$ following intravenous sotalol, but, since the data were acquired without cardiac pacing, it is likely that such a

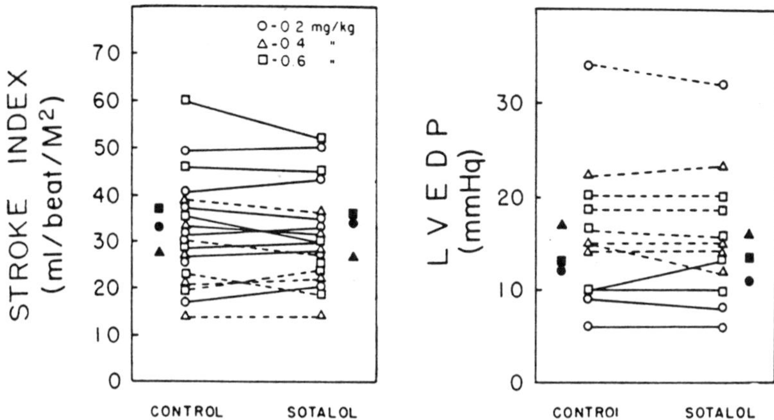


**Figure 4.** Effects of intravenously administered sotalol (0.2−0.6 mg/kg) in patients with heart failure. Note that unlike conventional beta blockers sotalol does not decrease stroke index or increase left ventricular end diastolic pressure. The net effect of the drug on cardiovascular hemodynamics is a balance bewteen the direct effect of the compound on myocardial contractility and those induced by beta blockade. (From Brooks H, Banas J, Meister S, et al: Sotalol-induced beta blockade in cardiac patients. *Circulation* 42:99, 1970. By permission of the authors and of the American Heart Association.)

reduction may have resulted from the blockade of cardiac beta adrenoceptors.

Although the available experimental and clinical data indicate that the hemodynamic effects of sotalol are less depressant than those after conventional beta antagonists, there is a need for further detailed studies to define various doses of the drug in patients with a varying spectrum of ventricular performance. It would be desirable to delineate the effects that result from the blockade of beta receptors and those that are modulated by the intrinsic properties of the compound.[24−29] For these reasons, it would be of importance to compare the hemodynamic effects of the racemic sotalol with those of the dextro-isomer devoid of beta blocking actions. It is known that cardiac failure may be exacerbated in a small number of patients given dl-sotalol. The absence of beta-blocking activity in the d-isomer would obviate this possibility if the latter compound has the same antiarrhythmic profile as the racemic mixture (see Chapter 9).

## Inotropic and Hemodynamic Effects of Amiodarone

Amiodarone is another Class III antiarrhythmic agent that is efficacious in a variety of supraventricular and ventricular tachyarrhythmias. Originally introduced as an antianginal drug with systemic and coronary vasodilating properties, amiodarone exerts complex pharmacologic effects on the heart and circulation.[30–33] Due to the relative insolubility of amiodarone, data on the intrinsic inotropic effects of this agent on isolated muscle are limited. Moreover, the hemodynamic effects in humans of the commerical intravenous preparation must be separated from those of the diluent, polysorbate or Tween 80, which also has significant hemodynamic effects.

Amiodarone has a broad pharmacodynamic profile (see Chapter 15) exhibiting coronary and peripheral vasodilator properties and catecholamine alpha- and beta-receptor blocking actions while exerting possible direct effects on myocardial contractility. Thus, the net in vivo effects on systemic hemodynamic and myocardial performance is likely a balance of cardiac and extracardiac actions of the drug.

Charlier et al.[33,34] demonstrated in anesthetized dogs a decrease in total vascular resistance and heart rate resulting from intrinsic effects of amiodarone in addition to noncompetitive alpha- and beta-adrenergic blockade. Petta and Zaccheo[35] and Singh et al.[36] confirmed these findings in open-chest anesthetized dogs using 2.5–10 mg/kg intravenous amiodarone in distilled water prepared by mild heating, thus eliminating the effects of the diluent present in many of the hemodynamic studies in humans. The mean data are summarized in Figure 5. Amiodarone increased coronary blood flow and coronary sinus oxygen content. There also was a decrease in left ventricular minute work, mean arterial pressure, left ventricular oxygen consumption, coronary vascular resistance, and total peripheral vascular resistance as well as heart rate. Left ventricular output was either unchanged or tended to increase. Singh et al.[36] demonstrated a dose-dependent depression of cardiac contractile force and reduction in LV $dp/dt_{max}$ by amiodarone; however, cardiac output was unchanged or increased and left ventricular end-diastolic pressure was increased only by the higher 10 mg/kg dose. The data indicated that only at high doses did the compound exert a significant negative inotropic effect in anesthetized animals.

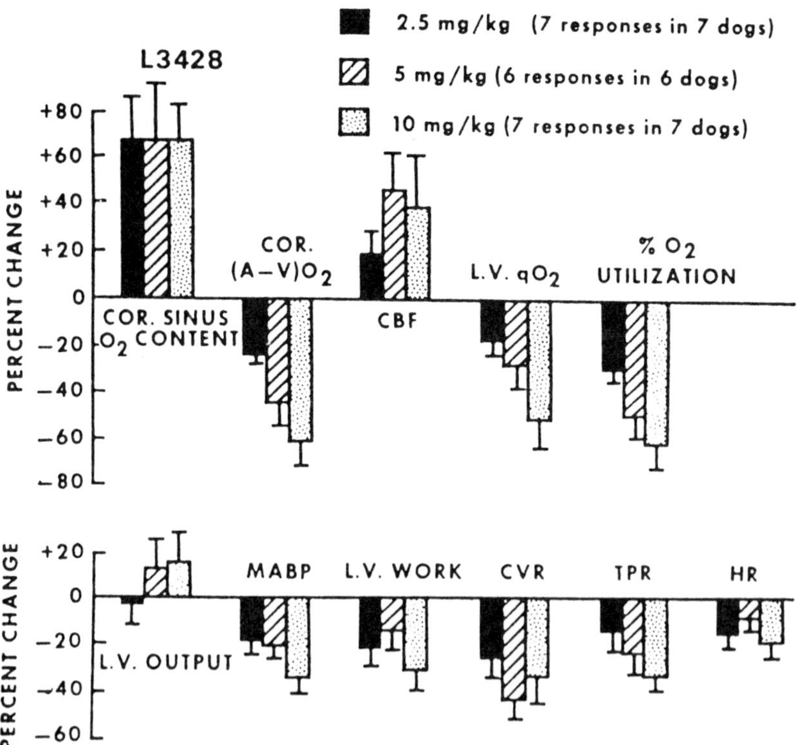


**Figure 5.** Effects of various doses of intravenous amiodarone (L3428) on hemodynamic variables in open-chest anesthetized dogs. The data (mean ± SD) shown represent percentage changes from control. CBF = coronary blood flow, MABP = mean arterial blood pressure, CVR = coronary vascular resistance, TPR = total peripheral resistance, HR = heart rate. The data are consistent with the drug's propensity to produce coronary and peripheral vasodilatation and to inhibit sympathetic excitation, as suggested by a decrease in heart rate despite peripheral vasodilation. (From Petta JM, Zaccheo VJ: Comparative profile of L3428 and other antianginal agents on cardiac hemodynamics. *J Pharmacol Exp Ther* 176:328, 1971. By permission of the authors of the journal.)

## Hemodynamic Effects of Amiodarone in Humans

When assessing the effects of amiodarone in humans, it is important to consider the dose, method of infusion, effects of the diluent in the intravenous form and the underlying level of ventricular function as well as the nature of the underlying heart disease. In most studies on the hemodynamic effects of the intravenous preparation, the commercial preparation using the diluent polysorbate 80 (Tween 80) was used. Gough et al.[37] demonstrated significant hypotensive and negative inotropic effects of this diluent, evidenced by a fall in LV $dp/dt_{max}$ in anesthetized dogs. Although the action of the diluent may not be of similar magnitude in humans, it is likely that negative inotropic effects occur in humans when commercially available amiodarone preparations are used.

Ourbak et al.[38] demonstrated a minimal reduction in heart rate and cardiac index and increased systemic resistance following intravenous amiodarone 5 mg/kg in patients with coronary artery disease. Using 7.5 mg/kg of intravenous amiodarone, Pfisterer et al.[39] also demonstrated significant negative inotropic effects acutely, with reduction in the left ventricular ejection fraction and an elevation in the pulmonary capillary wedge pressure. All hemodynamic effects were reversed, however, after 3 weeks of oral amiodarone (200−800 mg/day) treatment. Using 5 mg/kg intravenous amiodarone, Sicart et al.[40] and Cote et al.[41] demonstrated significant reductions in systemic resistance and blood pressure associated with reductions in the left ventricular end-diastolic pressure and an increase in cardiac index. Although contractility was not evaluated in these studies, a major negative inotropic effect was not likely in view of the increased cardiac output and lowered left ventricular end-diastolic pressure. Cote et al.[41] also confirmed in humans the significant coronary vasodilator effects of amiodarone demonstrating increased coronary flow despite a reduction in coronary perfusion pressure. Although it is difficult to separate the hemodynamic effects of amiodarone from those of the diluent in acute hemodynamic studies, it is clear that severe myocardial depression does not occur following intravenous amiodarone in patients with relatively preserved ventricular function. Bellotti et al;[42] using amiodarone dissolved in distilled water obviating the effects of the diluent, demonstrated significant myocardial depression for 1 hour following a 5 mg/kg dose infused over 5 minutes. After 1 hour 900−1050 mg were infused over the next 23 hours, at which time, evidence of left ventricular depression could not be detected although significant vasodilatory effects persisted. These patients all had baseline congestive heart failure as a result of Chagas' disease, and these results might not be representative of the effects of amiodarone in other settings of left ventricular dysfunction.

Kosinski et al.[43] studied the effects of acute and chronic (3−5 days) intravenous amiodarone in patients with varying levels of ventricular function. An initial 300 mg bolus of amiodarone was administered over 5 minutes and patients then received 1000 mg intravenously over 24 hours for 3–5 days. In this study, patients with a left ventricular ejection fraction greater than 0.35 experienced an increase in cardiac index in contrast with a 20 percent decrease in cardiac index in patients with an ejection fraction less than 0.35. Of note is the fact that 3 of 8 patients in the reduced ejection fraction group experienced clinically significant hemodynamic deterioration during intravenous infusion but were able to continue chronic oral amiodarone therapy without evidence of adverse hemodynamic effects. Similar findings were demonstrated by Schwartz et al.[44] with significant depression in cardiac index and stroke work index at 10 minutes after a 5 mg/kg infusion of intravenous amiodarone in patients with left ventricular ejection fractions less than 0.30. Marked hypotension necessitating discontinuation of amiodarone occurred in 2 patients during the intravenous infusion, emphasizing the need for caution when using intravenous amiodarone in patients with severely impaired ventricular function in whom sympathetic reflexes may be required to maintain cardiac compensation.

Several studies have demonstrated the anti-ischemic effects of amiodarone during exercise- or pacing-induced ischemia.[39,45] The reduction in myocardial oxygen demand due to the drug's vasodilating properties, despite its coronary vasodilating properties, appears to be the predominant anti-ischemic mechanism. In the setting of left ventricular dysfunction due to or exacerbated by ischemia, improved ventricular performance might result from the anti-ischemic effects of amiodarone.

In view of the predominant oral use of amiodarone it is noteworthy that adverse hemodynamic effects and reports of amiodarone-induced heart failure are infrequent despite large numbers of patients with significant left ventricular dysfunction maintained on chronic oral therapy.[46–52] When oral doses of 800–2000 mg/day were used to rapidly achieve a "therapeutic" serum concentration, no significant changes in cardiac output, pulmonary capillary wedge pressure, or arterial pressure were demonstrated, although heart rate was reduced approximately 10 percent.[49] Despite the fact that 12 of 18 patients had a history of heart failure, no adverse hemodynamic effects were demonstrated by doses of oral amiodarone, which produced significant reductions in ventricular ectopic activity. Their short-term observations are consistent with the results of multiple dose studies (Fig. 6), which have not demon-

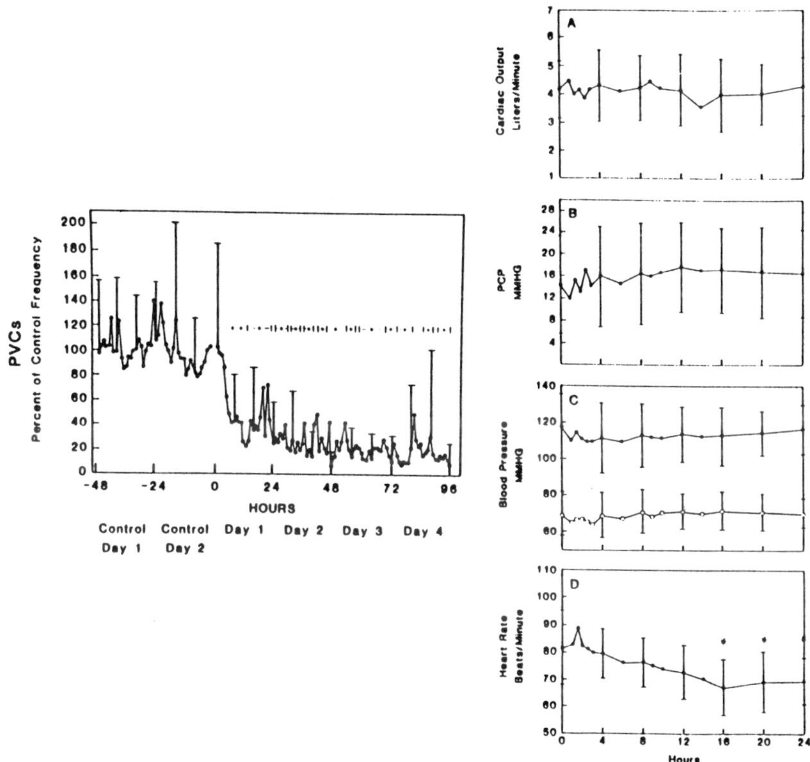

**Figure 6.** Changes in hemodynamic variables (right) and in ventricular ectopy (left) following high oral doses of amiodarone in patients with ventricular arrhythmias. Note that despite a significant suppression of ventricular ectopy, there were minimal changes in cardiac output, pulmonary capillary wedge pressure (PCP), or arterial pressure; heart rate tended to decrease towards the end of 24 hours of therapy. (From Mostow ND, Vrobel TR, Spielman SR, et al: Rapid suppression of complex ventricular arrhythmias with high-dose oral amiodarone. *Circulation* 73:1231, 1986. By permission of the authors and of the American Heart Association.)

strated any adverse effects of oral amiodarone on left ventricular ejection fraction.[50-53] Figure 7 illustrates the effects of long-term, steady state administration of oral amiodarone on left ventricular ejection fraction. There was no obvious depression in this index of ventricular function, even in patients with severely reduced baseline ejection fractions. It must be emphasized that, although congestive heart failure is rarely aggravated by chronic oral amiodarone treatment, this potential exists especially in pa-

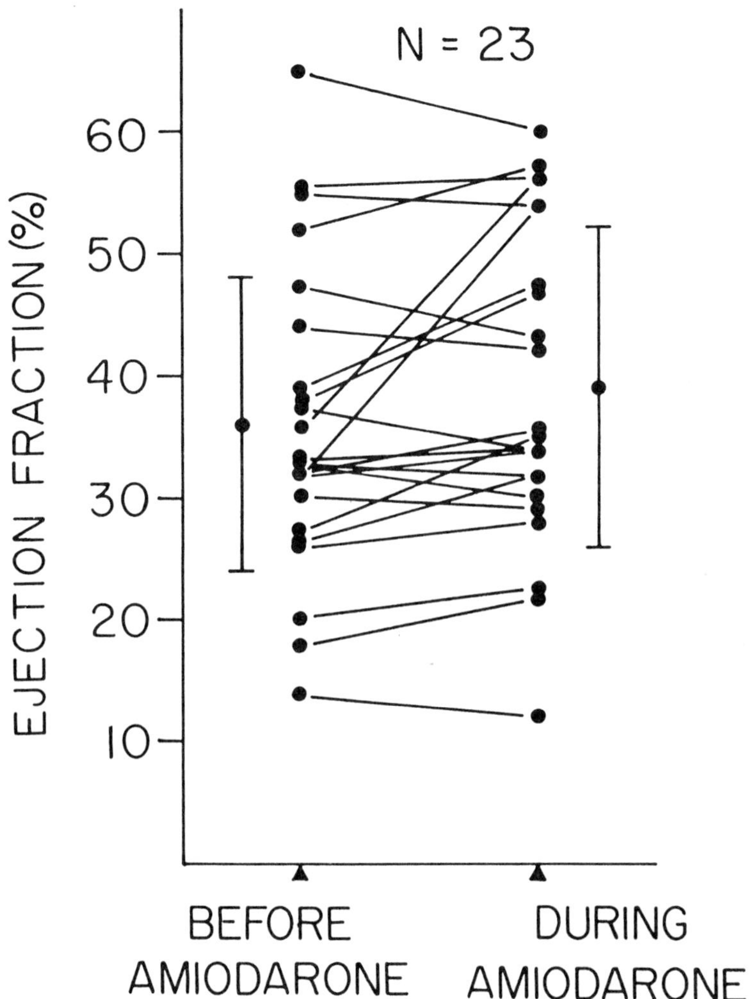


**Figure 7.** Effects on left ventricular ejection fraction (determined by radionuclide ventriculography) before and during steady state oral maintenance amiodarone administration. No significant effect is noted. (From Singh BN: Amiodarone: Historical development and pharmocologic profile. *Am Heart J* 106:788, 1983. By permission of the author and of the American Heart Association.)

tients dependent on augmented sympathetic drive, which may be blocked by the drug's noncompetitive beta-adrenergic blockade.[50]

Negative inotropic effects may be encountered in the setting of hypertrophic cardiomyopathy. Paulus et al.[54] determined the effects of long-term treatment with amiodarone on exercise hemodynamics and left ventricular relaxation (by echocardiography) in patients with hypertrophic cardiomyopathy before and after 5 weeks of 600 mg/day oral amiodarone. The drug produced a small but significant *increase* in left ventricular filling pressures at rest; exercise tolerance was reduced with a modest increase in ventricular filling pressures, although relaxation indexes were not altered. The data suggested an impairment of myocardial inactivation similar to that described in hypothyroidism. However, further data are needed to determine the propensity of amiodarone to induce clinically significant heart failure in patients with hypertrophic cardiomyopathy.

## Hemodynamic Effects of N-Acetylprocainamide (NAPA)

Available hemodynamic data on the antiarrhythmic NAPA are consistent with the concept that Class III agents, as a group, produce less myocardial depression than other classes. In isolated rabbit hearts, NAPA infusions of 40 µg/min or greater are required to produce myocardial depression, whereas significant depression is seen with procainamide infusion rates of 2 µg/min.[55] Lertora et al.[56] demonstrated in open-chest dogs that NAPA increased myocardial contractile force in contrast to the effects of procainamide, which decreased contractile force despite a greater decrease in arterial pressure. Lertora et al.[57] further demonstrated that NAPA doses of 12 mg/kg and 60 mg/kg increased contractile force 12 percent and 33 percent, respectively, while only the high dose produced significant chronotropic and hypotensive effects. The positive inotropic effect at the low dose was blocked by atropine and believed secondary to the vagolytic effects of NAPA, whereas that following the higher dose was probably mediated by catecholamine. Badke et al.[58] demonstrated a biphasic hemodynamic response following 10 and 20 mg/kg NAPA doses in conscious dogs with improved left ventricular performance early and negative inotropic effects 6 hours after the infusion. An initial catecholamine response with late sympathetic nervous system depression was suggested as the mechanism of this biphasic response.

In humans, oral NAPA decreases the PEP/LVET ratio,[59,60] although no evidence of a positive inotropic effect using systolic time intervals could be demonstrated after 1 year of therapy. In patients with primary cardiomyopathy, no effect of NAPA (3–6 g/day) on heart rate, blood pressure, or echocardiographic assessment of left ventricular performance was demonstrated at rest or during isometeric handgrip exercise.[61] In 14 patients with normal ventricular function, NAPA 18 mg/kg administered intravenously over 30 minutes decreased cardiac index 8 percent, LV $dp/dt_{max}$ 9 percent, and the pulmonary capillary wedge pressure 27 percent,[62] see Figure 8. Although a negative inotropic effect of NAPA cannot be excluded, the decrease in cardiac index and LV $dp/dt_{max}$ most likely results from arterial and venodilatation and reduced ventricular filling. Clinically, aggravation of heart failure by NAPA has not been reported.

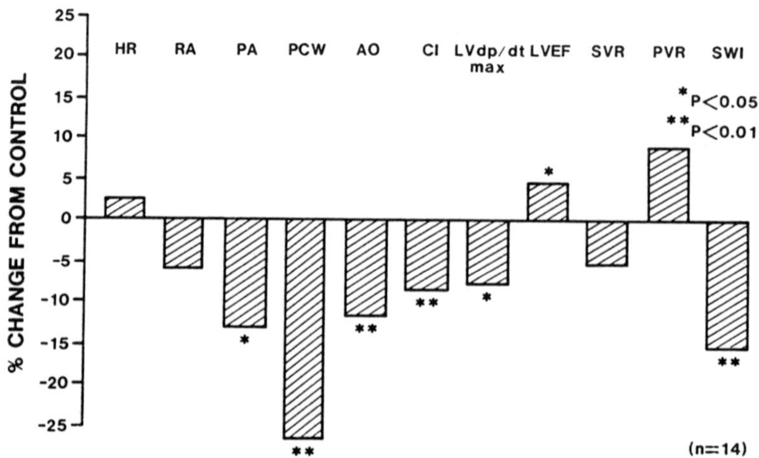


**Figure 8.** Hemodynamic effects of intravenously administered N-acetylprocainamide (NAPA) in patients undergoing diagnostic cardiac catheterization. The effects shown are expressed as percentage changes from control. HR = heart rate, RA = mean right atrial pressure, PA = mean pulmonary artery pressure, PCW = mean pulmonary capillary wedge pressure, AO = mean aortic pressure, CI = cardiac index, LVEF = left ventricular ejection fraction, SVR = systemic vascular resistance, PVR = pulmonary vascular resistance, SWI = strike work index. (From Josephson MA, Schwab M, Coyle K, et al: Effects of intravenous N-acetylprocainamide on hemodynamics and left ventricular function in man. *Am Heart J* in press. By permission of the authors and of the American Heart Association.)

## Conclusions

Theoretical considerations and experimental observations suggest a link between augmentation in myocardial contractility and in the lengthening of cardiac repolarization. Therefore, pharmacologic agents that prolong ventricular repolarization might be expected to exert a positive inotropic action in isolated cardiac muscle, an action that might influence their net hemodynamic effects. The data on the so-called Class III antiarrhythmic agents, which tend to act predominantly by lengthening cardiac repolarization, provide the framework for defining the potential differences in hemodynamic effects among various classes of antiarrhythmic compounds. The available clinical data suggest that as a group Class III agents (sotalol, amiodarone, NAPA, melperone) usually do not exert a significant depressant hemodynamic effect in doses that are therapeutically relevant. However, these agents are chemically and pharmacologically heterogeneous and their net hemodynamic effects are likely to represent a balance between their intrinsic myocardial actions and those that are due to their extracardiac actions. At least in the case of sotalol and amiodarone, the propensity to aggraviate failure in some patients does exist by virtue of their antiadrenergic actions.

*We are indebted to Lawrence Kimble for help in preparing this chapter and to the Medical Media Department for assistance with illustrations and photography.*

## References

1. Kennedy HL, Whitlock JA, Sprague MK, et al: Long-term follow-up of asymptomatic healthy subjects with frequent and complex ventricular ectopy. *N Eng J Med* 312:193, 1985.
2. Ruberman W, Weinblatt E, Goldberg JD, et al: Ventricular premature complexes and sudden death after myocardial infarction. *Circulation* 64:297, 1981.
3. Podrid PJ, Schoenberger A, Lown B: Congestive heart failure caused by oral disopyramide. *N Eng J Med* 302:614, 1980.
4. Kavaler F: Membrane depolarization as a cause of tension development in mammalian cardiac muscle. *Am J Physiol* 197:968, 1959.
5. Morad M, Trautwein W: The effect of the duration of the action potential on contraction in the mammalian heart muscle. *Pfuegers Archiv Ges Physiol* 299:66, 1968.

6. Kaumann AJ, Olson CB: Temporal relations between long-lasting aftercontractions and action potentials in cat papillary muscles. *Science* 161:293, 1968.
7. Platou ES: Class III antiarrhythmic action. Doctoral thesis, Norway, University of Tromsø, 1982.
8. Singh BN, Nademanee K: Control of cardiac arrhythmias by selective lengthening of repolarization: Theoretic considerations and clinical observations. *Amer Heart J* 109:421, 1985.
9. Aberg G, Dzedin T, Lundholm L, et al: A comparative study of some cardiovascular effects of sotalol (MJ 1999) and propranolol. *Life Sci* 8:353, 1969.
10. Blinks JR: Evaluation of the cardiac effects of several beta-adrenergic blocking agents *Ann NY Acad Sci* 139:673, 1967.
11. Singh BN: A study of the pharmacological actions of certain drugs and hormones with a particular reference to cardiac muscle. D. Phil. thesis, England, University of Oxford, 1971.
12. Gomoll AW, Braunwald E: Comparative effects of sotalol and propranolol on myocardial contractility. *Arch Int Pharmacodyn Ther* 205:338, 1973.
13. Parmley WW, Rabinowitz B, Chuck L, et al: Comparative effects of sotalol and propranolol on contractility of papillary muscles and adenyl cyclase activity of myocardial extracts of cat. *J Clin Pharmacol* 12:127, 1972.
14. Hoffmann RP, Grupp G: The effects of sotalol and propranolol on contractile force and atrioventricular conduction time of the dog heart in situ. *Chest* 55:229, 1969.
15. Goldstein RE, Hall CA, Epstein SE: Comparison of relative inotropic and chronotropic effects of propranolol, practolol and sotalol. *Chest* 64:619, 1973.
16. Puri PS, Bing RJ: Effects of myocardial contractility, hemodynamics and cardiac metabolism of a new beta-adrenergic blocking drug, sotalol. *Chest* 55:235, 1969.
17. Rogers GG, Rosendof C, Coull A, et al: Sotalol and infarct size after coronary ligation in the baboon. *J Cardiovasc Pharmacol* 5:28, 1985.
18. Brooks H, Banas J, Meister S, et al: Sotalol-induced beta-blockade in cardiac patients. *Circulation* 42:99, 1970.
19. Dexter L, Brooks H, Banas JS, et al: Effects of sotalol on myocardial function in dogs and patients with heart failure. *Pro Int Sym* (Rome), May 1974, 1:41. AG Snart, (ed). Amsterdam, Excerpta Medica.
20. Taylor SH: General review of the haemodynamic effects of beta-adrenoceptor blocking drugs. *Curr Ther Res* 28:83S, 1980.
21. Svedmyr N, Malmberg R, Haggendal E: The hemodynamic effects of sotalol (MJ 1999) and propranolol in man. *Pharmacologia Clinica* 2:82, 1970.
22. Thumala A, Hammermeister KE, Campbell WB, et al: Hemodynamic studies with sotalol in man, performed at rest, during exercise, and during right ventricular pacing. *Am Heart J* 82:439, 1971.
23. Hutton I, Lorimer AR, Hillis WS, et al: Hemodynamics and myocardial function after sotalol. *Br Heart J* 34:787, 1972.
24. Johnston GD, Finch MB, McNeill JA, et al: A comparison of the car-

diovascular effects of (+)-sotalol and (±)-sotalol following intravenous administration in normal volunteers. *Br J Clin Pharmacol* 20:507, 1985.

25. Kaumann AJ, Blinks JR: Beta-adrenoceptor blocking agents as partial agonists in isolated heart muscle. *Naunyn Schmiedebergs Arch Pharmacol* 311:237, 1980.

26. Kaumann AJ, McInerny TK, Gilmour DP, et al: Comparative assessment of beta-adrenoceptor blocking agents as simple competitive antagonists in isolated heart muscle. *Naunyn Schmiedebergs Arch Pharmacol* 311:219, 1980.

27. Lish PM, Weikel JH, Dungan KW: Pharmacological and toxicological properties of two new beta-adrenergic receptor antagonists. *J Pharmacol Exp Ther* 149:161, 1965.

28. Lish PM, Shelanski MV, LaBudde JA, et al: Inhibition of cardiac chronotropic action of isoproterenol by Sotalol (MJ1999) in rat, dog and man. *Curr Ther Res* 9:311, 1967.

29. Singh BN, Vaughan Williams EM: A third class of anti-arrhythmic action: Effects on atrial and ventricular intracellular potentials, and other pharmacological actions on cardiac muscle of MJ1999 and AH 3474. *Br J Pharmacol* 39:675, 1970.

30. Singh BN, Vaughan Williams EM: The effect of amiodarone, a new anti-anginal drug, on cardiac muscle. Br J Pharmacol 39:657, 1970.

31. Singh BN, Hauswirth O: Comparative mechanisms of action of antiarrhythmic drugs. *Am Heart J* 87:367, 1974.

32. Singh BN, Collett JT, Chew CYC: New perspectives in the pharmacologic therapy of cardiac arrhythmias. *Prog Cardiovasc Dis* 20:243, 1980.

33. Charlier R, Deltour G, Baudine A, et al: Pharmacology of amiodarone, an anti-anginal drug with a new biological profile. *Arzneim Forsch* 18:1408, 1968.

34. Charlier R: Cardiac actions in the dog of a new antagonist of adrenergic excitation which does not produce competitive blockade of adrenoceptors. *Br J Pharmacol* 39:668, 1970.

35. Petta JM, Zaccheo VJ: Comparative profile of L3428 and other antianginal agents on cardiac hemodynamics. *J Pharmacol Exp Ther* 176:328, 1971.

36. Singh BN, Jewitt DE, Downey JM et al: Effects of amiodarone and L8040, novel antianginal and antiarrhythmic drugs, on cardiac and coronary haemodynamics and on cardiac intracellular potentials. *Clin Exp Pharmacol Physiol* 3:427, 1976.

37. Gough WB, Zeiler RH, Barreca P, et al: Hypotensive action of commercial intravenous amiodarone and polysorbate 80 in dogs. *J Cardiovasc Pharmacol* 4:375, 1982.

38. Ourbak P, Rocher R, Aziza JP, et al: Effets hemodynamiques de l'jection intra-veineuse de chlorhydrate d'amiodarone chez le sujet normal et le coronarien. *Arch Mal Coeur* 69:293, 1976.

39. Pfisterer M, Burkart F, Muller-Brand J, et al: Important differences between short- and long-term hemodynamic effects of amiodarone in patients with chronic ischemic heart disease at rest and during ischemia-induced left ventricular dysfunction. *J Am Coll Cardiol* 5:1205, 1985.

40. Sicart M, Besse P, Choussat A, et al: Action hemodynamique de l'amiodarone intra-veineuse chez l'homme. *Arch Mal Coeur* 70:219, 1977.
41. Cote P, Bourassa MG, Delaye J, et al: Effects of amiodarone on cardiac and coronary hemodynamics and on myocardial metabolism in patients with coronary artery disease. *Circulation* 59:1165, 1979.
42. Bellotti G, Silva LA, Filho AE, et al: Hemodynamic effects of intravenous administration of amiodarone in congestive heart failure from chronic Chagas' disease. *Am J Cardiol* 52:1046, 1983.
43. Kosinski EJ, Albin JB, Young E, et al: Hemodynamic effects of intravenous admiodarone. *J Am Coll Cardiol* 4:565, 1984.
44. Schwartz A, Shen E, Morady F, et al: Hemodynamic effects of intravenous amiodarone in patients with depressed left ventricular function and recurrent ventricular tachycardia. *Am Heart J* 106:848, 1983.
45. Remme WJ, van Hoogenhuyze DCA, Krauss XH, et al: Acute hemodynamic and antiischemic effects of intravenous amiodarone. *Am J Cardiol* 55:639, 1985.
46. Singh BN: Amiodarone: Historical development and pharmacologic profile. *Am Heart J* 106:788, 1983.
47. Rotmensch HH, Belhassen B, Ferguson RK: Amiodarone-benefits and risks in perspective. *Am Heart J* 104:1117, 1982.
48. de Paola AAV, Horowitz LN, Spielman SR, et al: Amiodarone therapy in patients with sustained ventricular tachyarrhythmias: Observations on heart failure and the influence of ejection fraction. *Am J Cardiol* (in press 1987).
49. Mostow ND, Vrobel TR, Noon D, et al: Rapid suppression of complex ventricular arrhythmias with high-dose oral amiodarone. *Circulation* 73:1231, 1986.
50. Greene HL, Graham EL, Werner JA, et al: Toxic and therapeutic effects of amiodarone in the treatment of cardiac arrhythmias. *J Am Coll Cardiol* 2:1114, 1983.
51. Haffajee CI, Love JC, Alpert JS, et al: Efficacy and safety of long-term amiodarone in treatment of cardiac arrhythmias: Dosage experience. *Am Heart J* 106:935, 1983.
52. Valantine H, Dickie S, Lavender JP, et al: Lack of effect of amiodarone on impaired left ventricular function: Comparison with disopyramide. (abst) *Circulation* 72:III-167, 1985.
53. Haffajee CI, Love JC, Canada AT, et al: Clinical pharmacokinetics and efficacy of amiodarone for refractory tachyarrhythmias. *Circulation* 67:1347, 1983.
54. Paulus WJ, Nellens P, Heyndrick X, et al: Effects of long-term treatment with amiodarone on exercise hemodynamics and left ventricular relaxation in patients with hypertrophic cardiomyopathy. *Circulation* 74:544, 1986.
55. Kluger J, Drayer D, Reidenberg M, et al: The clinical pharmacology and antiarrhythmic efficacy of acetylprocainamide in patients with arrhythmias. *Am J Cardiol* 45:1250, 1980.
56. Lertora JJL, Glock D, Stec GP, et al: Effects of N-acetylprocainamide and procainamide on myocardial contractile force, heart rate, and blood pressure (40547). *Proc Soc Exp Biol Med* 161:332, 1979.
57. Lertora JJL, King LW, Donkor KA: The inotropic actions of N-

acetylprocainamide: Blockade and reversal by propranolol. *Angiology* 37:939, 1986.
58. Badke FR, Walsh RA, Crawford MH: Hemodynamic effects of N-acetylprocainamide compared with procainamide in conscious dogs. *Circulation* 64:1142, 1981.
59. Atkinson AJ, Lee WK, Quinn ML, et al: Dose-ranging trial of N-acetylprocainamide in patients with premature ventricular contractions. *Clin Pharmacol Ther* 21:575, 1977.
60. Lertora JJL, Atkinson AJ, Kushner W, et al: Long-term antiarrhythmic therapy with N-acetylprocainamide. *Clin Pharmacol Ther* 25:273, 1979.
61. Crawford MH, Ludden TM, Kennedy GT, et al: Hemodynamic effects of N-acetylprocainamide in heart disease. *Clin Pharmacol Ther* 31:459, 1982.
62. Josephson MA, Schwab M, Coyle K, et al: Effects of intravenous N-acetylprocainamide on hemodynamics and left ventricular function in man. *Am Heart J* 113:952, 1987.

# Chapter 6

# Pharmacokinetics of the Class III Antiarrhythmic Agents

Robert E. Kates, Ram Kannan, and Bramah N. Singh

As indicated elsewhere in this volume, control of cardiac arrhythmias by prolonging the action potential duration in a selective manner now has an increasing appeal. The agents that exert their salutary effects in this way appear to share certain pharmacologic effects. The pharmacokinetic characteristics of the Class III antiarrhythmic drugs—amiodarone, bretylium, N-acetylprocainamide (NAPA), and sotalol—form the basis of this chapter. Although these agents are grouped together based on their electropharmacologic actions, chemically, they are very different from one another (see Fig. 1) and have dissimilar physicochemical properties. In this review, the unique characteristics of each drug will be emphasized. The data discussed are likely to be relevant to their effective clinical application in the control of ventricular and supraventricular tachyarrhythmias.

## General Comparative Features

Both the cardiac effects[1,2] and the pharmacokinetic characteristics[3] of antiarrhythmic drugs are modulated by their solubility and molecular composition. Therefore, it is not unreasonable to anticipate that a group of drugs (such as the Class III antiarrhythmic agents) that produce qualitatively similar cardiac effects might have somewhat similar physicochemical properties and, conse-

---

From: *Control of Cardiac Arrhythmias by Lengthening Repolarization*, edited by Bramah N. Singh, MD, Futura Publishing Company Inc., Mount Kisco, NY, © 1988.

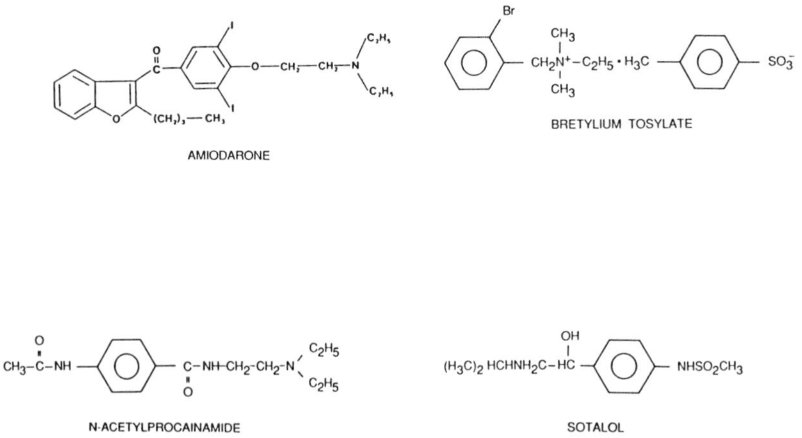

AMIODARONE

BRETYLIUM TOSYLATE

N-ACETYLPROCAINAMIDE

SOTALOL

**Figure 1.** Chemical structures of major Class III antiarrhythmic agents. Note their structural dissimilarities.

quently, similar pharmacokinetic characteristics. While bretylium, NAPA, and sotalol share some similarities, amiodarone clearly stands alone as a unique agent. Indeed, although classified as a Class III antiarrhythmic agent, even its electrophysiologic profile is considerably broader (see Chapter 14), as are its potency and efficacy as an antiarrhythmic agent in the clinical setting. In a listing of antiarrhythmic drugs based on solubility, amiodarone resides at an extreme end of the spectrum as one of the most highly lipid soluble antiarrhythmic compounds; bretylium, NAPA, and sotalol are at the opposite end of the spectrum representing the most polar, hydrophilic, agents.

As with other aspects of Class III agents, their absorption and bioavailability characteristics represent extremes. Sotalol and NAPA are almost completely absorbed, with bioavailability in the 90–100 percent range; amiodarone and bretylium are absorbed poorly and slowly, with very low availability.

With few exceptions, the drugs currently available for the treatment of cardiac rhythm abnormalities undergo extensive biotransformation in the liver and are highly dependent on metabolic processes for their deactivation and elimination. It is noteworthy that the three antiarrhythmic drugs that are the exceptions to this rule are all Class III agents. Sotalol, bretylium, and NAPA are eliminated almost entirely by renal excretion. Amiodarone, maintaining its uniqueness within this classification, is metabolized almost entirely.

These differences, which are emphasized further in the discussion of the properties of individual agents, are likely to be important in determining the pharmacokinetic characteristics of various compounds that act by lengthening repolarization.

The pharmacokinetics of NAPA and bretylium are discussed at length in Chapters 11 and 12. Only the salient features are presented here for completeness. The bulk of this chapter is devoted to the pharmacokinetics of sotalol and amiodarone. Each of the four drugs is discussed with respect to its fundamental pharmacokinetic features.

## Pharmacokinetics of Bretylium

Bretylium is highly soluble in aqueous media and only very slightly soluble in organic or lipophilic media. Bretylium is a halogenated quarternary ammonium compound, which is the most hydrophilic of the currently available antiarrhythmic agents. Its high degree of aqueous solubility is not surprising for a compound that permanently bears a positive charge. At a pH of 7.4, the octanol/buffer distribution coefficient of bretylium is only 0.1.[3] The intravenous formulation of bretylium contains the tosylate salt. Bretylium base is equivalent to 52 percent of bretylium tosylate by weight.

## Absorption and Metabolism

Bretylium is absorbed poorly and variably following oral administration. Anderson et al.[4] evaluated the bioavailability of bretylium tosylate (5 mg/kg) in 10 healthy volunteer subjects. They reported a low but variable bioavailability ranging from 11.6 percent to 32.1 percent (mean 22.6 percent). Peak plasma concentrations ranged from 38 to 143 ng/ml, and the time to peak level varied from 1 to 9 hours after ingestion. Garrett et al.[5] found similar results in a study conducted in normal volunteers. These investigators administered doses ranging from 100 to 400 mg and found no evidence of dose-dependent bioavailability.

Unlike amiodarone, bretylium is not metabolized. In one study, Anderson et al.[4] evaluated the route of elimination of bretylium in 10 normal volunteer subjects following intravenous administration. They reported that bretylium is completely eliminated in the urine as unchanged drug over a period of 2–3 days.

## Distribution and Elimination

Though bretylium is a highly polar compound, its volume of distribution (3–5 kg) suggests that it accumulates significantly in body tissues.[4,5] Very little has been reported concerning its tissue accumulation, but Anderson et al. have shown that bretylium does accumulate in the myocardium of dogs to levels about twelvefold greater than the plasma levels.[6]

In contrast to its tissue binding, bretylium does not bind significantly to plasma proteins. Anderson et al.[4] studied the binding of bretylium to human plasma proteins over the range of 0.03 µg/ml to 30 µg/ml, and found binding to be negligible at all levels. Garrett et al.[5] reported the binding of bretylium to plasma protein to be about 6 percent.

Unlike amiodarone, bretylium is eliminated from the body by renal excretion. Anderson et al.[4] studied the disposition kinetics of bretylium following both oral and intravenous administration to 10 healthy volunteer subjects. They found that within 48 hours, 100 percent of an intravenous dose is excreted in the urine; however, they found a significant difference in the renal clearance of bretylium following intravenous and oral administration. The renal clearance of bretylium following oral administration was 4.2 times the renal clearance after an intravenous dose. They concluded that the renal clearance of bretylium may be nonlinear at the high plasma levels achieved with intravenous administration.

These same investigators evaluated the plasma level time course of bretylium following administration of both oral and intravenous doses. They observed that the terminal log-linear decay phase was not evident in many of their subjects until 16–24 hours after drug administration. This suggests very slow tissue distribution. They reported average terminal elimination half-lives of 6 hours and 13.6 hours for the oral and intravenous doses, respectively. This conclusion, however, is not consistent with the findings of Garrett and et al.[5] These investigators performed an extensive evaluation of the pharmacokinetics of bretylium over a broad range of doses. In their study, they found the elimination half-life following either oral (10 hours) or intravenous (9 hours) administration to be similar.

Since bretylium is eliminated entirely via the kidneys, its clearance is reduced in renal failure. Josselson et al.[7] reported a significant relationship between the renal clearance of bretylium and creatinine clearance. Hemodialysis does not significantly increase the clearance of bretylium in anephric patients.

## Concentration–Response Relationships

Since the use of bretylium is restricted primarily to the emergency treatment of ventricular arrhythmias, therapeutic response and not a plasma level must guide dosage determination. In one study Woosley et al.[8] attempted to evaluate the relationship between the plasma levels of bretylium and clinical efficacy in patients treated with multiple oral doses for control of recurrent ventricular tachycardia. The minimum effective plasma concentrations they reported were in the range of 1.1 to 2.3 µg/ml. However, at these levels all patients experienced significant hypotension.

In an effort to study the relationships between plasma and myocardial levels of bretylium and its effect on the ventricular fibrillation threshold (VFT), Anderson et al.[6] studied this drug after intravenous administration in anesthetized dogs. They observed a significant delay in the time to the maximal effect, which occurred 3–6 hours after administration of a single intravenous bolus dose. While there was no relationship between the plasma levels and cardiac effects of bretylium, there was a clear relationship between the cardiac effects (e.g., a change in VFT) and the myocardial drug concentrations.

## N-Acetylprocainamide (NAPA)

Like bretylium, NAPA is very soluble in aqueous media but only slightly soluble in nonpolar organic solvents. NAPA is slightly more lipophilic than procainamide; at a pH of 7.4 its octanol/buffer partition coefficient is 0.31, compared to 0.11 for procainamide.[3] The pharmaceutical formulation of NAPA employed for clinical evaluation is the hydrochloride salt.

### Absorption and Elimination

NAPA appears to be absorbed rapidly and completely following oral administration. Peak concentrations are achieved within 1–3 hours after drug administration.[9] The absolute bioavailability of NAPA has been studied in 3 normal volunteer subjects. The results indicate almost complete absorption with values of 100 percent, 93 percent, and 82 percent for the subjects. Winkle et al.[9] studied the relationship between dose and mean steady-state plasma concentrations of NAPA during chronic administration. They found, for each patient, a linear relationship between dose and mean steady-state plasma concentration. However, a threefold range of intersubject variability was found.

Renal excretion also is the major route of elimination of NAPA. Following oral administration, 59–87 percent of a dose is excreted unchanged in the urine.[10,11] The routes of nonrenal elimination of NAPA have not yet been thoroughly elucidated. It has been shown that a small amount of NAPA is deacetylated back to procainamide. The only other metabolite of N-acetylprocainamide to be identified is desethyl-NAPA. In one study,[12] NAPA was administered intravenously to a normal volunteer subject, and urine was collected and analyzed. Less than 1 percent of the administered dose was eliminated as the desethylated compound; 2.8 percent of the dose was deacetylated, and 86.6 percent was excreted unchanged. They were unable to account for 10 percent of the administered dose.

NAPA, being a highly hydrophilic compound, does not have great affinity for tissues. The volume of distribution of NAPA is only 1–2 l/kg.[13] Consistent with its weak affinity for tissues, NAPA is bound only slightly to plasma proteins. Reidenberg et al.[14] studied the binding of NAPA to proteins in the plasma of normal subjects. Over the concentration range of 1–16 µg/ml, they found binding to be only about 10 percent.

The elimination of NAPA is characterized by a plasma disappearance half-life of 5–15 hours.[13] Following oral administration, 59–87 percent of a dose of NAPA is excreted unchanged in the urine. Stec et al. have reported the renal clearance of NAPA to be 199.5 ml/min in patients with normal renal function.[11] It appears that the renal clearance of NAPA is greater than the clearance of creatinine, indicating active secretion. Since clearance of NAPA is dependent on renal function, it decreases significantly in patients with renal function impairment. Several studies have found a strong direct correlation between creatinine clearance and both the renal and total body clearance of NAPA.[11,15,16] This linear relationship between the renal clearance of NAPA and creatinine clearance has been demonstrated in several patient populations, including individuals with normal renal function as well as those with end-stage renal failure.

## Concentration–Response Relationships

The relationship between plasma concentrations of NAPA and arrhythmia suppression has been studied by several investigators.[9,15,17] While there are considerable differences in the conclusions of the different studies, it appears that levels between 15 and 25 µg/ml most commonly are reported to be associated with significant PVC reduction. However, it should be noted that Winkle et al.[9] reported 1 patient who first responded to NAPA at a plasma level of 32.3 µg/ml. Unfortunately, NAPA has a very narrow therapeutic window between therapeutic and toxic concentrations. Winkle et al.[9] also reported side effects in 3 of 11 patients at plasma NAPA levels below 10 µg/ml. Roden et al.[17] estimated that there was a 50 percent risk of adverse effects when a therapeutic response had been achieved with NAPA. Clearly, further data are needed to define the toxic–therapeutic ratio, especially in different subsets of patients with ventricular arrhythmias.

## Pharmacokinetics of Sotalol

The pharmacokinetics of sotalol has been studied extensively in experimental animals and in humans. The clinical pharmacokinetic profile of the drug is shown in Table 1 and the major pharmacokinetic constants of the drug are compared with those of other beta-adrenoceptor blocking drugs in Table 2. It is the only available beta blocker that exhibits Class III electrophysiologic properties.

The solubility of sotalol is very similar to that of bretylium. Sotalol is very polar and, consequently, highly soluble in aqueous but not organic media. Sotalol has a pKa of 9.02 and at a pH of 7.4, its chloroform/water partition coefficient is only 0.03. Similarly, its octanol/water partition coefficient is low (discussed later), about 0.1.[3] Sotalol is a compound with an asymmetric center. The drug can be measured accurately in biological fluids by high-pressure liquid chromatography.[18,19]

## Drug Disposition and Plasma Concentrations

Schnelle and Garrett[20] studied the absorption, distribution, and excretion of sotalol in conscious dogs after intravenous as well as oral drug administration. They found unchanged sotalol to be excreted 90 percent in the urine with no protein binding, and the partition coefficient between plasma and red cells was unity. The graphic fit of the plasma levels following the intravenous administration in accordance with a two-compartment open-body model indicated a rapid distribution phase with a half-life of about 3.2 hours, followed by an elimination phase with a half-life of about

Table 1
Clinical Pharmacokinetic Profile of Sotalol

| | |
|---|---|
| Absorption rate | $T_{max}$: 2−3 hours |
| Extent of absorption | > 90% of dose |
| Bioavailability | 100% |
| Protein binding | 0% |
| Volume of distribution | 1.6−2.4 liters/kg |
| Elimination, Renal (unchanged) | > 75% |
| Biotransformation | 0% |
| Elimination half-life | 10−15 hours |
| Total body clearance | 0.11−0.4 liters/min |
| Pattern of elimination kinetics | First order |
| Kinetic model applicable | Open two compartment |
| Metabolites | None detected |
| Steady-state/dose ratio | Twofold |
| Therapeutic plasma range | 1−3 µg/ml |
| Dose schedule | One or twice daily |
| Special features | Accumulation in renal failure; kinetics unaffected by liver function. |

Source: Adapted from Sundquist H. Basic review and comparison of beta-blocker pharmacokinetics. *Curr Ther Res* 28:388, 1980.

4.8 hours. The data have been similar in humans although the distribution and elimination half-lives have been found to be very much longer. The distribution characteristics of sotalol are similar to those of NAPA. The volume of distribution of sotalol is only 1−2 l/kg, indicating only minor distribution to body tissue sites.[21] Sotalol, like bretylium, does not bind to plasma proteins to any significant extent.

## Absorption

Despite its highly polar nature, sotalol appears to be rapidly absorbed, with peak levels being achieved between 2.5 and 4 hours after administration. The absorption of sotalol in humans, however, occurs more slowly than that found for most other beta blockers.[21−24] The absorption of sotalol is not affected significantly by antacids[25] but it may be reduced by food[26] especially milk and milk products, which reduce bioavailability of the drug; it is possible that an interaction with calcium ions may be the major reason for the decreased drug absorption.

## Table 2
### Pharmacokinetic Parameters of Sotalol Compared to Those of Other Beta Blockers

| Beta Blocker | Daily dose (mg) | Absorption (%) | First-pass Effect (%) | Bioavailability (%) | Log Part Coeff-Octanol/water* | Elimination Half-Life (H) | Clearance (ml/min) | Parent Drug in Urine (%) | Protein Binding (%) |
|---|---|---|---|---|---|---|---|---|---|
| Acebutolol | 300 | 70 | 30 | 50 | 1.87 | 3−4 | 615 | 18 | 27 |
| Atenolol | 200 | 50 | <10 | 50 | 0.23 | 6−9 | 130 | 40 | 5 |
| Labetalol | 600 | >90 | 60 | 33 | — | 2−3 | 2700 | < 4 | 50 |
| Metoprolol | 300 | >90 | 50 | 50 | 2.15 | 3−4 | 1100 | 3 | 12 |
| Nadolol | 80 | 34 | 0 | 34 | 0.71 | 10−12 | 200 | 34 | 28 |
| Oxprenolol | 160 | 90 | 40 | 50 | 2.18 | 1−2 | 380 | 3 | 80 |
| Pindolol | 15 | >90 | 13 | 87 | 1.75 | 3−4 | 400 | 35 | 40 |
| Propranolol | 300 | >90 | 60 | 30 | 3.65 | 2−3 | 1000 | < 1 | 93 |
| Sotalol | 240 | >80 | 0 | >80 | −0.79 | 7−15 | 150 | 75 | 0 |
| Timolol | 30 | >90 | 25 | 75 | 2.10 | 2−5 | 660 | 5 | 10 |

*Data from Cruiskshank[37].

Source: Mier AJ: Pharmacokinetic comparison of pindolol with other beta-adrenoceptor blocking agents. *Am Heart J* 104:364, 1982.

The $t_{max}$ for single doses of 80 mg has been reported to be 2–3 hours, whereas values of about 1.5 hours have been found for many other beta antagonists. Sotalol is well absorbed, about 75 percent of the drug being excreted in the urine within 72 hours after single dose administration. The protein binding of the drug appears to be negligible.

The absolute bioavailability following sotalol on oral administration approaches 100 percent indicating negligible first-pass effect in the liver or metabolic transformation.[21] The plasma clearance of sotalol, unlike that of propranolol, is not dependent on liver enzyme metabolizing capacity[27] but it may be reduced by drinking alcohol.[28] No active metabolites of the drug have been identified.[29-31] The urinary excretion is solely by the process of glomerular filtration.[32]

The disposition kinetics of sotalol has been evaluated by several investigators in normal subjects[21,33] and patients.[34,35] For individuals with normal renal function, the half-life of sotalol is in the range of 9 to 18 hours. Pharmacokinetically, sotalol conforms to an open, linear two-compartment model[36] in which all processes of drug absorption, distribution, and elimination occur by first-order kinetics (see Table 3). After oral dosing with 160 mg of the drug, the peak plasma levels varied between 1.4 and 1.7 mg/liter at 2–3 hours after dosing. The total apparent volume of distribution was 1.5 times the body weight and the rate-limiting factor that controlled the terminal serum elimination half-life of sotalol was the apparent rate of diffusion of the drug from the central compartment.[32] As with bretylium and NAPA, the major route of elimination of sotalol is by renal excretion. Poirier et al. reported that about 90 percent of an administered dose of sotalol is excreted unchanged in the urine.[33] It appears that the balance of the administered dose is excreted into the feces.

## Lipophilicity, CNS Uptake, and Clearance

Numerous investigators have measured the partition coefficient in octanol/water to quantify the lipophilic versus hydrophilic properties of various beta blockers.[37] These properties, relative to other pharmacokinetic constants, are shown in Table 2. In anesthetized cats, Rendt et al.[38] reported that propranolol had the highest rate of penetration into the CSF with the highest brain–plasma uptake ratio (38.0). In contrast, sotalol, the most hydrophilic drug in the series that was studied, had the slowest CSF entry and the lowest brain–plasma ratio (0.52). These findings are in agreement

|               | **Table 3** |
| **Clinical Pharmacokinetic Profile of Amiodarone** | |
| --- | --- |
| Absorption rate | $T_{max}$: 2–12 hours (lag time 0.4–3 hrs) |
| Extent of Absorption | Poor and slow |
| Bioavailability | Variable (22–86%) |
| Protein Binding | 96.3 ± 0.6% |
| Volume of distribution | 1.3–65.8 l/kg (acute) |
| Elimination, Renal | Negligible renal excretion |
| Biotransformation | Hepatic and intestinal |
| Elimination half-life | 3.2–20.7 hrs (acute); *13.7–52.6 days (chronic) |
| Total body clearance | 0.10–0.77 l/min. |
| Pattern of elimination kinetics | First order |
| Metabolites | Major: Mono N-desethylamiodarone; Minor: bis-N-desethylamiodarone, deiodinated metabolites |
| Therapeutic plasma range | 1–2.5 μg/ml |
| Dose schedule | Once daily |
| Special factors | Slow onset and offset of action |

*A terminal elimination half life of 24.8 ± 11.7 days was reported by Holt et al.[82] after a 400 mg IV dose in 6 healthy volunteers.

with those found in humans. For example, in one study in which sotalol was measured in the plasma and the CSF after single doses of the drug, the CSF level was only 10 percent of that in the plasma.[23] However, there is some controversy as to whether sotalol or atenolol is the most hydrophilic of the beta blockers that have been studied in this regard. The most recent study has revealed that although the distribution coefficients of the two beta blockers are somewhat similar, that for atenolol was lower.[39] Ochs et al.[40] studied single-dose kinetics of oral propranolol, metoprolol, atenolol, and sotalol in relation to the lipophilic properties of these beta antagonists. They found that propranolol had the largest oral clearance and sotalol the least, with the in vitro lipid solubility of the compounds being highly correlated with their oral clearance, indicating that the physicochemical properties of beta blockers appeared to influence their intrinsic clearance after oral dosage.[40]

## Renal Insufficiency and Elimination Half-Life of Sotalol

Since sotalol is not metabolized in the liver, its pharmacokinetics is not affected by hepatic function. However, since it is excreted largely by the renal route, the serum levels of the drug for any given dose is likely to vary linearly with the creatinine clearance (Fig. 2). This has been demonstrated by a number of investigators.[24,34,41–43] For example, Berglund et al.[34] studied sotalol kinetics in normal subjects and in those with impaired renal function. In subjects with creatinine clearance equal to or greater than 39 ml/min/m$^2$, sotalol plasma clearance was 71 ± 31 ml/min/m$^2$, elimination half-life was 8.1 ± 3.4 hours, and renal clearance was 46 ± 26 ml/min/m$^2$. In patients with moderate impairment of renal function (creatinine clearance of 8–38 ml/min/m$^2$), the $t_{1/2}$ was 24.2 ± 7.5 hours with a plasma clearance of the drug of 24 ± 7 ml/min/m$^2$. In patients on dialysis, the $t_{1/2}$ was found to be 33.9 ± 27.1 hours. During dialysis, the elimination half-life was 5.8 ± 2.1 hours and was associated with a reduction of 56.7 ± 21 percent in plasma levels. These data indicate that in patients with moderately reduced renal function the initial dose of sotalol should

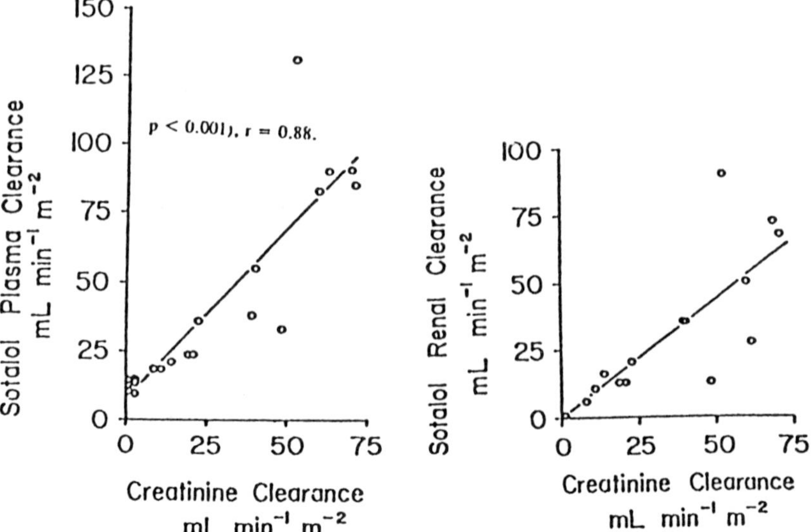


**Figure 2.** Relationship between creatinine clearance, sotalol plasma clearance (left panel) and sotalol renal clearance (right panel). Sotalol plasma clearance = 8.34 ± 1.22 [creatinine clearance] (p < 0.001; r = 0.88). Sotalol renal clearance = -0.75 ± 0.90 [creatinine clearance] (p < 0.001; r = 0.85). (From Blair AD, Burgess ED, Maxwell BM, et al: Sotalol kinetics in renal insufficiency. *Clin Pharmacol Ther* 29:457, 1981. By permission of the authors and of the Editor of *Clinical Pharmacology and Therapeutics*.)

be 160 mg/day and subsequent dose adjustment should be made in light of the clinical response and plasma drug levels. In cases with severely diminished renal function (e.g., GFR less than 25 ml/min/1.73m$^2$ BSA), the drug should be used with a great deal of caution with regular monitoring of serum drug levels. In cases of overdosage or excessively high serum drug levels with life-threatening effects, the studies of Blair et al.[43] indicate that hemodialysis rapidly may reverse the effects by reducing the serum drug concentrations.

## Pharmacokinetics of Sotalol in Pregnancy

Beta-blockers are used widely in the control of hypertension during pregnancy.[44] It has been reported that sotalol does not cross the placenta[45] in the pregnant ewe. However, O'Hare et al.[46] have shown that in humans the drug does cross the placenta rapidly. They found that the elimination half-life of the drug was approximately 14 hours, but was not affected by pregnancy,[46] which also had no effect on bioavailability. Erkkola et al.[47] found sotalol levels in the maternal circulation twice (four times in the case of propranolol) that in the umbilical cord. It appears that the more rapid clearance noted during pregnancy may be due to increases in renal plasma flow and glomerular filtration.[46]

## Effect of Age on Sotalol Pharmacokinetics

Limited data are available in this regard. Ishizaki et al.[48] compared the pharmacokinetics and pharmacodynamics of sotalol in young hypertensive versus elderly hypertensive subsets of patients. In the elderly patients, the terminal half-life of the drug was prolonged (11 versus 7 hours approximately), the total plasma clearance was reduced, and this was considered to be due primarily to reduced renal clearance of the drug (1.93 versus 4.10 ml/min/kg). There was also a decrease in the volume of distribution in the elderly. The increased serum levels of the drug in the elderly patients was attributed to a reduction in both the total plasma clearance and the volume of distribution, there being no evidence of impaired absorption of the drug. The authors found a significant correlation between the plasma drug levels and the reduction in the absolute values of exercise-induced increments in heart rate. It is of interest that while the plasma levels of the drug decayed by first-order kinetics, the pharmacodynamic actions declined by zero-order rate, indicating that the effects of the beta blocker outlasted its serum half-life.

## Pharmacokinetic and Pharmacodynamic Correlations

After a single oral sotalol dose of 400 mg, or after 400 mg daily doses for 8 days, Brown et al.[49] found an elimination half-life of 15.5 ± 1.2 and 17.7 ± 2.6 hours, respectively. They did not find a significant difference in the plasma concentrations between the two drug elimination curves. Thus, chronic therapy with the drug did not alter its kinetics. At the end of 3 hours after a dose of the drug, the exercise-induced tachycardia was attenuated by about 39 percent; at the end of 24 hours, just before the next dose, it was reduced by 20 percent. These observations therefore indicate that 400 mg sotalol per day provide an effective dosage regimen for sustained beta blockade for 24 hours. This is supported further by the studies of other investigators,[50,51] who found 15–18 percent reduction in exercise-induced tachycardia 24 hours after a dose of the oral drug. Harron et al.[52] determined the effects of varying doses of sotalol on exercise-induced tachycardia as a function of plasma concentration. The maximum effect occurred at 2 or 3 hours and was greater with each increasing dose, although the effect of 50 mg of the drug was negligible. The effects of 400 mg was significantly greater than that of 200 mg. All four doses (50 mg, 100 mg, 200 mg, 400 mg), reduced exercise-induced changes in heart rate at 24 hours. The data indicated that the effects of sotalol in blocking beta receptors occurred as a function of drug dose and plasma concentration as well as that of the elimination half-life.

Several studies have been conducted to evaluate whether a clinically useful relationship exists between plasma sotalol concentrations and its antiarrhythmic efficacy. Teo et al.[53] evaluated intravenous infusions of sotalol for the treatment of supraventricular tachycardias. Patients who responded to sotalol had an average ( ± SE) plasma concentration of 0.526 ± 0.088 µg/ml. Nonresponders, on the average, had slightly higher levels. No relationship between plasma sotalol concentratons and therapeutic effectiveness was observed. Nademanee et al.[54] reported plasma sotalol levels of 2.3 ± 0.8 (160 mg b.i.d.) and 3.1 ± 0.4 µg/ml (320 mg b.i.d.) in patients being treated chronically with sotalol for the treatment of ventricular tachycardia. No attempt was made, however, to relate plasma sotalol levels to antiarrhythmic efficacy. Recently, Creamer et al.[55] studied the acute and chronic effects of sotalol on ventricular repolarization in 8 patients. They observed serum sotalol concentrations in the range of 1–4 µg/ml, but found no correlation between any electrocardiographic intervals and sotalol levels. They reported, however, that there was a greater QT and JT prolongation after chronic oral sotalol therapy than after acute intravenous administration at corresponding serum drug levels. They concluded that this supported the possibility that an additional delayed tissue effect may be responsible.

Based on the available data, at present there are no criteria for interpreting sotalol plasma concentrations in relation to their clinical usefulness, but the utility for drug levels in averting the development of torsades de pointes is not excluded.

## Pharmacokinetics and Metabolism of Amiodarone

Although the electrophysiologic and hemodynamic characterists of amiodarone have been well documented,[56,57] information on its pharmacokinetics and disposition only recently have become available. Development of sensitive and specific liquid chromatographic methods for the measurement of amiodarone in serum and tissues[58–67] has aided in pharmacokinetic and metabolic studies of amiodarone. Most of these methods have the capability of quantitating the major metabolite of amiodarone, desethylamiodarone, in body fluids simultaneously with amiodarone. The salient pharmacokinetic constants of amiodarone are listed in Table 3.

The physicochemical properties of amiodarone previously have been described in detail by Bonati et al.[68] Amiodarone is an amphiphilic compound with both hydrophilic and hydrophobic regions. However, amiodarone is very poorly soluble in aqueous or polar media, but is highly soluble in chloroform and other nonpolar organic solvents. The $pK_a$ of amiodarone is 6.56 and its maximal lipid solubility occurs in the pH range of 3.5 to 5.5.[68] The pharmaceutical formulation of amiodarone contains the drug in the form of its hydrochloride salt.

## Absorption and Bioavailability

The absorption of amiodarone following oral administration is erratic,[69] and the time to reach peak plasma concentrations has been reported to vary from 2 to 12 hours.[60,69–71] After a single oral dose Kannan et al.[71] found that the metabolite appeared as early as after 30 minutes and had a $t_{max}$ of absorption similar to that of amiodarone (Fig. 3). The bioavailability of amiodarone has been reported to be highly variable, ranging from 22 percent to 85 percent, with an average of about 35 percent.[60,72] The available information on the bioavailability of amiodarone is shown in Table 4. Originally, it was thought that the large variation observed in bioavailability arose from the drug's poor water soluble properties.[68] But, in a recent report, Pourbaix et al.[73] showed that the bioavailability of an oral solution and a tablet formulation were similar, suggesting that the variation in bioavailability is probably due to interpatient differences in the first-pass effect of amiodarone rather than in its dissolution characteristics.

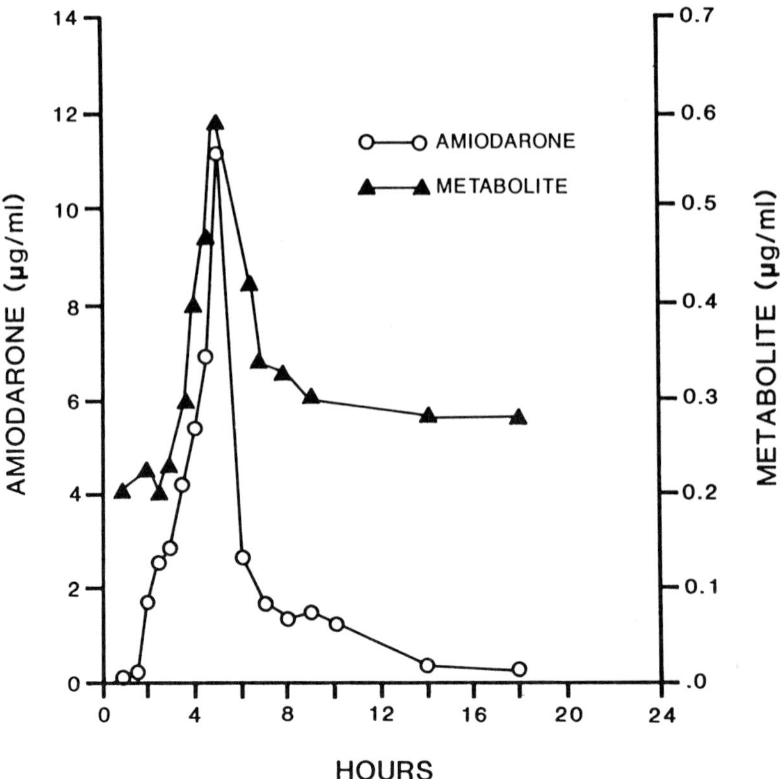


**Figure 3.** Serum concentrations of amiodarone and its metabolite after single oral administration of amiodarone (1400 mg) to a patient (After Kannan R, Nademanee K, Hendrickson J, et al: Amiodarone kinetics after oral doses. *Clin Pharmacol Ther* 31:438, 1982. By permission.)

## Metabolism

The metabolism of amiodarone has not been completely characterized. However, available evidence indicates that amiodarone is metabolized almost completely and only very minor amounts of the unchanged drug are excreted in either the urine or feces.[74-76] Several potential metabolites have been analyzed, but only desethylamiodarone has been identified positively in the blood of patients during oral therapy. This metabolite accumulates to steady-state concentrations that are comparable to those of the parent drug. Staubli et al.[77] evaluated the content of iodine containing compounds in sera from patients on chronic amiodarone therapy and reported that only 36 percent of total serum iodine is associated with amiodarone or desethylamiodarone; 64 percent is associated with unidentified amiodarone metabolites.

## Binding

Binding studies have been difficult to perform with amiodarone because of the drug's insolubility in physiological buffer solutions. Andreasen et al.[60] used ultrafiltration and equilibrium dialysis methods to show that amiodrone is strongly (96.3 ± 0.6 percent) bound to proteins in serum at a concentration of 10 $\mu$g/ml. About 60 percent of the whole blood concentration of amiodarone was found in red blood cells. Heger et al.[78] found that the amiodarone–metabolite ratio was different for red blood cells and extracellular fluid in patients on chronic amiodarone treatment. They suggested that red blood cell levels of the drug and the metabolite could serve as useful markers because of their good correlation to toxic effects.

Table 4
Bioavailability of Amiodarone

| Study | No. of Subjects | Mean ± SD % | Range % |
|---|---|---|---|
| Anastasiou et al.[63] | 4 | 35 ± 13 | 23–50 |
| Andreasen et al.[60] | 2 | 42 ± 19 | 22–80 |
| Holt et al.[82] | 6 | 35 ± 9 | 22–46 |
| Plomp et al.[84] | 7 | 31 ± 26 | 3–69 |
| Riva et al.[70] | 3 | 58 ± 33 | 22–86 |
| Pourbaix et al.[73] | 12 | 65 ± 22 | 22–104 |

In a recent communication Lalloz et al.[79] reported that amiodarone is bound mainly to albumin (62.1 percent) and to B-lipoprotein to a lesser extent (33.5 percent). More recent studies have shown that amiodarone is bound in almost equal proportions to albumin and $alpha_1$-acid glycoproteins.[80] The high molecular weight protein that Lalloz et al.[79] refer to as B-lipoprotein probably represents $alpha_1$-acid glycoprotein since it is known that these two proteins elute in the same region in the gel chromatographic method used by these authors. Kannan et al.[80] found that as in the case of amiodarone, desethylamiodarone also binds to albumin and $alpha_1$-acid glycoprotein. More definitive answers are likely to become available with the recent synthesis of labelled amiodarone.[81]

## Distribution and Tissue Accumulation

The distribution of amiodarone in the body is extensive, and an average volume of distribution of 66 l/kg has been reported.[82] Amiodarone is highly bound to body tissues, and several studies have been conducted to evaluate its tissue sites of accumulation. Broekhuysen et al.[69] administered 100 mg of $^{131}$I labelled amiodarone to 1 subject and measured regional isotope distribution by total body scanning. Analyses were performed daily for 6 days after administration. Radioactivity was observed to decrease slowly in lung, liver, heart, and kidney, while it remained almost constant in the limbs; radioactivity increased steadily over time in the thyroid gland. Recent studies in experimental animals[83,84] as well as in humans[85,86] support these earlier findings. Riva et al.[62] showed that after an intravenous dose of 50 mg/kg body weight to rats, amiodarone concentrations were higher in liver, kidney, and heart and lower in the brain. Adipose tissue was a major storage site for amiodarone with a fat−blood ratio of 1000 after 16 hours. In the rabbit, the myocardial amiodarone concentrations were 6−7 times that in serum 15 minutes after a single intravenous administration.[87] A much higher ratio (90:1) was found in the dog after an acute IV dose.[88] Kannan et al. recently examined the uptake of amiodarone in several tissues after chronic (6 week) administration.[83] Table 5 shows the mean concentrations of amiodarone and desethylamiodarone in various organs and the tissue to serum ratio for the drug and the metabolite. Fat had the highest concentration of amiodarone followed by lung, liver, and kidney. Desethylamiodarone concentrations were higher in liver, lung, and kidney. In a similar study in rats after repeated intra-peritoneal administration of amiodarone, Plomp et al.[84] found that the uptake of amiodarone by various tissues is dose-dependent. In contrast to data in rabbits and humans (discussed later), they found substantially lower concentrations of desethylamiodarone in tissues.

Haffajee et al.,[76] Holt et al.,[82] and Maggioni et al.[86] have determined amiodarone levels in post-mortem tissues of patients treated with amiodarone long term. Maggioni et al.[86] reported finding the highest levels in fat and lung, followed, in order, by the pancreas, liver, heart, and kidney. In a similar study, Holt et al.[82] reported post-mortem data from 9 patients; liver and fat contained the highest concentrations, followed by the lung, lymph node, myocardium, skeletal muscle, thyroid gland, and brain, in decreasing order. Interestingly, the concentrations of the desethyl metabolite (DEA) were higher than amiodarone in all tissues analyzed, except fat. A representative profile of tissue uptake is shown in Figure 4 taken from the work of Holt et al.[82] High levels of the drug and the metabolite have been reported in liver and lung biopsy samples in patients with hepatic and pulmonary toxicity.[89,90] The metabo-

---

### Table 5
### Amiodarone and Desethylamiodarone Concentrations in Serum and Tissues After Chronic Amiodarone Administration to Rabbits

| Tissue | Amiodarone (µg/g) | Desethylamiodarone (µg/g) | Amiodarone/ Desethylamiodarone Ratio |
|---|---|---|---|
| Fat | 55.98 ± 8.88 | trace | — |
| Lung | 23.03 ± 6.85 | 15.89 ± 4.41 | 1.51 ± 0.45 |
| Liver | 17.92 ± 7.43 | 18.56 ± 8.96 | 1.07 ± 0.58 |
| Muscle | 14.11 ± 5.28 | 2.67 ± 0.73 | 4.57 ± 0.70 |
| Spleen | 12.36 ± 4.20 | 10.49 ± 1.41 | 1.18 ± 0.27 |
| Kidney | 10.79 ± 1.69 | 6.81 ± 1.08 | 1.61 ± 0.33 |
| Bile[a] | 7.05 ± 2.68 | 5.28 ± 1.17 | 1.24 ± 0.25 |
| Ventricle | 6.90 ± 1.00 | 3.12 ± 0.43 | 2.37 ± 0.50 |
| Serum[a] | 1.42 ± 0.45 | 0.42 ± 0.20 | 3.95 ± 0.75 |
| Brain | trace[b] | trace[b] | — |

Note: All values are mean ± SE from 5–6 rabbits except for bile (n = 3).

[a]µg/ml.

[b]Amiodarone and desethylamiodarone were present in insignificant quantities in the brain.

Source: From Kannan R, Miller S, Singh BN: Tissue uptake and metabolism of amiodarone after chronic administration in rabbits. *Drug Metab Dispos* 13:646, 1985.

lite concentrations were two to three times higher than the parent drug indicating a possible relationship between the metabolite and toxicity. In specimens obtained during cardiac surgery, myocardium to serum ratio ranging from 20–60 for amiodarone and 100–260 for desethylamiodarone were found.[91,92] Zackary et al.[93] recently showed that the pigmented skin in chronically treated patients had concentrations of amiodarone and metabolite ten times that of nonpigmented skin. The significance of the presence of large amounts of the metabolite in tissues is not yet understood clearly.

Because of its toxic effects on the lung, the accumulation of amiodarone in the lungs of patients during chronic therapy has received considerable attention. High concentrations of amiodar-

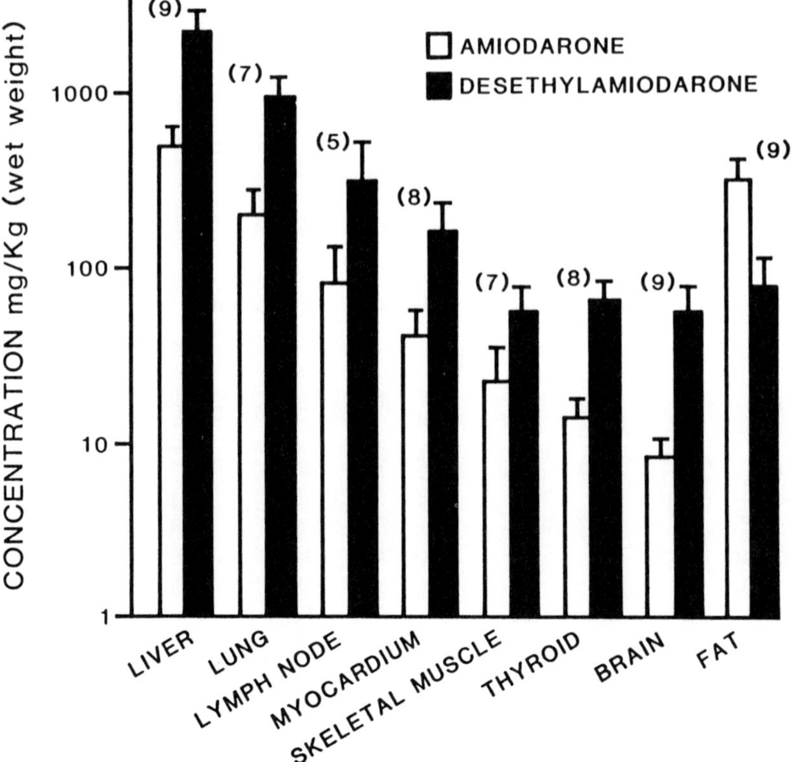


**Figure 4.** Amiodarone and desethylamiodarone concentrations in several post-mortem tissues. (From Holt DW, Tucker GT, Jackson PR, et al: Amiodarone pharmacokinetics. 13:646, 1985. By permission of the authors and of the American Heart Association.)

one and DEA (734 μg/g and 2551 μg/g, respectively) have been measured in lung biopsy samples from a patient with symptoms of pulmonary toxicity.[94] Recently, Camus and Mehendale[95] studied the uptake of amiodarone into isolated perfused rabbit and rat lungs. They observed that amiodarone accumulated extensively in lung tissue, and uptake was not saturable over the concentration range studied. They also observed that DEA accumulated in lung to a greater extent than did amiodarone.

## Tissue Drug Kinetics and Pharmacodynamic Correlation

Results on correlation of tissue levels to the pharmacological and electrophysiological effects of amiodarone have been conflicting (see also Chapter 14). Debbas et al.[91] showed that $QT_c$ prolongation correlated with plasma amiodarone levels better than with myocardial concentrations of amiodarone. On the other hand, Latini et al.[96] observed that the time course of amiodarone electrophysiologic effects after intravenous bolus administration in dogs followed its myocardial concentrations better than its blood concentrations. Yet in a recent study,[97] the prolongation of the ventricular refractory period during chronic amiodarone treatment did not correlate with myocardial amiodarone levels. Interestingly, the later study also revealed that the metabolite levels in the heart did not show any relationship to prolongation of the ventricular refractory period (in spite of increasing the desethylamiodarone concentration threefold by enzyme induction) indicating that the Class III action of amiodarone may not be related solely to desethylamiodarone. Further work is needed to clarify this issue. However, it is clear that a species difference exists in the myocardial accumulation of desethylamiodarone. While the metabolite to amiodarone ratio is low in rats,[97] rabbits,[95,98] and dogs,[88] Cantor et al.[99] noted in a clinical post-mortem study that desethylamiodarone accumulated in the myocardium to a much greater extent than amiodarone.

## Elimination Kinetics

As discussed earlier, bretylium, NAPA, and sotalol are eliminated primarily by renal excretion, while amiodarone is metabolized almost completely. Studies have been conducted in both normal volunteers and patients with cardiac arrhythmias to evaluate the pathways and kinetics of elimination of amiodarone. In this regard, the effects of the acutely versus chronically administered drug should be distinguished.

Riva et al.[70] collected urine for 72 hours after administering single 150 mg intravenous doses of amiodarone to 3 normal volunteers and found no unchanged drug excreted in the urine. Other investigators have reported similar findings supporting the conclusion that amiodarone is excreted only slightly, if at all, in the urine as unchanged drug.

The rate limiting step in the removal of amiodarone from the body appears to be the slow release of the drug from tissue-binding sites. Table 6 summarizes some of the pharmacokinetic parameters obtained by a number of laboratories. The terminal elimination half-life $(t_{1/2})$ after an intravenous administration varied over a wide range. The clearance accordingly was very low (0.14−0.69 l/min, Table 6). For example, Holt et al.[82] studied the pharmacokinetics in normal volunteers following administration of a single intravenous dose of 400 mg. They reported the clearance of amiodarone to be only 0.14 l/min. Similar results have been reported by others.

The elimination half-life of amiodarone after a single oral dose was found to be similar to that after a single intravenous dose. The metabolite, desethylamiodarone, appeared as early as 30 minutes after a loading oral dose and its elimination half-life was slightly longer than that of amiodarone.[71] Experiments in the rat,[62] rabbit,[87] and dog[88] have shown a rapid elimination $(t_{1/2} = 2−3$ hours) of amiodarone from serum after intravenous administration. There was a rapid uptake of amiodarone by the myocardial tissue with peak concentration at 10−15 minutes. The myocardial

## Table 6
### Pharmacokinetic Parameters of Amiodarone After Intravenous Bolus Administration

| No. of Subjects | Dose (mg) | $T\frac{1}{2}$ (h) | Clearance (l/min) | VD (l/kg) | Study |
|---|---|---|---|---|---|
| 3 | 150 | 17.4 | 0.60 | 12.9 | Riva et al.[70] |
| 8 | 150 | 4.3 | 0.2 | 1.3 | Anastasiou-Nana et al.[63] |
| 7 | 400 | 11 | — | — | Andreasen et al.[60] |
| 3 | 300 | 16.1 | 0.45 | 11.7 | Riva et al.[70] |
| 6 | 400 | 24.8 | 0.14 | 658 | Holt et al.[82] |

concentratons decreased as a function of time with an elimination pattern similar to that of serum levels. In spite of the fact that myocardial concentrations were several fold higher than in the serum throughout the kinetic study, no electrophysiologic changes were noted in both dog and rabbit studies.[87,88] Coumel and Bourain[100] described the rapid myocardial uptake as an "injectable like" effect that probably occurs due to fixation of drug to the cardiac tissue during the first few circulations. The beneficial antiarrhythmic effects of amiodarone after single IV[101] or single oral administration[102] reported by some authors could be due to such an effect or to effects such as adrenergic or calcium antagonism manifest acutely (see Chapter 14).

In contrast to the short half-life after acute administration, the elimination of amiodarone after long-term therapy is extremely slow. Elimination half-lives ranging from 13.7 days to 52.6 days have been reported (Table 7). A large interpatient variation exists in the elimination of amiodarone after cessation of therapy in chronically treated patients. In a recent report, Holt et al.[82] showed that the disappearance kinetics followed a complex multiexponential function with a terminal elimination phase of 44–107 days. The elimination half-life of the metabolite of amiodarone also was long and was not significantly different from that of the parent drug. Staubli et al.[75] recently showed that the elimination half-life of amiodarone (35–68 days), desethylamiodarone (31–110 days), and other iodinated metabolites (57–160 days) increased in that order in 23 patients receiving 2.5–8.6 mg/kg/day amiodarone for about a year.

Table 7

Serum Elimination Kinetics of Amiodarone in Chronically Treated Patients

| No. of Subjects | Daily Dose (mg) | Duration of maintenance dose (days) | Mean Terminal $t\frac{1}{2}$ (days) | Study |
|---|---|---|---|---|
| 1 | 300 | 8 months | 13.7 | Andreasen et al.[60] |
| 4 | 400–800 | 39 ± 13 | 29 | Kannan et al.[71] |
| 70 | 200–1200 | — | 52 | Harris et al.[112] |
| 8 | 200–600 | — | 52.6 | Holt et al.[82] |
| 3 | 200–1600 | 23.3 | 19.3 | Haffajee et al.[76] |
| 12 | 200–600 | 150–637 | 41.1 | Staubli et al.[77] |

## Dosage, Serum Concentrations, and Therapeutic Monitoring

In trying to evaluate the usefulness of amiodarone plasma levels for monitoring purposes, a number of considerations should be borne in mind. First, it has been shown that tissue equilibrium occurs slowly, and that the relationship between myocardial and plasma levels during nonequilibrium is different than what is achieved at steady-state; there is a poor correlation between the effects of the drug and the tissue and serum levels of the compound. Second, one must consider the potential contribution of the metabolite, desethylamiodarone. Since this metabolite accumulates extensively in both the plasma and the myocardium, it may be an important modulator of the clinical efficacy of amiodarone during chronic therapy with the parent compound. Animal studies have indicated its pharmacologic activity (see Chapter 14).

A linear correlation was found between the dosage of amiodarone and serum amiodarone concentrations by many laboratories.[82,89,103,104] A large loading dose (1200–1600 mg) generally is used to accelerate the onset of clinical efficacy.[105] The maintenance dose has ranged from 100–600 mg in most centers. An approach to optimal dosing is discussed in Chapter 21.

Table 8 shows the data on serum concentrations of amiodarone and desethylamiodarone with respect to daily maintenance dosage of 200, 400, and 600 mg from Holt et al.[82] The authors found a linear relationship between dose and mean amiodarone and desethylamiodarone levels. The mean amiodarone–desethylamiodarone ratio was 1.08 ± 0.33. Similar linear relationships between maintenance dose and serum amiodarone levels have been reported by Heger et al.[89] and Boppanna et al.[104]

### Table 8
### Relationship Between Plasma Concentrations of Amiodarone and Desethylamiodarone and the Daily Dosage of Amiodarone

| Daily Dose (mg) | Plasma Concentration (mg/l; mean ± SD) | | N |
|---|---|---|---|
| | Amiodarone | Desethylamiodarone | |
| 200 | 1.06 ± 0.43 | 1.04 ± 0.34 | 101 |
| 400 | 1.93 ± 0.80 | 1.79 ± 0.65 | 51 |
| 600 | 3.46 ± 1.50 | 2.79 ± 1.17 | 18 |

Source: Adapted from Holt DW, Tucker GT, Jackson PR, et al: Amiodarone pharmacokinetics. *Am Heart J* 106:840, 1983.

The therapeutic concentration range of amiodarone is not yet well defined although some general recommendations can be made from the available data. Haffajee et al.[76] reported a steady state serum concentration of 0.6–2.8 µg/ml in 96 patients with life-threatening ventricular arrhythmias and 77 patients with supraventricular tachyarrhythmias. Arrhythmia recurred in 9 patients when their serum levels decreased to less than 1.0 µg/ml. Mostow et al.[106] found a negative correlation between the serum amiodarone concentration and the number of premature ventricular complexes in 25 patients. In a recent report, Rotmensch et al.[107] showed that toxic side effects were more common in patients whose serum concentrations were higher than 2.5 µg/ml. Out of the 127 patients they studied, arrhythmia recurred in 47 percent with serum amiodarone concentrations less than 1.0 µg/ml. Preliminary data from Nademanee et al.[108] suggested that serum levels of desethylamiodarone may play an important role in monitoring efficacy and toxicity of amiodarone. Data from 18 patients on standardized amiodarone therapy (11 responders and 7 with chronic toxicity) indicated that (1) for efficacy, the metabolite should be $>$ 1.0 µg/ml; and (2) to avoid serious toxic effects, the metabolite should be $<$ 3.0 µg/ml. In addition, a good correlation was found between desethylamiodarone levels and serum $rT_3$, but no such correlation existed between serum amiodarone and $rT_3$. Recently, Fraser et al.[109] found that adverse side effects of amiodarone were related closely to serum desethylamiodarone concentrations. In 24 patients who had taken amiodarone for more than 1 year, the strongest correlation existed between side effects and desethylamiodarone levels. Preliminary data in 47 children[110] with cardiac arrhythmias showed that (1) unlike, in adults, the serum concentration of amiodarone and desethylamiodarone needed to achieve clinical efficacy was much lower; (2) there was no correlation between dosage or duration of therapy and serum amiodarone and desethylamiodarone levels; and (3) the major side effects of amiodarone in adults, viz. pulmonary toxicity and hepatic toxicity, were not found in children.

## Pharmacokinetic Monitoring of Amiodarone Side Effects

Although the nature and the range of frequency of unwanted side effects resulting from amiodarone usage now are widely appreciated, their avoidance by careful monitoring of pharmacokinetic parameters is not established. The incidence of side effects seems to vary from center to center and at least in part may be due to the difference in loading and maintenance dose regimens.[111–113] It is known that some of the side effects may result from excess dosage and others from an idiosyncratic reaction in a predisposed patient. This is established clearly in the case of altered thyroid state (see Chapter 15).

Only general recommendations can be made with regard to the use of serum drug levels in predicting toxicity. As stated earlier, serum amiodarone levels with an upper limit of 2.5 μg/ml were found to be safe in a number of studies. Rotmensch et al.[107] found that the risk of developing side effects was related to serum amiodarone levels and adverse reactions were more common in patients with serum levels exceeding 2.5 μg/ml except for pulmonary fibrosis, which occurred also at lower concentrations. On the other hand, Haffajee et al.[76] concluded from their investigation of 173 patients that serum levels do not predict the incidence of side effects. Nademanee et al.[108] found that desethylamiodarone and reverse $T_3$ were better indices for monitoring toxicity than serum amiodarone levels. Clearly, further work is needed to clarify the utility of serum amiodarone and metabolite levels in the therapeutic monitoring of amiodarone.

## Conclusions

The so-called Class III antiarrhythmic agents constitute a pharmacokinetically dissimilar group of agents. They share the common electrophysiologic property of prolonging the action potential duration in some or all cardiac tissues as the major mechanism of their antiarrhythmic actions. Amiodarone lies at an extreme end of the spectrum as one of the most highly lipid soluble antiarrhythmic compounds; bretylium, NAPA, and sotalol are at the opposite end of the spectrum, representing the most polar, hydrophilic agents. As with other aspects of Class III agents, their absorption and bioavailability characteristics also represent extremes. Sotalol and NAPA are absorbed almost completely, with bioavailability in the 90–100 percent range; amiodarone and bretylium are absorbed poorly and slowly, with low bioavailability.

The drugs currently available for the treatment of cardiac arrhythmias generally undergo extensive biotransformation in the liver and are highly dependent on metabolic processes for their deactivation and elimination. It is noteworthy that the three antiarrhythmic drugs that are the exceptions to this rule are all Class III agents. Sotalol, bretylium, and NAPA are eliminated almost entirely by renal excretion. Amiodarone, again remaining unique within this classification, is metabolized almost entirely resulting in at least one active metabolite—desethylamiodarone.

Pharmacokinetically, perhaps the simplest of the four compounds is sotalol; it is absorbed rapidly and fully, is not metabolized, and is excreted essentially unchanged in the urine. Its renal clearance varies with creatinine clearance. N-acetylprocainamide(NAPA) has been studied extensively in the pharmacokinetic laboratory, but there are limited data on correlations between its antiarrhythmic efficacy and its pharmacokinetic properties. Electrophysiologically, it is the simplest Class III agent. There appears to be an excellent correlation between the tissue kinetics of bretylium and its pharmacologic effects. Amiodarone is the most complex of antiarrhythmic agents, both electrophysiologically and pharmacokinetically. It is amphophilic in nature. It has a variable but exceedingly long elimination half-life and an ill-defined relationship between its serum, tissue, and membrane concentrations and its electrophysiologic and therapeutic effects. The delineation of the precise nature of the electrophysiologic and pharmacokinetic interactions of the compound is likely to provide newer insights into mechanisms for control of cardiac arrhythmias by lengthening repolarization.

# References


1. Courtney KR: Fast frequency-dependent block of action potential upstroke in myocardium. In R Fink (ed): *Molecular Mechanisms of Anesthesia.* New York, Raven Press, 1980.
2. Courtney KR: Structure-activity relations for frequency-dependent sodium channel block in nerve by local anesthetics. *J Pharmacol Exp Ther* 213:114, 1980.
3. Drayer DE: Clinical consequences of the lipophilicity and plasma protein binding of antiarrhythmic drugs and active metabolites in man. *Ann NY Acad Sci* 432:45, 1984.
4. Anderson JL, Patterson E, Wagner JG, et al: Oral and intravenous bretylium disposition. *Clin Pharmacol Ther* 28:468, 1980.
5. Garrett ER, Gren DR, Bialer M: Bretylium pharmacokinetics and bio-availabilities in man with various doses and modes of administration. *Biopharm Drug Disp* 3:129–164, 1982.

6. Anderson JL, Patterson E, Conlon M, et al: Kinetics of antifibrillatory effects of bretylium: Correlation with myocardial drug concentrations. *Am J Cardiol* 46:583, 1980.
7. Josselson J, Narang PK, Adir J, et al: Bretylium pharmacokinetics in renal insufficiency. *Clin Pharmacol Ther* 33:144, 1983.
8. Woosley RL, Stots B, Reele MD, et al: Pharmacologic reversal of hypotensive effect complicating antiarrhythmic therapy with bretylium. *Clin Pharmacol Ther* 32:313, 1982.
9. Winkle RA, Jaillon P, Kates RE, et al: Clinical pharmacology and antiarrhythmic efficacy of N-acetylprocainamide. *Am J Cardiol* 47:123, 1981.
10. Butcher JS, Strong JM, Lucas SV, et al: Procainamide and N-acetylprocainamide kinetics investigated simultaneously with stable isotope methodology. *Clin Pharmacol Ther* 22:447, 1977.
11. Stec GP, Atkinson AJ, Nevin MJ, et al: N-acetylprocainamide pharmacokinetics in functionally anephric patients before and after pertubation by hemodialysis. *Clin Pharmacol Ther* 26:618, 1979.
12. Stec GP, Ruo TI, Thenot JP, et al: Kinetics of N-acetylprocainamide deacetylation. *Clin Pharmacol Ther* 28:659, 1980.
13. Kates RE, Jaillon P, Rubenson DS, et al: Intravenous N-acetylprocainamide disposition kinetics in coronary artery disease. *Clin Pharmacol Ther* 28:52, 1980.
14. Reidenberg MM, Drayer DE, Ley M, et al: Polymorphic acetylation of procainamide in man. *Clin Pharmacol Ther* 17:722, 1975.
15. Atkinson AJ Jr, Krumlosky FA, Huang CM, et al: Hemodialysis for severe procainamide toxicity: Clinical and pharmacokinetic observations. *Clin Pharmacol Ther* 20:585, 1976.
16. Galeazzi RL, Sheiner LB, Lockwood T, et al: The renal elimination of procainamide. *Clin Pharmacol Ther* 19:55, 1981.
17. Roden DM, Reele SB, Higgins SB, et al: Antiarrhythmic efficacy, pharmacokinetics and safety of N-acetylprocainamide in human subjects: Comparison with procainamide. *Am J Cardiol* 46:463, 1980.
18. Lefebvre MA, Girault J, Saux MC, et al: Fluorimetric high performance liquid chromatographic determination of sotalol in biologic fluids. *J Pharm Sci* 68:1216, 1980.
19. Karkkainen S: High performance liquid chromatographic determination of sotalol in biological fluids. *J Chromatog* 336:313, 1984.
20. Schnelle K, Garrett ER: Pharmacokinetics of the beta-adrenergic blocker sotalol in dogs. *J Pharm Sci* 62:363, 1973.
21. Anttila M, Arstila M, Pfeffer M, et al: Human pharmacokinetics of sotalol. *Acta Pharmacol et Toxicol* 39:118, 1976.
22. Sundquist H, Anttila M, Arstila M: Antihypertensive effects of practolol and sotalol. *Clin Pharmacol Ther* 16:465, 1974.
23. Sundquist H: Basic review and comparison of beta-blocker pharmacokinetics. *Curr Ther Res* 28:388, 1980.
24. Meier J: Pharmacokinetic comparison of pindolol with other beta-adrenoceptor blocking agents. *Am Heart J* 104:364, 1982.
25. Kahela P, Antilla M, Sundquist H: Antacids and sotalol absorption. *Acta Pharmacol et Toxicol* 49:181, 1981.
26. Kahela P, Antilla M, Tikkanen R, et al: Effect of food and food con-

stituents and fluid volume on the bioavailability of sotalol. *Acta Pharmacol et Toxicol* 44:7, 1979.

27. Sotaniemi EA, Anttila M, Pelkonen O, et al: Plasma clearance of propranolol and sotalol and hepatic drug-metabolizing enzyme activity. *Clin Pharmacol Ther* 26:153, 1979.

28. Sotaniemi EA, Anttila M, Rautio A, et al: Propranolol and sotalol metabolism after a drinking party. *Clin Pharmacol Ther* 29:705, 1981.

29. Johnson G, Regardh CG: Clinical pharmacokinetics of beta-adrenoceptor blocking drugs. *Clin Pharmacol Ther* 27:593, 1979.

30. Lish PM, Weikel JH, Dungan KW: Pharmacological and toxicological properties of two new beta-adrenergic receptor antagonists. *J Pharmacol Exp Ther* 149:161, 1985.

31. Shand DG: Pharmacokinetic properties of the beta-adrenergic receptor blocking drugs. *Drugs* 7:39, 1984.

32. Sundquist H, Anttila MS, Simon A, et al: Comparative bioavailability and pharmacokinetics of sotalol alone and in combination with hydrochlorothiazide. *J Clin Pharmacol* 19:557, 1979.

33. Poirier JM, Aubry JP, Cheymol G, et al: Pharmacokinetic study of sotalol administered intravenously to healthy men. Application of high performance liquid chromatography. *Therapie* 36:465, 1981.

34. Berglund GG, Descamps R, Thomis JA: Pharmacokinetics of sotalol after chronic administration to patients with renal insufficiency. *Eur J Clin Pharmacol* 18:321, 1980.

35. Sundquist HK, Anttila M, Forsstrom J, et al: Serum levels and half-life of sotalol in chronic renal failure. *Ann Clin Res* 7:442, 1975.

36. Ritschel WA: Compilation of pharmacokinetic parameters of beta-adrenergic blocking agents. *Drug Intell Clin Pharm* 14:746, 1980.

37. Cruickshank JM: The clinical importance of cardioselectivity and lipophilicity in beta-blockers. *Am Heart J* 100:160, 1980.

38. Rendt RM, Greenblatt DJ, de Jong et al: Pharmacokinetics, central nervous system uptake and lipid solubility of propranolol, acebutolol and sotalol. *Cardiology* 71:307, 1984.

39. Taylor PJ, Cruickshank JM: Distribution coefficients of atenolol and sotalol. *J Pharm Pharmacol* 36:118, 1984.

40. Ochs HR, Greenblatt DJ, Arendt RM, et al: Single-dose kinetics of oral propranolol, metroprolol, atenolol and sotalol: Relation to lipophilicity. *Arzneimittel Forschung* 35:1580, 1985.

41. Singh BN, Deedwania P, Nademanee K: Sotalol: A review of Pharmacodynamics and therapeutic applications. *Drugs* 34:311, 1987).

42. Tjandramaga TB, Thomas J, Verbeeck R, et al: The effect of end-stage renal failure and hemodialysis on the elimination kinetics of sotalol. *Br J Clin Pharmacol* 3:259, 1976.

43. Blair AD, Burgess ED, Maxwell BM, et al: Sotalol kinetics in renal insufficiency. *Clin Pharm Ther* 29:457, 1981.

44. Lewis PJ, DeSwiet M, Chamberlian GVP, et al: The management of hypertension in the pregnant woman. In PJ Lewis (ed): *Therapeutic Problems in Pregnancy*. Lancaster, MTP Press, p 530, 1977.

45. Truelove JF, Van Petten GR, Willes RF: Action of several beta-adrenoceptor blocking drugs in the pregnant sheep and fetus. *Br J Pharmacol* 47:161, 1973.

46. O'Hare MF, Leahey W, Murnaghan GA, et al: Pharmacokinetics of sotalol during pregnancy. *Eur J Clin Pharmacol* 24: 521, 1983.
47. Erkkola R, Lamintausta R, Linkko P, et al: Transfer of propranolol and sotalol across the human placenta. *Acta Obstet Syn Scan* 61:31, 1982.
48. Ishizaki T, Hirayama H, Taware K, et al: Pharmacokinetics and pharmacodynamics in young normal and elderly hypertensive subjects: A study using sotalol as a model drug. *J Pharmacol Exp Ther* 212:173, 1980.
49. Brown HC, Carruthers SG, Kelly JG, et al: Observations on the efficacy and pharmacokinetics of sotalol after oral administration. *Europ J Clin Pharmacol* 9:49, 1979.
50. Johansson SR, McCall M, Wilhelmsson J, et al: Duration of action of beta-blockers. *Clin Pharmacol Ther* 27:593, 1980.
51. Leahy WJ, Neill JD, Varma MPS, et al: Comparison of the activity and plasma levels of oxprenolol, slow-release oxprenolol, long-acting propranolol and sotalol. *Europ J Clin Pharmacol* 17:419, 1980.
52. Harron DWG, Balnave K, Kinney CD, et al: Effects of exercise tachycardia during 48 hours of a series of doses of atenolol, sotalol and metoprolol. *Clin Pharmacol Ther* 29:295, 1981.
53. Teo KK, Harte M, Horgan JH: Sotalol infusion in the treatment of supraventricular tachyarrhythmias. *Chest* 87:113, 1985.
54. Nademanee K, Feld G, Hendrickson J, et al: Electrophysiologic and antiarrhythmic effects of sotalol in patients with life-threatening ventricular tachyarrhythmias. *Circulation* 72:555, 1985.
55. Creamer JE, Nathan AW, Shennan A, et al: Acute and chronic effects of sotalol and propranolol on ventricular repolarization using constant rate pacing. *Am J Cardiol* 57:1092, 1986.
56. Singh BN, Nademanee K, Ikeda N, et al: Pharmacology and electrophysiology of amiodarone: Experimental and clinical correlations. In G Breithardt, F Loogan (eds): *New Aspects in the Medical Treatment of Arrhythmias: Role of Amiodarone.* München, Wien, and Baltimore, Urban and Schwarzenberg p 46, 1983.
57. Zipes DP, Prystowsky EN, Heger JJ: Amiodarone: Electrophysiologic actions, pharmacokinetics and clinical effects. *J Amer Coll Cardiol* 3:1059, 1984.
58. Latini R, Tognoni G, Kates RE: Clinical pharmacokinetics of amiodarone. *Clin Pharmacokinet* 9:136, 1984.
59. Storey GCA, Holt P, Curry PVL, et al: High performance liquid chromatographic measurements of amiodarone and its desethylmetabolite: Methodology and preliminary observations. *Ther Drug Monit* 4:385, 1982.
60. Andreasen F, Agerback H, Bjerregaard P, et al: Pharmacokinetics of amiodarone after intravenous and oral administration. *Eur J Clin Pharmacol* 19:293, 1981.
61. Lesko LJ, Marion A, Canada AT, et al: High pressure liquid chromatography of amiodarone in biological fluids. *J Pharm Sci* 70:1366, 1981.
62. Riva E, Gerna M, Neyroz P, et al: Pharmacokinetics of amiodarone in rats. *J Cardiovasc Pharmacol* 4:270, 1982.
63. Anastasiou-Nana M, Levis GM, Moulopoulos SD: Pharmacokinetics

of amiodarone after intravenous and oral administration. *Int J Clin Pharmacol Ther Toxicol* 20:524, 1982.

64. Plomp TA, Engles M, Robles de Medina EO, et al: Simultaneous determination of amiodarone and its major metabolite desethylamiodarone in plasma, urine and tissues by high performance liquid chromatography. *J Chromatog* 273:379, 1983.

65. Brien JF, Jimmo S, Armstrong PW: Rapid high performance liquid chromatographic analysis of amiodarone and N-desethylamiodarone in serum. *Can J Physiol Pharmacol* 61:245, 1983.

66. Mostow NR, Noon DL, Myers LM, et al: Determination of amiodarone and its N-deethylated metabolite in serum by high performance liquid chromatography. *J Chromatog* 227:229, 1983.

67. Kannan R, Miller S, Singh BN: A sensitive HPLC method for the measurement of amiodarone and desethylamiodarone in serum and tissues and its application to disposition studies. *J Chromatog* 385:225, 1987.

68. Bonati M, Gaspari F, D'Aranno V, et al: Physicochemical and analytical characteristics of amiodarone. *J Pharm Sci* 73:829, 1984.

69. Broekhuysen J, Laurel R, Sion R: Recherches dans ler serie des benzfurannes XXXVII. Etude comparee du transit et du metabolisme de l'amiodarone chez diverses esperes animales et chez l'homme. *Arch Internat de Pharmacodynamie et de Therapie* 177:340, 1969.

70. Riva E, Gerna M, Latini R, et al: Pharmacokinetics of amiodarone in man. *J Cardiovasc Pharmocol* 4:264, 1982.

71. Kannan R, Nademanee K, Hendrickson J, et al: Amiodarone kinetics after oral doses. *Clin Pharmacol Ther* 31:438, 1982.

72. Tucker GT, Jackson RR, Storey GCA, et al: Bioavailability of amiodarone. *Eur J Clin Pharmacol* 26:533, 1984.

73. Pourbaix S, Berger Y, Desager JP, et al: Absolute bioavailability of amiodarone in normal subjects. *Clin Pharmacol Ther* 37:118, 1985.

74. Flanagan RJ, Storey GCA, Holt DW, et al: Identification and measurement of desethylamiodarone in blood plasma specimens from amiodarone-treated patients. *J Pharm Pharmacol* 34:638, 1982.

75. Staubli M, Troendle A, Schmid B, et al: Pharmacokinetics of amiodarone, desethylamiodarone and other iodine-containing amiodarone metabolites. *Eur J Clin Pharmacol* 29:417, 1985.

76. Haffajee CI, Love JC, Canada AT, et al: Clinical pharmacokinetics and efficacy of amiodarone for refractory tachyarrhythmia. *Circulation* 67:1347, 1983.

77. Staubli M, Bircher J, Galeazzi RL, et al: Serum concentrations of amiodarone during long term therapy: Relation to dose, efficacy and toxicity. *Eur J Clin Pharmacol* 24:485, 1983.

78. Heger JJ, Solow EB, Prystowsky EN, et al: Plasma and red blood cell concentrations of amiodarone during chronic therapy. *Am J Cardiol* 53:912, 1984.

79. Lalloz MEA, Byfield PGH, Greenwood RM, et al: Binding of amiodarone to serum proteins and the effects of drugs, hormones and other interesting ligands. *J Pharm Pharmacol* 36:366, 1984.

80. Kannan R, Takikawa R, Sugiyama R, et al: Binding studies on amiodarone and desethylamiodarone. Unpublished.

81. Savoie F, Diquet B, Savoie JC: Synthesis of $^{125}$[I] amiodarone and

its purification by high performance liquid chromatography. *J Chromatog* 261:305, 1983.

82. Holt DW, Tucker GT, Jackson PR, et al: Amiodarone pharmacokinetics. *Am Heart J* 106:840, 1983.
83. Kannan R, Miller S, Singh BN: Tissue uptake and metabolism of amiodarone after chronic administration in rabbits. *Drug Metab Dispos* 13:646, 1985.
84. Plomp TA, Wiersinga WM, Maes RAA: Tissue distribution of amiodarone and desethylamiodarone in rats after multiple intraperitoneal administration of various amiodarone dosages. *Drug Res* 35:122, 1985.
85. Adams PC, Nicholson MR, Storey GCA, et al: Amiodarone tissue distribution: relation to adverse effects. *Br Heart J* 49:297, 1983.
86. Maggioni AP, Maggi A, Volpi A, et al: Amiodarone distribution in human tissue after sudden death during Holter monitoring. *Am J Cardiol* 52:217, 1983.
87. Kannan R, Ikeda N, Wagner R, et al: Serum and myocardial kinetics of amiodarone and its deethylmetabolite after intravenous administration in rabbits. *J Pharmac Sci* 73:1208, 1984.
88. Latini R, Conolly SJ, Kates RE: Myocardial disposition of amiodarone in the dog. *J Pharmacol Exp Ther* 224:603, 1983.
89. Heger JJ, Prystowsky EN, Zipes DP: Relationship between amiodarone dosage, drug concentrations and adverse side effects. *Am Heart J* 106:981, 1983.
90. Heger JJ, Prystowsky EN, Jackman WM, et al: Amiodarone: Clinical efficacy and electrophysiology during long term therapy for recurrent ventricular tachycardia or ventricular fibrillation. *New Eng J Med* 305:539, 1981.
91. Debbas NMG, Bexton RS, du Cailar C, et al: Relation between myocardial amiodarone concentration and QT interval. *Br Heart J* 49:297, 1983.
92. Marchiset D, Egre A, Baille Y, et al: Taux myocardiques et plasmatiques de l'amiodarone et de son metabolite n-monodesthyle'. *Therapie* 38:107, 1983.
93. Zachary CB, Slater DN, Holt DW, et al: The pathogenesis of amiodarone-induced pigmentation and photosensitivity. *Br J Dermatol* 110:451, 1984.
94. Heger JJ, Prystowsky EN, Zipes DP: Relationship between amiodarone dosage, drug concentrations, and adverse side effects. *Am Heart J* 106:931, 1983.
95. Camus P, Mehendale HM: Pulmonary sequestration of amiodarone and desethylamiodarone. *J Pharmacol Exp Ther* 237:867, 1986.
96. Latini R, Connolly S, Kernoff R, et al: Amiodarone myocardial concentrations correlate better than plasma concentrations with electrophysiologic effects. *Circulation* 66 (Suppl II): 223, 1982.
97. Lambert C, Vermuelen M, Cardinal R, et al: Effect of the induction of amiodarone biotransformation on ventricular refractory periods in rats. *J Pharmacol Exp Ther* 238:307, 1986.
98. Ikeda N, Nademanee K, Kannan R, et al: Electrophysiologic effect of amiodarone: Experiments and clinical observation relative to serum and tissue drug concentrations. *Am Heart J* 108:890, 1984.

99. Cantor JR, Olman M, Cerreta JM, et al: Amiodarone induced pulmonary fibrosis in hamsters. *Exp Lung Res* 6:1, 1984.
100. Coumel PL, Bourain Y: Etude Clinique de effects, pharmacodynamiques et antiarrhythmiques de l'amiodarone. *J Agreges* 6:69, 1973.
101. Holt P, Curry P, Way B, et al: Intravenous amiodarone: An effective antiarrhythmic agent. *Am J Cardiol* 49:1001, 1982.
102. Faequet J, Nevet M, Grosgogeat Y, et al: L'influence de l'amiodarone sur le rythgme cardiaque et l'electrocardiogramme. *Therapie* 25:335, 1970.
103. Staubli M, Bircher J, Galeazzi RL, et al: Serum concentrations of amiodarone during long term therapy: Relation of dose efficacy and toxicity. *Eur J Clin Pharmacol* 24:485, 1983.
104. Boppanna VK, Belhassen B and Rotmensch HH: Clinical efficacy and serum concentrations of amiodarone. *Clin Pharmacol Ther* 33:A23, 1983.
105. Siddoway LA, McAllister CB, Wilkinson GR, et al: Amiodarone dosing: A proposal based on its pharmacokinetics. *Am Heart J* 106:951, 1983.
106. Mostow NR, Rakita L, Vrobel TR, et al: Amiodarone: Correlation of serum concentration with suppression of complex ventricular ectopic activity. *Am J Cardiol* 54:569, 1984.
107. Rotmensch HH, Belhassen B, Swanson BN, et al: Steady state serum amiodarone concentrations: Relationships with antiarrhythmic efficacy and toxicity. *Ann Int Med* 101:463, 1984.
108. Nademanee K, Kannan R, Wagner R, et al: Role of amiodarone, desethylamiodarone and reverse $T_3$ serum levels in monitoring antiarrhythmic efficacy and toxicity: Superiority of $rT_3$ and desethylamiodarone levels. *Circulation* 68(Suppl III):278, 1983.
109. Fraser AG, Stephens MR, Newcombe RG, et al: Association of serum desethylamiodarone concentration with adverse effects of amiodarone. *Br Heart J* 50:276, 1984.
110. Kannan R, Yabek S, Garson A. Jr, et al: Relationship between amiodarone efficacy and serum drug levels in children. II World Congress of Pediatric Cardiology, New York, June 2–6, 1985, Abstract 069.
111. Fogoros RN, Anderson KP, Winkle RA, et al: Amiodarone: Clinical efficacy and toxicity in 96 patients with recurrent drug refractory arrhythmias. *Circulation* 68:88, 1983.
112. Harris L, McKenna WJ, Rowland E, et al: Side effects of long-term amiodarone therapy. *Circulation* 67:45, 1983.
113. Nademanee K, Singh BN, Hendrickson JA, et al: Amiodarone in refractory life-threatening ventricular arrhythmias. *Ann Int Med* 98:577, 1983.

# Chapter 7

# Electrophysiologic and Antiarrhythmic Effects of Sotalol with Particular Reference to the Control of Ventricular Arrhythmias

Koonlawee Nademanee and
Bramah N. Singh

Introduced in the early 1960s as a specific beta-adrenergic blocking agent,[1] MJ1999 or sotalol has been somewhat slow in gaining recognition as a therapeutic agent in cardiovascular disorders. It is now known that the drug is devoid of membrane stabilizing or local anesthetic properties, intrinsic sympathomimetic actions, or cardioselectivity.[2,3] Although Singh and Vaughan Williams[3] and Singh and Hauswirth[4] drew attention to the drug's unique electrophysiologic properties many years ago, it is only in the last few years that its broad spectrum antiarrhythmic properties increasingly has become recognized.[5-8] Sotalol is now regarded as an important Class III antiarrhythmic agent for the control of supraventricular and ventricular arrhythmias. Its in vitro electrophysiologic effects, its hemodynamic properties and pharmacokinetic properties have been discussed elsewhere in this volume (Chapters 3, 5, and 6). In this chapter, we will discuss the electrophysiologic basis for its antiarrhythmic and antifibrillatory actions and will review the evidence currently available for its

From: *Control of Cardiac Arrhythmias by Lengthening Repolarization*, edited by Bramah N. Singh, MD, Futura Publishing Company Inc., Mount Kisco, NY, © 1988.

emerging role in the control of supraventricular and ventricular tachyarrhythmias.

## Pharmacodynamic Properties

Two distinct properties of sotalol are the major determinants of its net pharmacodynamic and therapeutic effects: beta blockade and the lengthening of the duration of the cardiac action potential. The commercially available preparation is the racemic mixture of d- and l-sotalol, the dextro-isomer having less than one-fiftieth the activity of the levo-compound.[9]

In isolated tissues, sotalol shifts the agonist dose-response curve in a parallel fashion to the right.[10-12] In the formal analysis of the differences between propranolol and sotalol as beta antagonists, $pA_2$ values for propranolol of about 8.4 and 6.4 for sotalol have been reported, reflecting a marked difference in the relative potencies of the two beta blockers.[10,13] However, this two-hundred−fold difference in the blocking actions of the two compounds has not always been demonstrated. Some studies (see Aberg et al.[14]) have shown that sotalol in vitro was one-tenth to one-fiftieth as potent as propranolol. The marked difference in the vitro and in vivo blocking potencies of sotalol is not understood completely but has been attributed to a low lipid solubility, which is balanced by good absorption and high metabolic stability of the drug.

In intact anesthetized animals and in conscious humans the potency ratio between sotalol and propranolol appears to be 1:3 or 1:2−3.[13,14] However, sotalol exerts a nonadrenergically mediated positive inotropic effect,[9,10,14,15] albeit a weak one, which may influence the precise determination of its beta-blocking propensity against standard agonists such as isoprenaline as well as the drug's net hemodynamic actions (see Chapter 5).

## Electrophysiological Basis for Antiarrhythmic Actions

It is now clear that sotalol is not simply "another beta blocker."[16-18] The initial electrophysiologic studies[3] established that the drug increased the duration of the action potential in a concentration-dependent fashion with an associated lengthening of the effective and absolute refractory periods. Recent observations have confirmed by voltage clamp analysis[19] that the compound has no significant effect on the fast sodium channel in concentrations in which it markedly prolongs the action potential duration. Studies with the dextro-and levo-isomer also have confirmed that the property of lengthening of the cardiac action potential duration is not related to its antiadrenergic action.[9]

The experimental data are consistent with the clinical observations, which showed that the intravenous injection of the dextro-isomer of sotalol had little or no beta-blocking effect compared to the racemic mixture; however, the repolarization effects (i.e., on the $QT_c$ interval of the electrocardiogram) of the dextro-isomer and the racemic compound were comparable over the same drug dose range.[20]

## Antiarrhythmic Correlates of the Electrophysiologic Effects

There have been numerous experimental[3,11,21-25] and clinical[26-31] reports that have documented a broad range of antiarrhythmic effects in the case of dl-sotalol. Indeed, the spectrum of effects of the compound in arrhythmias is wider than that of conventional beta blockers.[3] In a model of post-myocardial infarction arrhythmias in conscious dogs Cobbe et al.[26] found that ventricular arrhythmias were prevented by sotalol in 11 of 19 (58 percent) studies compared with 1 of 14 (7 percent) with metoprolol, which does not lengthen the action potential duration. The salutary effect of sotalol could be correlated with a lengthening of the refractory period of the infarct zone, metoprolol having no effect on this parameter, indicating that the antiarrhythmic effect of sotalol was not mediated solely through beta blockade. These observations are also consistent with the findings of Marshall et al.[32] who found that sotalol given intravenously significantly increased the ventricular fibrillation threshold (VFT) of both normal and ischemic myocardium in the anesthetized rat, whereas metoprolol had no effect on the VFT in the normal myocardium and merely prevented the fall in VFT after coronary artery occlusion. Again, these findings are indicative of the antifibrillatory and antiarrhythmic actions of sotalol in a variety of animal models as emphasized by Patterson et al.[24,25] The major effect appears to be mediated through the lengthening of the action potential duration. Although our data clearly have shown that the dextro-isomer is equipotent with the levo-isomer and with the racemic compound in prolonging the effective refractory period, the data dealing with the antiarrhythmic actions of d-sotalol are limited. However, Lynch et al.[23] recently found that 8 mg/kg intravenous cumulative doses of the l- as well as the d-isomer suppressed the induction of ventricular tachycardia in their conscious-dog ischemic model of sudden death in 50 percent of the animals. At this dose, only the l-sotalol exerted an antiadrenergic effect, such as lengthening of the PR interval of the surface EKG, but both isomers produced equivalent increases of 15–20 percent in the ventricular effective refractory period. Culling et al[33] found that the drug prevented ventricular arrhythmias associated with myocardial ischemia and reperfusion in the isolated buffer-perfused model of the guinea-pig heart. In this preparation ischemia was produced by reduction of flow to 10 percent for 30 minutes followed by reperfusion. It is noteworthy however that the beneficial effect on the arrhythmia could not be accounted for by alterations in the measured electrophysiologic parameters such as refractoriness or the time course of the monophasic action potentials. It also should be emphasized that during myocardial ischemia sotalol has been shown to elevate myocardial pH in the dog heart[34] and the drug's effect on its so-called Class III action is not negated by elevated extracellular potassium.[35] Finally, there are data to suggest that the antifibrillatory effects of sotalol are not confined to ventricular tissue. Bertrix et al.[36] measured the fibrillation threshold in the dog ventricle and atria concurrently with the amplitude and duration of the monophasic action potential, effective refractory period, the conduction time in the contractile fibers, and the fibrillation rate once fibrillation had been triggered. Sotalol increased the fibrillation threshold in association with increases in the duration of the action potential and the effective refractory period. There was a slowing of the fibrillation rate but *without* a change in conduction time. It is of interest that the overall changes were more striking in the case of the atria (than in the ventricle) in which vulnerability to fibrillation had been enhanced by acetylcholine. Sotalol antagonized the changes induced by acetylcholine. The experimental data thus provide a compelling basis for antiarrhythmic and antifibrillatory effects in a broad spectrum of supraventricular and ventricular arrhythmias.

The expanding clinical experience with sotalol as an antiarrhythmic agent is in line with the experimental findings. For example, unlike conventional beta-blocking drugs, dl-sotalol has been found to be effective in lengthening the anterograde effective refractory period of the bypass tracts in the Wolff-Parkinson-White (WPW) syndrome[16,31] and to prevent the reinduction of ventricular tachycardia in experimental animals[26] and in humans.[5,6,38] These observations suggest that the additional antiarrhythmic actions of dl-sotalol as compared to those of other beta blockers may be due to its propensity to lengthen repolarization and refractoriness in cardiac muscle. The in vitro electrophysiologic data on the effects of the two isomers[9] on the refractory period of cardiac muscle are consistent with these in vivo experimental findings and with the preliminary clinical experience with intravenously administered d-sotalol in humans.[40,41]

## Clinical Electrophysiologic Effects

The clinical effects of sotalol are in accord with the experimental data. Electrophysiologic studies using the intravenous drug have established that sotalol lengthens the monophasic action potential in atria and ventricles in humans[42−44] and increases the effective refractory period in atria, ventricle, AV node, and bypass tracts while prolonging the intranodal but not the infranodal conduction time.[5,6,16,37,45,46] These properties differ from those of conventional beta blockers, which have little or no effect on atrial, ventricular, and bypass tract effective refractory period (ERP).[47] The results of our studies[6] are concordant in this regard. Intravenous sotalol lengthened the ERP in atria ($+24.6$ percent; $p < 0.01$), AV node ($+24.9$ percent; $p < 0.01$), and ventricle ($+14.9$ percent; $p < 0.01$); it significantly lengthened sinus node recovery time, $QT_c$, and AH but not the HV interval. There also was lengthening of the effective refractory period of the His-Purkinje system following the intravenous administration of sotalol in patients undergoing programmed electrical stimulation of the heart.[48] Very similar overall electrophysiologic data have been reported by Touboul et al.,[45] overall effects being accountable in terms of a summated effect of beta-blockade and those due to the lengthening of the action potential duration without a change in depolarization.

## Comparison of Sotalol and Propranolol, Acute versus Chronic Effects

Creamer et al.[49] compared the acute and the chronic effects of propranolol and sotalol in conventional equi-active beta-blocking doses of the two antagonists in 8 patients with permanent programmable pacemakers. They found sotalol to prolong the $QT_c$ interval by 6.5 percent following intravenous sotalol and by 11.5 percent after 4 weeks of oral therapy. There was no change in the QRS duration, and the entire increase in repolarization therefore was due to a lengthening of the JT interval. The prolongation of the QT and JT intervals were related to the plasma concentrations of the drug, but a significant relationship was not established in this study. It was of interest that the QT lengthening was greater during chronic therapy despite somewhat lower serum levels of the drug. Following propranolol therapy, there was no change in the QT or JT intervals and, although there was a minor tendency for the $QT_c$ to increase following chronic therapy, this did not reach statistical significance. Thus, the data provide further confirmation that the lengthening of the $QT_c$ induced by sotalol is not due to its antiadrenergic property. The study of Creamer et al.[49] further showed that neither drug had an effect on the pacing threshold of the ventricle following intravenous drug administration.

These overall findings clearly indicate a combination of beta-blocking (Class II) and Class III actions, a combination that is likely to confer on sotalol a broad spectrum antiarrhythmic effect and a side effect profile that are essentially predictable on the basis of these two fundamental actions. Although the complete spectrum of the antiarrhythmic actions of sotalol has not been completely delineated,[5,6,7,8,27,28,50] the available data allow certain general conclusions regarding the drug's overall clinical utility.

## The Role of Sotalol in Cardiac Arrhythmias

The major importance of sotalol as an antiarrhythmic agent has focused on its broad-spectrum electrophysiologic properties, especially as the prototype of the so-called Class III antidysrhythmic compounds.[3,11] The fact that the compound is a beta blocker that lengthens the action potential duration and refractoriness enhances the overall clinical utility of the compound.

### The Utility of Sotalol in Supraventricular Arrhythmias

As yet, this issue has not been addressed specifically by controlled studies. However, since sotalol is a beta blocker, it is likely to be as effective as conventional beta blockers in suppressing atrial extrasystoles and other ectopic atrial tachycardias, in slowing sinus tachycardia and the ventricular response in atrial flutter and fibrillation, in terminating reentrant supraventricular tachycardia, and in controlling the recurrence of a proportion of such arrhythmias during prophylactic drug administration. It remains to be demonstrated whether sotalol's associated property of lengthening action potential duration will make the compound unique in this regard, compared to conventional beta blockers. The recent data of Teo et al.[51] nevertheless are very encouraging in so far as sotalol infusion led to a 100 percent conversion of paroxysmal supraventricular tachycardia.

There are situations in which one might expect sotalol to be more effective than conventional beta-blocking agents in the control of supraventricular arrhythmias. First, preliminary experience suggests that, unlike most beta blockers, intravenously administered sotalol will convert[51] significant numbers of patients with atrial fibrillation (33 percent conversion) and flutter (86 percent conversion) into sinus rhythm and that it is effective in maintaining the stability of sinus rhythm once this has been restored either by pharmacologic or electrical conversion. Second, orally administered sotalol is likely to be more effective than conventional beta blockers in preventing recurrences of paroxysmal supraventricular tachycardias involving both AV nodal reentry and accessory pathways. From the knowledge of the electrophysiology of the compound, one might expect the agent to be of particular value in the control of atrial flutter and fibrillation in the Wolff-Parkinson-White syndrome. However, at present, there are limited data on the use of dl-sotalol in supraventricular tachyarrhythmias, and even less on the antiarrhythmic effects of d-sotalol.

## Atrial Flutter and Fibrillation

Fogelman et al.[28] gave 20 mg of intravenous sotalol to 5 patients with atrial flutter; in none was sinus rhythm restored, but in all the ventricular response was slowed. The atrial rate was also slowed with a mean of 334/minute to 311/minute, 60 minutes after the end of drug injection. The mean ventricular response was reduced from 167/minutes to 127/minutes. In the case of atrial fibrillation 3 of the 5 patients with acute onset of the arrhythmia given intravenous sotalol (20 mg) converted to sinus rhythm with a slowing of the ventricular response in the remaining two. Sinus rhythm was restored in 0 of the 9 patients with chronic atrial fibrillation but the ventricular response was reduced from 127 to 94 beats/minute, in 2 patients there was a mild acceleration of the ventricular response. The dose of the drug used by Prakash et al.[27] varied between 9 and 50 mg intravenously followed by 20 to 80 mg orally every 6 hours. The drug produced conversion to sinus rhythm in 1 of 4 patients, there was a decrease in the ventricular response in the other 3 patients but an increase in the AV block. In the 3 cases of atrial fibrillation in this series sotalol decreased the ventricular response without producing conversion to sinus rhythm. It should be emphasized that the sotalol doses used by Fogelman et al.[28] or Prakash et al.[27] were small in light of the subsequent experience with sotalol dosage, since currently 1.5 mg/kg of the drug is now being used in controlling acute arrhythmias. Thus, further studies are needed to define a dose–response relationship in the acute conversion of atrial flutter and fibrillation by sotalol in subsets of patients with varying left atrial size and chronicity of the arrhythmias. Moreover, it will be of interest to determine how effective the drug might be in maintaining sinus rhythm following electrical or chemical conversion from atrial flutter and fibrillation.

## Sotalol in Preventing Atrial Flutter and Fibrillation After Cardiopulmonary Bypass Surgery

Campbell et al.[52] compared the effects of disopyramide and digoxin to those of sotalol by a randomized study. In the sotalol group, the drug was given 1 mg/kg intravenously as a bolus followed by 0.2 mg/kg intravenously over 12 hours; in the other group disopyramide was given 2 mg/kg as an intravenous bolus with 0.4 mg/kg/hour for 10 hours in addition to 0.75 mg digoxin intravenously. In each group 17 out of 20 patients reverted to sinus or junctional rhythm within 12 hours. However, the time to conversion was significantly shorter in the case of sotalol.

In another preliminary study, the effects of metoprolol and sotalol were evaluated in 151 patients undergoing coronary artery bypass surgery:[53] 39 were treated with metoprolol, 41 with sotalol, and 50 served as controls. In the metoprolol group, 15.3 percent developed supraventricular tachyarrhythmias compared to 2.4 percent of the sotalol group. Of the 18 patients in the control group developing an arrhythmia, 10 patients received sotalol and 4 metoprolol for arrhythmia conversion. The time to conversion was strikingly shorter after sotalol than after metoprolol. This study indicates the possible superiority of sotalol over conventional beta blockers in the treatment of atrial arrhythmias complicating bypass surgery.

## Sotalol in Supraventricular Tachycardia (PSVT)

The effects of sotalol in all varieties of paroxysmal supraventricular tachycardias (reentrant or ectopic) have not been fully defined. Fogelman et al.[28] found that 5 of 6 (83 percent) patients with PSVT converted to sinus rhythm after 20 mg of intravenous sotalol, between 21 seconds and 10 minutes. In the other patient, the tachycardia slowed from a rate of 203 beats/minute to 169 beats/minute. Prakash et al.[27] also found 4 of their 6 patients with PSVT converting to sinus rhythm following 10 to 20 mg of intravenous sotalol. It should be emphasized that the doses of sotalol used in these two studies were small and probably led to no more than beta blocking plasma drug concentrations. Moreover, the precise diagnosis of the PSVT could not be ascertained from these studies. Recently, in controlled studies in which electrophysiologic evaluation was used to determine the nature of the PSVT, Rizos et al.[31] found that sotalol was more effective in preventing inducible supraventricular tachycardia than metoprolol. In this study, the effects of intravenous sotalol (1.5 mg/kg; plasma concentration 2.1 $\pm$ 1.1 µg/ml) was compared to those of 0.15 mg/kg (plasma concentration, 67 $\pm$ 15 ng/ml) of intravenous metoprol in 17 patients with either atrioventricular reentrant PSVT or atrioventricular reciprocating PSVT. Sotalol prevented inducible PSVT in 10 of 17 patients (59 percent) and metoprolol in 4 (28 percent), a difference that was significant (p $<$ 0.05). Thus, qualitatively, metoprolol had the same but less potent effect than sotalol emphasizing that the two drugs share the common property of beta blockade but sotalol has the additional property of lengthening refractroriness as a result of lengthening the action potential duration. In this case, this was particularly evident in the bypass tracts of the heart.

## Sotalol and the Wolff-Parkinson-White Syndrome

As mentioned earlier, sotalol lengthens the effective refractory period of the bypass tract, but the study of Rizos et al.[31] showed no effects in the case of metoprolol. Manz et al.[54] also studied the effects of intravenous sotalol (80 mg) in 11 patients with the Wolff-Parkinson-White syndrome and in 9 patients with the atrioventricular reentrant PSVT. Sotalol lengthened the effective refractory period of the right atrium and the right ventricle with a depression of conduction in the AV node and the accessory tracts in the anterograde as well as the retrograde directions. The rate of the reentrant tachycardia was slowed from $182 \pm 29$ beats/min to $153 \pm 14$ beats/min and the ventricular rate during atrial fibrillation slowed from $148 \pm 14$ beats/min to $112 \pm 12$ beats/min. Their data showed that sotalol exerted a depressant effect in all parts of the reentrant circuit including the atrium, ventricle, atrioventricular node, and the accessory tracts of the heart. These data indicate that the drug is effective in reentrant PSVT with or without the bypass tracts. However, little data are available on the long-term effects of the drug and on the dose–response relationships in the various forms of PSVT. Uncontrolled data[29] indicate that the drug, given prophylactically, may be of value in a variety of supraventricular tachyarrhythmias, but there are no comparative studies of the relative potencies of conventional agents and sotalol in this regard.

It is likely that intravenous sotalol may slow the ventricular response in atrial flutter and fibrillation and prevent their relapses during chronic therapy in the setting of the Wolff-Parkinson-White syndrome. Blanc et al.[55] determined the effects of orally administered sotalol 160 mg/daily in 5 patients and 320 mg/daily in 1 patient for 27–80 days (plasma levels, 0.33 to 2.3 µg/ml) in preexcitation tachycardia. The anterograde effective refractory period of the bypass tract increased from $258 \pm 61$ to $318 \pm 33$ msec. The increase in the effective refractory period occurred even in patients with the shortest periods before the drug was given. These observations indicate that the drug is likely to be effective in preventing the rapid ventricular response to atrial fibrillation in patients with the WPW syndrome as well as in preventing reciprocating tachycardias. It clearly will be of importance to compare the effects of the drug in this setting with Class I antiarrhythmic agents such as quinidine, disopyramide, and procainamide, on the one hand, and with Class III agents such as N-acetylprocainamide and particularly amiodarone on the other.

## Sotalol in Ventricular Arrhythmias

Increasing data over the last ten years have indicated that in the control of ventricular arrhythmias, the spectrum of activity of sotalol is wider than that of conventional beta-blocking drugs. The initial studies focussed on relatively crude evaluations of the potency of the drug in suppressing premature ventricular contractions in small numbers of patients;[27,28,30,36] more recent studies have employed larger numbers of patients to determine the effects of the drug not only on the suppression of premature ventricular contractions[57-59] but also in those with life-threatening ventricular tachyarrhythmias, including ventricular fibrillation.[5-8] Such studies provide evidence that sotalol is a major agent for the control of ventricular arrhythmias.


## Premature Ventricular Contractions

The earlier studies indicated that sotalol had the potential to suppress premature ventricular contractions[27,28] but the dose of the drug used in this study was small and the numbers of patients limited.

Myburgh et al.[30] reported that in "optimally" titrated doses sotalol reduced premature ventricular contractions by about 86 percent in 20 patients with ischemic heart disease. Similar results from an uncontrolled study in 5 patients were reported by Stroobandt and Kesteloot.[56] In this study 40–100 mg of sotalol was administered intravenously in patients with exercise-induced ventricular ectopics. Sotalol reduced singles, couplets, and triplets occurring during maximal exercise and in the recovery phase. The sotalol plasma levels following the injection of 100 mg of the drug were between 3.7 and 4.75 µg/ml (mean 4.2 µg/ml). This dose of the drug was well tolerated, there being no arrhythmogenic effects.

Of particular interest are the studies of Mary-Rabine et al.[59] They studied the long-term effects of oral sotalol 80–160 mg/day on symptomatic ventricular ectopy in 8 patients with ischemic heart disease, 1 with congestive cardiomyopathy, and 1 with "atypical" chest pain without having evidence of structural heart disease. Serial Holter recordings were obtained before sotalol was started and then after 3 and 6 months of drug therapy. Initially, a significant suppression of ectopy was obtained in 9 of the 10 patients; subsequently efficacy was maintained in 50 percent of the patients, the effect including suppression of ventricular couplets as well as premature beats with R on T phenomenon. However, in all these studies it is not clear whether the antiarrhythmic responses could be accounted for by the beta blocking effects of sotalol or whether its effect on refractoriness might have contributed. No direct comparison with other beta blocking agents was made. The results of a multicenter, double-blind, placebo-controlled study comparing the effects of propranolol and sotalol are pending.[60]

Lidell et al.[58] compared the efficacy of oral sotalol (160–640 mg/day) and procainamide (1 gm t.i.d. to 1.5 g t.i.d.) in patients with premature ventricular arrhythmias open randomized, and a crossover study (to procainamide) in 33 patients with chronic stable premature ventricular contractions. Lidell et al.[58] showed that the drug produced over 75 percent reduction of PVCs in 67 percent of the patients (see Fig. 1); procainamide was effective in 39 percent. When PVCs were reduced significantly both drugs induced a comparable reduction in runs of nonsustained ventricular tachycardia. Nine patients responded to both agents and 7 to neither. In 5 patients, sotalol produced side effects, whereas procainamide produced adverse reactions in 12. These data suggest that the role of sotalol in patients with PVCs with and without heart disease should be investigated.

A recent multicenter, placebo-controlled study involving 57 patients demonstrated a significant suppressant effect of sotalol on PVCs.[60] During the placebo administration, the mean PVC count was $532 \pm 76$/hour on 48-hour Holter recordings; 320 mg/day of sotalol reduced it by 76 percent ($p < 0.0001$) and 640 mg/day of the drug by 83 percent ($p < 0.0001$). Twenty-two of the 37 (59 percent) of the sotalol-treated patients had arrhythmia reduction equal to or greater than 75 percent versus 2 of 19 (11 percent) during the placebo phase. Sotalol reduced the median frequency of couplets by 94 percent ($p < 0.0001$) and ventricular tachycardia runs by 89 percent ($p < 0.001$).

Another blind, placebo-controlled study reported by Burckhardt et al.[57] demonstrated the efficacy of sotalol in suppressing premature ventricular contractions. Fourteen patients with history of remote myocardial infarction and high-density, stable premature ventricular contractions were given 320 mg of sotalol or a matching placebo; Holter recordings were obtained at baseline and again after 7 and 14 days of therapy. In 6 of the 14 patients, the total number of premature ventricular contractions decreased by 50 percent, there being a greater degree of suppression of the higher grades of ventricular ectopy. There were no adverse reactions and the left ventricular ejection fraction measured by radionuclide ventriculography was unchanged ($43.8 \pm 4.0$ percent on placebo versus $44.6 \pm 3.9$ percent on sotalol). No consistent effect was noted between an antiarrhythmic effect and the prolongation of the $QT_c$ interval of surface electrocardiogram.

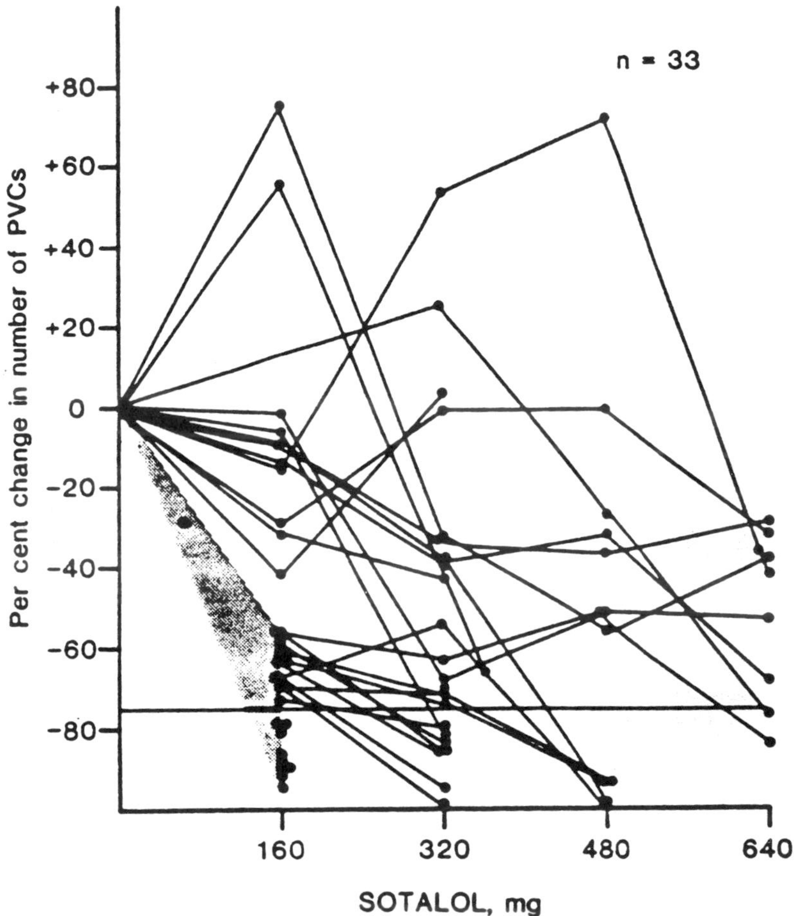


**Figure 1.** Responses (percentages) of premature ventricular contractions (PVCs) to increasing doses of sotalol in 33 patients. Placebo PVC value = 0. (From Lidell C, Rehnquist N, Sjogren A, et al: Comparative efficacy of oral sotalol and procainamide in patients with chronic ventricular arrhythmias: A multicenter study. *Am Heart J* 109:970, 1985. By permission of the authors and of the American Heart Association.)

The recent study by Wang et al.[62] examined the significance of the lengthening of cardiac repolarization in affecting the changes in heart rate and arrhythmia suppression induced by sotalol. They studied 17 patients under baseline conditions and following an incremental dose regimen protocol under serum plasma level control. The doses used were 160 mg, 320 mg, 640 mg, and 960 mg per day given in one or two daily doses. Beta blockade was quantified by examining the effects of sotalol on exercise-induced tachycardia. Eleven of the 17 patients derived an antiarrhythmic response, 70–100 percent reduction of premature ventricular contractions (Fig. 2), at a wide range of plasma concentrations. The responders included 8 patients who had failed conventional beta-blocker therapy. It was found that the concentration of sotalol at which $QT_c$ prolongation was noted (2.55 μg/ml) was greater than that (0.80 μg/ml) producing 50 percent reduction in exercise-induced increases in heart rate. In this study, sotalol was well tolerated but 1 patient developed torsades de pointes 3 hours after a 640 mg dose of the drug. The data of Wang et al.[62] show that the

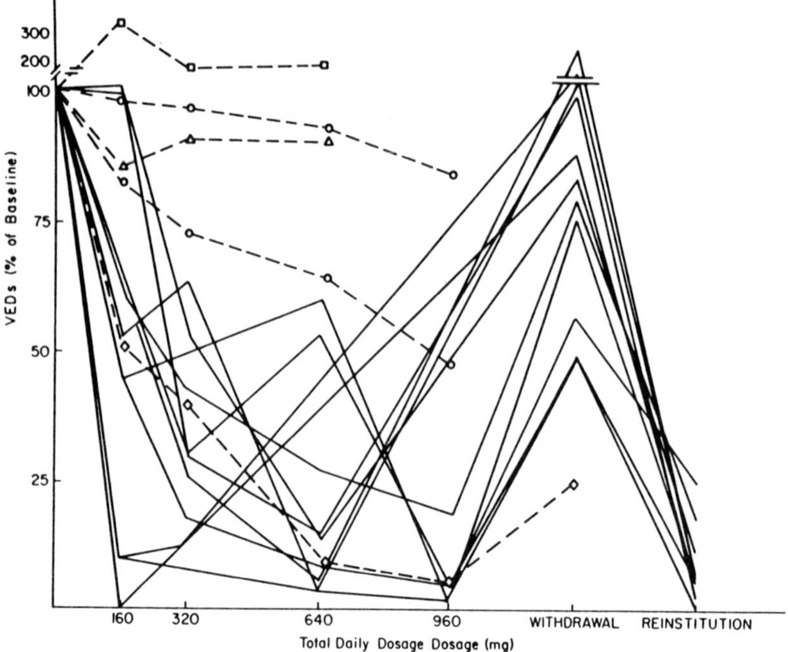


**Figure 2.** Sotalol dose–response curve relation between dosages and frequency of ventricular ectopic depolarizations (VEDs). The 11 confirmed responders are indicated by solid lines. Of the other patients, 1 (triangle) had torsades de pointes, 1 (square) had gastrointestinal side effects, and 2 (circles) failed to respond to the maximal dosage. In 1 other patient, response was not confirmed, and 1 patient was excluded from the study because of a highly variable baseline arrhythmia frequency. (From Wang T, Bergstrand RH, Thompson KA, et al: Concentration-dependent pharmacologic properties of sotalol. *Am J Cardiol* 57:1160, 1986. By permission of the authors and the journal.)

beta blocking effects occur at lower drug concentrations than those that increase repolarization and refractoriness (Fig. 3).

## Sotalol in Patients with Complex PVCs After Myocardial Infarction

It is now well established that the presence of complex PVCs following acute myocardial infarction enhances the incidence of sudden death in these patients, especially if they have reduced myocardial infarction (MI). Whether the suppression of such PVCs leads to reduction in sudden death remains an unresolved issue. In a recent preliminary study, Spielman et al.[63] randomly assigned post-MI patients into three groups for drug therapy: sotalol (320 mg twice daily), timolol (10 mg twice daily), and encainide (50 mg three times daily). The study patients all had left ventricular ejection fraction equal to or below 40 percent and all had evidence of complex PVCs documented on 24-hour Holter recordings. Encainide (n = 17) induced 70 percent or greater reduction in PVCs in 12 out of 15 patients, sotalol (n = 17) in 7 of 11, and timolol (n = 18) in 0 out of 8 patients. Within 4 days of the trial, 1 patient (5 percent) on timolol died suddenly, as did 1 on encainide and 6 on sotalol. These data are difficult to interpret statistically as there was no concurrent control, the dose of sotalol was high, and no plasma drug determinations were available. Clearly, further studies are needed to define the role of sotalol in an appropriate dose regimen in the survivors of acute myocardial infarction with complex ventricular ectopy in the setting of reduced ventricular ejection fraction.

## Sotalol in Life-Threatening Ventricular Arrhythmias

Although there have been sporadic reports as to the efficacy of sotalol in the control of recurrent ventricular tachycardia, there have been few systematic studies.[5,6] Senges et al.[5] performed electrophysiologic testing in 18 patients before and after intravenous sotalol (1.5 mg/kg) using double-stimuli for the induction of ventricular tachycardia/fibrillation. In this study, sotalol prevented reinduction of the tachycardia in 12 of 18 (67 percent) patients. The effect on inducibility was not related systematically to the lengthening of the $QT_c$ interval. Nine of the 12 patients with preventable VT-VF were placed on oral sotalol and 4 patients were placed on another regimen. In these 13 patients, successful long-term effects

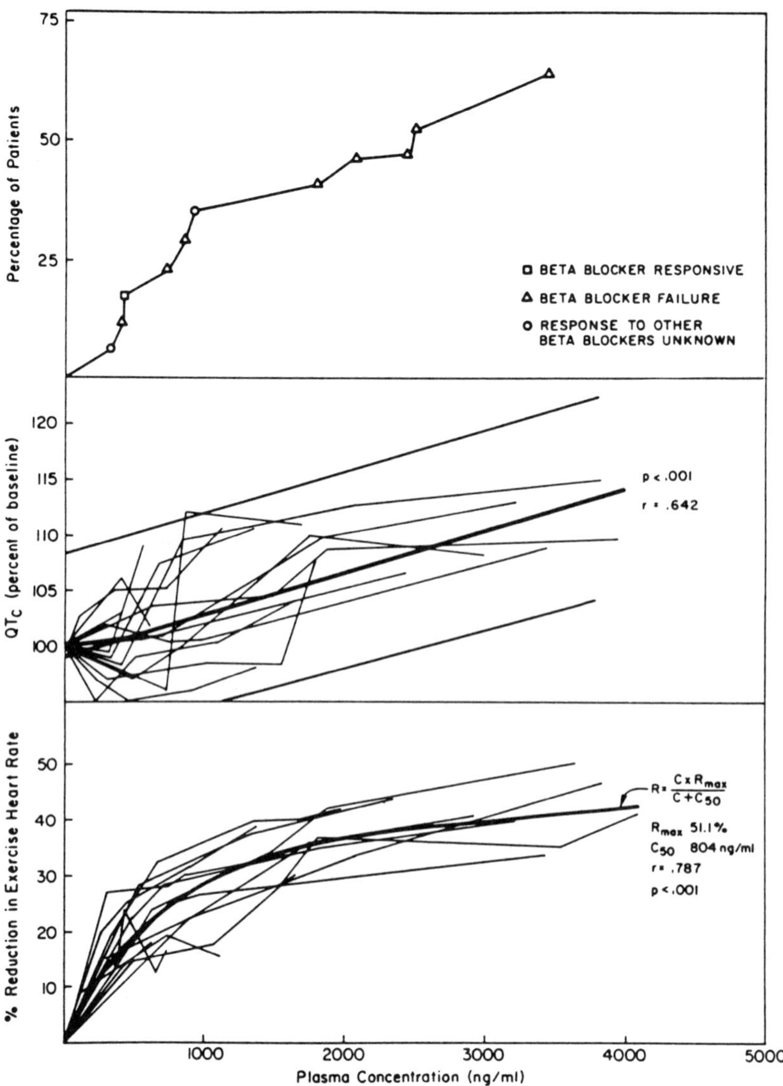


**Figure 3.** Relations among plasma sotalol and responses: Top, percentage of patients responding. Middle, percentage of $QT_c$ prolongation. The lower 95 percent confidence limit rises above baseline at a sotalol concentration of 2555 ng/ml. Bottom, percentage reduction(R) in exercise heart rate. $R_{max}$ = maximal modeled reduction; $C_{50}$ = concentration(C) producing 50 percent of $R_{max}$. (From Wang T, Burkhardt RH, Thompson KA, et al: Concentration-dependent pharmacologic properties of sotalol. *Am J Cardiol* 57:1160, 1986. By permission of the authors and the journal.)

were found in 12 patients and partial responses in 1 patient over a mean follow-up period of 16 (range 8 to 24) months. In 3 patients, heart failure or sinus node dysfunction developed during the early months of treatment. The authors concluded that the overall anti-arrhythmic response exhibited by sotalol was not typical of beta blockers and related the observed effects of the drug to its property of prolonging the cardiac action potential duration. These data are supported by our own experience.[6]

We investigated the effects of the drug in preventing inducible ventricular tachycardia and its long-term effects in controlling the recurrent arrhythmia on chronic oral sotalol therapy. The study population consisted of 37 patients who clinically had manifested sustained symptomatic recurrent ventricular tachycardia and/or ventricular fibrillation. There were 36 men and 1 woman with a mean age of 58 (range 25 to 72) years. No patient had a reversible cause of the ventricular arrhythmias or recent myocardial infarction (i.e., in the 4 weeks immediately prior to the study). Except for 1 patient, who had sarcoidosis, all others had coronary artery disease. The mean left ventricular ejection fraction measured either by contrast or radionuclide ventriculography for 23 patients was $33.0 \pm 14.0$ percent. Patients in whom there was a contraindication to beta blockade or who had evidence of decompensated cardiac failure were excluded from entry into the study. Two patients in whom ventricular tachycardia could not be induced during the control study were excluded from analysis (discussed later). All patients except 1 had failed on or had not tolerated one or more (mean number, $2.76 \pm 1.3$) conventional antiarrhythmic drugs. In 2 patients with recurrent and frequent ventricular tachycardia/fibrillation that had not responded to intravenous lidocaine, procainamide, and bretylium tosylate, intravenous sotalol was given but electrophysiologic studies were not done either before or after the drug administration because of clinical exigencies.

In the two patients the drug was effective in controlling incessant ventricular tachycardia or fibrillation. An example is illustrated in Figure 4.

Thirty-five patients underwent electrophysiologic (EP) testing, 33 were found to have inducible ventricular tachycardia or fibrillation. Sotalol (after 1.5 mg/kg intravenously) prevented VT/VF reinduction in 15 (45.5 percent). Twenty-five of the 33 (15 EP positive, 10 EP negative) were given oral sotalol (dose range 160 b.i.d. to 460 mg b.i.d.).

The clinical outcome of patients with inducible versus nonin-

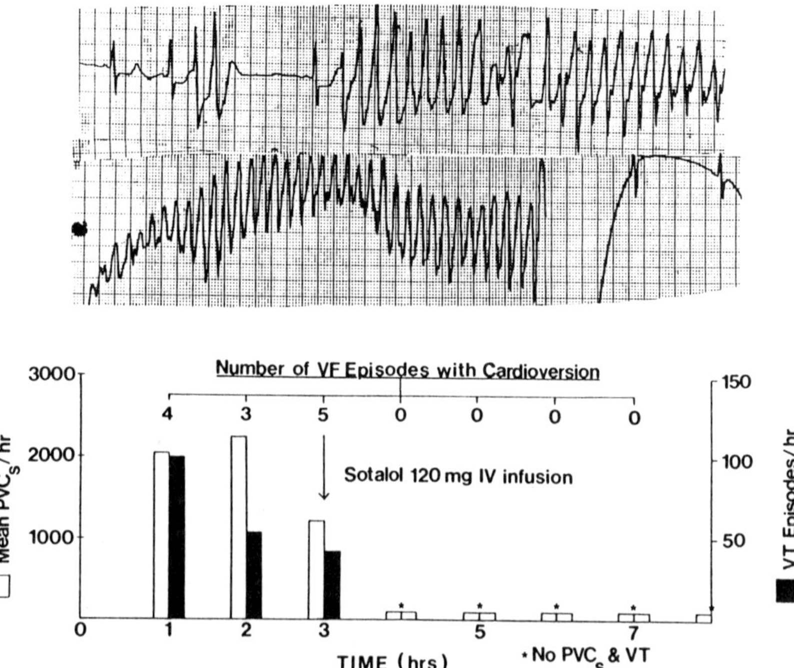



**Figure 4.** Effects of intravenous sotalol in a patient with recurrent VT/ VF resistant to lidocaine, procainamide, and bretylium. The upper panel shows the characteristic patterns of incessant ventricular tachyarrhythmias uncontrolled by conventional antiarrhythmic therapy. The lower panel shows the changes in the total PVC counts and ventricular tachycardia episodes before and after the intravenous injection of sotalol. Note that after sotalol was given, there were no further recurrences of VT/VF. (Based on data from Nademanee K, Feld G, Hendrickson JA, et al: Electrophysiologic and antiarrhythmic effects of sotalol in patients with life-threatening ventricular tachyarrhythmias. *Circulation* 72:555, 1985. By permission of the authors and American Heart Association.)

ducible VT/VF after IV sotalol relative to the subsequent administration of oral sotalol is summarized graphically in Figure 5. It is evident that in the patients in whom IV sotalol (see Fig. 6) prevented inducible VT/VF (n = 15), the arrhythmia could be controlled in 13 (86.7 percent) by oral sotalol; the drug failed early (within the first month) in 1 and appeared to aggravate it in another. During chronic therapy (longer than 1 month), arrhythmia recurred in 2 (at 8 and 8.4 months, respectively), and side effects precluded the continued use in an additional 2 patients. Eight patients remained free of arrhythmia and without side effects during

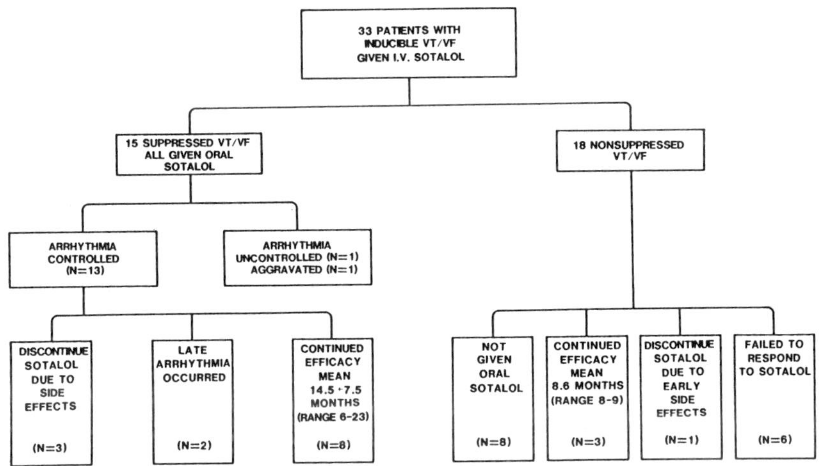


**Figure 5.** Flow diagram demonstrating the clinical outcome of patients on oral sotalol relative to the effects of the intravenous drug on the inducibility of VT/VF in patients with life-threatening ventricular tachyarrhythmias undergoing electrophysiologic studies. (Based on data from Nademanee K, Feld G, Hendrickson JA, et al: Electrophysiologic and antiarrhythmic effects of sotalol in patients with life-threatening ventricular tachyarrhythmias. *Circulation* 72:555, 1986.)

a mean follow-up period of 14.5 ± 7.5 (range 2 to 23) months. In 18 patients in whom sotalol failed to suppress VT/VF, oral sotalol was given in 10 but not in the other 8, because they did not have significant PVCs on baseline ambulatory EKG recordings. Of the 10 patients who were given oral sotalol in spite of the inducible VT after IV sotalol, 6 had recurrent VT/VF and 1 had a limiting side effect. The remaining 3 patients have been free of arrhythmias (mean follow-up 8.6 months, range 8 to 9). For the patients treated with oral sotalol 160 mg/b.i.d., the mean plasma levels were 2.3 ± 0.8 $\mu$g/ml (n = 6) and levels of 3.1 ± 0.4 $\mu$g/ml (n = 3) were found for those treated with 320 mg/b.i.d.

## Holter versus Electrophysioloic Testing in Predicting Long-Term Outcome of Sotalol Therapy

In 21 patients, 24-hour Holter recordings could be obtained before as well as during steady-state therapy with oral sotalol. The mean data (see Fig. 7) showed that sotalol reduced the total PVC count by 73 percent (p < 0.01), paired PVCs by 89 percent (p <

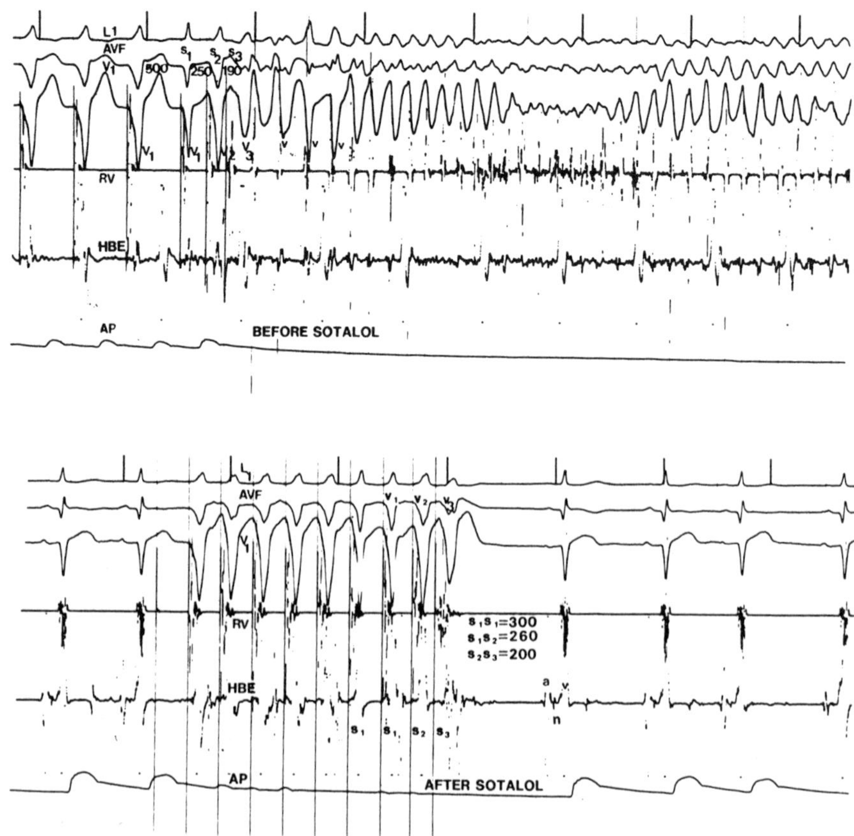


**Figure 6.** An example of the prevention of inducible (by programmed electrical stimulation of the heart) ventricular tachycardia (VT) by intravenous (1.5 mg/kg) sotalol. Double stimuli were used to produce the VT. Note that after sotalol, VT is no longer inducible. (Based on data from Nademanee K, Feld G, Hendrickson JA, et al: Electrophysiologic and anti-arrhythmic effects of sotalol in patients with life-threatening tachyarrhythmias. *Circulation* 72:555, 1986.)

0.01), and VT beats by 95 percent (p < 0.01). In 11 of the 21 patients, sotalol reduced total PVCs by at least 85 percent, and paired PVCs and VT beats by at least 90 percent (Group A). In the other 10 patients, sotalol did not significantly suppress spontaneously occurring arrhythmias (Group B). Group A (11 patients) included 9 patients in whom VT could not be reinduced and 2 in whom VT remained inducible. By contrast, VT remained inducible in 8 of 10 patients in Group B. Analysis by the Fisher's exact test

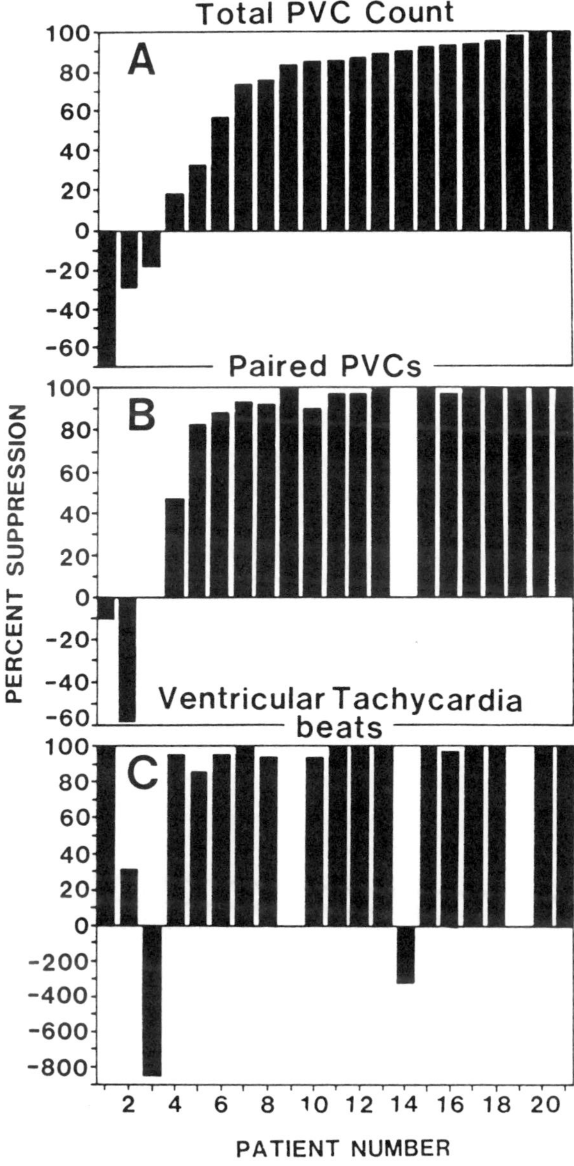


**Figure 7.**   Effects of orally administered sotalol on the total, paired, and repetitive ventricular ectopic beats in 21 patients with life-threatening ventricular tachyarrhythmias. Note that sotalol is more effective in suppressing complex premature ventricular contractions (PVCs) than the total PVCs. (Based on data from Nademanee K, Feld G, Hendrickson JA, et al: Electrophysiologic and antiarrhythmic effects of sotalol in patients with life-threatening tachyarrhythmias. *Circulation* 72:555, 1986.)

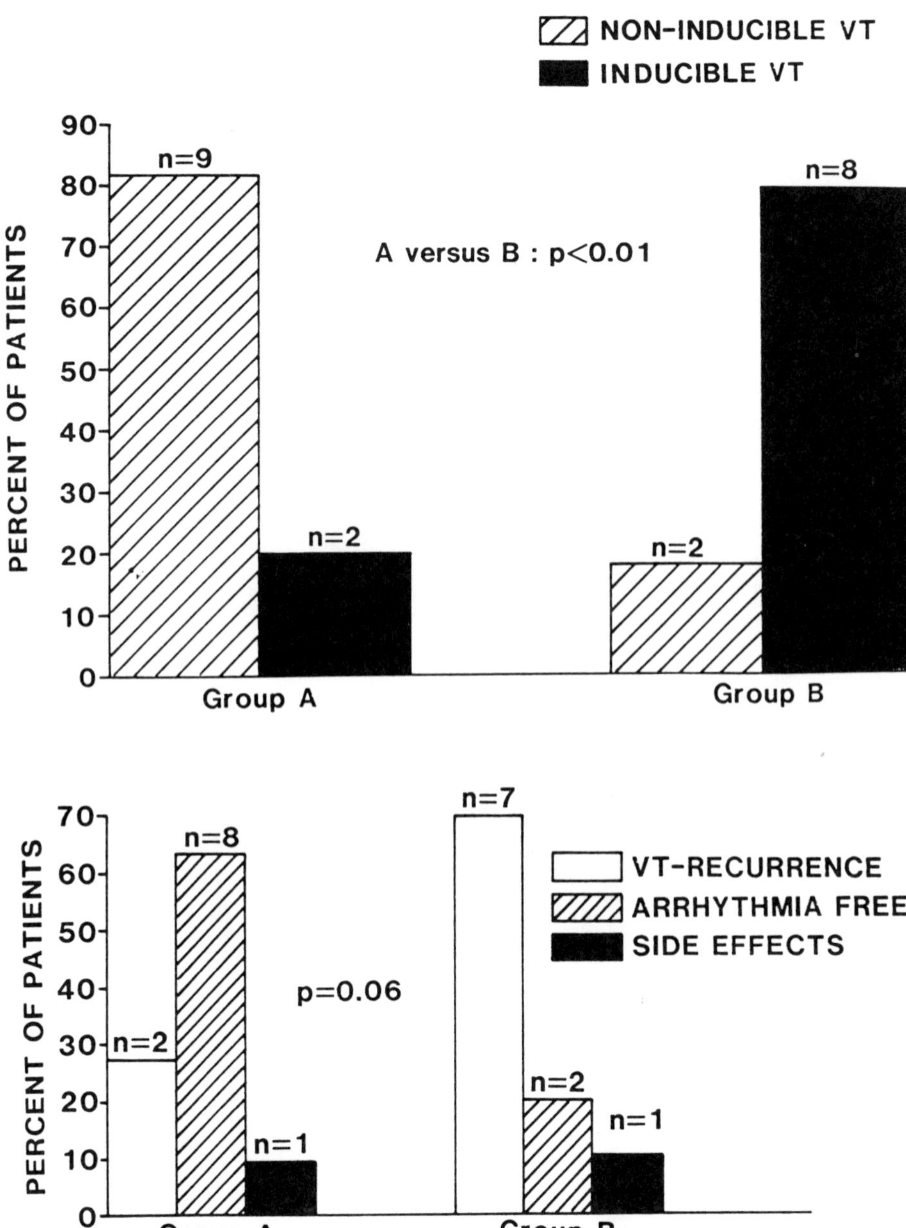


**Figure 8.** The relationship between the effects of intravenous sotalol on the inducibility of VT/VF and the degree of suppression by the oral drug of the spontaneously occurring ventricular arrhythmias in the same patients.

(Fig. 8) showed that Group A had a significantly greater number of patients with noninducible VT than Group B (p < 0.01). Moreover, in Group A only 2 patients (18 percent) who had recurrent VT/VF, whereas there were 7 in Group B (70 percent; p < 0.06). Two patients in group A and 1 patient in group B had significant side effects necessitating discontinuation of the drug.

In the study of Nademanee et al.,[6] intravenous sotalol prevented the reinduction of VT/VF in 45.5 percent, a figure that generally is higher than those reported for the so-called membrane-active or Class I compounds.[46,63] There is little data on this issue for other Class III agents except for amiodarone, which has been reported to prevent reinduction of VT/VF after chronic therapy in 8 to 50 percent[64] of cases. However, Senges et al.[5] recently showed that, in their hands, intravenous sotalol prevented VT/VF reinduction in 12 of 18 patients (67 percent), which is a somewhat higher success rate than that in our own series, in which 15 of 33 patients became noninducible after intravenous sotalol. Nine of their 12 patients, subsequently treated with oral sotalol over a long-term, remained in complete or partial control over a mean follow-up period of 16 months. Our own data on chronic oral therapy are similar. Although the numbers of patients in our series have been limited, there is a trend indicating the clinical utility of electrophysiologic testing in predicting long-term effectiveness of oral sotalol in controlling VT/VF. Our data, as well as those of Senges et al.[5] have dealt with the predictive value of intravenous sotalol response. The possibility that a greater predictive accuracy might be attained by

---

Group A patients: Administration of sotalol resulted in 85 percent suppression of total PVCs and 90 percent suppression of paired PVCs and beats of ventricular tachycardia. Group B: Sotalol did not have these effects. Note that the number of patients in whom sotalol prevented reinduction of VT/VF was significantly higher in Group A than in Group B. The differences in the clinical outcome in patients relative to the degree of suppression of spontaneously occurring arrhythmias during Holter monitoring. The separation of patients into Groups A and B by the same criteria as in A. The difference between the two groups is of borderline significance. The data presented in this figure suggest that the prevention of inducible VT/VF by intravenous sotalol and the suppression of spontaneously occurring arrhythmias by oral sotalol are both predictive of long-term clinical outcome of prophylactic sotalol therapy in patients with ventricular tachyarrhythmias. (From Nademanee K, Feld G, Hendrickson JA, et al: Electrophysiologic and arrhythmic effects of sotalol in patients with life-threatening tachyarrhythmias. *Circulation* 72:555, 1986. By permission of the authors and of the American Heart Association.)

the use of oral drug testing with respect to the inducibility of ventricular tachycardia/fibrillation cannot be excluded.

Our data also demonstrate that orally administered sotalol is moderately effective in suppressing PVCs, particularly complex and repetitive forms. In over 50 percent of the patients, the drug was found to suppress at least 85 percent of total PVC counts and nearly abolish complex forms (paired PVCs and VT beats), a feature that was statistically concordant with drug-induced prevention of VT/VF induction by programmed electrical stimulation of the heart in the same patients. A comparison of the effects of sotalol demonstrated here with those of conventional beta blockers[46] suggests that the major antiarrhythmic effects of the drug in patients with life-threatening VT/VF might be mediated through its nonadrenergic properties. Further resolution of this issue is likely to be accomplished by a direct comparison of the antiarrhythmic effects of the dextro-isomer of the compound with those of the racemate.

## Sotalol Versus Procainamide Comparison in Life-Threatening Ventricular Arrhythmias

A recent double-blind, randomized, multicenter study compared the effects of intravenous and oral procainamide.[38] Patients who had recurrent VT/VF underwent electrophysiologic study with programmed electrical stimulation of the heart. Patients who had inducible VT/VF were selected randomly to receive either procainamide (n = 49) or sotalol (n = 54) in a blinded fashion (using a third-party blinder). Intravenous procainamide (plasma level, 7.8 ± 2.3 µg/ml) prevented induction VT/VF reinduction in 11 patients (22 percent) and sotalol (plasma level 2.14 ± 40 µg/ ml) in 18 patients (33 percent), but the difference was not statistically significant. The repeat electrophysiologic studies on the oral drug regimens included mean plasma levels of 11 ± 5 µg/ml for procainamide and 2.73 ± 0.98 µg/ml for sotalol. In the procainamide series, the oral drug was ineffective in preventing the arrhythmia in 2 patients: 1 developed side effects on the oral drug, 1 had a proarrhythmic effect (torsades de pointes). In 1 patient, the reason for the withdrawal from the study could not be ascertained. In 6 (12 percent) of the total patients selected randomly, procainamide was effective and the patients could be discharged from the hospital. In the sotalol series, the oral drug was not effective in preventing

VT/VF reinduction in 6, side effects developed in 1, torsade de pointes in 2, and in 1 patient acute myocardial infarction developed as a concurrent clinical event. Eight patients (15 percent) in the sotalol series were under satisfactory control and could be discharged from the hospital on the drug. Long-term follow-up revealed that only 3 patients in the procainamide series and 6 patients in the sotalol series continued to take the drug with an adequate control of the arrhythmia. This multicenter study has indicated that, in the treatment of life-threatening ventricular arrhythmia, the overall efficacy of sotalol and procainamide was comparable. However, further controlled data are needed to determine the differences in the overall utility of the two agents in the long-term management of malignant ventricular arrhythmias.

## Comparison of the Efficacy of Sotalol with Amiodarone

Limited data are available on the effects of sotalol compared to those of other Class III agents. Greze et al.[65] studied 23 men and 11 women with high-density premature ventricular contractions. All antiarrhythmic agents had been withdrawn 10 days before the enrollment into the study. Amiodarone was given 400 mg/day for 5 days out of 7; sotalol was given 160 mg twice daily. The effects of the drugs were judged on the basis of PVC suppression. In 11 patients, sotalol and amiodarone proved equally effective, in 5 amiodarone was superior to sotalol and the converse was true in another 5. The study had a crossover design. The data from this study needs to be interpreted with caution, as neither drug was titrated to a steady-state effect and a crossover effect from amiodarone may have affected the overall efficacy of sotalol.

Burckhardt et al.[66] studied 6 patients who had been on amiodarone 200–400 mg/day for repetitive PVCs for a mean period of 12 months. Amiodarone was withdrawn and weekly Holter recordings were obtained until there was evidence of the recurrence of repetitive PVCs. Sotalol was then started at a dose of 160–320 mg/day. In 1 patient, sotalol had to be stopped because of insomnia and recurrence of angina; amidoarone was reintroduced but the patient died suddenly 2 days later. In the remaining 5 patients, repetitive PVCs were controlled by sotalol as determined by Holter recordings 7 days after the initiation of therapy. The effect was maintained for a mean follow-up period of 8.4 months. More data are needed in this subset of patients as well as in patients with life-threatening ventricular arrhythmias controlled on amiodarone and then switched over to sotalol.

## Sotalol in Survivors of Acute Myocardial Infarction

It has now been well established that beta blockers given prophylactically to the survivors of acute myocardial infarction prolong survival and reduce the frequency of reinfarction.[67] In the case of sotalol the data is less decisive. Julian et al.[68] compared the effects of 320 mg of sotalol daily (in two divided doses) with those of placebo in patients surviving acute myocardial infarction. Treatment was initiated 5–14 days after infarction in 1456 patients (60 percent randomly chosen to receive sotalol and 40 percent to receive placebo). The follow-up period was 12 months. The mortality rate was 7.3 percent in the sotalol group versus 8.9 percent in the placebo group; the 18 percent lower mortality in the sotalol group, however, did not reach statistical significance. In contrast, the reinfarction rate was 41 percent lower in the sotalol group ($p < 0.05$). It should be emphasized that although the incidence of sudden death was not reduced significantly by sotalol in this study, the overall trend clearly is indicative of the salutary effect of the beta blocker in this setting and is in line with the results of other more comprehensive studies involving other beta blockers.[68] Because of the well-demonstrated Class III antiarrhythmic action, one might have expected a more striking effect on sudden death in the case of sotalol. However, the mechanism of sudden death reduction by beta blockers in the survivors of acute infarction is unclear and may not be mediated via a primarily antiarrhythmic action.[67] Alternatively, only a small fraction of patients following acute infarction have electrical instability and complex premature ventricular ectopic beats. The suppressant effect of sotalol on arrhythmias in this subset of patients is unlikely to have a discernible impact on the overall mortality in clinical trials in which patients have not been preselected for testing the effects of sotalol on cardiac arrhythmias.

## Dose and Administration

Sotalol is available in an intravenous as well as oral formulation. Doses of the drug between 0.2 mg/kg and 1.5 mg/kg given intravenously have been used in patients with normal as well as depressed ejection fraction with impunity. As in the case of all beta blockers, slow administration of the drug is recommended.

The lowest single doses of the drug shown to have an antiarrhythmic effect is about 80 mg. However, the lowest minimum effective dose for orally administered sotalol has not been defined. It is likely to be 80 mg twice daily. However, recent studies have indicated that the most commonly used initial dose is 160 mg given twice daily; the dose may be increased every 3 to 4 days to a maximum of 480 mg twice daily, although the efficacy and safety of such a high dose has not been evaluated critically. Barring exceptional circumstances, we cannot recommend daily doses exceeding 640 mg daily. The use of the higher doses should be used in conjunction with careful monitoring of the electrocardiographic changes, serum drug levels, and careful attention to the possibility of concomitant hypokalemia. This is particularly important when diuretics are used concomitantly with sotalol.

In patients with reduced renal function, a careful adjustment of drug dose and dosing interval is necessary. For example, in cases of moderate impairment of renal function, the initial dose should not exceed 160 mg/day and subsequent dose adjustment should be made on the basis of clinical response and serum drug levels. In patients with severely compromised renal function (e.g., GFR reduced below 25 ml/min/1.73 $m^2$ BSA) sotalol should be avoided or be used with a great deal of caution with frequent monitoring of serum drug levels and the electrocardiogram.

## Side Effects

The adverse reactions due to sotalol may be attributed to its beta-blocking actions and those to its propensity to lengthen the $QT_c$ interval of the electrocardiogram. The incidence of side effects due to beta blockade is similar to that exhibited by other beta antagonists: tiredness, lassitude, impotence, depression, headache. Rare cases of retroperitoneal fibrosis, as in the case of other beta blockers, have been reported.[69] As in the case of hydrophilic beta blockers, such as atenolol, the effects of sotalol on the EEG, sleep patterns, and performance in psychologic tests have been found to be equivocal and suggest little or no CNS activity of the compound.[70] The cardiovascular effects include AV block, bradycardia, hypotension, and exacerbation of heart failure although the incidence of the latter is lower than that for other beta blockers.[5,6] The development of polymorphic ventricular tachycardia or torsades de pointes as a complication of sotalol therapy is unrelated to its beta blocking actions.

During intravenous sotalol administration rarely are there significant hemodynamic disturbances in doses up to 1.5 mg/kg.[5,6] In the study by Nademanee et al.[6] in 4 patients, distal AV block developed transiently following intravenous injection of sotalol. In the same study, involving oral drug administration, lethargy, weakness, and fatigue developed in 4 patients, depression in 1, aggravation of heart failure in 1, severe bradycardia in 2, decreased libido and impotence in 2, and dry mouth in 1. In 4 patients, the side effects were sufficiently severe to necessitate drug discontinuation. The left ventricular ejection fraction determined by radionuclide ventriculography in 10 patients before oral sotalol was given was $33.1 \pm 14.0$ percent; on sotalol it was $42.6 \pm 16.0$ percent. The side effects due to sotalol reported by Senges et al.[5] were similar to those reported by Nademanee et al.[6]

## Sotalol-Induced $QT_c$ Prolongation Torsades de Pointes

The subject of the potential mechanisms of torsade de pointes developing as a complication of Class III agents is discussed in Chapter 23. Here, we review the cases that have been reported in the literature[71-86] and draw general conclusions from the observations.

Prolongation of $QT_c$ interval may occur with sotalol in therapeutic doses both during intravenous injections[5,6] and during oral drug administration, short term as well as long term. Moreover, Neuvonen et al.[76-80] have reported a correlation between the serum sotalol concentration and prolongation of the $QT_c$ interval. Initially, severe ventricular arrhythmia, including ventricular tachycardia and fibrillation, was reported in 5 of 6 cases of sotalol poisoning[79] and correlated with the prolongation of the QT interval and serum sotalol concentration. In a recent report, McKibben et al.[71] reported a series of 13 patients who developed syncope and prolonged QT interval while taking therapeutic doses of sotalol. Polymorphous ventricular tachycardia was observed in 12 patients and criteria typical of torsades de pointes were present in 10 patients. Most (12 of 13) patients in this series had been treated with sotazide, a combination of sotalol and hydrochlorothiazide with or without or with inadequate potassium supplementation. Serum potassium concentrations were reduced in 8 patients. Four patients were taking other drugs (3 on disopyramide and 2 on tricyclic antidepressants) known to cause prolongation of QT interval. The QT interval returned to normal in all patients after withdrawal of the drugs and correction of the hypokalemia. Most other cases of torsades de pointes following sotalol therapy have (Fig. 9) occurred with overdosage,[77,79,83,85] although uncommonly cases have been reported in the context of so-called therapeutic serum concentrations.[82] These results indicate that even in therapeutic doses sotalol can induce life-threatening ventricular arrhythmia, particularly when given in combination with hydrochlorothiazide[85] without potassium supplementation. However, when the dose of the drug is kept low and patients are monitored carefully the incidence of torsade is low.[5,6]

The proarrhythmic effect of sotalol is most likely to occur in instances of renal failure, hypokalemia, bradycardia, at high concentrations of the drug, and in situations in which there is preexisting lengthening of the $QT_c$ interval.[86-90] Whether a combination of Class Ia antiarrhythmic agents and sotalol may lead to torsades de pointes has not been demonstrated, but it is prudent that such a combination therapy be undertaken with caution until its safety and efficacy has been established. It is recommended that careful attention should be paid to assure a normal serum potassium level in all patients being treated with sotalol.

Torsades de pointes developing during sotalol therapy may be treated by withdrawal of the drug, administration of isoprenaline, ventricular pacing,[90] and the correction of serum electrolyte disturbances. Antiarrhythmic agents that the prolong $QT_c$ interval should be avoided.


## Conclusions

The role of sotalol as a therapeutic agent should be considered in light of its property as a nonselective beta antagonist with a less depressant effect on myocardial performance than conventional beta blockers and the fact that the compound selectively prolongs myocardial refractoriness by lengthening the action potential duration in all cardiac tissues. By reason of its combined beta blocking activity (Class II antiarrhythmic action) and its property of homogeneously prolonging the action potential duration in myocar-

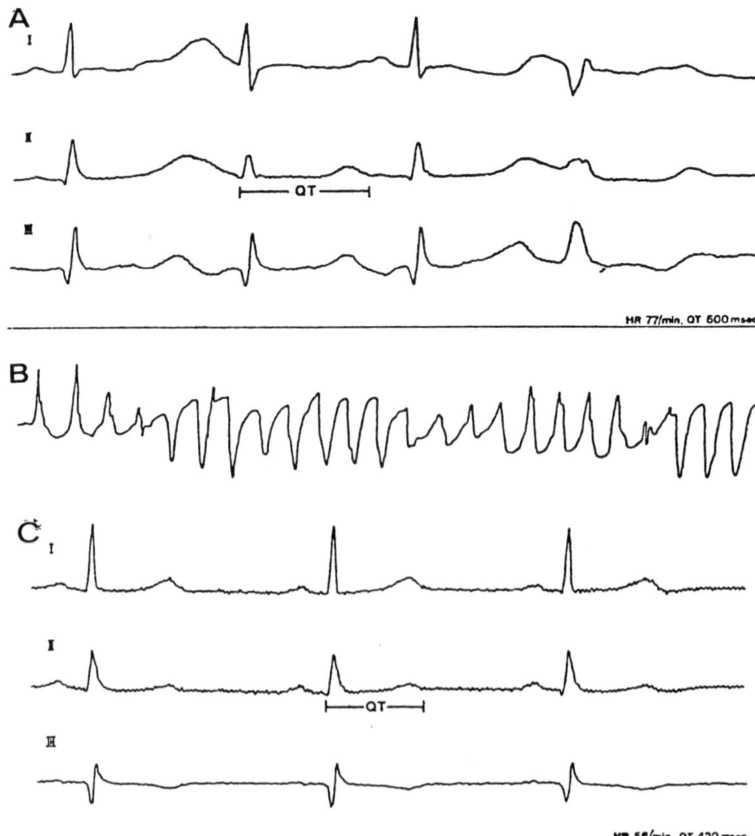


**Figure 9.** Electrocardiographic recordings illustrating the unusually striking lengthening of the $QT_c$ interval and the development of torsades de pointes in a patient treated with sotalol. A: Changes in the EKG at admission to hospital, with the hospital administering sotalol, following which the patient developed recurrent syncope. B. A strip of EKG demonstrating torsades des pointes follows panel A. This arrhythmia complicated the marked lengthening of the $QT_c$ induced by sotalol. C: Return of the $QT_c$ lengthening to normal following discontinuation of sotalol. C: Improvement in the $QT_c$ interval following withdrawal of sotalol and a period of ventricular pacing. (From Totterman KJ, Tutro H, Pellinen T: Overdrive pacing as treatment of sotalol-induced ventricular tachyarrhythmias (torsades des pointes). *Acta Med Scand* (Suppl) 668:28, 1982. By permission of the authors and the Editor of *Acta Med Scand*.)

dial tissues (a Class III action), the compound is likely to have a wide spectrum of action in ventricular and supraventricular arrhythmias, a spectrum of activity that would differ from that of conventional beta blocking drugs. The difference is particularly marked in the case of ventricular arrhythmias.

The available data indicate that sotalol is an effective antiarrhythmic compound for a significant number of patients with life-threatening VT/VF refractory to conventional antiarrhythmic drugs. Sotalol appears to have a low arrhythmogenic potential and, since it has a rapid onset of action with a predictable long-term outcome on the basis of intravenous electrophysiologic testing, it appears to be a significant advance in the acute and the prophylactic management of ventricular tachyarrhythmias. The relative lack of the propensity to depress ventricular function, predictable pharmacokinetics, and side effect profile with a low arrhythmogenic potential make sotalol a promising approach for the control of a broad spectrum of disorders of cardiac rhythm.

---

*The research behind this chapter was supported by grants from the Medical Research Service of the Veterans Administration and the American Heart Association of the Greater Los Angeles Affiliate (789 G1-1).*

# References

1. Lish PM, Weikel JH, Dungan KW: Pharmacological and toxicological properties of two new beta-adrenergic receptor antagonists. *J Pharmacol Exp Ther* 149:161, 1965.
2. Singh BN, Collett JT, Chew CYC: New perspectives in the pharmacologic therapy of cardiac arrhythmias. *Prog Cardiovasc Dis* 20:243, 1980.
3. Singh BN, Vaughan Williams EM: A third class of antiarrhythmic action: Effects on atrial and ventricular intracellular potentials, and other pharmacological actions on cardiac muscle of MJ1999 and AH 3676. *Br J Pharmacol* 39:675, 1970.
4. Singh BN, Hauswirth O: Comparative mechanisms of action of antiarrhythmic drugs. *Am Heart J* 87:367, 1974.
5. Senges J, Lengfelder W, Jauernig R, et al: Electrophysiologic testing of therapy with sotalol for sustained ventricular tachycardia. *Circulation* 69:577, 1984.
6. Nademanee K, Feld G, Hendrickson JA, et al: Electrophysiologic and antiarrhythmic effects of sotalol in patients with life-threatening ventricular tachyarrhythmias. *Circulation* 72:555, 1985.
7. Singh BN, Nademanee K: Control of cardiac arrhythmias by selective

lengthening of repolarization: Theoretic considerations and clinical observations. *Am Heart J* 109:421, 1985.

8. Singh BN, Nademanee K: Control of arrhythmias by lengthening cardiac repolarization: Unique role of sotalol. In *Advances in Cardiology: Unique Role of Sotalol.* Oxford, Medicine Publishing Foundation, p 15, 1985.

9. Kato R, Yabek S, Ikeda N, et al: Electrophysiologic effects of dextro- and levo-isomers of sotalol in isolated cardiac muscle. *J Amer Coll Cardiol* 7:116, 1986.

10. Blinks JR: Evaluation of the cardiac effects of several beta-adrenergic blocking agents. *Ann NY Acad Sci.* 139:673, 1967.

11. Singh BN: A study of the pharmacological actions of certain drugs and hormones with a particular reference to cardiac muscle. D. Phil. thesis, England, University of Oxford, 1971.

12. Kofi Ekue JM, Lowe DC, Shanks RG: Comparison of the effects of propranolol and MJ1999 on cardiac beta-adrenoceptors in man. *Brit J Pharmacol* 38:546, 1970.

13. Lewis MJ, Grey AC, Henderson AH: Inotropic beta-blocking (pA$_2$) and partial agonist activity of propranolol, sotalol and acebutolol. *Eur J Pharmacol* 86:71, 1983.

14. Aberg G, Dzedin T, Lundholm L, et al: A comparative study of some cardiovascular effects of sotalol (MJ 1999) and propranolol. *Life Sci* 8:353, 1969.

15. Kaumann AJ, Olson CB: Temporal relationship between long-lasting aftercontractions and action potentials in cat papillary muscles. *Science* 163:293, 1968.

16. Nathan AW, Hellestrand KJ, Bextan RS, et al: Electrophysiological effects of sotalol—just another B-blocker? *Br Heart J* 47:575, 1982.

17. Bennett D: Acute prolongation of myocardial refractoriness by sotalol. *Br Heart J* 47:521, 1982.

18. Bextan RS, Camm AJ: Drugs with Class III antiarrhythmic action. *Pharmacol Ther* 17:315, 1982.

19. Carmeliet E: Electrophysiologic and voltage clamp analysis of effects of sotalol on isolated cardiac muscle and Purkinje fibers. *J Pharmacol Exp Ther* 232:817, 1985.

20. Johnston GD, Finch MB, McNeil JA, et al: A comparison of the cardiovascular effects of (+)-sotalol and (±)-sotalol following intravenous administration in normal volunteers. *Br J Clin Pharmacol* 20:507, 1985.

21. Schmid JR, Hanna C: A comparison of the antiarrhythmic actions of two new synthetic compounds, iproveratril and MJ1999, with quinidine and pronethalol. *J Pharmacol Exp Ther* 156:331, 1967.

22. Kaumann A, Aramendia P: Prevention of ventricular fibrillation induced by coronary ligation. *J Pharmacol Exp Ther* 164:326, 1968.

23. Lynch JJ, Wilber DJ, Montgomery DG, et al: Antiarrhythmic and antifibrillatory actions of the levo- and dextro- rotatory isomers of sotalol. *J Cardiovasc Pharmacol* 6:1132, 1984.

24. Patterson E, Lynch JJ, Lucchesi BR: The antiarrhythmic and antifibrillatory actions of the beta-adrenergic receptor antagonist, d,1-sotalol. *J Pharmacol Exp Ther* 230:519, 1984.

25. Patterson E, Lucchesi, BR: Antifibrillatory properties of the beta-

adrenergic receptor antagonists, nadolol, sotalol, atenolol and propranolol in the anesthetized dog and rabbit cardiac tissue. *Pharmacology* 28:121, 1984.

26. Cobbe SM, Hoffman E, Ritzenhoff A, et al: Action of sotalol on potential re-entrant pathways and ventricular tachyarrhythmias in conscious dogs in the late post-myocardial infarction phase. *Circulation* 68:865, 1983.

27. Prakash R, Parmley WW, Allen HN, et al: Effect of sotalol on clinical arrhythmias. *Am J Cardiol* 29:397, 1972.

28. Fogelman F, Lightman SL, Sillett RW, et al: The treatment of cardiac arrhythmias with sotalol. *Eur J Clin Pharmacol* 5:72, 1972.

29. Simon A, Berman E: Long-term sotalol therapy in patients with arrhythmias. *J Clin Pharmacol* 19:547, 1979.

30. Myburgh DP, Goldman AP, Cartoon J, et al: The efficacy of sotalol in suppressing ventricular ectopic beats. *Afr Med J* 56:295, 1979.

31. Rizos I, Senges J, Jauernig R, et al: Differential effects of sotalol and metoprolol on the induction of paroxysmal supraventricular tachycardia *Am J Cardiol* 53:1022, 1984.

32. Marshall RJ, Muir AW, Winslow E: Effects of antiarrhythmic drugs on ventricular fibrillation thresholds of normal and ischemic myocardium in the anesthetized rat. *Brit J Pharmacol* 78: 165, 1983.

33. Culling W, Penny WJ, Sheridan DJ: Effects of sotalol on arrhythmias and electrophysiology during myocardial ischemia and reperfusion. *Cardiovasc Res* 18:397, 1984.

34. Izumi T, Sakai K, Abiko Y: Effects of sotalol on ischemic myocardial pH in the dog heart. *Arch Pharmacol* 318:340, 1982.

35. Cobbe SM, Manley BS: Effects of elevated extraceullar potassium concentrations on the Class III antiarrhythmic action of sotalol. *Cardiovasc Res* 19:69, 1985.

36. Bertrix L, Timour-Chah Q, Lang J, et al: Protection against ventricular and atrial fibrillation by sotalol. *Cardiovasc Res* 20:358, 1986.

37. Ward DE, Camm AJ, Spurrell RAJ: The acute cardiac electrophysiological effects of intravenous sotalol hydrochloride. *Clin Cardiol* 2:185, 1979.

38. The Sotalol Multicenter Study Group: A multicenter, double-blind evaluation of procainamide and sotalol by programmed electrical stimulation in patients with life-threatening ventricular arrhythmias. In press, 1988.

39. Rowland E, Perrins J, Donaldson RM, et al: The clinical electrophysiologic effects of d-sotalol—a new Class III antiarrhythmic drug. (abstract) *J Am Coll Cardiol* 5:498, 1984.

40. McComb JM, McGowan JB, McGovern BA, et al: Comparison of the electrophysiologic properties of d- and dl-sotalol. (abstract) *J Am Coll Cardiol* 5:438, 1985.

41. Schwartz J, Wynn J, Maza S, et al: Antiarrhythmic properties of d-sotalol in patients with ventricular tachycardia determined by programmed electrical stimulation. *J Am Coll Cardiol* 7:93A, 1986.

42. Edvaardsson N, Hirsch L, Emmanuelsson H, et al: Sotalol-induced delayed ventricular repolarization in man. *Eur Heart J* 1:335, 1980.

43. Edvaardsson N, Olsson B: Effects of acute and chronic beta-receptor

blockade on ventricular repolarization in man. *Br Heart J* 45:628, 1981.

44. Echt DS, Berte LE, Clusin WT, et al: Prolongation of the human cardiac monophasic action potential by sotalol. *Am J Cardiol* 50:1082, 1982.

45. Touboul P, Atallah G, Kirkorian G, et al: Clinical electrophysiology of intravenous sotalol, a beta blocking drug with class III antiarrhythmic properties. *Am Heart J* 107:888, 1984.

46. Dumoulin P, Weissenburger J, Poirier JM, et al: Etude des effets electrophsyiologiques du sotalol intraveineux. Relation avec les concentrations plasmatiques. *Arch Mal du Coeur et des Vaisseaux* 78:562, 1985.

47. Horowitz LN, Josephson ME, Kastor JA: Intracardiac electrophysiologic studies as a method for the optimization of drug therapy in chronic ventricular arrhythmias. *Prog Cardiovasc Dis* 23:81, 1980.

48. Nademanee K, Feld G, Noll E, et al: Effect of sotalol, Class III antiarrhythmic agent on conduction and refractoriness of the His-Purinje system in man. *J Am Coll Cardiol* 5(2):438, 1985.

49. Creamer JE, Nathan AW, Shennan A, et al: Acute and chronic effects of sotalol and propranolol on ventricular repolarization using constant rate-pacing. *Am J Cardiol* 57:1092, 1986.

50. Attuel P, Do-Gnoc D, Friocourt P, et al: Sotalol more than a beta blocker: A clinical reality. In *Advances in Cardiology: The Unique Role of Sotalol.* Oxford, Medicine Publishing Foundation, p 45, 1985.

51. Teo KK, Harte M, Morgan JH: Sotalol infusion in the treatment of supraventricular tachyarrhythmias. *Chest* 87:113, 1985.

52. Campbell TJ, Gavaghan TD, Morgan JJ: Intravenous sotalol for the treatment of atrial fibrillation and flutter after cardiopulmonary bypass. Comparison with disopyramide and digoxin in a randomized trial. *Br Heart J* 54:86, 1985.

53. Janssen JH: Prevention and treatment of supraventricular tachycardia early following coronary artery bypass surgery. *Angiology* 36:575, 1985.

54. Manz M, Kuhl AJ, Luderitz B: Sotalol bei supraventrikularer tachycardie elektrophysiologische messungen bein Wolff-Parkinson-White syndrom und AV-Knoten-Reentrytachykardie. *Kardiologie* 74:500, 1985.

55. Blanc JJ, Boschat J, Ollivier JP, et al: Effets du sotalol per os sur la conduction des voies accessoires auriculo-ventriculaires. *Arch des Maladies du Coeur et des Vaisseaux* 78:1097, 1985.

56. Stroobandt, R, Kesteloot H: Efficacy of intravenous sotalol on ventricular arrhythmias occurring during maximal exercise stress testing. *Arch Int Pharmacodyn* 264:290–297, 1983.

57. Burckhardt D, Pfisterer M, Hoffmann A, et al: Effects of the beta-adrenoceptor blocking agent sotalol on ventricular arrhythmias in patients with chronic ischemic heart disease. *Cardiology* 70 Suppl 1:114, 1983.

58. Lidell C, Rehnquist N, Sjogren A, et al: Comparative efficacy of oral sotalol and procainamide in patients with chronic ventricular arrhythmias: A multicenter study. *Am Heart J* 109:970, 1985.

59. Mary-Rabine L, Soumagne D, Stiels B: Long-term sotalol therapy in patients with ventricular arrhythmias. *Acta Cardiol* 2:89, 1986.

60. Deedwania PC, the Multicenter Sotalol Study Group: Comparative efficacy of sotalol and propranolol in the suppression of premature ventricular contractions (Unpublished).
61. Anderson JL, Askins JC, Gilbert MG: Multicenter trial of sotalol for suppression of frequent, complex ventricular arrhythmias: A double-blind, randomized, placebo-controlled evaluation of two doses. *J Amer Coll Cardiol* 8:752, 1986.
62. Wang T, Bergstrand RH, Thompson KA, et al: Concentration-dependent pharmacologic properties of sotalol. *Amer J Cardiol* 57:1160, 1986.
63. Spielman SR, Kay HR, Morganroth J, et al: Drug therapy in high risk patients following acute myocardial infarction. The results of timolol, encainide and sotalol trial. *Circulation* 72:III-14, 1985.
64. Duff HJ, Mitchell LB, Wyse DG: Antiarrhythmic efficacy of propranolol: Comparison of low and high serum concentrations. *J Amer Coll Cardiol* 8:959, 1986.
65. Greze M, Berteau P, Dequidt M, et al: Etude comparative de l'activite du sotalol et de l' amiodarone dans le traitement des troubles du rythme ventriculaire em ambulatoire. *Semains des Hopitaux* 61:3105, 1985.
66. Burckhardt D, White AR, Hoffman A: Replacement of amiodarone by sotalol for repetitive ventricular premature beats. *Amer Heart J* 107:167, 1984.
67. Singh BN, Venkatesh N: Prevention of myocardial reinfarction and sudden death in the survivors of acute myocardial infarction: Role of prophylactic beta-blockade. *Amer Heart J* 107:189, 1984.
68. Julian DG, Jackson FS, Prescott RJ, et al: Controlled trial of sotalol for one year after myocardial infarction. *Lancet* 1:1142, 1982.
69. Laakso M, Arvala I, Tervonen S, et al: Retroperitoneal fibrosis associated with sotalol. *Br Med J* 285:1085, 1982.
70. Bender W, Greil W, Ruther E, et al: Effects of the beta-adrenoceptor blocking agent sotalol on CNS: Sleep, EEG, and psychophysiologic parameters. *J Clin Pharmacol* 143:505, 1979.
71. McKibben JK, Pocock WA, Barlow JB, et al: Sotalol, hypokalemia, syncope and torsades de pointes. *Br Heart J* 51:157, 1984.
72. Kontopoulos A, Filindris A, Manoudis F, et al: Sotalol-induced torsade de pointes. *Postgrad Med J* 57:321, 1981.
73. Laakso M, Pentikainen PH, Lampainen E: Sotalol, Prolonged Q-T interval, and ventricular tachyarrhythmias. *Ann Clin Res* 13:439, 1981.
74. Laakso M, Pentikainen PJ, Pyorala K: Sotalol and QTc interval. *Lancet* 2:1168, 1981.
75. Laakso M, Pentikainen PH, Pyorola K, et al: Prolongation of the Q-T interval caused by sotalol—possible association with ventricular tachyarrhythmias. *Eur Heart J* 2:355, 1981.
76. Laakso M, Pentikainen PJ, Rehnberg S: Sotalol-induced prolongation of the QT interval and attacks of unconsciousness. *Int J Clin Pharmacol Toxicol* 22:487, 1984.
77. Neuvonen PJ, Elonen E, Tarssanen L: Sotalol intoxication, two patients with concentration–effect relationships. *Acta Pharmacol et Toxicol* 45:52, 1979.

78. Neuvonen PJ, Elonen E, Tanskanen A, et al: Sotalol and prolonged QTc interval. *Lancet* 2:426, 1981.
79. Neuvonen PJ, Elonen E, Vuorenmaa T, et al: Prolonged Q-T interval and ventricular tachyarrhythmias; common features of sotalol intoxication. *Eur J Clin Pharmacol* 20:85, 1981.
80. Neuvonen PH, Elonen E, Tanskanen A, et al: Sotalol prolongation of the QTc interval in hypertensive patients. *Clin Pharmacol Ther* 7:25, 1982.
81. Neuvonen PH, Elonen E, Tanskanen A, et al: Sotalol prolongation of the QTc interval in hypertensive patients. *Clin Pharmacol Ther* 32:25, 1982.
82. Krapf R, Gertsch M: Torsades de pointes induced by sotalol despite therapeutic concentrations. *Br Med J* 290:1784, 1985.
83. Montagna M, Groppi A: Fatal sotalol poisoning. *Arch Toxicol* 43:221, 1980.
84. Kuck KH, Kunze KP, Roewer N, et al: Sotalol-induced torsade de pointes. *Amer Heart J* 107:179, 1984.
85. Elonen E, Neuvonen PJ, Tarssanen L, et al: Sotalol intoxication with prolonged QT interval and severe tachyarrhythmias. *Br J Med* 1:1184, 1979.
86. Bennett JM, Gourassas J, Konstatibides S: Torsade de pointes induced by sotalol and hypokalemia. *South Afr Med J* 68:591, 1985.
87. Castro M, Descamps R, Thomis JA: Electrocardiographic changes after long-term treatment with sotalol in hypertensive patients. *Intern J Clin Pharmacol Ther Toxicol* 20:88, 1982.
88. Belton P, Sheridan J, Mulcahy R: A case of sotalol poisoning. *Irish J Med Sci* 151:126, 1982.
89. Skehan JD, Barnes JN, Drew PJ, et al: Hypokalemia-induced by a combination of a beta-blocker and a thiazide. *Br Med J* 284:83, 1982.
90. Totterman KJ, Turto H, Pellinen T: Overdrive pacing as treatment of sotalol-induced ventricular tachyarrhythtmias (torsade des pointes). *Acta Med Scand* (Suppl) 668:28, 1982.

# Chapter 8

# Preclinical Studies on the Antiarrhythmic and Antifibrillatory Effects of Sotalol and Its Optical Isomers

## Benedict R. Lucchesi and Joseph J. Lynch

Antiarrhythmic agents such as quinidine, procainamide, disopyramide, and other members of the Class I group of antiarrhythmic drugs long have been known to possess the ability to depress the "fast inward sodium current" and to result in a decrease in conduction velocity along with an increase in the duration of the action potential duration. The relative significance of the alterations in depolarization and repolarization in mediating the associated antidysrhythmic effects has not been clear, despite a detailed appreciation of the ability of these agents to alter the cardiac action potential, as recorded by intracellular microelectrodes. The availability of agents that increase the phase of cardiac repolarization without exerting a marked effect upon myocardial conduction velocity has permitted the critical evaluation of changes in repolarization in achieving an antiarrhythmic effect as well as an antifibrillatory action with or without associated antiarrhythmic activity both in experimental animal and human clinical studies.

The properties of *dl*-sotalol and its *dextro-* rotatory isomer, *d*-sotalol, have been of special interest in this context. The racemic compound is a unique beta-adrenergic receptor antagonist that causes a prolongation of the cardiac membrane action potential, while exhibiting no effect upon the rate of myocardial depolariza-

From: *Control of Cardiac Arrhythmias by Lengthening Repolarization*, edited by Bramah N. Singh, MD, Futura Publishing Company Inc., Mount Kisco, NY, © 1988.

tion. The d-sotalol exhibits the same cardiac electrophysiologic properties, but possesses only a limited capacity to produce beta-adrenergic receptor blockade. The resolution of the racemic compound into its respective dextro- and levo- optical isomers, has provided the investigator with an opportunity to examine the significance of beta-adrenergic receptor blockade as opposed to the direct electrophysiologic effect of the compound, with respect to achieving an antiarrhythmic/antifibrillatory action in experimental models of cardiac arrhythmogenesis as well as in clinical settings, in which life-threatening cardiac arrhythmias pose a threat to a favorable prognosis. The focus of this chapter is to examine the relative efficacy of the racemic or isomeric d-sotalol, in an experimental animal model, in which well-defined end-points of arrhythmogenesis permit the identification of whether a test drug possesses antiarrhythmic and/or antifibrillatory activity.

## Electrophysiologic Considerations

Single-cell microelectrode recordings from cardiac muscle and Purkinje fiber preparations have provided evidence that sotalol and its optical isomers produce prolongation of the action potential duration and refractory period without producing significant changes in the resting membrane potential, the rate of rise, or the amplitude of the action potential.[1-5]

As first reported by Lathrop,[4] on the basis of effective concentrations calculated to produce a 50 percent maximal increase in the Purkinje fiber action potential duration, d-sotalol, appeared to be one to three times more potent than either l-sotalol or the racemic mixture. The results would suggest that the electrophysiologic effects and possibly the antiarrhythmic actions of sotalol are related primarily to its ability to prolong the action potential duration rather than to its beta-adrenergic receptor blocking activity. On the other hand, Kato et al.[5] reported that equimolar concentrations of the d- and the l- optical isomers of sotalol produce nearly identical electrophysiologic effects and that the potency of the isomers did not differ from that of the racemate. The lengthening of the action potential duration produced by sotalol can not be attributed to beta-adrenergic receptor blockade since the dextro-isomer is devoid of this pharmacologic property at a concentration of $10^{-5}$ M. Voltage clamp experiments[3] have indicated that the lengthening of the action potential duration by sotalol may be due to a substantial reduction in the plateau of the outward potassium current in association with a small decrease in the background current. In the absence of catecholamines, d- and l-sotalol exerted identical effects on the action potential and voltage currents. A reduction in the $V_{max}$ during the upstroke of the action potential, concomitant with a shortening of the action potential duration, was observed only at elevated concentrations of sotalol. This event, as would be expected, was associated with a substantial inhibition of the tetrodotoxin-sensitive fast inward sodium current.[5] The drug failed to produce a direct effect on the slow inward current. As suggested by Kato et al.,[5] the lengthening of the phase of repolarization will delay the inactivation of the slow calcium channel, which will tend to augment myocardial contractility. This latter effect is more likely to occur with the dextro-isomer of sotalol since the positive inotropic action would not be attenuated by the associated negative inotropic effect related to beta-adrenergic receptor inhibition.

Studies by Brachmann et al.[6] in the in situ ischemic canine heart demonstrated that d-sotalol increased refractoriness of the ventricular myocardium in both the normal and ischemic regions. The observed change in the ventricular refractory period was greater in the ischemically damaged myocardium in the infarct zone as compared to the normally perfused myocardial region.

## Experimental and Clinical Antiarrhythmic Studies

Early animal studies demonstrated that racemic sotalol possessed antiarrhythmic actions in common with other beta-adrenergic receptor antagonists. In anesthetized dogs, sotalol suppressed experimentally induced atrial arrhythmias.[7,8] Racemic sotalol partially protected the anesthetized guinea pig against the induction of cardiac arrhythmias due to ouabain[8] and reduced the incidence of ventricular fibrillation in anesthetized as well as conscious dogs subjected to coronary artery ligation.[9,10]

In view of its Class III antiarrhythmic actions, sotalol received early attention as an antiarrhythmic agent in limited clinical trials, where it was demonstrated to exhibit moderate efficacy in patients with supraventricular and ventricular arrhythmias.[11-14] Recent studies by Senges et al.[15] have provided evidence that sotalol is effective in the prophylaxis against sustained ventricular tachycardia in a high proportion of the patients studied. Eighteen patients with sustained ventricular tachycardia were subjected to electrophysiologic testing using programmed electrical stimulation for the induction of ventricular tachycardia. Sotalol prevented the induction of ventricular tachycardia in 12 of 18 patients. Long-term prophylaxis against the spontaneous development of ventricular tachyarrhythmias was found in 8 of 9 patients placed on an oral dosing regimen with sotalol.

The reported efficacy of amiodarone, a Class III antiarrhythmic agent,[16-20] to reduce the incidence of repetitive episodes of ventricular tachycardia and ventricular fibrillation has led to an increased awareness of other pharmacologic agents with related electrophysiologic actions, such as sotalol. The primary focus has been on the prevention of lethal ventricular arrhythmias both experimentally and clinically. The availability of the dextro- and levo-rotatory isomers of sotalol would provide an opportunity to determine if the beneficial effects of sotalol could be ascribed entirely to beta-adrenergic receptor blockade or to its direct electrophysiologic effects, manifest by prolongation of the effective refractory period of the ventricular myocardium. The question of whether sotalol and its optical isomers possess antiarrhythmic and antifibrillatory properties similar to those of amiodarone and other reported Class III drugs has been addressed in our laboratory studies. Our in vivo experimental results demonstrate that sotalol and its isomers prolong the duration of the myocardial effective refractory period, prolong the $QT_c$ interval, and provide significant protection against the development of lethal ventricular arrhythmias in a canine model of sudden coronary death. Furthermore, the ability of both isomers of sotalol to exert similar protective effects against the development of ventricular fibrillation is strong evidence that beta-adrenergic receptor blockade is not the sole determinant in the observed antifibrillatory action.

## Evaluation of Potential Antifibrillatory Drugs in an Animal Model of Sudden Coronary Death

### Experimental Models

A major problem in the identification of potentially effective antifibrillatory drugs for the prevention of sudden coronary death has been the lack of a suitable animal model. Most of the data on the electrophysiological properties of the current antiarrhythmic drugs have been derived from the in vitro studies on normal cardiac muscle from a variety of animal species. Within recent years some effort has been made to employ ischemically injured tissue in electrophysiological studies in vitro.[21,22] The description of the mechanisms for arrhythmias and conduction disturbances has been based primarily on electrophysiological data obtained with isolated heart muscle or intact hearts studied many hours or days after ischemic injury. In many instances, investigators have used intact animal preparations in which cardiac arrhythmias are induced through the administration of digitalis glycosides or other cardiotoxic arrhythmogenic agents. Other approaches involve maneuvers that modify autonomic nervous system outflow to the heart in the presence of acute myocardial ischemia.[21,23] Several methods have been developed for producing animal models with chronic myocardial ischemic injury in which ventricular arrhythmias develop spontaneously or in response to programmed electrical stimulation.[24,28] Despite the effort to design a more relevant animal model for the assessment of potential antifibrillatory agents, none suffice with respect to providing the opportunity to examine the electrophysiological events preceding the development of ventricular fibrillation or to study pharmacological interventions for the prevention of life-threatening arrhythmias. Table 1 lists the experimental methods most frequently employed for the assessment of potential antiarrhythmic agents. It is obvious that most of the models do not address the specific issue involving the prevention of life-threatening or lethal ventricular arrhythmias, such as ventricular tachycardia and/or ventricular fibrillation. In the clinical setting, these fatal rhythm disorders occur spontaneously and without warning in a myocardium that has been subjected to an earlier event of ischemic injury, so as to provide the proper substrate in which to generate and sustain an electrophysiologic disturbance that can lead to ventricular fibrillation.

## Canine Model for Programmed Electrical Stimulation and of Sudden Coronary Death

The ideal animal model for the study of pharmacological interventions for the prevention of life-threatening ventricular arrhythmias should be based on the knowledge that the incidence of primary ventricular fibrillation is maximal in the first few minutes after an acute ischemic event and thereafter decays exponentially, and that the majority of patients who experience ventricular fibril-

---

**Table 1**
**Experimental Methods for the Study of Antiarrhythmic Agents**

| Method of Arrhythmia Induction | Method |
| --- | --- |
| Chemical/Drug Application | Aconitine |
| | Hydrocarbon-catecholamine |
| | Barium Chloride |
| | Veratrum alkaloids |
| | Calcium Chloride |
| | Quabain or other digitalis glycosides |
| Electrical Stimuli Applied Directly to the Heart | Ventricular fibrillation threshold |
| | Repetitive ventricular response |
| | Programmed electrical stimulation |
| Enhancement of Neuronal Activity | Application of stimuli to the lateral ventrical of the brain |
| | Electrical stimulation of cardiac sympathetic nerves |
| | Psychic stress |
| Myocardial Ischemic Injury | Acute interruption of regional coronary artery blood flow (Harris one- or two-stage procedure) |
| | Acute interruption of coronary artery blood flow followed by reperfusion ("mottled-infarct") |
| | Acute regional ischemia superimposed on a previously infarcted myocardium (ischemia at a distance) |

---

lation do so without acute myocardial infarction as the precipitating event.

We have described a conscious canine model[29] that is susceptible to the induction of ventricular tachyarrhythmias by programmed electrical stimulation and that possesses the characteristics stated earlier so that ventricular fibrillation (sudden coronary death) develops in response to a transient ischemic event that is superimposed on a ventricular myocardium with a previous history of ischemic injury.

Figure 1 illustrates the basic features involved in the surgical preparation of the canine model we have employed in our assessment of the antifibrillatory potential of sotalol and its optical isomers. The left anterior descending coronary artery is isolated at the tip of the left atrial appendage, and the left circumflex coronary artery is isolated approximately 1 cm from its origin. A 19 or

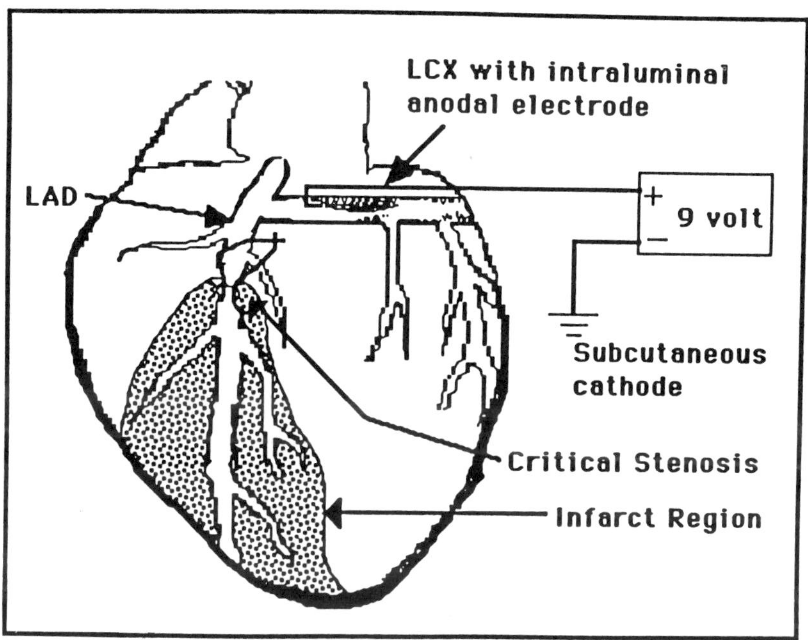


**Figure 1.** Schematic diagram showing the instrumentation of the canine heart and the experimental induction of myocardial ischemic injury by occlusion and reperfusion of the left anterior descending coronary artery. A critical stenosis is maintained on the vessel throughout the period of reperfusion. The shaded area represents the myocardial region in the infarct-related artery, which on gross examination has the characteristic appearance of a "mottled infarct." A wire electrode is inserted in the circumflex coronary artery so that the bared end is in intimate contact with the endothelial surface. Subsequent application of an anodal current by means of a 9 V nickel-cadmium battery leads to an area of injury on the luminal surface of the vessel and platelet deposition and thrombus formation at the site of injury.

20 gauge hypodermic needle is placed parallel to the left anterior descending coronary artery and a suture is passed around both the vessel and the needle. The suture is tied securely and the needle is withdrawn, leaving in place a critical stenosis. The artery is then occluded by means of a snare formed from a loop of silicone rubber tubing passed through a polyethylene tube. Blood flow through the left anterior descending coronary artery is restored after 2 hours of regional ischemia. The myocardium regionally ischemic and reperfused myocardial tissue undergoes irreversible cellular injury and necrosis and has the characteristic appearance of a "mottled in-

farct" when examined visually after histochemical delineation of the reperfused myocardial region.

An epicardial bipolar electrode (1 mm diameter silver electrodes embedded 3 mm apart in acrylic) is sutured to the left atrial appendage for atrial pacing. A bipolar, plunge electrode (25 gauge, insulated stainless steel wire, 5 mm in length, 2 mm apart) is sutured into the interventricular septum adjacent to the right ventricular outflow tract for the determination of the ventricular excitation threshold, the ventricular effective refractory period, and for the introduction of ventricular extrastimuli during programmed electrical stimulation. Two stainless steel bipolar plunge electrodes are used to measure the ventricular activation times. One bipolar electrode is implanted in the distribution of the left anterior descending coronary artery distal to the site of occlusion, while a second is implanted in the left circumflex coronary artery distribution. As illustrated in Figure 1, a 3 mm section of bared, insulated, 30 gauge silver wire is inserted through the wall of the circumflex coronary artery so that the electrode is in contact with the endothelial surface. Silver disc electrodes are implanted subcutaneously for monitoring the electrocardiogram. The surgical incision is closed and the animal is allowed to recover from surgical anesthesia and studied on subsequent days.

## Programmed Electrical Stimulation of the Canine Heart During the Subacute Phase of Myocardial Infarction

### *Effects of dl-Sotalol*

The presence of myocardial electrical instability is determined with the use of programmed electrical stimulation using single, double, and triple premature ventricular stimuli delivered to the ventricular septum. Electrical instability is revealed by electrically inducible ventricular arrhythmias as manifested by nonsustained ventricular tachycardia, or ventricular fibrillation. When examined 4 days after myocardial infarction, 90 percent (n = 30)[29] of the animals had electrically inducible ventricular arrhythmias in response to the stimulation protocol (Figure 2, Table 2). Neither nonsustained nor sustained tachyarrhythmias could be induced by programmed electrical stimulation in sham-operated dogs that had been subjected to the placement of a critical stenosis about the left anterior descending coronary artery, but in which myocardial infarction was not induced. Thus, a tachyarrhythmia could not be

## PROGRAMMED   ELECTRICAL   STIMULATION

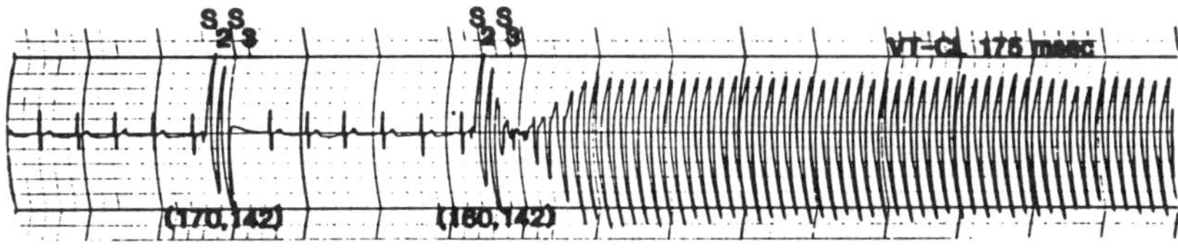

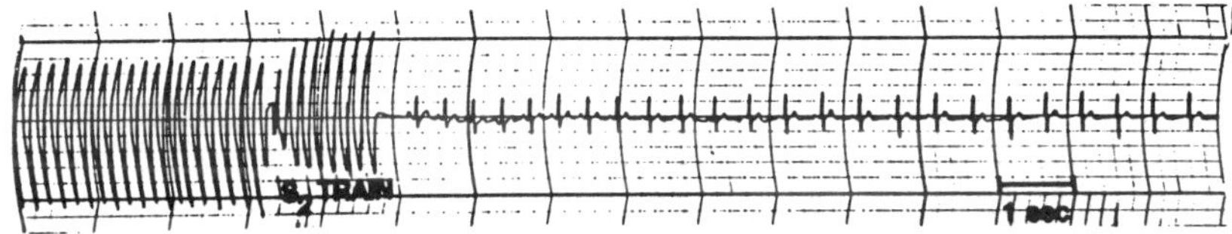

**Figure 2.**   Programmed electrical stimulation of the canine heart in the subacute phase of anterior wall myocardial infarction. The electrocardiographic tracing in the upper panel was recorded 4 days after the occlusion-reperfusion of the left anterior descending coronary artery and the induction of an anterior wall infarct. Application of appropriately programmed electrical stimuli ($S_2S_3$ 160, 142 msec) to the region of the right ventricular outflow track is followed by the abrupt onset of a sustained monophasic ventricular tachyarrhythmia with a ventricular tachycardia cycle length (VT–CL) of 175 msec. In the lower panel, the tachyarrhythmia is terminated by the application of a train of stimuli applied to the region of the right ventricular outflow track ($S_2$ train) followed by the resumption of sinus rhythm.

### Table 2
Incidence of Myocardial Electrical Instability in Response to Programmed Electrical Stimulation in the Conscious Noninfarcted Sham Controls and in the Conscious Canine Four Days After Experimentally Induced Myocardial Infarction

| | Control Group | | Myocardial Infarction Group | |
|---|---|---|---|---|
| | *n* | % | *n* | % |
| Not inducible | 10 | 100 | 3 | 10 |
| Nonsustained ventricular tachycardia | — | — | 16 | 53 |
| Sustained ventricular tachycardia | — | — | 7 | 23 |
| Ventricular fibrillation | — | — | 4 | 13 |

induced by electrical provocation in the noninfarcted heart, suggesting that the region of injury (mottled infarct) provides the "myocardial substrate" required for the initiation and the maintenance of the reentry pathway.

In the assessment of the antiarrhythmic effects of sotalol and its optical isomers, the dogs were studied 4–7 days after occlusion-reperfusion of the anterior descending coronary artery and the development of anterior wall myocardial infarction. While unsedated and resting in a sling, programmed electrical stimulation of the heart was carried out, both before and after the intravenous administration of dl-sotalol in cumulative doses of 2, 4, and 8 mg/kg. During the predrug evaluation, each of the nine animals responded to provocative electrical stimulation as summarized in Figure 3.

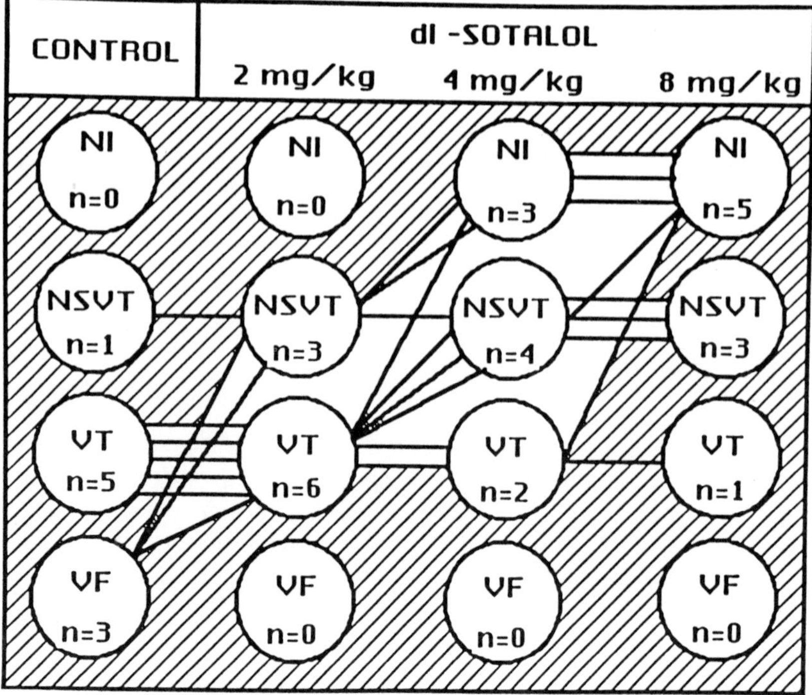


**Figure 3.** Programmed electrical stimulation in the postinfarcted canine heart and the effect of dl-sotalol administration. The electrical testing procedure was conducted in 9 conscious dogs 4–7 days after experimental myocardial infarction. The results are shown before and after cumulative dosages of dl-sotalol of 2, 4, and 8 mg/kg. Nl = noninducible; NSVT = nonsustained ventricular tachycardia; VT = sustained ventricular tachycardia; VF = ventricular fibrillation.

One animal developed nonsustained ventricular tachycardia, 5 animals had sustained ventricular tachycardia, and 3 dogs had a brief period of ventricular tachycardia followed by the onset of ventricular fibrillation that required electrical defibrillation to restore sinus rhythm. As illustrated in Figure 3, the administration of dl-sotalol was accompanied by a dose-dependent decrease in the susceptibility to the induction of rapid ventricular tachyarrhythmias by programmed electrical stimulation as compared to the predrug trial. In the predrug control state, 8 of the 9 animals responded to programmed electrical stimulation with either sustained ventricular tachycardia (n = 5) or ventricular fibrillation (n = 3). After 8 mg/kg of dl-sotalol, 5 dogs would not respond to programmed electrical stimulation and 3 developed nonsustained ventricular tachycardia; only 1 animal developed sustained ventricular tachycardia in response to electrical testing.

The administration of dl-sotalol in the stated doses was associated with a marked increase in the ventricular refractory period (Table 3). The change in the refractory period was manifest as an increase in the ventricular tachycardia cycle length in those animals in which programmed stimulation after dl-sotalol resulted in sustained or nonsustained ventricular tachyarrhythmia. Epicardial composite electrodes sutured on the noninjured as well as the ischemically injured myocardium permitted the recording of continuous electrical diastolic activity in response to premature ventricular stimuli. Ventricular tachyarrhythmias were induced in the predrug treatment state, when the activation delay within the ischemic zone exceeded 150 msec. The administration of dl-sotalol did not decrease the duration of the continuous electrical activity

### Table 3
#### Programmed Electrical Stimulation: Ventricular Refractory Periods and Ventricular Tachycardia Cycle Lengths

| | Ventricular Refractory Period (msec) | Ventricular Tachycardia Cycle Length (msec) |
|---|---|---|
| Predrug | 156 ± 5 | 175 ± 11 |
| dl-Sotalol | | |
| 2 mg/kg | 185 ± 6** | 194 ± 10* |
| 4 mg/kg | 192 ± 7** | 195 ± 9* |
| 8 mg/kg | 191 ± 7** | 188 ± 7 |

*P < 0.05
**P < 0.01 versus predrug

between ventricular complexes; however, it did prevent the electrical induction of the tachyarrhythmia when given in doses of 4–8 mg/kg (Fig. 4).

Figure 5 depicts an observation made in several dogs that had been subjected to anterior wall myocardial infarction and examined at a later date with programmed electrical stimulation before and after having received dl-sotalol. Provocative electrical stimuli delivered to the heart in the course of programmed stimulation

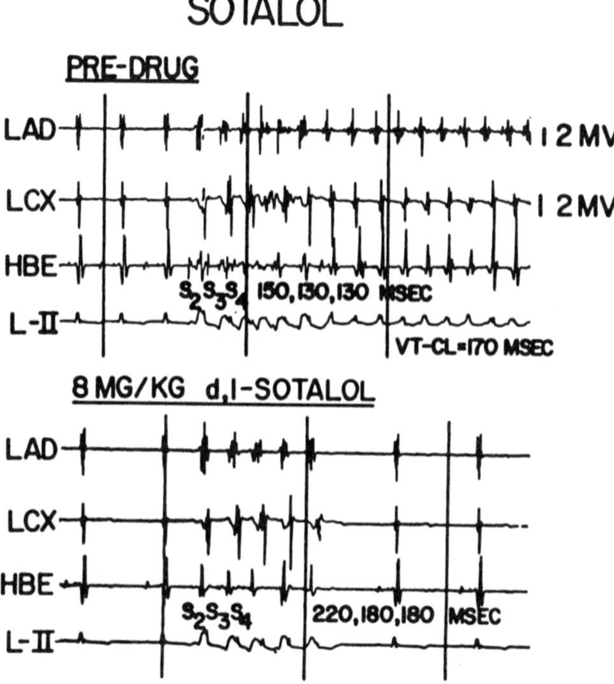


**Figure 4.** Programmed electrical stimulation of the postinfarcted canine heart before (upper panel) and after the administration of dl-sotalol (8 mg/ kg IV). The tracings from top to bottom in each panel are LAD = composite electrogram recorded from ischemically injured ventricular myocardium in the left anterior descending coronary artery distribution; LCX = composite electrogram recorded from remote myocardial region in the distribution of the left circumflex coronary artery; HBE = His bundle electrogram; L-II = lead II electrocardiogram; VT–CL = ventricular tachycardia cycle length.

In the predrug test period, three premature ventricular stimuli produced a sustained ventricular tachycardia (VT–CL 170 msec). The stimulation protocol was repeated after the administration of dl-sotalol and shown in the lower panel. The application of three premature ventricular stimuli is no longer able to induce a ventricular tachyarrhythmia.

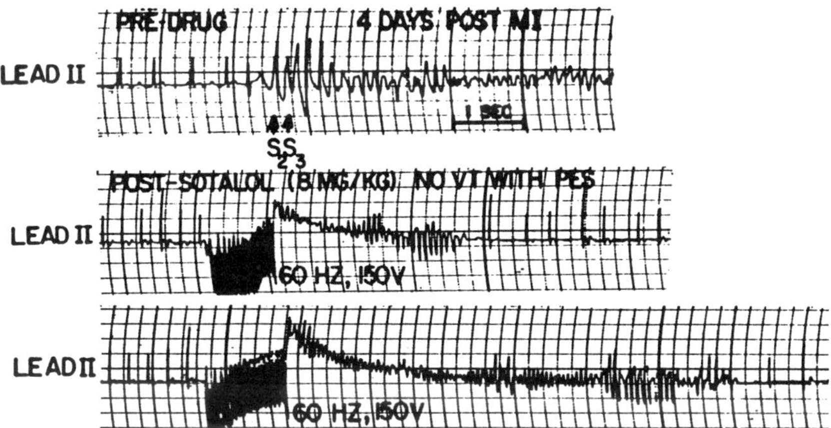


**Figure 5.** Spontaneous defibrillation in the presence of dl-sotalol. In the upper panel, the introduction of two premature ventricular stimuli with coupling intervals of 270 and 170 msec produced a polymorphous ventricular tachycardia (VT) that degenerated into ventricular fibrillation. After the administration of dl-sotalol, 8 mg/kg, programmed electrical stimulation failed to produce ventricular tachyarrhythmia (not illustrated). The application to the region of the right ventricular outflow tract of a 60 Hz train of current of 150 volt intensity produced ventricular fibrillation, which spontaneously converted to sinus rhythm. The induction of ventricular fibrillation was repeated as shown in the third panel with the spontaneous recovery occurring as before. A total of four episodes of electrically induced ventricular fibrillation with spontaneous recovery was conducted in this particular animal. Such events of spontaneous recovery from ventricular fibrillation in the postinfarcted canine heart seldom occur, therefore, suggesting that dl-sotalol has the potential to induce "chemical defibrillation."

testing led to the development of ventricular fibrillation, which was converted by electrical countershock. After the administration of 8 mg/kg of dl-sotalol, programmed electrical stimulation failed to produce ventricular arrhythmias (not illustrated). However, trains of 60 Hz stimuli at 150 V produced ventricular fibrillation that terminated spontaneously on repeated occasions, followed in each instance by the return of normal sinus rhythm. Thus, dl-sotalol pretreatment appears to be associated, in some instances, with the ability of the heart to return spontaneously to sinus rhythm after the onset of ventricular fibrillation.

## Effects of d-Sotalol

The responses of postinfarction canine hearts to programmed electrical stimulation before and after d-sotalol are summarized graphically in Figure 6. The administration of d-sotalol (8 mg/kg intravenously every 8 hours for 24 hours) suppressed the induction of ventricular tachyarrhythmia by programmed stimulation in 6 of 9 dogs tested and increased the cycle length (reduced the rate) of the induced tachyarrhythmia in 2 of the remaining 3 animals. When compared to a saline-treated control group of dogs in the subacute phase of anterior wall myocardial infarction, the overall rate of complete suppression of the induction of ventricular tachycardia was greater with d-sotalol (6/9 or 67 percent than obtained in the saline-treated control group (1/11 or 9 percent).

It is of importance to note that d-sotalol, in the dose employed in these studies did not produce an impressive degree of beta-adrenergic receptor blockade. Inhibition of beta-adrenergic recep-

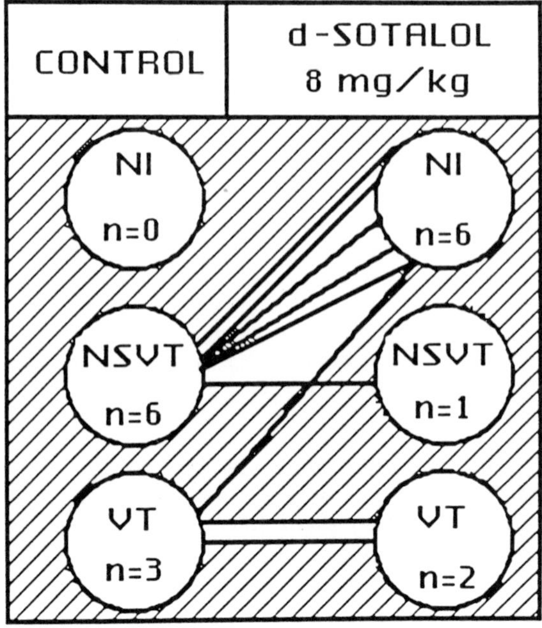


**Figure 6.** The effects of d-sotalol administered in a dose of 8 mg/kg every 8 hours for 4 doses upon the responses of the postinfarcted canine heart to programmed electrical stimulation. Before treatment with d-sotalol each of 9 dogs responded to programmed electrical stimulation by displayingg either nonsustained ventricular tachycardia (NSVT) or sustained ventricular tachycardia (VT). After the completion of the sotalol dosing regimen, only 3 of the 9 dogs remained responsive to provocative electrical stimulation.

tor responsiveness was determined by assessing the heart rate and blood pressure responses to isoproterenol before and after the administration of d-sotalol. The selective increase in the ventricular myocardial refractory period in conjunction with the prolongation of the paced QT and $QT_c$ intervals (general indices of action potential duration) suggest that the direct Class III electrophysiologic actions of d-sotalol contribute to the antiarrhythmic actions of the isomer in the postinfarction canine model. In contrast, the unimpressive degree of beta-adrenergic receptor blockade produced by d-sotalol in our studies, as well as the previously demonstrated lack of efficacy of the beta-adrenoceptor antagonists metoprolol[30] and nadolol[31] against the induction of ventricular tachycardia by programmed electrical stimulation in the postinfarcted canine heart, argue against the importance of specific receptor blockade in the suppression of electrically induced ventricular tachycardia.

## Prevention of Ventricular Fibrillation by Sotalol and its Optical Isomers

### *Effects of dl-Sotalol*

Anodal electrical stimulation of the intimal surface of the left circumflex coronary artery produced intimal injury and phasic alterations in coronary artery blood flow in each of 15 control animals. Electrocardiographic evidence of acute myocardial ischemia developed 130 ± 21 minutes after application of the anodal current to the vessel wall. The appearance of ST-segment changes was followed by the development of premature ventricular depolarizations, ventricular tachycardia, and ventricular fibrillation in 14 of 15 control animals. Thus, the conscious dog in the postinfarcted state displays a high incidence of sudden death when the heart is subjected to a transient ischemic event in a myocardial distribution remote from the infarct artery. The development of ventricular fibrillation in the canine model of sudden coronary death could be reduced significantly by pretreatment with dl-sotalol.

Treatment with dl-sotalol did not appear to alter the time to the development of the first electrocardiographic signs of regional myocardial ischemia secondary to the induction of anodal current injury in the left circumflex coronary artery. Pretreatment with dl-sotalol did prevent the development of sinus tachycardia and QT segment prolongation, which invariably accompanies acute myocardial ischemia in the control group. Drug treatment did not alter the development of epicardial activation delays, as the maximum observed delays were equal in control, 176 /pm 5 msec (n = 6), and sotalol, 172 ± 11 msec (n = 5), treated animals. In the drug treated animals, the progressive vessel wall injury resulted in thrombotic occlusion of the circumflex coronary artery and the appearance of fragmentation in the epicardial composite electrograms recorded from the acutely ischemic region remote from the previous myocardial infarct. The fragmentation and delay in activation was associated with the appearance of ventricular premature depolarizations and eventually ventricular tachycardia and ventricular fibrillation. Dogs pretreated with dl-sotalol displayed the same development of fragmentation and delay of activation in the composite electrode recordings from the acutely ischemic myocardial region supplied by the left circumflex coronary artery. However, despite the fact that continuous diastolic electrical activity in the ischemic myocardium exceeded the QT duration of the lead II electrocardiogram, it was not accompanied by disturbances in ventricular rhythm. The administration of dl-sotalol significantly reduced the incidence of ventricular fibrillation in the conscious dog and increased survival at 24 hours after anodal current application was initiated (Fig. 7). At the end of 24 hours from the onset of anodal current application to the circumflex coronary artery, 14/15 control animals in contrast to 7/20 drug-treated animals had developed ventricular fibrillation. The experimental protocol demonstrates the significant beneficial effect of dl-sotalol in preventing the onset of spontaneous ventricular fibrillation in the conscious canine model of sudden coronary death. Table 4 summarizes the pertinent features with respect to the incidence of ventricular fibrillation, infarct mass as a percent of the left ventricle, and thrombus mass in the circumflex coronary artery determined at the conclusion of the study protocol 24 hours after applying the anodal current to the circumflex coronary artery for the purpose of inducing transient ischemic events and ultimate thrombotic occlusion of the vessel.

*Effects of d-Sotalol*

Immediately after the posttreatment assessment of the ability of d-sotalol or its vehicle to influence the induction of ventricular tachycardia by programmed electrical stimulation (discussed earlier), an anodal current of 150 μA was applied to the intimal surface of the left circumflex coronary artery in each of 8 dogs in two treatment groups (saline control and sotalol). The times to develop-

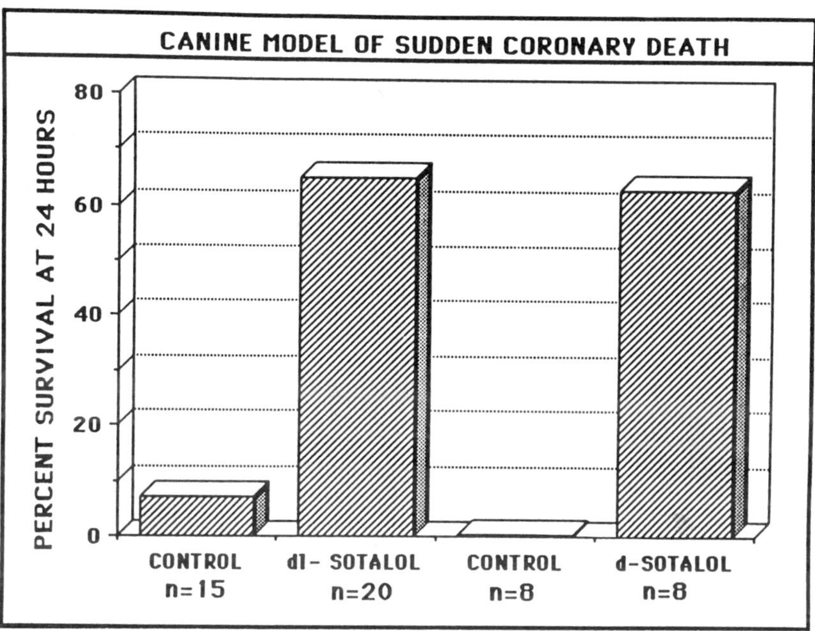


**Figure 7.** The effects of dl-sotalol and d-sotalol upon survival for 24 hours in a canine model of sudden coronary death. Both the racemate form of the drug and the dextro-rotatory optical isomer have the potential to reduce the incidence of ventricular fibrillation in the postinfarcted canine heart subjected to a superimposed transient ischemic event in a myocardial region remote from the previous infarct. In contrast, saline treated control animals had a significantly higher incidence of sudden death due to ventricular fibrillation when compared to their respective drug-treated groups.

ment of electrocardiographic evidence of posterolateral ischemia in the two groups were comparable. The reflex tachycardia in response to the acute ischemic event due to interruption in the circumflex coronary artery blood flow as well as the size of the anterior wall infarct did not differ between the two groups.

The responses of d-sotalol and vehicle pre-treated dogs to posterolateral ischemia in a region remote from a previous anterior wall infarction are compared graphically in Figure 7. Pretreatment with the vehicle afforded minimal protection against the spontaneous onset of ventricular fibrillation. In the vehicle-treated group, 7 of the 8 dogs developed ventricular fibrillation within $13 \pm 6$ minutes after the appearance of electrocardiographic evidence of myocardial ischemia in the non-infarct-related region, as assessed

Table 4
Conscious Canine Model of Sudden Coronary Death

| Parameter | Vehicle (n = 15) | dl-Sotalol (n = 20) |
|---|---|---|
| Incidence of sudden ventricular fibrillation | 14/15 | 7/20 |
| Infarct size (% of left ventricular) | | |
| Left anterior descending region | 19 ± 3 | 18 ± 3 |
| Left circumflex region | — | 19 ± 3 |
| Thrombus mass in circumflex coronary artery (mg) | 13 ± 3 | 20 ± 4 |

| Parameter | Vehicle (n = 8) | dextro-Sotalol (n = 8) |
|---|---|---|
| Incidence of sudden ventricular fibrillation | 7/8 | 1/8 |
| Survival at 24 hours | 0/8 | 5/8 |
| Infarct size (% of left ventricle) | | |
| Left anterior descending region | 22 ± 3 | 19 ± 3 |
| Left circumflex region | — | 23 ± 4 |
| Thrombus mass in circumflex coronary artery (mg) | 5 ± 2 | 11 ± 3 |

| Parameter | Vehicle (n = 10) | levo-Sotalol (n = 10) |
|---|---|---|
| Incidence of sudden ventricular fibrillation | 8/10 | 2/10 |
| Survival at 24 hours | 1/10 | 4/10 |
| Infarct size (% of left ventricle) | | |
| Left anterior descending region | 22 ± 3 | 19 ± 2 |
| Left circumflex region | — | 23 ± 3 |
| Thrombus mass in circumflex coronary artery (mg) | 14 ± 2 | 20 ± 5 |

by alterations in the ST segment of the lead II electrocardiogram. The 1 remaining animal died of ventricular fibrillation 108 minutes after the onset of regional ischemia.

Pretreatment with d-sotalol (8 mg/kg intravenously every 8 hours, 4 doses over 24 hours) provided significant protection against the spontaneous development of ventricular fibrillation occurring in response to ischemia in the region remote from a previous myocardial infarction. In the d-sotalol treated group only 1 of 8 dogs developed ventricular fibrillation within the first 60 minutes of ischemia and 5 dogs survived the entire 24-hour protocol. In contrast, in the control group 7 of the 8 dogs experienced a sudden onset of ventricular fibrillation upon the development of ischemia with the remaining animal dying at a later point, so that after 24 hours none of the animals were alive. In the d-sotalol treated group, 5 of the 8 animals were still alive after 24 hours, despite the presence of a subacute anterior wall myocardial infarction and a recent infarct that had developed in the posterolateral wall as a result of the formation of an occlusive thrombus in the left circumflex coronary artery secondary to anodal current injury. The data are summarized in Table 4, which also summarizes our results with the levo- optical isomer of sotalol. The l-sotalol is associated with the development of beta-adrenergic receptor blockade and was observed to have effects upon the induction of arrhythmias by programmed electrical stimulation and the development of sudden coronary death very similar to those of the dextro- rotatory form of the drug.[32,33] There is a marked similarity with respect to d- and l-sotalol upon the recorded electrophysiologic parameters in the postinfarcted canine heart and the ability to prevent the spontaneous development of ventricular fibrillation. These observations provide additional support to the concept that beta-adrenergic receptor blockade makes a minor contribution to the prevention of sudden coronary death in the experimental animal model and suggests that the beneficial action of sotalol and its optical isomers is a result of its direct electrophysiologic properties.

The rapid progression from the onset of posterolateral wall ischemia to the development of ventricular fibrillation in the control group precludes the opportunity for the myocardial tissue to undergo irreversible alterations and evidence of myocardial infarction. As indicated in Table 4, the thrombus mass in the left circumflex coronary artery at the time of death is too small to achieve total occlusion of the vessel and ventricular fibrillation is the result of a transient ischemic event being superimposed upon an already damaged myocardium that provides the appropriate substrate for initiating and sustaining a reentrant mechanism, which leads to the spontaneous development of ventricular fibrillation. In contrast are the observed changes in the hearts from the d-sotalol treated animals, in which an occlusive thrombus mass was present in the circumflex coronary artery. Since the d-sotalol treated animals survived to the end of the study protocol, there was ample time for an occlusive thrombus to form in the left circumflex coronary artery. The resulting period of prolonged ischemia in the region of distribution of the left circumflex coronary vessel led to the development of myocardial infarction and necrosis averaging $23.3 \pm 3.9$ percent of the left ventricle. The mass of infarcted myocardium in the circumflex region, combined with the anterior wall infarcted region of 18.9 ± 2.9 percent, amounted to over 42 percent of the left ventricular wall being compromised by the presence of necrosis in the animals treated with d-sotalol. Despite the large loss of functional myocardium, 5 of the 8 animals in the d-sotalol treated group survived the 24-hour study period. The ability to achieve an antifibrillatory effect without the presence of beta-adrenergic receptor blockade in the functionally compromised heart suggests that d-sotalol may have a distinct advantage over the racemic form of the drug in those clinical situations where life-threatening arrhythmias are present in patients with a compromised ventricular function secondary to ischemic heart disease.

*Studies with d-Sotalol in Experimental Atrial Flutter*

Our observations with d-sotalol in the canine sudden death model are consistent with those of Feld et al.[34] in experimental atrial flutter produced in the open-chest anesthetized dog in which the atrial arrhythmia was induced by rapid electrical pacing after producing a crush injury in the intercaval regional to establish a region of conduction block. In this experimental setting, which is believed to represent a reentrant arrhythmia, d-sotalol (2 mg/kg) restored normal sinus rhythm in 14 of 15 animals (93 percent). Quinidine (10 mg/kg) was less effective displaying a conversion rate of 9 of 15 (60 percent), whereas lidocaine (1.5 mg/kg, followed with an infusion of 0.03 mg/kg/min) converted only 2 of 10 (20 percent) animals with sustained flutter. The previous administration of d-sotalol prevented the reinduction of the atrial flutter in 53 percent, quinidine protected 27 percent, whereas lidocaine was relatively ineffective in preventing the redevelopment of atrial flutter (Fig. 8).

The major determinant of the observed beneficial effect of a pharmacologic intervention in the prevention and/or conversion of atrial flutter, was the ability to prolong the refractory period of atrial tissue without an observed change in conduction velocity.


## Discussion

Ventricular tachyarrhythmias can be produced in the dog by programmed electrical stimulation 3–14 days after experimental myocardial infarction,[26,29,32,33] The efficacy of antiarrhythmic agents against ventricular arrhythmias produced by provocative

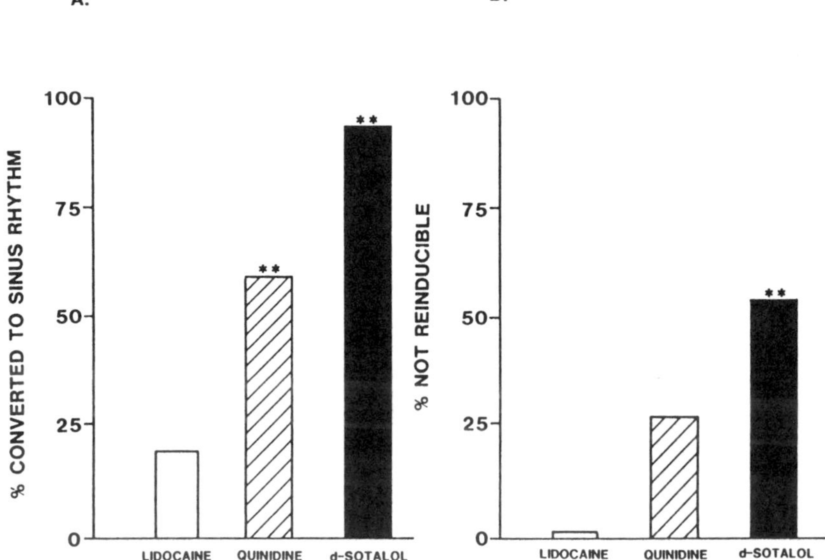



**Figure 8.** Effects of d-sotalol, quinidine, and lidocaine on the conversion and prevention of reinduction of atrial flutter. A: Percentage of dogs converted to sinus rhythm by each drug. B: Percentage of dogs in which reinduction was prevented by each drug. Note that d-sotalol and quinidine compared with placebo produced a significant frequency of conversion of atrial flutter to sinus rhythm, but only d-sotalol prevented reinduction in a significant number of dogs. In converting and suppressing atrial flutter, d-sotalol was most effective (p<.01 and p<.02, respectively). Significance of the conversion or suppression frequency compared with placebo: ** indicates p < .01.

electrical stimulation in the experimental animal may reflect more accurately the ability of a drug to prevent ventricular fibrillation in humans than do other currently accepted animal models. In the conscious canine subjected to programmed electrical stimulation during the subacute phase of myocardial infarction, dl-sotalol prevented the induction of sustained ventricular tachycardia. The beneficial actions of dl-sotalol were observed to occur without a significant change in the epicardial activation delay, measured from normal and ischemically injured ventricular myocardium. An important observation regarding the electrophysiological effects of dl-sotalol relates to its ability to increase the effective refractory period of the normal zone ventricular myocardium.

The similar electrophysiologic effects observed with dl-, the levo- rotatory sotalol, and the non-beta-adrenergic receptor blocking dextro-isomer supports the concept that specific receptor inhibition can not account for the action of the racemic compound and of that of the levo-isomer. In the postinfarcted (anterior wall infarct) canine heart in which ventricular fibrillation occurs spontaneously in response to a transient ischemic event in the distribution of the left circumflex coronary artery (remote from the previous infarct), both optical isomers of sotalol as well as its racemic form significantly reduce the incidence of ventricular fibrillation despite no significant alteration in the rate of development of posterolateral ischemia and no difference in the extent of anterior wall myocardium that had undergone irreversible damage and infarction (mottled infarct).

The results of our studies with dl-sotalol and its optical isomers indicate that direct Class III electrophysiologic actions underlie the antiarrhythmic and antifibrillatory actions. In theory, agents that prolong the duration of the cardiac action potential, thereby increasing myocardial refractoriness, might terminate a reentrant arrhythmia by providing refractory tissue to an advancing wave of depolarization.[2] Cobbe et al.[30] have suggested that dl-sotalol may act selectively to increase refractoriness in depressed myocardial areas, thereby suppressing potential reentrant circuits. Patterson et al.[35] have noted that dl-sotalol, through its ability to increase the refractoriness of normal zone ventricular myocardium, might serve to establish an "entrance block" of critically premature ventricular extrastimuli or continuous diastolic electrical activity from acutely ischemic zones into surrounding myocardial areas. These electrophysiologic changes would prevent activation or the establishment of a reentrant pathway. Conversely, increased refractoriness of nonischemic ventricular myocardium might block the "exit" of continuous diastolic electrical activity from acutely ischemic zones, thereby preventing the development of tachyarrhythmias.[35]

Cobbe et al.[36] have examined the effects of dl-sotalol in the isolated, arterially perfused interventricular septum of the rabbit heart. In the control state, dl-sotalol increased the action potential duration and the mean effective refactory period. However, when the heart muscle preparation was made ischemic ("global") by arresting the perfusion to the coronary bed, the action potential duration decreased more rapidly in the sotalol-treated preparations than in the controls. The initial difference between the sotalol and control groups was abolished after 24 minutes of ischemia. In the sotalol-treated group, the effective refractory period shortened rapidly during ischemia and was significantly less than in the control group after 30 minutes. Ischemia was associated with the development of postrepolarization refractoriness in the control group, but not in the dl-sotalol treated group. The authors concluded that the Class III antiarrhythmic effects of dl-sotalol gradually withdraw during ischemia and that sotalol slows the rate of rise of extracellular potassium concentration in acute ischemia, which may explain its antiarrhythmic effect.

Although it is difficult to translate the events from a perfused septal preparation to the intact heart, it is of interest to note that our own[35] interpretation of the antiarrhythmic and antifibrillatory actions of dl-sotalol and its isomers is not inconsistent with the observations of Cobbe et al.[36] In the presence of sotalol, the intact heart when subjected to regional ischemia would exhibit a decrease in the refractory period and action potential duration. These electrophysiologic alterations would be confined to the ischemic region. The electrophysiologic effects of sotalol would be expected to persist within the nonischemic myocardium and would continue to participate in establishing a region of exit block that surrounds the ischemic zone, preventing the spread of continuous electrical activation from the electrically depressed myocardium into the surrounding regions, and thereby establishing a reentry rhythm. Furthermore, the ability of sotalol to prevent postrepolarization refractoriness within the ischemic zone would add to its antiarrhythmic effect by preventing or delaying conduction block within the depressed region. It must be recalled that in most instances of sudden coronary death in patients with coronary artery disease, recent myocardial infarction and necrosis is not the precipitating event. The most likely precipitating cause is a transient ischemic episode being superimposed on an already damaged myocardium, one that possesses electrical instability as manifested by the presence of premature ventricular complexes and/or episodic bouts of ventricular tachycardia. The conversion of the nonfatal but electrophysiologically unstable heart rhythm to fatal ventricular fibrillation may be the result of regional electrophysiologic changes associated with an acute ischemic event occurring in a myocardial region remote from the earlier zone of injury or infarction.[37]

## Clinical Correlations

The clinical antiarrhythmic efficacy of sotalol has been evaluated by Senges et al.[15,38] These authors demonstrated that sotalol prevented the initiation of sustained ventricular tachycardia in 12 of 18 (67 percent) patients with the results of short-term testing being predictive of the absence of recurrent ventricular tachycardia in all 9 patients in whom sotalol was selected for long-term oral therapy for an average of 16 months. Similar observations have been provided in the publication by Nademanee et al.,[39] in which it is reported that the intravenous administration of sotalol was effective in preventing reinduction of ventricular tachycardia/ventricular fibrillation in patients with refractory recurrent life-threatening arrhythmias who were undergoing evaluation with electrophysiologic testing. In addition, the suppression of spontaneously occurring arrhythmias by the oral drug was observed, leading the authors to conclude that sotalol provides a significant advance in the short- and long-term management of life-threatening ventricular tachyarrhythmias (also see Chapter 7).

Preliminary reports[40,41] have appeared in which it is demonstrated that d-sotalol, like the racemic form of the drug, possesses antiarrhythmic properties, but these are unrelated to the presence of beta-adrenergic receptor blockade. Schwartz et al.[40] reported that d-sotalol prevented the induction of ventricular tachycardia in 10 patients undergoing programmed electrical testing as compared to a control group of 10 patients who continued to respond to programmed stimulation. Seven of the 10 patients who were protected by d-sotalol at the time of electrical testing were discharged on oral d-sotalol (200−400 mg twice daily). One patient died 1 month after discharge due to acute myocardial infarction and 1 patient had a cardiac arrest. The remaining 5 patients were alive 5 ± 3 months after discharge. Rowland et al.[41] examined the electrophysiological effects of d-sotalol in patients undergoing investigation for arrhythmia. There were no changes in intracardiac conduction intervals or in the AV nodal effective refractory period. Prolongation of the monophasic membrane action potential was accompanied by a lengthening of the ventricular effective refractory period and an increase in the $QT_c$ interval. In 2 patients with inducible ventricular tachycardia, the administration of d-sotalol prevented reintroduction of the tachyarrhythmia by electrical stimulation. The clinical antiarrhythmic actions of d-sotalol were observed to occur in the absence of an alteration in AV nodal function suggesting that the immediate effects are not achieved by beta-adrenergic receptor antagonism.

Presently, amiodarone and bretylium are the only Class III antiarrhythmics approved for clinical use in the United States. Amiodarone, in particular has been employed for the chronic management of patients with life-threatening arrhythmias and has been documented to possess the ability to suppress a wide variety of tachyarrhythmias. One major drawback to the use of amiodarone, despite its demonstrated antidysrhythmic efficacy, is its potential to produce major organ toxicity. In contrast, the potential adverse effects due to the administration of sotalol are most likely the result of concomitant beta-adrenergic receptor antagonism, which would be less pronounced or absent with the use of the d-isomer. On the basis of experimental and clinical studies, sotalol and/or its dextro- optical isomer appear to offer promise as an approach to the management of patients who are at risk of sudden coronary death.

## Conclusions

We appreciate the difficulty in extrapolating from the animal experiment to the clinical situation, particularly in the area of cardiac rhythm disorders and ischemic heart disease as they relate to sudden coronary death caused by ventricular fibrillation. However, it has become obvious that most antiarrhythmic drugs have pre-clinical development in in vitro and/or in vivo models, which have little relevance to the clinical situation of sudden coronary death. The animal model being used in our laboratory allows the investigator to evaluate the efficacy of a drug in response to provocative electrical procedures as well as against the spontaneous development of ventricular fibrillation. This approach should provide expanded opportunities to study and evaluate potential pharmacologic interventions intended specifically for the prevention of ventricular fibrillation. In the final analysis, however, the ultimate utility of any therapeutic intervention will depend upon an appropriate clinical protocol in patients who are at risk of developing sudden and unexpected life-threatening arrhythmias and/or ventricular fibrillation. The challenge, although great, may be realized more readily by selecting potential candidate drugs for clinical evaluation based upon more relevant animal models with appropriate spontaneously developing, electrophysiologic end-points (ventricular tachycardia/fibrillation) that mimic those known to exist in a patient population known to be at an increased risk of sudden coronary death.

## References

1. Singh BN, Vaughan Williams EM: A third class of anti-arrhythmic action. Effects on atrial and ventricular intracellular potentials, and

other pharmacological actions on cardiac muscle, of MJ 1999 and AH 3474. *Br J Pharmacol* 39:675, 1970.

2. Strauss HC, Bigger JT, Hoffman BF: Electrophysiological and beta-receptor blocking effects of MJ-1999 on dog and rabbit cardiac tissue. *Circ Res* 24:661, 1970.

3. Carmeliet E: Electrophysiologic and voltage clamp analysis of the effects of sotalol on isolated cardiac muscle and Purkinje fibers. *J Pharmacol Exp Therap* 232:817, 1985.

4. Lathrop DA: Electromechanical characterization of the effects of racemic sotalol and its optical isomers on isolated canine ventricular trabecular muscles and Purkinje strands. *Can J Physiol Pharmacol* 63:1506, 1985.

5. Kato R, Ikeda N, Yabek SM, et al: Electrophysiologic effects of the levo- and dextrorotatory isomers of sotalol in isolated cardiac muscle and their *in vivo* pharmacokinetics. *J Am Coll Cardiol* 7:116, 1986.

6. Brachmann J, Senges J, Aidonidis I, et al: Antiarrhythmic class III effects of d-sotalol in conscious dogs with subacute myocardial infarction. *J Amer Coll Cardiol* 5:466A, 1985.

7. Stanton HC, Kirchgessner T, Parmenter K: Cardiovascular pharmacology of two new beta-adrenergic receptor antagonists. *J Pharmacol Exp Ther* 149:174, 1965.

8. Schmid JR, Hanna C: A comparison of the antiarrhythmic action of two new synthetic compounds, iproveratril and MJ1999, with quinidine and pronethalol. *J Pharmacol Exp Ther* 156:331, 1967.

9. Kaumann AJ, Aramendia P: Prevention of ventricular fibrillation induced by coronary ligation. *J Pharmacol Exp Ther* 164:326, 1968.

10. Khan MI, Hamilton JL, Manning GW: Protective effect of beta-adrenoceptor blockade in experimental coronary occlusion in conscious dogs. *Am J Cardiol* 30:832, 1972.

11. Prakash R, Parmley WW, Allen HN, et al: Effect of sotalol on clinical arrhythmias. *Am J Cardiol* 29:397, 1972.

12. Fogelman F, Lightman SL, Sillett RW, et al: The treatment of cardiac arrhythmias with sotalol. *Eur J Clin Pharmacol* 5:72, 1972.

13. Simon A, Berman E: Long term sotalol therapy in patients with arrhythmias. *J Clin Pharmacol* 19:547, 1979.

14. Myburgh DP, Goldman AP, Cartoon J, et al: The efficacy of sotalol in suppressing ventricular ectopic beats. *South Afr Med J* 56:295, 1979.

15. Senges J, Lengfelder W, Jauernig R, et al: Electrophysiologic testing in assessment of therapy with sotalol for sustained ventricular tachycardia. *Circulation* 69:577, 1984.

16. Nademanee K, Hendrikson JA, Cannon DS, et al: Control of refractory cardiac arrhythmias with amiodarone. *Am Heart J* 101:759, 1981.

17. Nademanee K, Hendrickson J, Kannan R, et al: Antiarrhythmic efficacy and electrophysiologic actions of amiodarone in patients with life-threatening ventricular arrhythmias: Potent suppression of spontaneously occurring tachyarrhythmias versus inconsistent abolition of induced ventricular tachycardia. *Am Heart J* 103:950, 1982.

18. Singh BN: Amiodarone: Historical development and pharmacologic profile. *Am Heart J* 106:788, 1983.

19. Nademanee K, Singh BN, Cannom DS, et al: Control of sudden recur-

rent arrhythmic deaths: Role of amiodarone. *Am Heart J* 106:895, 1983.
20. Peter T, Hamer A, Mandel WJ, et al: Evaluation of amiodarone therapy in the treatment of drug-resistant cardiac arrhythmias: Long-term follow-up. *Am Heart J* 106:943, 1983.
21. Winslow E: Methods for the detection and assessment of antiarrhythmic activity. *Pharmacol Ther* 24:401, 1984.
22. Wit AL: Cellular electrophysiological mechanisms for re-entry in the distal Purkinje system after ischemia or infarction. In HE Kulbertus (ed.): *Re-entrant Arrhythmias.* Baltimore, University Park Press, 1976, p 210.
23. Szekeres L: Methods for evaluating antiarrhythmic agents. In A Schwartz (ed.): *Methods in Pharmacology,* vol. 1. New York, Appleton-Century-Crofts, 1971, p 151.
24. El-Sherif N, Hope R, Sherlag BJ, et al: Reentrant arrhythmias in the late myocardial infarction period. 2. Pattern of initiation and termination of reentry. *Circulation* 55:702, 1977.
25. El-Sherif N, Scherlag BJ, Lazzara R, et al: Reentrant ventricular arrhythmias in the late myocardial infarction period. 1. Conduction characteristics in the infarction zone. *Circulation* 55:686, 1977.
26. Karaguezian HS, Fenoglio JJ, Weiss MB, et al: Protracted ventricular tachycardia induced by premature stimulation of the canine heart after coronary artery occlusion and reperfusion. *Circ Res* 44:833, 1979.
27. Myerburg RJ, Gelband H, Nilsson K, et al: Long-term electrophysiological abnormalities resulting from experimental myocardial infarction in cats. *Circ Res* 41:73, 1977.
28. Schwartz PJ, Vanoli E: Cardiac arrhythmias elicited by interaction between acute myocardial ischemia and sympathetic hyperactivity: A new experimental model for the study of antiarrhythmic drugs *J Cardiovasc Pharmacol* 3:1251, 1981.
29. Patterson E, Holland K, Eller BT, et al: Ventricular fibrillation resulting from ischemia at a site remote from previous myocardial infarction. A conscious canine model of sudden coronary death. *Am J Cardiol* 50:1414, 1982.
30. Cobbe SM, Hoffman E, Ritzenhoff A, et al: Action of sotalol on potential reentrant pathways and ventricular tachyarrhythmias in conscious dogs in the late postmyocardial infarction phase. *Circulation* 68:865, 1983.
31. Patterson E, Lucchesi BR: Antifibrillatory actions of nadolol. *J Pharmacol Exp Ther* 223:144, 1982.
32. Lynch JJ, Wilber DJ, Montgomery DG, et al: Antiarrhythmic and antifibrillatory actions of the levo- and dextrorotatory isomers of sotalol. *J Cardiovas Pharmacol* 6:1132, 1984.
33. Lynch JJ, Coskey LA, Montgomery DG, et al: Prevention of ventricular fibrillation by dextrorotatory sotalol in a conscious canine model of sudden coronary death. *Am Heart J* 109:949, 1985.
34. Feld GK, Venkatesh N, Singh BN: Pharmacologic conversion and suppression of experimental canine atrial flutter: Differing effects of d-sotalol, quinidine, and lidocaine and significance of changes in refractoriness and conduction. *Circulation* 74:197, 1986.

35. Patterson E, Lynch JJ, Lucchesi BR: The antiarrhythmic and antifibrillatory actions of the beta-adrenergic receptor antagonist, d,l-sotalol. *J Pharmacol Exp Ther* 230:519, 1984.
36. Cobbe SM, Manley BS, Alexopoulos D: The influence of acute myocardial ischaemia on the Class III antiarrhythmic action of sotalol. *Cardiovas Res* 19:661, 1985.
37. Schuster EH, Bulkley BH: Ischemia at a distance after acute myocardial infarction: A cause of early post-infarction angina. *Circulation* 62:509, 1980.
38. Senges J, Lengfelder W, Jauernig R, et al: Electrophysiologic testing in assessment of therapy with sotalol for sustained ventricular tachycardia. *Circulation* 69:577, 1984.
39. Nademanee K, Feld G, Hendrickson J, et al: Electrophysiologic and antiarrhythmic effects of sotalol in patients with life-threatening ventricular tachyarrhythmias. *Circulation* 72:555, 1985.
40. Schwartz J, Wynn J, Maza S, et al: Antiarrhythmic properties of d-sotalol in patients with ventricular tachycardia determined by programmed electrical stimulation. *J Am Coll Cardiol* 7:93A, 1986.
41. Rowland E, Perrins EJ, Donaldson RM, et al: The clinical electrophysiological effects of d-sotalol—A new class III antiarrhythmic drug. *J Am Coll Cardiol* 5:498, 1985.

# Chapter 9

# Pharmacologic Basis for the Antiarrhythmic Actions of N-Acetylprocainamide

Gregory K. Feld and
Bramah N. Singh

Numerous antiarrhythmic compounds undergo biotransformation in the body resulting in pharmacologically active metabolites. However, none has been developed as a discrete antiarrhythmic agent for therapeutic use. Many years ago, it was found that when procainamide undergoes N-acetylation, the resulting metabolite N-acetylprocainamide (NAPA, Fig. 1) exhibits properties that differ significantly from those of the parent compound.[1-9] First, NAPA has little or no propensity to induce systemic lupus erythematosus or other immunologically mediated side effects.[9,10] Second, the pharmacokinetics of the metabolite differ in the duration of elimination half-life and in a predominantly renal route of excretion.[10,11] Third, NAPA appears to have a less negative inotropic effect than procainamide.[12,13] Finally, and most important, unlike procainamide, NAPA has little effect on cardiac conduction and exerts an essentially Class III antiarrhythmic action.[14] The purpose of this chapter is to review the pharmacologic properties of NAPA compared to those of procainamide with a particular reference to the effect of NAPA in lengthening cardiac repolarization relative to its effect on experimentally induced cardiac arrhythmias.

From: *Control of Cardiac Arrhythmias by Lengthening Repolarization*, edited by Bramah N. Singh, MD, Futura Publishing Company Inc., Mount Kisco, NY, © 1988.

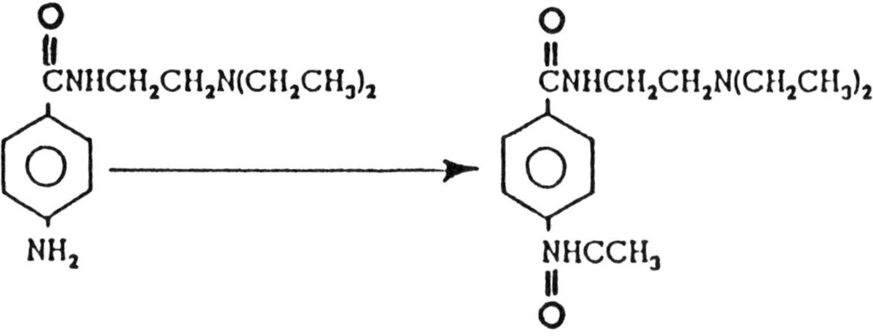


**Figure 1.** The chemical structures of procainamide and its metabolite N-acetylprocainamide.

## Electrophysiologic Effects of N-Acetylprocainamide

### In Vitro Observations

In studies by Refsum et al.[6] in isolated perfused (Ringer's solution, $K^+$ 5.3 mEq/l) rat atrium, NAPA was noted to increase atrial rate, atrial contractile force, and work index, whereas procainamide exerted a predominantly negative inotropic effect. These effects of NAPA generally were seen only at concentrations above 100 µg/ml. The atrial threshold current was increased only minimally by NAPA even at concentrations up to 1000 µg/ml, whereas it was increased by procainamide. The maximum following frequency (an index of effective refractory period) of the atrium was prolonged up to 25 percent by NAPA at concentrations up to 1000 µg/ml, whereas it was prolonged up to 60 percent by procainamide at a concentration of 500 µg/ml. Similar findings were reported by Minchin et al.[5] in the isolated perfused rabbit atrium at concentrations of NAPA and procainamide above $1.5 \times 10^{-4}$.

In isolated perfused (Tyrode's solution, $K^+$ 4.0 mM) canine Purkinje fibers, Bagwell et al.[3] observed that NAPA, in concentrations of 10 and 20 mg/l, significantly increased the action potential duration at 50 percent repolarization ($APD_{50}$ +24 percent) and at 90 percent repolarization ($APD_{90}$ +22 percent) and decreased the spontaneous depolarization rate (−33 percent). There were no consistent effects on the maximum diastolic potential, action potential amplitude, or dV/dT. In contrast, procainamide produced a significant depressant effect on dV/dT ($-13$ percent) and a lesser prolongation of $APD_{50}$ ($+12$ percent) and $APD_{90}$ ($+11$ percent) compared to NAPA. In this study the tissue concentrations of NAPA were significantly greater than those of procainamide at identical bath concentrations.

Similar electrophysiologic effects of NAPA were observed in isolated perfused canine Purkinje fibers and ventricular muscle by Dangman et al.[4] NAPA, at concentrations up to 40 mg/ml, did not produce significant changes in membrane resting potential, membrane responsiveness, action potential amplitude, or dV/dT (Fig. 2). At concentrations up to 40 mg/ml NAPA prolonged the action potential duration measured at $-60$ mV during repolarization ($APD_{-60mV}$) by $+14$ percent in ventricular muscle and by $+19$ percent in Purkinje fiber (Fig. 3). In contrast to the studies of Bagwell et al.,[3] significant effects on normal and abnormal (barium-induced) automaticity were not observed in Purkinje fibers (i.e., phase 4 depolarization and spontaneous rates were not consistently altered). Purkinje fibers exposed for several hours to high concentrations of NAPA ($> 40$ mg/l) developed two possible toxic effects defined by the authors as (1) slight depolarization with accelerated automaticity of sudden onset; and (2) early afterdepolarizations, although these observations were not consistently reproducible (Fig. 4). The salient features of the in vitro electrophysiologic effects of NAPA and procainmide are summarized in Table 1.

## In Vivo Canine Preparations

In anesthetized dogs Amlie et al.[1] observed that NAPA at doses of 25 mg/kg and 50 mg/kg produced slight increases in sinus cycle length, interatrial conduction time, and QRS duration, particularly at the higher concentration (see Table 2). These changes, with the exception of the sinus cycle length, were significantly less than those produced by procainamide at similar concentrations, however. NAPA had little or no effect on atrioventricular and His-Purkinje conduction times, in contrast to procainamide which prolonged both. Both NAPA and procainamide significantly prolonged the ventricular and atrial effective and functional refractory periods in a dose-dependent fashion. NAPA and procainamide also prolonged the atrioventricular node effective and functional refractory periods in the dog, although such changes have not been observed

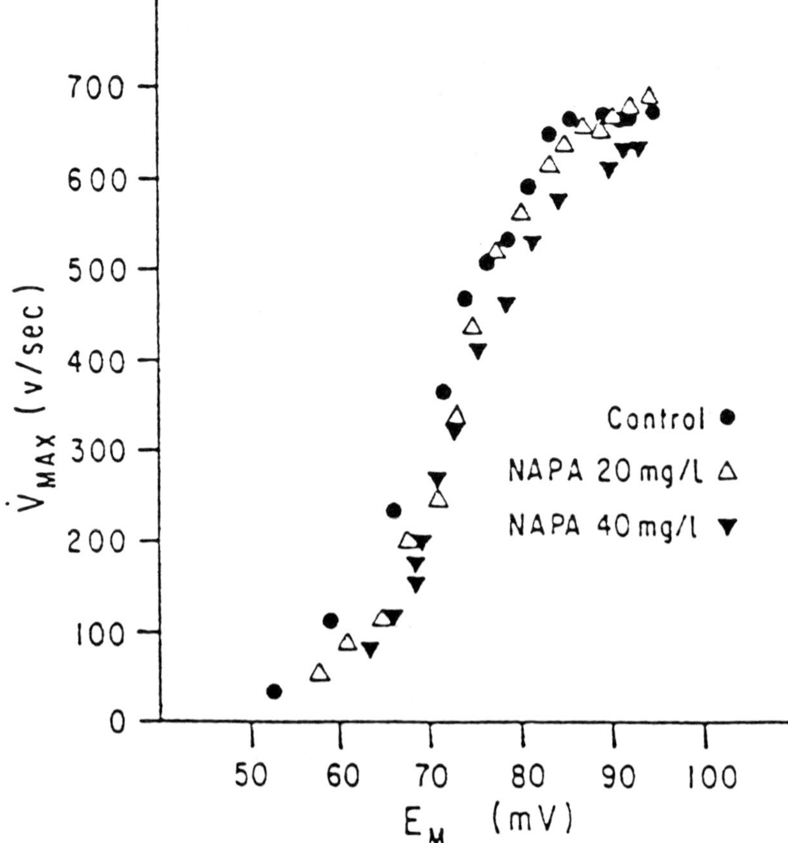


**Figure 2.** Relationship between membrane potential at the onset of phase 0 and maximum rate of depolarization during phase 0 ($V_{max}$) for a canine Purkinje fiber under control conditions and after equilibrium with each of two concentrations of NAPA. The drug had no effect on membrane responsiveness consistent with lack of effect on the fast sodium channel. (From Dangman KH, Hoffman BF: In vivo and in vitro antiarrhythmic and arrhythmogenic effects of N-acetylprocainamide. *J Pharmacol Exp Ther* 217(3):815, 1981. By permission of the authors and the journal.)

in humans.[14] Similar findings were reported by Jaillon and Winkle[2] in chloralose-anesthetized dogs, in which incremental boluses and infusions of NAPA and procainamide were given. Serum concentrations varying from 2 to 50 µg/ml for procainamide and 7 to > 100 µg/ml for NAPA were found.

In each case, the predominant effects of NAPA were on repol-

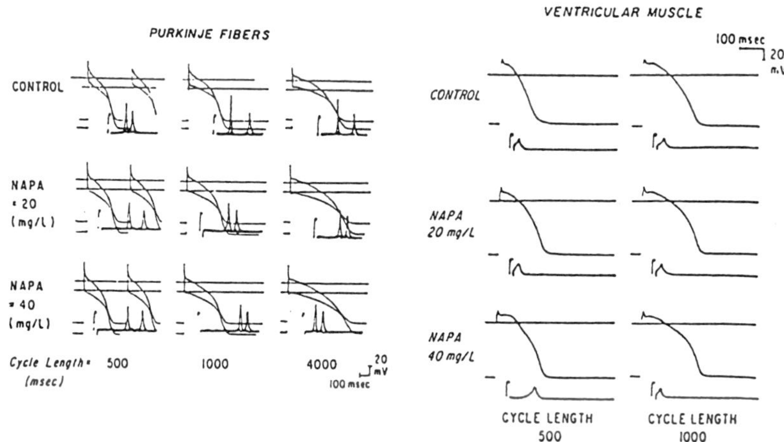



**Figure 3.** Transmembrane action potentials recorded from sites in preparations of canine Purkinje fibers and left ventricular endocardial muscle cells. Each panel shows transmembrane action potentials with related zero reference lines and, below, traces of the first time derivative of phase 0 of the transmembrane potential ($V_{max}$). These traces are preceded by a calibration of 400 V/sec and 200 V/sec, respectively. Calibration of voltage and time are as indicated. From left to right, the frames show the effect of stimulating the preparation at increasing cycle lengths of 500, 1000, and 4000 msec; from top to bottom, control conditions and steady-state effects of NAPA in concentrations of 20 and 40 mg/l. (From Dangman KH, Hoffman BF: In vivo and in vitro antiarrhythmic and arrhythmogenic effects of N-acetylprocainamide. *J. Pharmacol Exp Ther* 217(3):851, 1981. By permission of the authors and the journal.)

arization ($QT_c$) and refractoriness (atrial, ventricular, and AV nodal), whereas procainamide produced similar effects, in addition to prolonging conduction (AH, HV, and QRS intervals). Both drugs produced slight but statistically insignificant slowing of the heart rate. Procainamide again was noted to have greater potency in prolonging the AV node, atrial, and ventricular refractory periods.

Findings similar to those of Amlie et al.[1] and Jaillon and Winkle[2] were observed in our laboratory in anesthetized dogs (see Table 3). Following 30 mg/kg NAPA, a significant increase in atrial effective (+27 percent) and functional (+22 percent) refractory periods and in $QT_c$ (+16 percent) were found. The interatrial conduction time during sinus rhythm and rapid atrial pacing (cycle length 150 msec) and the QRS duration were not changed significantly from control.

Thus, NAPA exhibits typical Class III electrophysiologic effects, exemplified by prolongation of the atrial and ventricular ac-

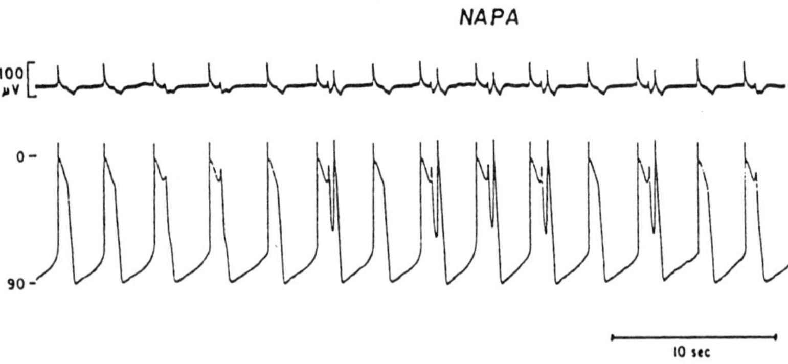


**Figure 4.** Extracellular recordings of early afterdepolarizations (EAD) induced by NAPA, 80 mg/l for 30 minutes. Lower trace shows transmembrane action potentials recorded from a fiber showing 0, 1, or 2 EADs after each action potential. EADs have variable amplitudes; note that these are reflected in the extracellular recordings in the upper trace. Voltage calibrations are shown at the left, time calibrations on the lower right. (From Dangman KH, Hoffman BF: In vivo and in vitro antiarrhythmic and arrhythmogenic effects of N-acetylprocainamide. *J Pharmacol Exp Ther* 217(3):851, 1981. By permission of the authors and the journal.)

tion potential duration and refractory periods, without depression of conduction velocity, dV/dT, action potential amplitude, membrane responsiveness, or membrane resting potential. These effects are produced without significant negative inotropic effects. The effects of NAPA on automaticity are somewhat variable but with little effect on most indices. The variable or biphasic heart rate response in vivo may be related to the effects of NAPA on the sympathetic nervous system rather than a direct effect on automaticity.[15] The development of abnormal automaticity and early afterdepolarizations at toxic levels of NAPA may have clinical relevance in terms of arrhythmogenic effects, such as the development of torsade de pointes (see Chapter 23).

## Antiarrhythmic Effects of NAPA in Experimental Arrhythmia Models

### Observations in Ventricular Arrhythmias

In studies by Minchin et al.[5] on the effects of NAPA on ouabain-induced ventricular fibrillation in the rabbit, a significant pro-

Table 1
Summary of the in Vitro Electrophysiologic Effects of N-Acetylprocainamide Compared to Procainamide in Cardiac Tissues.

| | N-Acetylprocainamide | Procainamide |
|---|---|---|
| **Atrium:** | | |
| Stimulation threshold | 0 | + + (45%) |
| Refractory period | + + (25%) | + + (50%) |
| **Ventricle:** | | |
| RMP | 0 | 0 |
| APA | 0 | − |
| MR | 0 | − |
| dV/dT | 0 | − |
| $APD_{-60mV}$ | + + (14%) | + + |
| **Purkinje Fiber** | | |
| RMP | 0 | 0 |
| APA | 0 | − |
| MR | 0 | − |
| Automaticity | 0 | − |
| dV/dT | 0 | − (14%) |
| $APD_{50}$ | + + (23%) | + + (9−12%) |
| $APD_{90}$ | + + (23%) | + + (11−21%) |

APA = action potential amplitude; APD = action potential duration at 50 percent or 90 percent repolarization or at −60 MV during repolarization; MR = membrane responsiveness; RMP = resting membrane potential; dV/dT = maximum rate of rise (volt/sec) of phase 0 of action potential, 0 = no change; + + = increased; − = decreased. The data from references 3, 4, 5 are summarized.

longation from control (12.3 ± 0.9 min to 17.3 ± 2.0 min) of the time to onset of ventricular fibrillation was observed after NAPA, particularly at the high dose of 75 mg/kg. The antiarrhythmic effects of NAPA thus were similar to those produced by procainamide at a dose of only 25 mg/kg.

In the dog, Bagwell et al.[3] noted that NAPA effectively suppressed ouabain-induced ventricular tachycardia for at least 30 minutes, although the dose required (140 to 210 mg/kg) was 3.5 times that required for procainamide (40 to 60 mg/kg). In the dog, ventricular ectopic beats induced by single-stage ligation of the left anterior descending coronary artery were significantly suppressed by NAPA for up to 30 minutes at a dose of 200 mg/kg, but the effects were variable when given in doses of 50−100 mg/kg.[3,4] In a study by Reynolds et al. NAPA pretreatment (20 mg/kg) also was

**Table 2**

**Summary of the in Vivo Electrophysiologic Effects of N-Acetylprocainamide Compared to Procainamide.**

|  | N-Acetylprocainamide | Procainamide |
|---|---|---|
| Heart rate | +/− | +/− |
| AH interval | +/− | ++ (29%) |
| Interatrial conduction | +/− | ++ |
| HV interval | 0 | ++ (44%) |
| QRS duration | +/− | ++ (17%) |
| $QT_c$ interval | ++ (23%) | ++ (12%) |
| Atrial ERP | ++ (47%) | ++ (28%) |
| Ventricular ERP | ++ (27%) | ++ (23%) |

AH = atrio-His interval; HV = His-ventricular interval; $QT_c$ = corrected QT by Bazett's formula; ERP = effective refractory period, 0 = no change; ++ = increased; +/− = variable or insignificant change. The data from references 1, 2, and 7 are summarized.

**Table 3**

**Electrophysiologic Effects of N-Acetylprocainamide and Recainam in Anesthetized Dogs with Induced Atrial Flutter**

| EP Parameter | Control | NAPA (n=15) | % | Control | Recianam (n=10) | % |
|---|---|---|---|---|---|---|
| QRS | 50±9 | 50±8 | (2) | 56±6 | 64±5 | (14)** |
| $QT_c$ | 320±31 | 369±37 | (16)** | 308±21 | 326±26 | (6)* |
| AERP | 127±14 | 161±15 | (27)** | 120±10 | 154±10 | (28)** |
| AFRP | 148±12 | 181±16 | (22)** | 143±9 | 171±26 | (20)** |
| Ct | 29±8 | 29±7 | (−1) | 26±8 | 39±13 | (50)** |
| Ct-150 | 44±7 | 46±8 | (6) | 53±9 | 89±12 | (70)** |
| AFcl | 151±21 | 170±23 | (13)** | 138±10 | 215±14 | (56)** |
| RRmin | 240±71 | 256±48 | (7) | 251±14 | 255±72 | (1) |

The data are means ± 1 standard deviation in milliseconds. All parameters were measured during sinus rhythm before and after drugs with the exception of atrial flutter cycle length and minimum RR inverval during atrial flutter. The values in parentheses represent the percent change of mean values from controls. The asterisks represent the statistical significance of the mean differences from controls: *p < 0.05, **p < 0.01. The drug doses were N-acetylprocainamide 30 mg/kg over 30 minutes and recainam 10 mg/kg over 20 minutes, then 10 mg/kg/hour constant infusion. AFcl = maximum atrial flutter cycle length; AERP = atrial effective refractory period; AFRP = atrial functional refractory period; CT = right to left atrial conduction time; CT-150 = Ct during rapid atrial pacing at a cycle length of 150 milliseconds; eP = electrophysiologic; $QT_c$ = $QT_a$ corrected; RRmin = minimum observed RR interval.

noted to reduce the incidence of ventricular fibrillation by 37 percent in dogs undergoing acute single-stage coronary ligation.[16]

## Observations in Atrial Arrhythmias

In a canine model of atrial flutter produced by intercaval crush in our laboratory,[17] NAPA 30 mg/kg was significantly more effective in conversion of atrial flutter to sinus rhythm in 10 of 15 dogs or 66 percent, in comparison to the new Class I antiarrhythmic agent recainam, which converted only 2 of 10 or 20 percent (Fig. 5). NAPA (Table 3) produced only a slight prolongation of the interatrial conduction time (+6 percent) during rapid atrial pacing (cycle 150 msec) and slowing of the atrial flutter rate (+13 percent) before conversion, in comparison to recainam, which markedly prolonged interatrial conduction (+70 percent) and atrial flutter rate

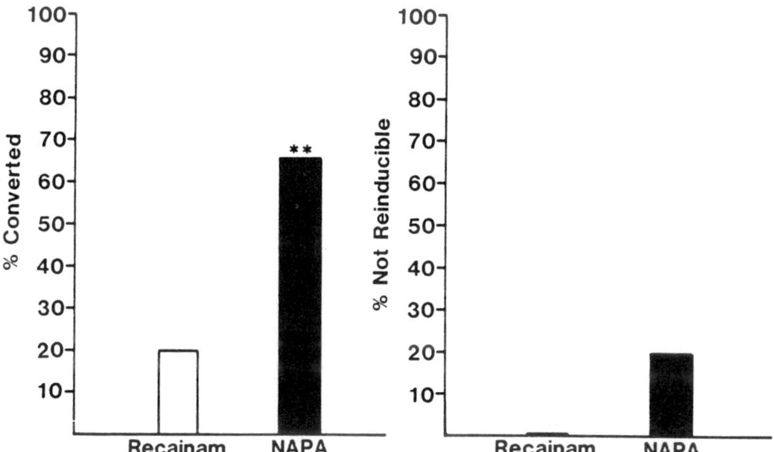

**Figure 5.** The effects of N-acetylprocainamide and recainam on the conversion and the prevention of reinduction of canine atrial flutter. Left panel shows the percentage of dogs converted to sinus rhythm by each drug. Right panel shows the percentage of dogs in which reinduction was prevented by each drug. Note that only NAPA produced a significant frequency of conversion of atrial flutter to sinus rhythm; neither drug prevented reinduction in a significant number of dogs. The asterisks represent the significance of the conversion or suppression frequency compared to placebo:**p < 0.05. From Feld G, Venkatesh N, Singh BN: Effects of N-acetylprocainamide and recainam in the pharmacologic conversion and suppression of experimental canine atrial flutter: Significance of changes in refractariness and conduction. *J Cardiovasc Pharmacol* in press, 1987.

(+56 percent). Both NAPA and recainam produced a similar prolongation of atrial refractoriness (see Table 3).

In dogs with chronic heart block, NAPA produced only slight slowing of the junctional pacemaker rate (narrow complex QRS, His-Purkinje rhythm) at doses of 50–100 mg/kg.[4] In these animals, ventricular premature depolarizations including single, coupled, and ventricular tachycardia beats were observed after doses of 50–100 mg/kg, including 3 deaths from malignant arrhythmias in the 11 dogs studied.[4]

Thus, NAPA in doses of 20–200 mg/kg exerts significant antiarrhythmic effects in experimental ouabain- and ischemia-induced ventricular arrhythmias in the rabbit and dog and in a canine model of atrial flutter, with few adverse hemodynamic effects. Potentially dangerous arrhythmogenic effects of NAPA may be produced at doses greater than 50 mg/kg, particularly in the presence of preexisting bradycardia (see Chapter 23).

## Mechanism of Antriarrhythmic Action of NAPA

The predominant electrophysiologic effect and probable mechanism of antiarrhythmic action of NAPA appears to be its ability to prolong the cardiac action potential duration, with a resultant prolongation of the voltage-dependent refractoriness in the atrium and ventricle.[1–6] Its lack of significant effects on dV/dT and conduction velocity, action potential amplitude, membrane responsiveness, and automaticity suggest that changes in these parameters play little role in the antiarrhythmic action of NAPA.[1–6] However, it is possible that under pathologic conditions such as ischemia, NAPA may produce changes in certain electrophysiologc parameters that it does not produce in normal tissue (e.g., greater depression of conduction velocity or automaticity) and that these changes might play a role in its antiarrhythmic action.[18] The additional effects of tissue hypoxia or ischemia on the electrophysiologic effects of NAPA have not been studied but warrant further investigation.

The interruption or prevention of reentrant arrhythmias by NAPA may be due to its selective prolongation of refractoriness with the resultant narrowing of the excitable gap and block of the excitation wave[17,19] in the case of arrhythmias due to reentry involving an anatomic obstacle to conduction (Fig. 5). In the case of slowing of the tachycardia by NAPA without interruption or prevention of the arrhythmia, a number of mechanisms need to be considered. The slowing may occur from a reduction of the frequency of depolarization produced by abnormal automaticity as observed by Dangman et al.;[4] it may arise from the development of use-dependent or ischemia-induced effects of NAPA on conduction velocity,[18,20] if the arrhythmia is due to reentry around or through an anatomic obstacle; alternatively, it may result from the prolongation of refractoriness if the mechanism of the tachycardia is the leading-circle type of reentry (Fig. 5), as proposed by Allessie et al.[19] Finally, it is possible that a combination of two or more of these effects might be operative in the slowing of tachycardia under the influence of NAPA.

## Clinical Correlates and Conclusions

Although the precise mechanism of antiarrhythmic action of NAPA may not be elucidated fully and deserves further study, the available evidence indicates that the predominant effect appears to be the prolongation of the atrial and ventricular action potential duration and voltage-dependent refractoriness. As a result, NAPA might be expected to have an antiarrhythmic activity in a variety of clinical arrhythmias including atrial fibrillation or flutter, atrial tachycardia due to interatrial reentry, ventricular ectopic beats and ventricular tachycardia or fibrillation. It is less likely to be effective in sinus node or atrioventricular nodal reentrant tachycardias and atrial or ventricular arrhythmias due to enhanced automaticity. Its utility in supraventricular tachycardias associated with an accessory atrioventricular pathway may be significant in that most antiarrhythmic agents that prolong atrial and ventricular refractoriness also prolong accessory pathway refractoriness. The evolving clinical experience with ventricular arrhythmias is discussed elsewhere in this volume (see Chapter 12). It is concluded that the electrophysiologic profile of NAPA with a dominant effect on cardiac repolarization and without a significant autonomic interaction constitutes an important pharmacologic probe to determine the antiarrhythmic and arrhythmogenic correlates of the lengthening of the cardiac action potential.

## References

1. Amlie JP, Nesje OA, Frislid K, et al: Serum levels and electrophysiologic effects of N-acetylprocainamide as compared with procainamide in the dog heart in situ. *Acta Pharmacol Toxicol* 42:280, 1978.

2. Jaillon P, Winkle RA: Electrophysiologic comparative study of procainamide and N-acetylprocainamide in anesthetized dogs: Concentration–response relationships. *Circulation* 60(6):1385, 1979.
3. Bagwell EE, Walle T. Drayer DE, et al: Correlation of the electrophysiologic and antiarrhythmic properties of the N-acetyl metabolite of procainamide with plasma and tissue drug concentrations in the dog. *J Pharmacol Exp Ther* 197(1):38, 1976.
4. Dangman KH, Hoffman BF: In vivo and in vitro antiarrhythmic and arrhythmogenic effects of N-acetylprocainamide. *J Pharmacol Exp Ther* 217(3):851, 1981.
5. Minchin RF, Ilett KF, Paterson JW: Antiarrhythmic potency of procainamide and N-acetylprocainamide in rabbits. *Eur J Pharmacol* 47:51, 1976.
6. Refsum H, Frislid K, Lunde PKM, et al: Effects of N-acetylprocainamide as compared with procainamide in isolated rat atrial. *Eur J Pharmacol* 33:47, 1975.
7. Feld GK, Singh BN: N-acetylprocainamide (NAPA): Pharmacologic properties and therapeutic applications of a new antiarrhythmic compound. *Arrhythmia Clin* 1(3):10, 1984.
8. Singh BN, Feld G, Nademanee K: Arrhythmia control by selective lengthening of cardiac repolarization: Role of N-acetylprocainamide, active metabolite of procainamide. *Angiology* 37:930, 1986.
9. Kluger J, Leech S, Reidenberg MM, et al: Long-term antiarrhythmic therapy with acetylprocainamide. *Am J Cardiol* 48:1124, 1981.
10. Roden DM, Reele SB, Higgins SB, et al: Antiarrhythmic efficacy, pharmacokinetics and safety of N-acetylprocainamide in human subjects: Comparison with procainamide. *Am J Cardiol* 46:463, 1980.
11. Winkle RA, Jaillon PA, Kates RE, et al: Clinical pharmacology and antiarrhythmic efficacy of N-acetylprocainamide. *Am J Cardiol* 47:123, 1981.
12. Lertora JJL, Clock D, Stec P, et al: Effects of N-acetylprocainamide and procainamide on myocardial contractile force, heart rate and blood pressure. *Proc Soc Exp Biol Med* 161:332, 1979.
13. Badke FR, Walsh RA, Crawford MH, et al: Hemodynamic effects of N-acetylprocainamide compared with procainamide in conscious dogs. *Circulation* 64(6):1142, 1981.
14. Sung RJ, Juma Z, Saksena S: Electrophysiologic properties and antiarrhythmic mechanisms of intravenous N-acetylprocainamide in patients with ventriculr dysrhythmias. *Am Heart J* 105(5):811, 1983.
15. Eudeikis JR, Henthorn TK, Lertora JJL, et al: Kinetic analysis of the vasodilator and ganglionic blocking actions of N-acetylprocainamide. *J Cardiovasc Pharmacol* 4(2):303, 1982.
16. Reynolds RD, Kamath BL: N-acetylprocainamide and ischemia-induced ventricular fibrillation in the dog. *Eur J Pharmacol* 59:115, 1979.
17. Feld GK, Venkatesh N, Singh BN: Pharmacologic conversion and suppression of experimental canine atrial flutter: Differing effects of d-sotalol, quinidine and lidocaine and the significance of changes in refractoriness and conduction. *Circulation* 74(1):197, 1986.

18. Lazzara R, Hope RR, El-Sherif N, et al: Effects of lidocaine on hypoxic and ischemic cardiac cells. *Am J Cardiol* 41:872, 1978.
19. Allessie MA, Bonke FIM, Schopman FJG: Circus movement in rabbit atrial muscle as a mechanism of tachycardia. *Circ Res* 41(1):9, 1977.
20. Mason JW, Hondeghem LM, Katzung B: Block of inactivated sodium channels and of depolarization-induced automaticity in guinea pig papillary muscle by amiodarone. *Circ Res* 55(3):277, 194.

# Chapter 10

# N-Acetylprocainamide: Pharmacokinetics and Plasma-Level Effect Correlations

Arthur J. Atkinson, Jr., Tsuen Ih Ruo, and Antoni A. Piergies

The pharmacokinetics of N-acetylprocainamide (NAPA) have been studied extensively and have been the subject of a number of recent reviews.[1,2] In fact, it was a pharmacokinetic study that provided the crucial impetus for developing NAPA as an antiarrhythmic drug in its own right.[3] In this study, we found that the elimination-phase half-life of NAPA is more than twice that of procainamide in normal subjects and proposed that patient compliance and antiarrhythmic response might be improved if NAPA were used to circumvent the inconvenience of the frequent dosing schedule that has been recommended for procainamide.[4]

On the other hand, few formal studies have been conducted to correlate NAPA pharmacokinetics with therapeutic or toxic responses to this drug. This review will summarize the salient features of NAPA pharmacokinetics (see Table 1) and pharmacodynamics in order to provide a clinically useful approach for optimizing NAPA therapy.

*This work was supported in part by grants GM-22371 and GM-07842 from the National Institute of General Medical Sciences, and RR-00048 from the Division of Research Resources, National Institutes of Health.*

| Table 1 | |
| :-- | :-- |
| **Clinical Pharmacokinetic Profile of N-Acetylprocainamide** | |
| *Bioavailability* | |
| Time to reach peak levels | 2 hrs |
| Extent of absorption | 85% |
| *Distribution* | |
| Plasma protein binding | 10% |
| RBC/Plasma partition ratio | 1.6 |
| Initial distribution space | 0.11 l/kg |
| Total distribution volume | |
| $V_d$ (ss) | 1.5 l/kg |
| $V_d$ (area) | 1.8 l/kg |
| *Elimination* | |
| Elimination-phase half-life | 6.2 hrs* |
| Elimination clearance | |
| Total elimination clearance | 234 ml/min* |
| Renal clearance | 200 ml/min* |
| Nonrenal clearance | 34 ml/min |
| Percent renal excretion | 85%* |
| Metabolites | (See Figure 2) |
| *Dosing* | |
| Dose schedule | Every 8 hrs |
| Accumulation factor | 1.7* |
| Usual range of therapeutic plasma levels | 10–30 μg/ml |

*Critically dependent on status of renal function

## Pharmacokinetics of NAPA

### Absorption

NAPA absorption initially was studied in 3 normal subjects using a novel stable isotope method in which an intravenous dose of [13]C-labelled NAPA was administered simultaneously with an oral formulation.[5] Eighty-five percent of the oral NAPA dose was absorbed and peak NAPA plasma concentrations were reached in 45–90 minutes. Rodman et al. estimated that NAPA absorption also was 85 percent complete in 7 patients who received repeated oral NAPA doses.[6] However, there was considerable interpatient and intrapatient variability in absorption rate, and other investigators have noted that between 1.3 and 4.0 hours may be required to reach peak NAPA plasma levels in patients given oral NAPA doses.[7,8]

## Distribution

The three-compartmental pattern of NAPA distribution, shown schematically in Figure 1, is most apparent when intravenous doses of this drug are administered rapidly. In one study, the intravenous NAPA dose was injected over 10 minutes and the initial distribution space, $V_C$ in Figure 1, was found to average 7.5l.[9] When estimated $V_C$ was corrected for preferential partitioning of

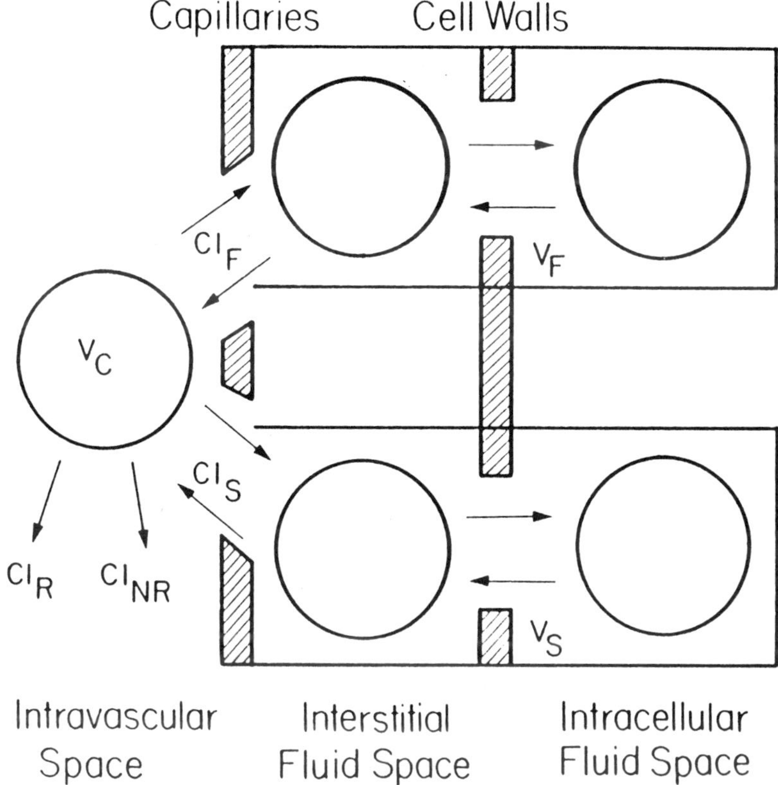


**Figure 1.** Model of NAPA distribution and elimination kinetics. After an oral or parenteral dose, NAPA initially enters the intravascular space ($V_C$). Transcapillary exchange limits the rate of NAPA distribution to the rapid ($V_F$) and slow ($V_S$) equilibrating peripheral model compartments as determined by the intercompartmental clearances ($Cl_F$ and $Cl_S$). These clearances depend on blood flow to each compartment as well as on properties of NAPA transfer through capillary walls but transfer from interstitial to intracellular fluid spaces is too rapid to be distinguished kinetically. NAPA is cleared from the body by renal ($Cl_R$) and nonrenal ($Cl_{NR}$) mechanisms. (From Atkinson AJ Jr, Ruo TI: Pharmacokinetics of N-acetylprocainamide. *Angiology* 37:959, 1986. By permission of the publisher.)

NAPA into erythrocytes (RBC), it was in close agreement with expected intravascular space.[10] This indicates that the transcapillary exchange is the rate-limiting step in NAPA distribution and, in conjunction with other studies of the multicompartmental distribution of urea and inulin,[11] suggests that the two peripheral model compartments reflect the kinetic heterogeneity of interstitial fluid space. Since transcapillary exchange is determined by blood flow as well as by movement across capillary walls, it can be anticipated that hemodynamic changes will affect the kinetics of NAPA distribution.[10]

NAPA is not bound extensively to plasma proteins and the percent bound ranges from 8 to 11 percent over a concentration range of 1 to 16 μg/ml.[12] The RBC−plasma partition ratio for NAPA is $1.62 \pm 0.05$[13] and NAPA also distributes preferentially into tissues, accounting for the fact that its 1.5 l/kg steady-state distribution volume exceeds estimates of total body water. In terms of an equivalent single compartment model, the NAPA distribution volume ($V_{d(area)}$) that relates elimination clearance to elimination half-life is 1.8 l/kg.

## Elimination

NAPA elimination is an apparent first-order process, as indicated by pharmacokinetic studies[3,5,9] and the directly proportional relationship between NAPA dose and steady-state plasma level.[8,14] Isolated anomalies that have yet to be confirmed or explained are that the "oral" clearance of NAPA declined after repeated doses[14] and, in a single patient, an increased NAPA dose was associated with a disproportionately large increase in plasma level.[15] In normal subjects, average values for NAPA elimination clearance and elimination-phase half-life are 234 ml/min and 6.2 hours, respectively.[9] However, the elimination-phase half-life may appear to be longer when NAPA is administered orally, because this drug has a slow terminal absorption rate.[5,14]

In normal subjects, the renal clearance of NAPA averages 200 ml/min and individuals with normal renal function can be expected to excrete approximately 85 percent of administered NAPA doses unchanged in the urine.[9] Accordingly, the rate of NAPA elimination is critically dependent on renal function and the elimination-phase half-life is prolonged in functionally anephric patients to approximately 42 hours.[13] However, estimation of approximate dose reductions for patients with impaired renal function is facilitated by the fact that there is a reasonably consistent relationship between creatinine clearance $(Cl_{Cr})$ and NAPA renal clearance $(Cl_R)$[13,15] and $Cl_R$ can be estimated from the equation: $Cl_R = 1.7\ Cl_{Cr}$.

Since $Cl_R$ exceeds glomerular filtration rate, there is net renal tubular secretion of NAPA and this can be competitively inhibited by concurrent therapy with cimetidine.[15] On the other hand, renal excretion of NAPA is relatively unaffected by changes in urine flow rate or pH.[16]

Nonrenal clearance of NAPA averages 34 ml/min or 0.49 ml/min/kg in normal subjects[13] and, in contrast to the nonrenal clearance of procainamide,[17] is unimpaired in functionally anephric patients.[13] N-Dealkylation[18,19] and deacetylation[20] pathways of NAPA metabolism have been identified (Fig. 2). Although deacetylation accounts for only 3 percent of NAPA elimination, this pathway has an important bearing on the immunologic safety of NAPA therapy.[20,21] Several investigators have described patients with the procainamide-induced lupus syndrome, who were subsequently treated successfully with NAPA.[22–24] However, in 1 of the patients reported by Kluger et al., arthralgias returned during NAPA therapy at a time when NAPA levels were 48 µg/ml and procainamide levels were 1.6 µg/ml.[24] These symptoms subsided

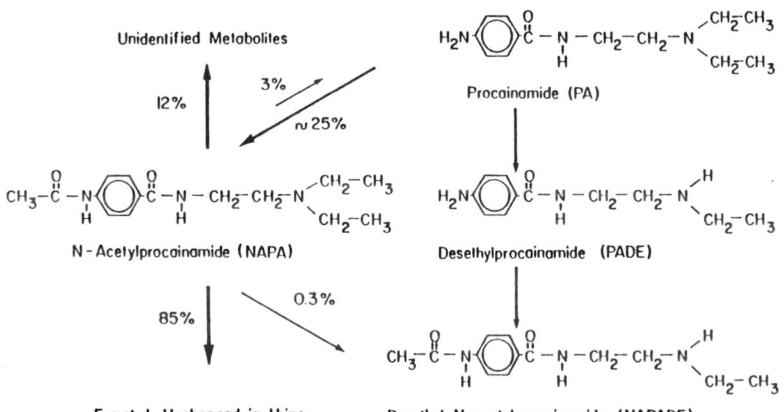


**Figure 2.** Pathways of NAPA metabolism and elimination. The relative contribution of each pathway is shown for normal subjects as a percentage of total NAPA elimination. There is interconversion of NAPA and procainamide and rapid acetylators convert back to NAPA approximately 25 percent of procainamide that is formed by deacetylation. (From Atkinson AJ Jr, Ruo TI: Pharmacokinetics of N-acetylprocainamide. Angiology, 37: 959, 1986. By permission of the publisher.)

when the NAPA dose was reduced and NAPA and procainamide levels fell to 27 μg/ml and 0.7 μg/ml, respectively. This suggests that insufficient procainamide was being formed at this point by deacetylation to exceed the apparent toxic dose threshold necessary to trigger lupus-like symptoms. Because procainamide concentrations during NAPA therapy appear to increase proportionally with NAPA plasma concentrations and dosage, NAPA deacetylation may limit the utility of NAPA in some patients who require high plasma levels of this drug for arrhythmia suppression.[20]

## Plasma-Level Effect Correlations

## Therapeutic Response

Several investigators have evaluated the antiarrhythmic efficacy of NAPA in placebo-controlled, dose-ranging studies of hospitalized patients.[8,23,25,26] Reduction in premature ventricular complex (PVC) frequency was chosen as the therapeutic end-point, even though it has not been shown that suppression of PVCs reduces the risk of sudden death. The different conclusions that were reached regarding the efficacy of NAPA therapy appear primarily to reflect different response criteria selected by various investigators, rather than marked differences in the extent of PVC suppression associated with NAPA therapy. Taken together, these reports indicate that NAPA reduced PVC frequency by 50 percent or more in about half of the patients that were studied.

Even among patients in whom NAPA therapy effectively suppresses ventricular arrhythmias, there is considerable variation in the NAPA plasma concentrations that are required. Temporal variation in PVC frequency has precluded rigorous kinetic analysis of the correlation between NAPA plasma levels and antiarrhythmic response in individual patients.[27] However, we obtained monthly ambulatory 24-hour electrocardiographic recordings while treating 4 patients with NAPA for 3–4 years.[28] These patients had clinically stable heart disease and we were able to demonstrate that they did not develop tolerance to the antiarrhythmic effects of this drug. Variation in patient compliance over the course of this study also made it possible for us to determine a threshold NAPA plasma concentration for each patient that generally was required to suppress PVC frequency to a significant extent (Fig. 3). This threshold averaged 21 μg/ml (range, 12 to 35 μg/ml). These

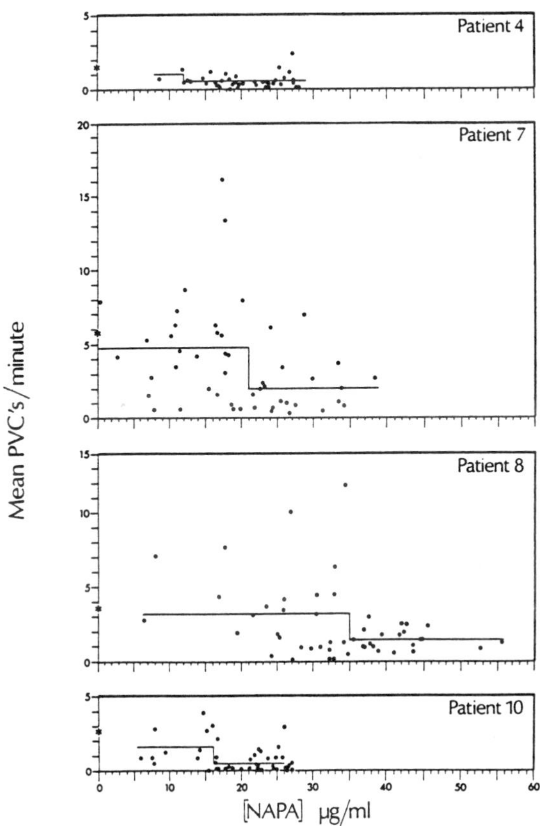


**Figure 3.** Relationship between plasma NAPA concentration and PVC frequency in ambulatory patients. The line is drawn to show mean PVC frequencies when NAPA levels were either below or above the apparent threshold required for antiarrhythmic response. Asterisks indicate the mean of placebo period observations, which were made every 6 months when each patient was hospitalized. (From Atkinson AJ Jr, Lertora JJL, Kushner W, et al: Efficacy and safety of N-acetylprocainamide in long-term treatment of ventricular arrhythmias. *Clin Pharmacol Ther* 33:565, 1983. By permission of the publisher.)

results agree with the experience of other investigators, who have found that therapeutic responses usually do not occur until NAPA plasma concentrations exceed 10 µg/ml[8,24]

Our results also suggest that the NAPA concentration–therapeutic response relationship may have the approximate shape of a step function and that there is little further gain in antiarrhythmic efficacy when plasma levels are increased much beyond the threshold values. In contrast, lower plasma NAPA levels, averaging only 10.5 µg/ml (range, 2 to 22 µg/ml), appeared to be maximally effective when our patients initially were hospitalized to evaluate their response to NAPA. Thus the level of patient activity appears to affect the correlation between NAPA plasma concentration and extent of PVC suppression. On the other hand, programmed electrical stimulation has been helpful in our experience for identifying a NAPA plasma level that is likely to be effective during subsequent long-term therapy.

## Other Effects

The relationship between NAPA plasma concentration and QT interval duration has been studied because NAPA is a Class III antiarrhythmic drug that appears to act primarily by prolonging cardiac repolarization and lengthening action potential duration.[29] In most patients there is a 2.4 msec lengthening of the corrected QT interval for every µg/ml increment in plasma NAPA concentration. This QT interval response was not exaggerated in a patient who subsequently developed NAPA-induced torsade de pointes.[27] However, an exaggerated response was observed in a patient with frequent PVCs and ventricular tachycardia that were neither suppressed nor exacerbated by NAPA therapy.[30] Thus, it appears that the relationship between NAPA plasma concentration and QT interval prolongation cannot be used to predict clinical response to this drug.

Although NAPA does not have the negative inotropic effects shared by procainamide and many other Class I antiarrhythmic drugs,[31] intravenous doses of NAPA may cause hypotension because NAPA is similar to procainamide in blocking sympathetic ganglionic transmission, thereby causing vasodilation by reducing vasoconstrictor tone.[32] Studies in dogs and a normal subject suggest that intravenous administration of NAPA will acutely lower mean arterial pressure by 0.4 mm Hg for every µg/ml increment in plasma NAPA concentration.[33] However, more pronounced hypotension would be expected in patients whose intravascular volume is depleted or whose vasomotor tone is impaired, and Sonnhag and Karlsson reported that NAPA reduced systolic blood pressure by at least 30 mm Hg in 2 of 10 patients who received rapid NAPA infusions that brought plasma NAPA levels to approximately 15 µg/ml in 10 minutes.[34] This effect should not cause hypotension during continued NAPA therapy but appears responsible for afterload reduction and a reduced ratio of PEP/LVET during long-term NAPA therapy of patients whose stroke volume was compromised.[28]

Other clinical effects correlate even less predictably with plasma NAPA levels. For example, gastrointestinal toxicity has been reported with NAPA levels ranging from 10.6 to 37.9 µg/ml (mean, 22.5 µg/ml).[35] With continued therapy, patients may develop tolerance to NAPA-induced nausea and some have been treated successfully with NAPA levels between 30 and 40 µg/ml.[8,28]

## Individualization of NAPA Therapy

Initial Dose Estimates

We have proposed 10–30 µg/ml as a tentative therapeutic range for plasma NAPA concentrations and, in the absence of more specific guidelines from electrophysiologic testing, have recommended 20 µg/ml as an initial target NAPA plasma level.[2] The upper limit of this range may be unnecessarily conservative and is set to avoid the immunologic risks that may be associated with procainamide cumulation when NAPA levels are higher. In some patients, the benefits of effective arrhythmia control certainly may outweigh these risks.

If the need for arrhythmia control is urgent, or if a loading dose is needed as part of a protocol for programmed electrical stimulation, a 17-mg/kg intravenous NAPA-HCl dose (15 mg/kg NAPA base) has been well tolerated when infused over 30 minutes and usually provides peak NAPA plasma levels of approximately 30 µg/ml (range, 25 to 36 µg/ml).[13,30]

Renal function is the most important patient characteristic to consider in initiating maintenance therapy with NAPA and creatinine clearance should be either measured directly or estimated by a standard method, such as the equation developed by Cockroft and Gault.[36] This equation can be used to estimate creatinine clearance in men as

$$Cl_{Cr} = \frac{(140 - age)\ (wt\ in\ kg)}{72(serum\ Cr\ in\ mg/dl)}$$

For women, this estimate should be reduced by 15 percent. The to-

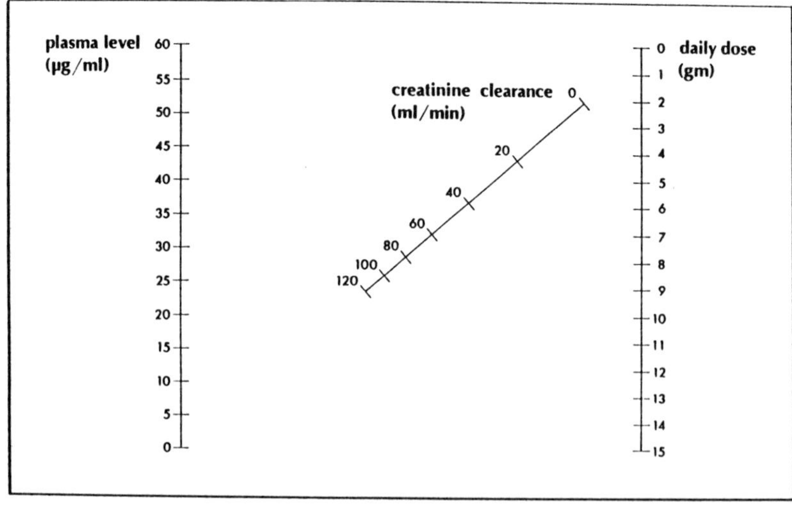


**Figure 4.** Nomogram for estimating an initial NAPA dose for patients with impaired renal function. Target plasma NAPA level and creatinine clearance are connected with a straightedge and total daily oral dose is read from the scale at the right. This estimate includes the assumption that absorption of oral NAPA doses is 85 percent complete. (From Atkinson AJ, Jr., Stec GP, Lertora JJL, et al: Impact of active metabolites on monitoring plasma concentration of therapeutic drugs. *Ther Drug Monitor* 2:19, 1980.

tal daily dose needed to maintain the target plasma level either can be calculated directly using the approach developed by Dettli[37] or estimated from the nomogram shown in Figure 4.[38] One-third of this total dose usually is administered every 8 hours, but a longer dosing interval may be feasible for patients whose creatinine clearance is less than 50 ml/min.

Age is another important patient factor that is not only associated with reductions in creatinine clearance but lowers the expected ratio of NAPA to creatinine clearance from 1.8 at age 50 to 1.4 at age 80.[39] A 25 percent reduction in NAPA dose requirement also should be anticipated for patients requiring concurrent cimetidine therapy, because cimetidine inhibits renal tubular secretion of NAPA.[15] On the other hand, coronary artery disease does not slow NAPA clearance more than expected from patient age and creatinine clearance.[40]

## Subsequent Therapy

After NAPA therapy is started, plasma levels will reach 90 percent of their eventual steady-state level in 3.3 elimination-phase half-lives, less if an initial loading dose was given. Plasma levels measured after this time can be used to check the accuracy of initial dose estimates, to establish a reference for subsequent evaluation of patient compliance, and to guide dose adjustment, using the proportional relationship between NAPA dose and plasma level. When NAPA plasma levels have been included in the protocol for programmed electrical stimulation, it may be important to verify that NAPA therapy is providing plasma levels similar to those found effective during electrophysiologic testing. "Valley" or "trough" samples obtained just before a NAPA dose should be used for routine plasma level monitoring, because NAPA concentrations in these samples are not as affected by variability in absorption rate as are concentrations in samples obtained when NAPA levels are estimated to be at their peak.[2]

Should dose-related toxicity necessitate a rapid reduction in NAPA plasma levels, hemoperfusion appears to be the method of choice and has been reported to provide an average NAPA plasma clearance of 144.8 ml/min in a dialysis patient who developed NAPA levels of 56 μg/ml while on procainamide therapy.[41] By comparison, NAPA plasma clearance averaged only 41.3 ml/min when this patient was dialyzed with an EX-23 coil dialyzer but was somewhat higher, averaging 97.2 ml/min (range, 94.0 to 104.6 ml/min), in 4 functionally anephric patients during routine hemodialysis therapy with a CDAK 2.5 large surface area dialyzer.[13] If more than 3 hours of hemoperfusion therapy is needed, the resin cartridge may become saturated with NAPA and may need to be changed.

## References


1. Connolly SJ, Kates RE: Clinical pharmacokinetics of N-acetylprocainamide. *Clin Pharmacokinet* 7:206, 1982.
2. Atkinson AJ Jr, Ruo TI: Pharmacokinetics of N-acetylprocainamide. *Angiology* 37:959, 1986.
3. Strong JM, Dutcher JS, Lee W-K, et al: Pharmacokinetics in man of the N-acetylated metabolite of procainamide. *J Pharmacokinet Biopharm* 3:223, 1975.
4. Koch-Weser J, Klein SW: Procainamide dosage schedules, plasma concentrations and clinical effects, *JAMA* 215:1454, 1971.

5. Strong JM, Dutcher JS, Lee W-K, et al: Absolute bioavailability in man of N-acetylprocainamide determined by a novel stable isotope method. *Clin Pharmacol Ther* 18:613, 1975.
6. Rodman JH, Hurst A, Gaarder T, et al: N-acetylprocainamide kinetics and clinical response during repeated dosing. *Clin Pharmacol Ther* 32:378, 1982.
7. Lee W-K, Strong JM, Kehoe RF, et al: Antiarrhythmic efficacy of N-acetylprocainamide in patients with premature ventricular contractions. *Clin Pharmacol Ther* 19:508, 1976.
8. Winkle RA, Jaillon P, Kates RE, et al: Clinical pharmacology and antiarrhythmic efficacy of N-acetylprocainamide. *Am J Cardiol* 47:123, 1981.
9. Dutcher JS, Strong JM, Lucas SV, et al: Procainamide and N-acetylprocainamide kinetics investigated simultaneously with stable isotope methodology. *Clin Pharmacol Ther* 22:447, 1977.
10. Stec GP, Atkinson AJ Jr: Analysis of the contributions of permeability and flow to intercompartmental clearance. *J Pharmacokinet Biopharm* 9:167, 1981.
11. Bowsher DJ, Avram MJ, Frederiksen MC, et al: Urea distribution kinetics analyzed by simultaneous injection of urea and inulin: Demonstration that transcapillary exchange is rate limiting. *J Pharmacol Exp Ther* 230:269, 1984.
12. Reidenberg MM, Drayer DE, Levy M, et al: Polymorphic acetylation of procainamide in man. *Clin Pharmacol Ther* 17:722, 1975.
13. Stec GP, Atkinson AJ Jr, Nevin MJ, et al: N-acetylprocainamide pharmacokinetics in functionally anephric patients before and after perturbation by hemodialysis. *Clin Pharmacol Ther* 26:618, 1979.
14. Ludden TM, Crawford MH: N-acetylprocainamide kinetics after single and repeated oral doses. *Clin Pharmacol Ther* 31:343, 1982.
15. Somogyi A, McLean A, Heinzow B: Cimetidine-procainamide pharmacokinetic interaction in man: Evidence of competition for tubular secretion of basic drugs. *Eur J Clin Pharmacol* 25:339, 1983.
16. Galeazzi RL, Sheiner LB, Lockwood T, et al: The renal elimination of procainamide. *Clin Pharmacol Ther* 19:55, 1976.
17. Gibson TP, Atkinson AJ Jr, Matusik E, et al: Kinetics of procainamide and N-acetylprocainamide in renal failure. *Kidney Int* 12:422, 1977.
18. Ruo TI, Thenot J-P, Stec GP, et al: Plasma concentrations of desethyl N-acetylprocainamide in patients treated with procainamide and N-acetylprocainamide. *Ther Drug Monitor* 3:231, 1981.
19. Ruo TI, Morita Y, Atkinson AJ Jr, et al: Identification of desethyl procainamide in patients: A new metabolite of procainamide. *J Pharmacol Exp Ther* 216:357, 1981.
20. Stec GP, Ruo TI, Thenot J-P, et al: Kinetics of N-acetylprocainamide deacetylation. *Clin Pharmacol Ther* 28:659, 1980.
21. Lertora JJL, Atkinson AJ Jr, Kushner W, et al: Long-term antiarrhythmic therapy with N-acetylprocainamide. *Clin Pharmacol Ther* 25:273, 1979.
22. Stec GP, Lertora JJL, Atkinson AJ Jr, et al: Remission of procainamide-induced lupus erythematosus with N-acetylprocainamide therapy. *Ann Intern Med* 90:800, 1979.
23. Roden DM, Reele SB, Higgins SB, et al: Antiarrhythmic efficacy, pharmacokinetics and safety of N-acetylprocainamide in human subjects: Comparison with procainamide. *Am J Cardiol* 46:463, 1980.

24. Kluger J, Drayer DE, Reidenberg MM, et al: Acetylprocainamide therapy in patients with previous procainamide-induced lupus syndrome. *Ann Intern Med* 95:18, 1981.
25. Atkinson AJ Jr, Lee W-K, Quinn ML, et al: Dose-ranging trial of N-acetylprocainamide in patients with premature ventricular contractions. *Clin Pharmacol Ther* 21:575, 1977.
26. Kluger J, Leech S, Reidenberg MM, et al: Long-term antiarrhythmic therapy with acetylprocainamide. *Am J Cardiol* 48:1124, 1981.
27. Chow MJ, Piergies AA, Bowsher DJ, et al: Torsade de pointes induced by N-acetylprocainamide *J Am Coll Cardiol* 4:621, 1984.
28. Atkinson AJ Jr, Lertora JJL, Kushner W, et al: Efficacy and safety of N-acetylprocainamide in long-term treatment of ventricular arrhythmias *Clin Pharmacol Ther* 33:565, 1983.
29. Dangman KH, Hoffman BF: In vivo and in vitro antiarrhythmic and arrhythmogenic effects of N-acetyl procainamide. *J Pharmacol Exp Ther* 217:851, 1981.
30. Piergies AA, Ruo TI, Jansyn EM, et al: Effect kinetics of N-acetylprocainamide-induced QT interval prolongation (abstract) *Clin Pharmacol Ther* 42:107, 1987.
31. Lertora JJL, Glock D, Stec GP, et al: Effects of N-acetylprocainamide and procainamide on myocardial contractile force, heart rate, and blood pressure. *Proc Soc Exp Biol Med* 161:332, 1979.
32. Reynolds RD, Gorczynski RJ: Comparison of the autonomic effects of procainamide and N-acetylprocainamide in the dog. *J Pharmacol Exp Ther* 212:579, 1980.
33. Eudeikis JR, Henthron TK, Lertora JJL, et al: Kinetic analysis of the vasodilator and ganglionic blocking actions of N-acetylprocainamide. *J Cardiovasc Pharmacol* 4:303, 1982.
34. Sonnhag C, Karlsson E: Comparative antiarrhythmic efficacy of intravenous N-acetylprocainamide and procainamide. *Eur J Clin Pharmacol* 15:311, 1979.
35. Roden DM, Reele SB, Higgins SB, et al: Antiarrhythmic efficacy, pharmacokinetics and safety of N-acetylprocainamide in human subjects: Comparison with procainamide. *Am J Cardiol* 46:463, 1980.
36. Cockcroft DW, Gault MH: Prediction of creatinine clearance from serum creatinine. *Nephron* 16:31, 1976.
37. Dettli L: Individualization of drug dosage in patients with renal disease. *Med Clin North Am* 58:977, 1974.
38. Atkinson AJ Jr, Stec GP, Lertora JJL, et al: Impact of active metabolites on monitoring plasma concentrations of therapeutic drugs. *Ther Drug Monitor* 2:19, 1980.
39. Reidenberg MM, Camacho M, Kluger J, et al: Aging and renal clearance of procainamide and acetylprocainamide. *Clin Pharmacol Ther* 28:732, 1980.
40. Kates RE, Jaillon P, Rubenson DS, et al: Intravenous N-acetylprocainamide disposition kinetics in coronary artery disease. *Clin Pharmacol Ther* 28:52, 1980.
41. Braden GL, Fitzgibbons JP, Germain MJ, et al: Hemoperfusion for treatment of N-acetylprocainamide intoxication. *Ann Intern Med* 105:64, 1986.

# Chapter 11

# Clinical Electrophysiologic and Antiarrhythmic Effects of N-Acetylprocainamide: Role as a Class III Antiarrhythmic Agent

Ruey J. Sung and Mitchell D. Silver

N-acetylprocainamide (NAPA) is the major metabolite of procainamide in human subjects[1] and has antiarrhythmic properties independent of its parent compound.[2-5] NAPA is considered to have therapeutic advantages over procainamide because of (1) low prevalence of drug-induced systemic lupus erythematosus,[6] and (2) long elimination half-life twice that of procainamide.[7] Theoretical considerations and preliminary clinical data suggest that the drug is likely to have minimal negative inotropic effects. The purpose of this chapter is to review electrophysiologic properties and antiarrhythmic mechanisms of NAPA and to discuss its potential role as an antiarrhythmic agent in clinical use.

## Electrophysiologic Considerations

The in vitro and in vivo electrophysiologic effects of NAPA have been discussed critically in Chapter 10. For completeness, the salient features are emphasized here.

In isolated Purkinje fibers, the predominant electrophysiologic effect of NAPA is prolongation of action potential duration.[3] A re-

From: *Control of Cardiac Arrhythmias by Lengthening Repolarization*, edited by Bramah N. Singh, MD, Futura Publishing Company Inc., Mount Kisco, NY, © 1988.

duction of automaticity associated with a decrease in the slope of phase 4 depolarization can only be seen at very high NAPA concentrations. NAPA exerts no effect on the resting membrane potential, amplitude and maximal upstroke of phase 0 of the action potential, and membrane responsiveness in canine Purkinje fibers and ventricular muscle cells. These findings are in accordance with Class III antiarrhythmic electrophysiologic action. In the presence of toxic NAPA concentrations, a "secondary plateau" appears during phase 3 of the action potential, which is associated with the occurrence of early afterdepolarizations and spontaneous action potentials,[8] probably the basis of torsade des pointes (see Chapter 24).

NAPA increases the effective and functional refractory periods of right atrial and ventricular muscle in the dog heart.[5,9] The atrioventricular (AV) nodal functional refractory period also increases over a wide range of plasma drug concentrations without a significant increase in His-Purkinje and AV nodal conduction time. The effect on QRS duration is minimal, although the $QT_c$ interval increases. NAPA exerts no significant effect on sinus nodal recovery or intraventricular conduction times. Thus, the overall clinical electrophysiologic effects of NAPA is consistent with a Class III action in cardiac muscle.

NAPA decreases the incidence of arrhythmias following coronary occlusion and ouabain administrations in pentobarbital-anesthetized dogs (140−220 mg/kg).[3] Antiarrhythmic effects have also been shown in choloroform and hypoxia-induced ventricular fibrillation in mice, and in atrial and ventricular arrhythmias within 24 hours of myocardial infarction in dogs.[8] It is postulated that NAPA's antiarrhythmic action is related to its ability to modify refractoriness and conduction in the ischemic zone, thereby abolishing reentrant impulses. The effect on abnormal automaticity is relatively weak or nonexistent.[8]

## Clinical Electrophysiologic Effects

The clinical electrophysiologic effects of NAPA are consistent with those reported in experimental in vitro and in vivo settings. In a group of 10 patients undergoing diagnostic cardiac catheterization, Jaillon et al. studied electrophysiologic effects of intravenous NAPA on atrioventricular conduction.[10] They administered NAPA at a total dose of 105 mg/kg body weight with one loading infusion over 15 minutes and one maintenance infusion of 30 minutes achieving plasma NAPA concentrations of 12.0 to 32.2 mcg/ ml. They demonstrated that NAPA did not significantly affect sinus cycle length, sinus nodal recovery time, conduction intervals (AH, HV, PR, and QRS), AV nodal functional refractory period, or AV nodal Wenckebach cycle length, but it significantly prolonged the $QT_c$ intervals and the atrial and ventricular effective refractory periods.

In a group of 16 patients with various forms of symptomatic ventricular arrhythmias, Sung et al. performed electrophysiologic studies before and after intravenous infusion of NAPA at 20 mg/kg body weight over 20 minutes, achieving plasma concentrations of $24 \pm 3.2$ to $35.5 \pm 4.5$ mcg/ml.[11] They also found that NAPA did not significantly change sinus cycle length and atrioventricular conduction times (PA, AH, HV, and QRS), but it significantly lengthened the $QT_c$ intervals during sinus rhythm. Similar to procainamide, NAPA prolonged atrial and ventricular refractory periods (Fig. 1), but unlike procainamide, it had negligible effects on atrioventricular nodal conduction, presumably due to its lack of vagolytic effects. They cautioned, however, that NAPA did exert depressant effects on the His-Purkinje system as revealed by incremental atrial pacing and programmed atrial extrastimulation in 9 of the 16 patients (Fig. 2), and therefore should be administered cautiously to patients, particularly those with preexisting His-Purkinje system disease. The data raises the possibility that NAPA may exert an inhibitory effect on fast sodium channels in depolarized fibers, a possibility that should be explored further in relevant experimental and clinical models.

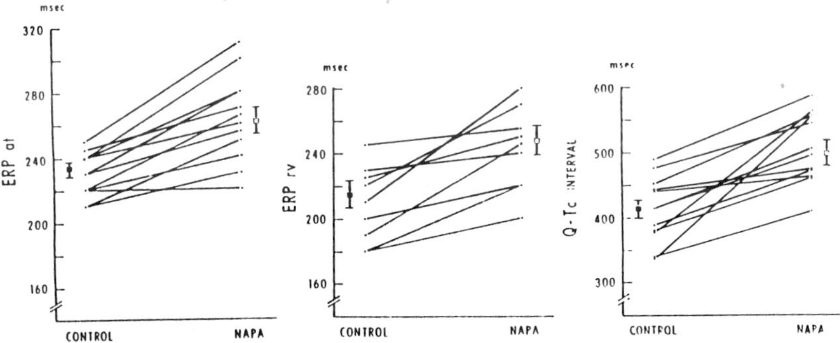

**Figure 1.** Prolongation of atrial and ventricular refractoriness and the $QT_c$ interval by N-acetylprocainamide. $ERP_{at}$ = effective refractive period of the atrium; $ERP_{rv}$ = effective refractory period of the right ventricle; NAPA = N-acetylprocainamide.

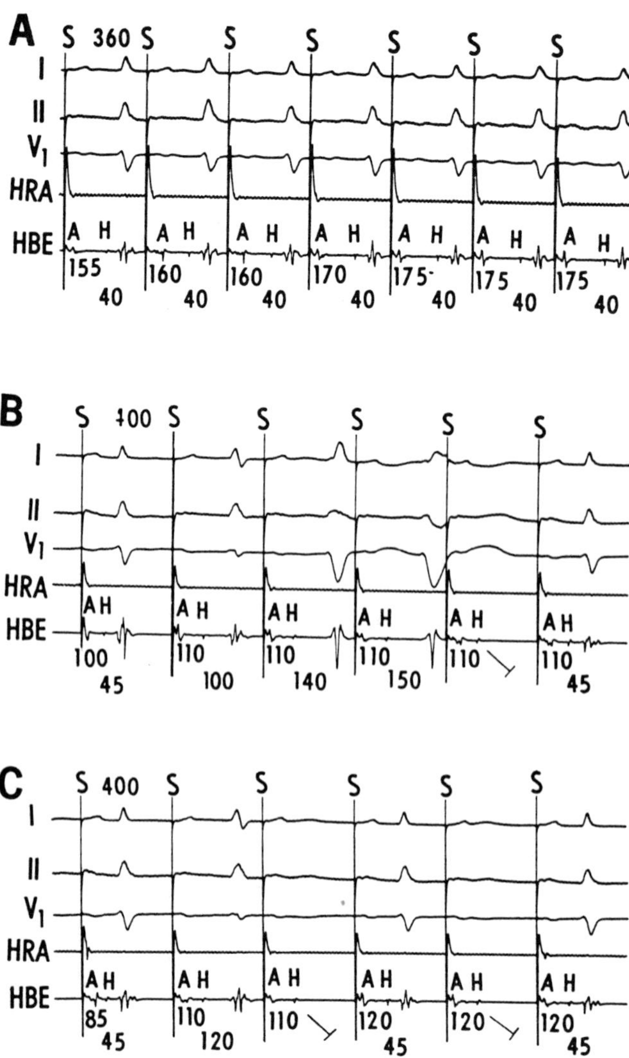



**Figure 2.** NAPA-induced conduction disturbance in the His-Purkinje system. A: During atrial pacing at a cycle length of 360 msec, AV conduction is 1:1. The corresponding AV nodal conduction time (AH interval) ranges from 155 to 175 msec, and His-Purkinje system conduction time (HV interval) is 40 msec. B: Following NAPA infusion, the atrium is

## Anti-Arrhythmic Effects of NAPA

At present there are limited data on the use of NAPA both in patients with inducible ventricular tachyarrhythmias as in those with simple or complex PVCs. With respect to ventricular arrhythmias in the same series of patients, Sung et al. noted that NAPA infusion abolished ventricular ectopy in only 3 of the 7 patients who exhibited frequent ventricular premature beats (Fig. 3). In 8 patients with inducible bundle-branch reentry manifested as repetitive ventricular responses, NAPA abolished reentry in 1 patient, narrowed and shifted the reentry zone rightward in 2 patients, and widened the reentry zone in 5 patients (Fig. 4). In the 2 patients with slow ventricular tachycardia (accelerated idioventricular rhythm), NAPA had no antiarrhythmic effects, and in the 2 patients with inducible sustained ventricular tachycardia, NAPA slowed the rate of ventricular tachycardia in 1 patient and abolished that inducibility in the other patient (Fig. 5). Sung et al., thus, concluded that NAPA was not uniformly effective for suppression of ventricular arrhythmias.[11] Recently, in a series of 15 patients with a history of sustained ventricular tachycardia, Somberg et al.[12] found that NAPA had a protection rate of 50 percent induction of ventricular tachycardia.

In this study, 15 patients with a history of cardiac arrest were evaluated using programmed electrical stimulation to determine antiarrhythmic efficacy. The arrhythmia induction was measured alone before and after intravenous NAPA 18 mg/kg given over 20 minutes. The mean left ventricular ejection fraction was 33 ± 6 percent.

Before NAPA was given, all patients had inducible ventricular

---

driven at a cycle length of 400 msec. Note development of 5:4 AV block below the level of the His bundle. This is preceded by prolongation of the His-Purkinje conduction time associated with progression of bundle-branch block–development of incomplete right bundle-branch block (second QRS complex), incomplete left bundle-branch block (third QRS complex), and complete left bundle-branch block (fourth QRS complex). C: Further progression of 3:2 and 2:1 AV block in the His-Purkinje system. In this illustration and in Figures 3 and 4, ECG leads I, II, and $V_1$ are simultaneously recorded with high right atrial (HRA) and His bundle electrographic (HBE) leads. S = stimulus; A = atrial electrogram; H = His bundle deflection. (From Sung RJ, Juma Z, Saksena S: Electrophysiologic properties and antiarrhythmic mechanisms of intravenous N-acetylprocainamide in patients with ventricular dysrhythmias. *Am Heart J* 105:811, 1983. By permission of the American Heart Association.)

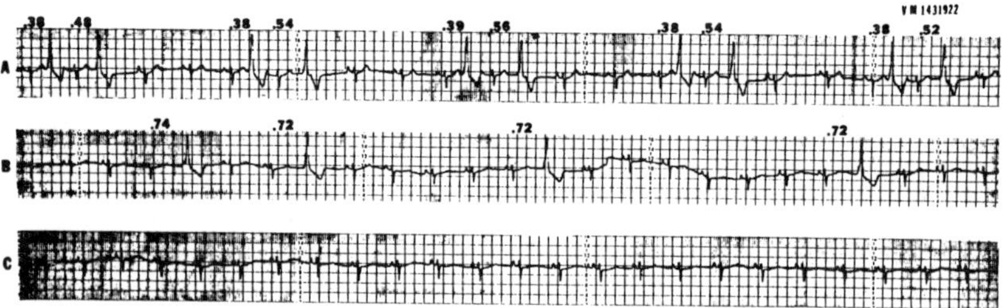

**Figure 3.** Suppression of ventricular premature beats with intravenous NAPA. A: Frequent ventricular premature beats before NAPA infusion. B: A decrease in the frequency of ventricular premature beats with marked lengthening of the ventricular premature coupling interval during NAPA infusion. C: Complete suppression of ventricular premature beats after NAPA infusion. Numerical numbers in Panels A and B are ventricular premature coupling intervals expressed in seconds. (From Sung RJ, Juma Z, Saksema S: Electrophysiologic properties and antiarrhythmic mechanisms of intravenous N-acetylprocainamide in patients with ventricular dysrhythmias. *Am Heart J* 105:811, 1983. By permission of the American Heart Association.)

tachycardia (VT). Eleven patients (73 percent) had nonsustained VT induced (12 to 30 seconds) and 4 patients (27 percent) had sustained VT that was terminated with defibrillation in two patients (13 percent) and pacing techniques in two (13 percent). Following NAPA, there was no significant change in mean arterial pressure, heart rate, PR interval, QRS duration, AH, or HV intervals. Ventricular tachycardia was reinduced in 9 patients (60 percent) at a slower mean rate of 233 beats/min ($p < 0.05$). As might be expected, NAPA prolonged the effective refractory period for the first extrastimulus from 235 to 286 msec ($p < .001$). The mean serum NAPA level in the protected groups was 15.7 $\pm$ 4 µg/ml.

In this series, 6 patients were discharged from the hospital on oral NAPA. Three did well with clinical or electrocardiographic (on Holter) recurrence of VT on long-term follow-up. These 3 had a mean NAPA level of 30 $\pm$ 12 µg/ml. One patient out of the 6 was dischanged from hospital by his primary care physician before NAPA levels could be determined; the patient expired 2 days later. Two of the remaining patients who were on NAPA had breakthrough VT on Holter monitoring and NAPA therapy was discontinued. The patients who continued to take NAPA had minor side effects, which included nausea and dizziness. Clearly, further systematic and controlled data are needed to define the role of NAPA in life-threatening ventricular arrhythmias.

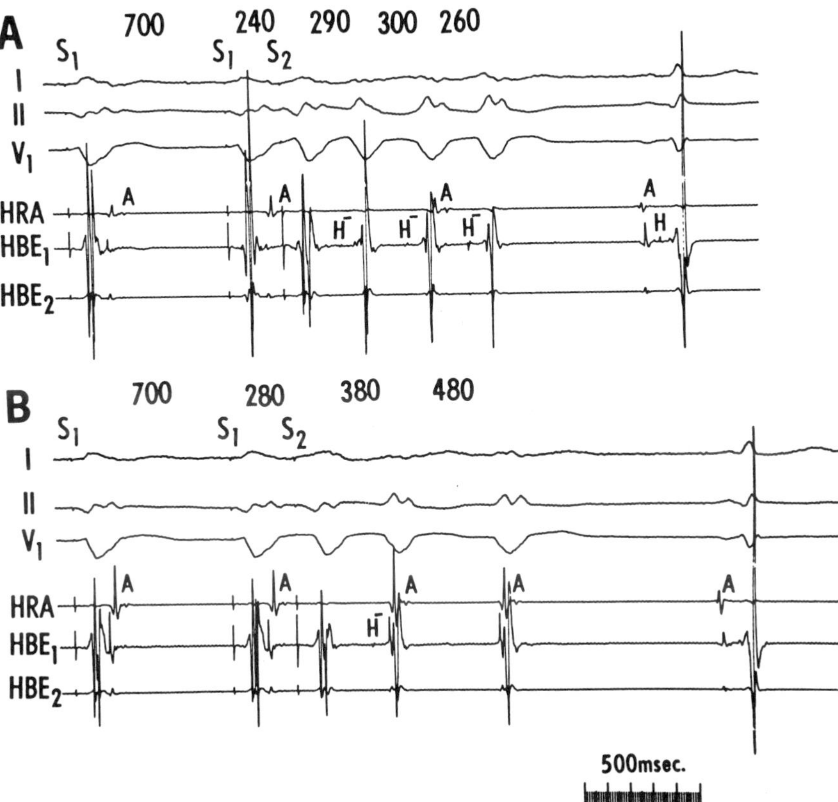



**Figure 4.** Effects of NAPA on repetitive ventricular response due to re-entry within the His-Purkinje system. A: Right ventricle is driven at a cycle length ($S_1$ to $S_1$) of 700 msec. A ventricular premature beat ($s_2$) with a premature coupling interval ($S_1$ to $S_2$) of 240 msec induces repetitive ventricular responses. The zone of repetitive ventricular responses ranges from ventricular premature coupling intervals ($S_1$ to $S_2$) of 220−240 msec. B: Following NAPA infusion, the right ventricle is driven at the same cycle length of 700 msec. The zone of repetitive ventricular response is shifted to the right and ranges from premature coupling intervals ($S_1$ to $S_2$) of 230−280 msec. Thus, the zone of repetitive ventricular response is widened from 20 to 50 msec. In addition, the cycle length of repetitive response is lengthened from between 260 and 300 msec (Panel A) to between 380 and 480 msec (Panel B) following NAPA infusion. (From Sung RJ, Juma Z, Saksena S: Electrophysiologic properties and antiarrhythmic mechanisms of intravenous N-acetylprocainamide in patients with ventricular dysrhythmias. *Am Heart J* 105:811, 1983. By permission of the American Heart Association.)

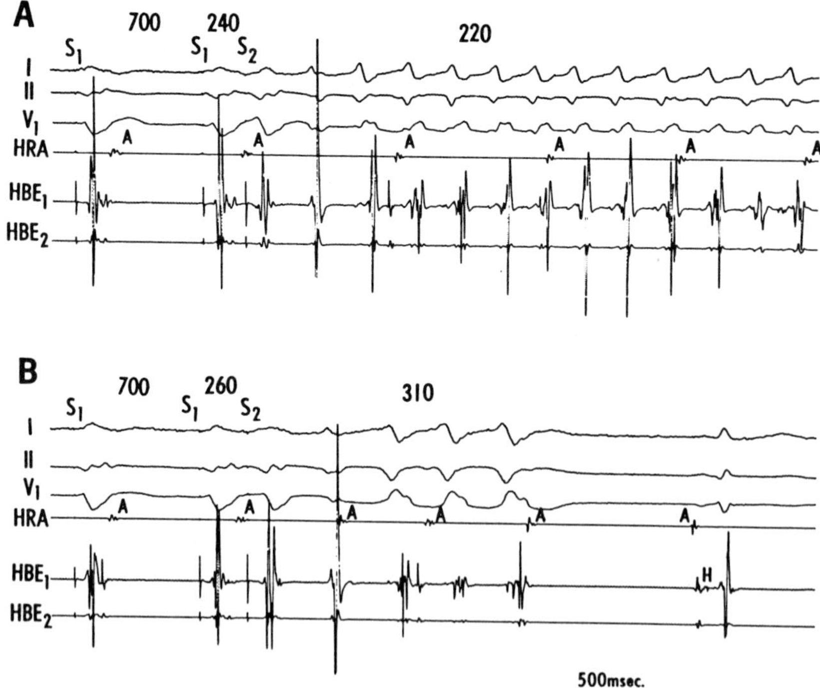

**Figure 5.** Suppression of induction of sustained ventricular tachycardia with intravenous NAPA. A: Before NAPA infusion, the right ventricle is driven at a cycle length ($S_1$ to $S_2$) of 700 msec. A ventricular premature beat ($S_2$) with premature coupling interval ($S_1$ to $S_2$) of 240 msec elicits a paroxysm of sustained ventricular tachycardia at a cycle length of 220 msec. B: After NAPA infusion, the right ventricle is driven at the same cycle length ($S_1$ to $S_2$) of 700 msec. A ventricular premature beat ($S_2$) elicits a short burst of nonsustained ventricular tachycardia at a cycle length of 310 msec. (From Sung RJ, Juma Z, Saksena A: Electrophysiologic properties and antiarrhythmic mechanism of intravenous N-acetylprocainamide in patients with ventricular dysrhythmias. *Am Heart J* 105:811, 1983. By permission of the American Heart Association.)

## Clinical Trials with NAPA

NAPA has been shown clinically to demonstrate antiarrhythmic efficacy when administered orally or intravenously.[13–17] Several studies have shown a decrease in ventricular ectopy in short-term NAPA therapy; but long-term assessment of the drug efficacy, in protection against ventricular tachycardia, ventricular fibrillation, or sudden death, remains to be investigated. NAPA prolongs atrial refractoriness and, thus, also may be useful in the treatment of atrial arrhythmias.

In a placebo-controlled, dose-ranging trial in 10 patients, 4 of whom had ventricular tachycardia, Atkinson et al. showed that oral NAPA effectively suppressed PVCs in 8 patients and caused a paradoxical increase in one.[13] Results were equivocal in the remaining patient. Klunger et al. studied 16 patients with ventricular arrhythmias and demonstrated that oral NAPA decreased the frequency of arrhythmias by greater than 75 percent in 9 patients with plasma levels of NAPA ranging from 10 to 24 mcg/ml.[14] Winkle and Jaillon[15] were able to achieve a 90 percent reduction in ventricular ectopy in only 2 of the 11 patients treated with oral NAPA. Redefining a *drug responder* as a 70 percent decreases in ectopy did not alter the overall results of the study. In 19 of 29 patients who had ventricular arrhythmias that initially were suppresssed by oral NAPA therapy, Kluger et al. found that only 6 patients had a persistent 70 percent reduction of PVCs over a 1−3 year follow-up period, and that 8 withdrawals were due either to death or recurrence of arrythmias.[14] They concluded that NAPA had limited long-term efficacy. Roden et al. studied 23 patients in an oral NAPA trial designed to test dose-response relation in a randomized crossover fashion.[17] All patients initially had chronic, high-frequency premature ventricular beats, with 11 of them having a history of ventricular tachycardia. Only 7 patients had a 70 percent reduction in frequency of ventricular ectopic activity during oral NAPA therapy. The plasma NAPA concentrations associated with efficacy ranged from 9.4 to 19.5 mcg/ml. The less-than-optimal results of these studies could be attributed to the fact that many of these patients previously had been refractory to other conventional antiarrhythmic agents.

The salient features of the data from the four studies mentioned are summarized in Table 1 and 2. The studies demonstrate that oral NAPA is effective in diminishing the frequency of ventricular premature beats and ventricular tachycardia in certain patients. In these studies, a 50 percent reduction in ventricular ectopic frequency occurred approximately one-half of the time, with a 70 percent reduction occurring one-third of the time. The range of plasma NAPA was 10−40 mcg/ml in these studies, with a mean plasma concentration of 20−35 mcg/ml. Most patients tolerated oral doses of 2−7 grams per day, and side effects frequently responded to a decrease in the daily dosage. True tachyphylaxis had

Table 1

Characteristics of Study Populations with PVCs Treated with
Oral NAPA

| | Atkinson et al.[13] | Kluger et al.[14] | Roden et al.[17] | Winkle and Jaillon[15] | Total |
|---|---|---|---|---|---|
| Men/Women | 9/0 | 14/3 | 14/9 | 9/2 | 46/14 |
| Age (mean $\pm$ SD) | 62 $\pm$ 10 | 58 $\pm$ 16 | 53 $\pm$ 11 | 58 $\pm$ 11 | 56 $\pm$ 11 |
| Weight (mean $\pm$ SD) | 80 $\pm$ 14 | 68 $\pm$ 17 | 73 $\pm$ 16 | — | 72 $\pm$ 16 |
| Initial mean AVC/min (mean $\pm$ SD) | 10.2 $\pm$ 9.3 | 5.9 $\pm$ 5.9 | 10.6 $\pm$ 7.7 | 7.1 $\pm$ 6.4 | 8.45 $\pm$ 7.3 |

Note: Based on studies form 60 patients in four centers in which the effects of NAPA on PVCs were investigated. PVCs = premature ventricular contractions.

Source: Adapted from Feld GK, Singh BN: Pharmocologic properties and therapeutic applications of NAPA. *Arrhythmia Clin* 1(3): 10, 1984.

Table 2

Effect of NAPA on PVC Suppression in Relation to Dose and Plasma–Drug Concentration

| | | Mean NAPA Dose (g/day) | Mean Plasma–NAPA Concentration ($\mu$/ml) | PVC supression | |
| Investigator | Number Patients | | | 50% or More | 75% or More |
|---|---|---|---|---|---|
| Atkinson et al.[13] | 10 | 6.4 | 21.03 | 6(60%) | 5(50%) |
| Kluger et al.[14] | 16 | 5.38 | 22.47 | 11(68%) | 9(56%) |
| Roden et al.[17] | 23 | 6.20 | 23.02 | 11(48%) | 8(35%) |
| Winkle and Jaillon[15] | 11 | 4.86 | 21.47 | 4(36%) | 2(18%) |
| Totals (mean $\pm$ SD) | 60 | 5.71 $\pm$ 0.72 | 22.01 $\pm$ 9.1 | 32(55 $\pm$ 19%) | 24(41 $\pm$ 18%) |

Note: Data based on effects in 60 patients with PVCs treated with oral NAPA.

Source: Feld GK, Singh BN: Parmocologic properties and therapeutic applications of NAPA. *Arrhythmia Clin* 1(3):10, 1984.

not been documented with NAPA therapy, although a substantial mortality due to arrhythmia recurrence did occur.

## Adverse Effects

Intravenous infusion of NAPA may cause mild nausea and transient hypotension.[10,11] Side effects of chronic oral NAPA therapy mainly are confined to the gastrointestinal tract and central nervous system. These include nausea, vomiting, diarrhea, constipation, anorexia, nonspecific stomach discomfort, dizziness, insomnia, nervousness, blurred vision, depression, and paresthesias.[14-17] Coombs' positive hemolytic anemia, allergic vasculitis, and agranulocystosis also have been reported. The incidence and nature of side effects in 60 patients involved in various clinical trials are shown in Table 3.

Polymorphic ventricular tachycardia (torsades de pointes) with and without ventricular fibrillation has been reported during NAPA therapy.[19-21] All cases were associated with QTC prolon-

Table 3
Side Effects Induced by N-Acetylprocainamide

| System | Adverse Reaction | Number of Patients |
|---|---|---|
| Central nervous system | Light headaches | 7 |
| | Dizziness | 5 |
| | Insomina | 5 |
| | Nervousness | 5 |
| | Blurred vision | 7 |
| | Tingling of extremities | 1 |
| | Depression | 1 |
| | Sleepiness | 1 |
| Gastrointestinal | Nausea | 16 |
| | Stomach discomfort | 5 |
| | Anorexia | 4 |
| | Diarrhea | 5 |
| | Vomiting | 4 |
| | Constipation | 1 |
| Cardiovascular | Increased PVCs | 2 |

Note: Data based on 60 patients.
Source: Adapted from Feld GK, Singh BN: Pharmocologic properties and therapeutic applications of NAPA. *Arrhythmia Clin* 1(3):10, 1984.

gation without electrolyte abnormalities, and the patients were treated with combinations of cardioversion, isoproterenol, lidocaine, right atrial pacing, and discontinuation of NAPA therapy. Polymorphic ventricular tachycardia without ventricular fibrillation occurred with NAPA levels of 29–32 mcg/ml and a procainamide level of 4.1 mcg/ml.[19] Torsades de pointes with degeneration to ventricular fibrillation was seen in 2 patients with plasma NAPA levels of 15.0 mcg/ml[19] and 32.8 mcg/ml.[21] This life-threatening complication appears to be related to either serum NAPA concentration or a proarrhythmic drug effect.

Development of ANA positivity while on NAPA therapy is uncommon,[13] and the reported incidence of NAPA-induced systemic lupus erythematosus is negligible. Most patients with active procainamide-induced systemic lupus erythematosus at the time of initiating NAPA therapy experience a resolution of symptoms.[16,17] Exacerbation of systemic lupus erythematosus in remission is uncommon and appears to be secondary to deacetylation of NAPA with return to the chemical structure of the parent compound.[9,16]

## Summary and Conclusions

NAPA possesses electrophysiologic properties that in part differ from those of procainamide. NAPA lengthens the QTC interval and prolongs atrial and myocardial refractoriness, but it has no effect on AV nodal and His-Purkinje conduction during sinus rhythm. Unlike procainamide, it does not prolong infranodal conduction or widen QRS duration. NAPA's antiarrhythmic mechanisms are similar to those of procainamide, especially in terms of effects on repolarization. NAPA suppresses ventricular premature beats and slows the rate of ventricular tachycardia, but clinical trials have shown that NAPA has a less-than-optimal success rate in controlling ventricular arrhythmias, and its efficacy against malignant ventricular arrhythmias for prevention of sudden death remains uncertain. A direct comparison of its antiarrhythmic effects with those of the parent compound have not been reported. The emerging experimental data suggest that NAPA may be effective in the conversion and prophylaxis of atrial flutter and fibrillation.

The side-effect profile of NAPA is similar to that of procainamide. The major difference is that drug-induced systemic lupus erythematosus occurs rarely, and NAPA can be used safely to treat patients with procainamide-induced systemic lupus erythematosus in the acute period. Deacetylation to the parent compound may be responsible for the negligible incidence of systemic lupus erythematosus as well as the recurrence of drug allergy to procainamide. Torsades de pointes, an acutely life-threatening complication related to $QT_c$ prolongation is uncommon but its precise incidence is not defined fully. The available data, although limited, suggest that further clinical evaluation of NAPA as a Class III antiarrhythmic compound merits consideration in ventricular as well as supraventricular arrhythmias.

# References


1. Dreyfuss J, Bigger JT Jr, Cohen AI, et al: Metabolism of procainamide in rhesus monkey and man. *Clin Pharmacol Ther* 13:366, 1972.
2. Elson J, Strong JM, Lee WK, et al: Antiarrhythmic potency of N-acetylprocainamide. *Clin Pharmacol Ther* 17:134, 1975.
3. Bagwell EE, Wall T, Drayer DE, et al: Correlation of the electrophysiological and antiarrhythmic properties of the N-acetyl metabolite of procainamide with plasma and tissue drug concentrations in the dog. *J Pharmacol Exp Ther* 197:38, 1976.
4. Minchin RF, Llett KF, Patterson JW: Antiarrhythmic potency of procainamide and N-aceprocainamide in rabbits. *Eur J Pharmacol* 47:51, 1978.
5. Jaillon P, Winkle RA: Electrophysiologic comparative study of procainamide and N-acetylprocainamide in anesthetized dogs: Concentration–response relationships. *Circulation* 60:1385, 1979.
6. Kluger J, Drayer DE, Reidenberg MM, et al: Acetylprocainamide therapy in patients with previous procainamide-induced lupus syndrome. *Ann Int Med* 95:18, 1981.
7. Dreyfuss J, Ross JJ Jr, Schreiber ED: Absorption, excretion, and biotransformation of procainamide-$C^{14}$ in the dog and rhesus monkey. *Arzneim Forsch* 21:948, 1971.
8. Dangman KH, Hoffman BF: In vivo and in vitro antiarrhythmic and arrhythmogenic effects of N-acetyl procainamide. *J Pharm Exp Ther* 217:815, 1981.
9. Amlie JP, Nesje OA, Frislid K, et al: Serum levels and electrophysiological effects of N-acetylprocainamide as compared with procainamide in the dog heart in situ. *Acta Pharmacol Toxical* 42:280, 1978.
10. Jaillon P, Rubenson D, Peters F, et al: Electrophysiologic effects of N-acetylprocainamide in human beings. *Am J Cardiol* 47:1134, 1981.
11. Sung RJ, Juma Z, Saksena S: Electrophysiologic properties and antiarrhythmic mechanisms of intravenous N-acetylprocainamide in patients with ventricular dysrhthmias. *Am Heart J* 105:811, 1983.
12. Somberg J, Wynn J, Miura D, et al: Antiarrhythmic actions of N-acetylprocainamide (NAPA) in patients with sustained ventricular tachycardia. *Angiology* 37:972, 1987.

13. Atkinson AJ, Lee WL, Quinn ML, et al: Dose-ranging trial of N-acetylprocainamide in patients with premature ventricular contractions. *Clin Pharmacol Ther* 21:575, 1977.
14. Kluger J, Drayer D, Reidenberg M, et al: The clinical pharmacology and antiarrhythmic efficacy of acetylprocainamide in patients with arrhythmias. *Am J Cardiol* 45:1250, 1980.
15. Winkle RA, Jaillon P: Clinical pharmacology and antiarrhythmic efficacy of N-acetylprocainamide. *Am J Cardiol* 47:123, 1981.
16. Kluger J, Leech S, Reidenberg MM, et al: Long term antiarrhythmic therapy with acetylprocainamide. *Am J Cardiol* 48:1124, 1981.
17. Roden DM, Reele SB, Higgins SB, et al: Antiarrhythmic efficacy, pharmacokinetics and safety of N-acetylprocainamide in human subjects: Comparison with procainamide. *Am J Cardiol* 46:463, 1980.
18. Feld GK, Singh BN: Pharmocologic properties and therapeutic applications of NAPA. *Arrhythmia Clin* 1(3):10, 1984.
19. Olshansky B, Martins J, Hunt S: N-acetylprocainamide causing torsades de pointes. *Am J Cardiol* 50:1439, 1982.
20. Chow MJ, Piergies AA, Bowsher DJ, et al: Torsades de pointes induced by N-acetylprocainamide. *J Am Coll Cardiol* 4:621, 1984.
21. Herre JM, Thompson JA: Polymorphic ventricular tachycardia and ventricular fibrillation due to N-acetyl procainamide. *Am J Cardiol* 55:227, 1985.

# Chapter 12

# Adrenergic Neurone-Blocking Drugs as Class III Antiarrhythmic Agents: Focus on Bretylium

Jeffrey L. Anderson

Although adrenergic neurone-blocking drugs initially were introduced as antihypertensive agents, in recent years they increasingly have been recognized for their antiarrhythmic and especially antifibrillatory properties. The relationship between their antiarrhythmic actions and their adrenergic neurone-blocking effects has not been elucidated completely. Members of this class also lengthen cardiac action potential duration, a Class III action.

Bretylium tosylate is the prototype of such adrenergic neurone-blocking drugs possessing antiarrhythmic activity.[1,2] Its quaternary ammonium structure is unique among antiarrhythmic compounds (Fig. 1). Its pharmacologic and electrophysiologic actions also are distinctive and complex. Bretylium was introduced for the treatment of hypertension in 1959, but soon became obsolete for this purpose, because it was erratically absorbed and patients developed tolerance to its antihypertensive effects.[3,4] By serendipity, Bacaner later noticed (1966) that bretylium possessed potent antifibrillatory activity in experimental cardiac preparations.[5] These observations led to bretylium's evaluation as an antiarrhythmic agent.[6] Acceptance of bretylium's unique therapeutic potential was gradual before marketing approval finally came in 1978.[7] Despite over 20 years of laboratory and clinical evaluation,

From: *Control of Cardiac Arrhythmias by Lengthening Repolarization*, edited by Bramah N. Singh, MD, Futura Publishing Company Inc., Mount Kisco, NY, © 1988.

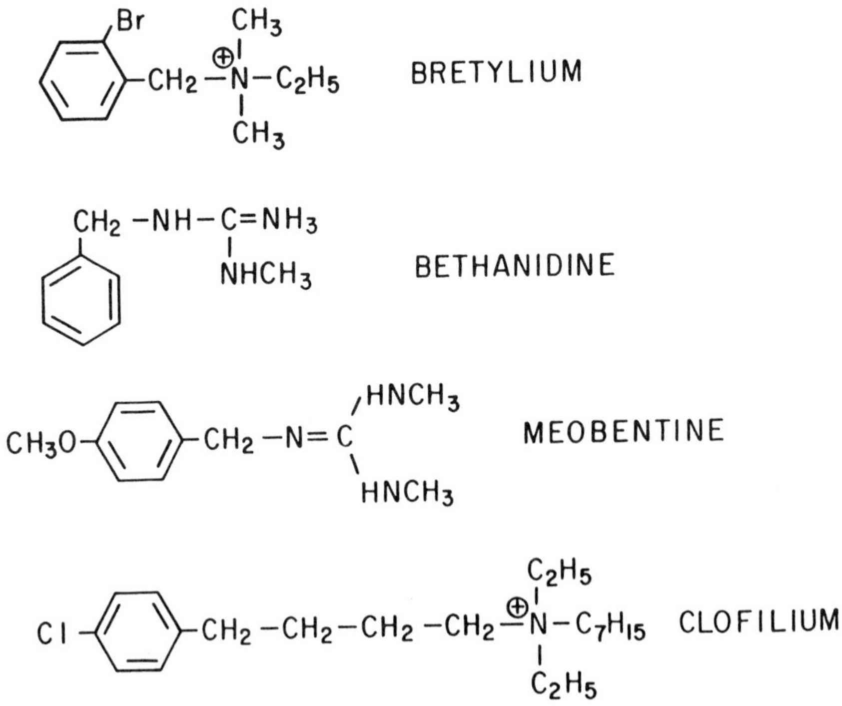

BRETYLIUM

BETHANIDINE

MEOBENTINE

CLOFILIUM

**Figure 1.** Chemical structure of bretylium and related compounds.

bretylium's antiarrhythmic mechanisms and its clinical role remain incompletely defined and continue to be debated. Bretylium is approved as a first-line agent in the prophylaxis and therapy of ventricular fibrillation.[8] It is indicated as a second-line agent in the treatment of other life-threatening arrhythmias, such as ventricular tachycardia.[8] This report updates previous reviews on bretylium,[9-12] emphasizing information from recent experimental and clinical studies, and comments on preliminary experience with related investigational agents such as bethanidine, meobentine, and clofilium (Figure 1).

## Bretylium's Properties as an Antiarrhythmic Agent

### Hemodynamic Effects

Intravenous injection of bretylium leads to a biphasic cardiovascular response in both animals and humans.[13-15] An initial release of norepinephrine from adrenergic nerve endings, accompanied by an increase in heart rate and arterial pressure, is followed within 15–30 minutes by reductions in vascular resistance, heart rate, and blood pressure, a manifestation of sympathetic neuronal blockade. These antiadrenergic effects usually predominate during chronic therapy. Competitive inhibition of acetylcholinesterase recently has been suggested as one potential mechanism for bretylium's induction of norepinephrine release.[16] The sympathetic ganglionic blockade caused by bretylium results from interference with the release of neurotransmitter stores in nerve terminals but not neurotransmitter depletion. Bretylium also prevents reuptake of norepinephrine, but has no effect on postganglionic adrenergic receptor function.[13,14] Ganglionic blockade may be associated with hypersensitivity to circulating catecholamines.

In an early hemodynamic study in patients with recent myocardial infarction, bretylium led to an initial rise in both systolic and diastolic blood pressures averaging 100 mmHg and heart rate averaging 24 beats/min.[15] Later, blood pressure declined 26/14 mmHg, and heart rate, 6–14 beats/min below control levels. No significant changes were observed in right atrial pulmonary artery and pulmonary capillary wedge pressures, cardiac index, stroke volume index, and stroke-work index. Adrenergic stimulant effects dominated at 5–10 minutes, after which ganglionic blockade become evident, with maximal effects occurring by 1 hour. Subsequent clinical experience has confirmed these conclusions.

The effects of bretylium on cardiac contractility are unlike those of other antiarrhythmic agents.[17,18] Early after drug administration, a positive inotropic effect is observed. This effect is due to norepinephrine release and can be abolished by beta-receptor blockade.[18] Later, contractility returns to control levels. This initial positive inotropic response may be viewed as therapeutically desirable[6] or not,[19] depending on the clinical circumstance.

A recent canine study raises concerns about potential deleterious effects of bretylium on hemodynamic recovery from ventricular fibrillation.[20] In anesthetized control animals, cardioversion after 1 minute of induced ventricular fibrillation was followed within 2 minutes by return of normal arterial pressure. However, after bretylium (10 mg/kg), cardioversion from ventricular fibrillation was accompanied at 2 minutes by electromechanical dissociation in 13 of 16 dogs. A stable blood pressure could not be restored in 6 of these animals, despite cardiopulmonary resuscitation and the administration of epinephrine and bicarbonate. Clofilium (discussed later), a related compound that does not cause sympathetic effects, did not alter hemodynamic recovery after cardioversion. The effects of bretylium on sympathetic nervous system function appeared to adversely affect the hemodynamic outcome after resuscitation from ventricular fibrillation. The revelance of these observations to the clinical setting is uncertain.

## Electrophysiology

The electrophysiologic actions of intravenously administered bretylium consist of indirect and direct effects that are complex and time dependent. Indirect effects result from early adrenergic stimulant and later antiadrenergic actions.[9] Direct effects are characterized by lengthening of action potential and refractory period duration.[1,2] The relative importance to bretylium's clinical activity of direct versus indirect effects has been difficult to assess. However, indirect (sympathetic) effects appear to be more important to its acute antifibrillatory effects; direct effects appear central to its chronic antiarrhythmic actions, but may contribute to its early effects.

The Vaughan Williams classification of antiarrhythmic drug action recognizes bretylium as the prototype of a distinct class of agents (Class III), based on its direct cellular electrophysiologic effects.[1,21] Bretylium does not affect membrance diastolic (resting) potential, rate or amplitude of membrance depolarization (phase 0), membrane responsiveness, or conduction velocity, distinguishing it from quinidinelike antiarrhythmics.[22] Spontaneous Purkinje fiber automaticity is unaffected by bretylium's direct action. In isolated canine Purkinje and ventricular muscle fibers, bretylium characteristically produces prolongation of the action potential and the effective refractory period without altering their relationship.[23,24] Bretylium also lengthens the action potential duration and refractory period in atrial tissue.[25] Prolongation affects primarily the plateau (phase 2) of the action potential.[23,24] These actions of bretylium do not depend on interactions with endogenous catecholamines.[18,23,24,26] This profile differs from that of traditional (Class I) antiarrhythmics, which cause an increase in the ratio of effective refractory period and action potential duration.[1,21,25]

Until recently, there has been little data regarding the question of which repolarizing currents mediate the lengthening of action potential duration induced by bretylium. Whereas Class I agents block sodium channel ionic conductance, it recently has been suggested that bretylium and related compounds may cause blockade of potassium channel conductance. Bacaner et al.[27] suggested that suppression of ventricular fibrillation by antiarrhythmic agents may correlate with their ability to block potassium channels in nerve and cardiac membranes. Bretylium, bethanidine, and meobentine were much more active than lidocaine and procainamide in blocking potassium channels. Potassium channel blockade appeared to take place on the outside of cardiac membranes. This action was postulated to cause an effective decrease in the electrical size of the heart, reducing the propensity to ventricular fibrillation.

Bretylium also differs from several other antiarrhythmics because of its consistent effects on action potential duration in both Purkinje and ventricular myofibers. In a comparative study, Varro et al.[28] found that all five Class I drugs tested (lidocaine, mexiletine, flecainide, disopyramide, quinidine) shortened the plateau phase of the action potential in Purkinje fibers, whereas bretylium and sotalol prolonged action potential duration. Prolongation was greater at longer cycle lengths. In ventricular muscle, Class I agents variably shortened (lidocaine, mexiletine) or lengthened (flecainide, disopyramide, quinidine) action potential duration. Bretylium and sotalol consistently lengthened the ventricular action potential (see also Chapter 3). Disparate effects on action potential duration in Purkinje versus ventricular muscle may be a potential cause of arrhythmogenic activity of some Class I agents (see Chapter 3).

In an alternative drug classification scheme[29] bretylium serves as a class prototype by virtue of its indirect, adrenergic neuronal activity, broadly analogous to Class II actions. Bretylium causes a transient increase in spontaneous Purkinje fiber automaticity within 10–15 minutes of drug administration, the result of sympathetic activity.[28] Depressed membrane responsiveness of Purkinje and ventricular muscle may transiently return toward normal (hyperpolarization) after bretylium, also as a result of initial release of endogenous norepinephrine.[28]

*Bretylium's Action in Hypoxic and Infarcted Myocardium.*

In order to elucidate the antiarrhythmic mechanism of action of bretylium, Cardinal and Sasyniuk[30] studied differential drug effects in normal versus infarcted regions of Purkinje tissue and ventricular muscle in canine endocardial preparations. Infarction prolonged the action potential in the surviving Purkinje network, leading to substantial disparity between normal and infarcted regions. As a result, slow conduction, unidirectional block, and reentrant behavior were observed in response to premature impulses propagating from normal to infarcted regions. Bretylium reduced this disparity in action potential duration by causing greater prolongation in normal than in infarcted tissue (Fig. 2). A more homogeneous electrophysiologic substrate resulted, minimizing the electrophysiologic conditions required for reentry. The maximal effects of bretylium were delayed for at least 1 hour, consistent with direct rather than indirect (adrenergic) actions.

Nishimura and Watanabe[31] have provided experimental evidence for a beneficial effect of the catecholamine release action of

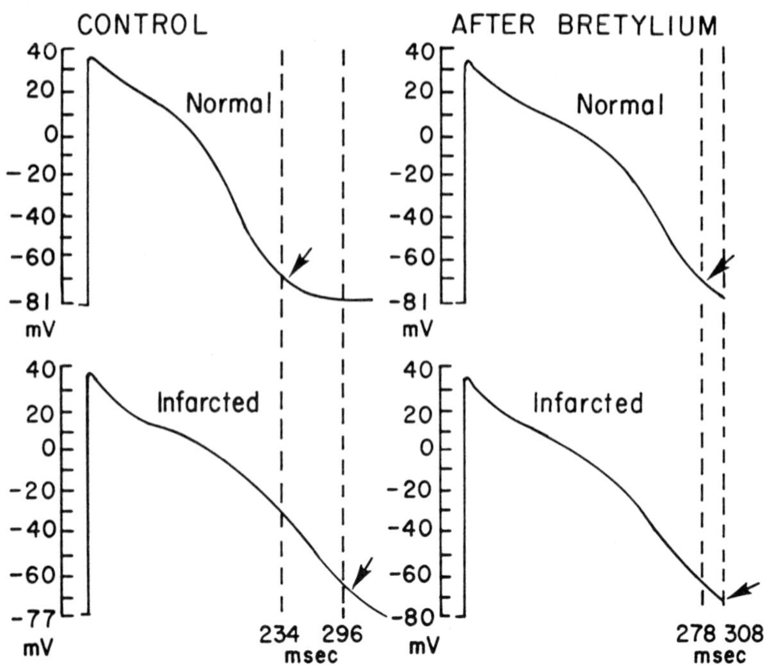



**Figure 2.** Relative duration of action potentials in normal and infarcted canine Purkinje fibers, before and after bretylium. (Adapted from data from Cardinal R, Sasyniuk BI: Electrophysiological effects of bretylium tosylate on subendocardial Purkinje fibers from infarcted canine hearts. *J Pharmacol Exp Ther* 204:159, 1978.)

bretylium in hypoxic mycardium. In normal canine Purkinje fibers, bretylium (20 mcg/ml) caused expected increases in action potential and effective refractory period durations without affecting membrane diastolic potential or rate of depolarization. In hypoxic fibers, bretylium antagonized the effects of hypoxia, which decreases action potential duration and amplitude, membrane diastolic potential, and rate of depolarization. However, hypoxic changes in Purkinje fibers pretreated with reserpine, which depletes endogenous catecholamines, were not reversed by bretylium, except that the action potential was prolonged. It was concluded that antiarrhythmic effects of bretylium in hypoxic, depressed myocardium probably are due to both (1) increased rate of membrane depolarization (with normalization of conduction velocity), caused by membrane hyperpolarization, a result of catecholamine release (an indirect effect of bretylium), and (2) prolongation of action potential duration and refractory period (a direct effect, since it occurred in reserpinized preparations).

The electrophysiologic effects of bretylium were evaluated in an intact canine model of coronary occlusion and reperfusion by Gibson et al.[32] Bretylium reduced the early decrease in ventricular refractory period caused by acute coronary occlusion and prevented the abrupt overshoot in refractory period which normally occurred upon reperfusion. The effects were more pronounced after chronic (24 hour) than acute (1 hour) bretylium therapy, consistent with a delayed, direct drug effect. Significant reperfusion arrhythmias also were prevented by chronic therapy. It was concluded that a reduction in the dispersion of cardiac refractory periods between normal and ischemic (occluded/reperfused) tissue may be an important mechanism of bretylium's antiarrhythmic action.

A decrease in the inhomogeneity of myocardial refractoriness also may be another antiarrhythmic effect of bretylium in certain other arrhythmia models. In canine hearts with quinidine-induced long QT intervals, bretylium was found to decrease the temporal dispersion of the effective refractory period in the right ventricle and to reverse the decrease in ventricular fibrillation threshold that accompanied high-dose quinidine administration.[33] Such an action is likely to be mediated by catecholamine release.

Bretylium lengthens action potential duration without depressing conduction time or excitability of normally occurring impulses in normal canine Purkinje and ventricular muscle.[34,35] The effects of bretylium on conduction of premature impulses during acute ischemia and reperfusion have been studied extensively by Fujimoto et al.[36] in an anesthetized dog model. Bretylium (10 mg/kg, then 2 mg/min) caused no significant change (compared with control) in the delayed conduction of premature impulses in ischemic muscle. However, it delayed premature impulse conduction in normal zones, thus lessening the disparity in conduction times between normal and ischemic heart. Conduction of these impulses from the normal zone across the ischemic zone border also was delayed. Moreover, increases in the excitability threshold induced by ischemia largely were prevented. These observations were viewed as supporting an antiarrhythmic role for bretylium in acute ischemia, based on its differential effects on conduction.

*Clinical Electrophysiologic Effects of Bretylium*

Studies on the electrophysiologic effects of bretylium in humans generally has been limited to observations within 30–90 min of administration.[37,38] They suggest that indirect (adrenergic) effects predominate early after administration. Anderson et al.[37] studied the electrophysiologic effects of bretylium (5 mg/kg/15 min, then 1.5 mg/min) in 10 patients undergoing cardiac catheterization or electrophysiologic study (Table I).[37] Prolongation of the ventricular refractory period, expected on the basis of bretylium's direct myocardial effects, did not occur during the 90-minute period of observation. Instead, a small but significant shortening was noted. Bretylium's indirect (adrenergic) effects thus may be of clinical importance, because therapeutic drug effects in the treatment of ventricular fibrillation typically occur within 10–15 minutes. Alternatively, early direct effects may be limited to diseased areas and not evident globally. Thus, the complexity of bretylium's observed electrophysiologic actions complicate the assessment of the mechanism(s) responsible for its clinical actions.

## Experimental Antiarrhythmic/Antifibrillatory Activity

## Effects on Ventricular Fibrillation Threshold

The observation by Bacaner and other early workers that bretylium reduces the propensity for experimental induction of ventricular fibrillation was the primary stimulus for development of the drug as an antiarrhythmic agent.[5,39–41] The increases in the electrical threshold for induction of ventricular fibrillation in both normal and ischemic myocardium after bretylium exceeded those

Table 1
Serial Electrophysiologic Effects of Bretylium in Ten Cardiac Patients

| Measurement | Control (0 min) | Bretylium[a] | |
| --- | --- | --- | --- |
| | | 15–30 min | 75–90 min |
| Heart rate (bpm) | 69 ± 11 | 83 ± 19[b] | 83 ± 13[b] |
| Corrected sinus node recovery time (msec) | 258 ± 105 | 269 ± 125 | 281 ± 84 |
| Effective refractory periods (msec) | | | |
|   Atrial | 260 ± 23 | 248 ± 23 | 239 ± 25 |
|   Atrioventricular nodal | ≤344 ± 85 | ≤342 ± 148 | ≤308 ± 70[c] |
|   Right ventricular | 262 ± 21 | 246 ± 22 | 249 ± 21[b] |
| Functional refractory period (msec) | | | |
|   Atrioventricular nodal | 450 ± 76 | 436 ± 133 | 419 ± 77[c] |
| Mean blood pressure (mmHg) | 94 ± 11 | 121 ± 16[b] | 101 ± 19 |

Note: The data shown are means ± SD. Changes in intracardiac intervals (PA, AH, and HV) and in surface ECG itnervals (PR, QRS, and QTc) were not significant.

[a]Dose was 5 mg/kg/15 min (loading), then 1.5 mg/min (maintenance). Serum bretylium concentrations averaged 1.5 ± 0.4 mcg/ml at 15 min and 1.3 ± 0.4 mcg/ml at 75 min.

[b]$p < 0.01$ vs control (paired t test).

[c]$p < 0.05$ vs control (paired t test).

Source: Adapted from Anderson JL, Brodine WN, Patterson E, et al: Electrophysiologic effects of bretylium in man. Correlation with plasma bretylium concentrations. *J. Cardiovasc Phamacol* 4:871, 1982.

after standard antiarrhythmic agents.[39] Guanethidine, another ganglionic blocker, had no effect on the fibrillation threshold. The unusual potential for bretylium to cause occasional chemical defibrillation when administered early after the onset of arrhythmias also was noted in some animal and clinical studies.[39,42,43]

The effects of bretylium on ventricular fibrillation threshold (VFT) are dose, time, and model dependent.[44,45] Increases in fibrillation threshold are observed more consistently and are of greater relative magnitude in studies using the stimulus-train[44,45] than the single extrastimulus method.[45] Anderson et al. determined the kinetics of the antifibrillatory effect of bretylium and correlated these with myocardial and serum concentrations of drug in an open-chest canine study.[44] Ventricular effective refractory period rose gradually after both low (2 mg/kg) and higher dose (6 mg/kg) injections to peak at 3 hours (12 percent increase) (Fig. 3). Substantial and prolonged increases in VF

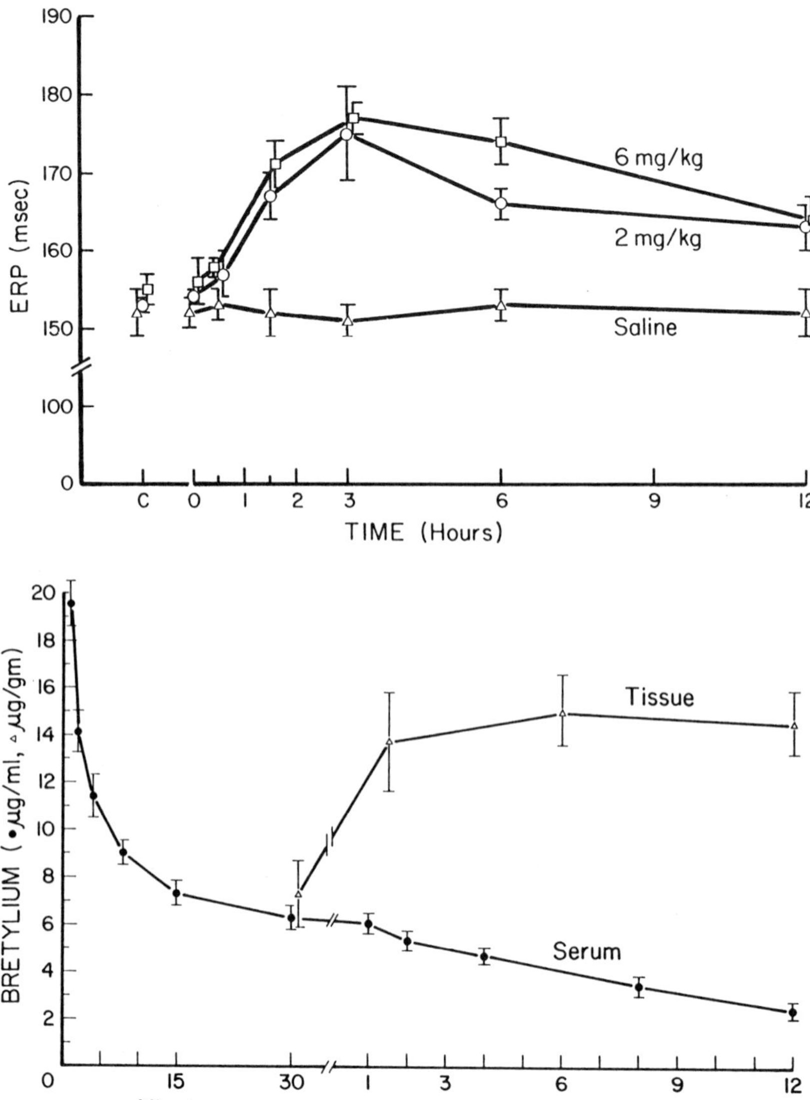



**Figure 3.** A: Temporal effects on ventricular effective refractory period of low (2 mg/kg) and higher (6 mg/kg) doses of breylium in dogs. B: Parallel temporal measurements of bretylium concentrations in serum and myocardium (after 6 mg/kg). (From Anderson JL, Patterson E, Conlon M, et al: Kinetics of antifibrillatory effects of bretylium: Correlation with myocardial drug concentrations. *Am J Cardiol* 46:583, 1980. By permission of the author and publisher.)

threshold were observed with both doses under both control conditions and transient regional ischemia (Fig. 4). Following low doses of drug, peak effect was delayed until 3 hours. Following higher drug doses, marked effects were evident within 2 minutes, although complete protection from VF induction during regional ischemia (to 50 mA current) was delayed until 1 hour and then persisted for 6–12 hours. Bretylium serum concentrations decreased rapidly after injection, whereas myocardial concentration increased gradually, peaking in parallel with antiarrhythmic effects between 1.5 and 6 hours.

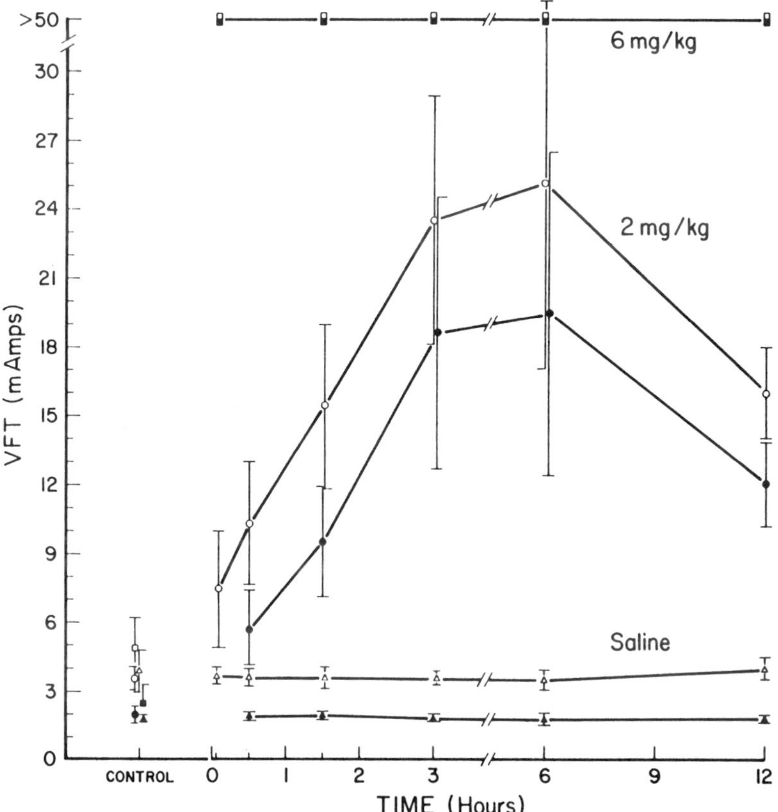


**Figure 4.** Temporal effects on ventricular fibrillation threshold (train method) of low (2 mg/kg) and higher (6 mg/kg) doses of bretylium in dogs. (From Anderson JL, Patterson E, Conlon M, et al: Kinetics of antifibrillatory effects of bretylium: Correlation with myocardial drug concentrations. *Am J Cardiol* 46:583, 1980. By permission of the author and publisher.)

Chow et al. compared the antifibrillatory effects of lidocaine and bretylium immediately after cardiopulmonary resuscitation.[46] Lidocaine in toxic doses (>6 mcg/ml) elevated VF threshold within 5 minutes, but effects were transient. Bretylium (5 mg/kg) elevated VF threshold more gradually (within 5–10 min), but effects persisted.

Frame and Wang[47] raised the issue of whether adrenergic neuronal interaction was important for the antifibrillatory effect of bretylium. In anesthetized, open-chest dogs, bretylium (5 mg/kg) caused rapid increases in VF thresholds, which peaked at 1 hour and persisted for over 3 hours. Complete adrenergic blockade was observed within 30 minutes. Increases in effective refractory period were small and variable. When the access of bretylium to adrenergic neurons was prevented by antagonism of the presynaptic amine transport pump with desipramine or chemical sympathectomy with 6-hydroxydopamine, the antifibrillatory effect was absent. When blockade of adrenergic neurotransmission by bretylium was reversed by d-amphetamine, VF threshold also decreased. Thus, interaction with adrenergic neurons appeared to be an important determinant in the elevation of VF threshold after bretylium.

Euler and Scanlon[45] observed a complete inhibition of sympathetic neuronal transmission within 15 min of 10 mg/kg bretylium in association with model-dependent elevations of VF threshold. They also interpreted their results as supporting an antiadrenergic mechanism of VF threshold effect. The demonstration that beta-blockers elevate VF threshold also has been considered as supportive evidence for an antiadrenergic basis for antifibrillatory effects early after bretylium administration.[45,48]

*Experimental Prophylactic Effects Against Ventricular Fibrillation and Tachycardia*

Patterson, et al.[49] have developed a canine model of sudden ischemic cardiac death (see Chapter 8) presenting many features of the clinical syndrome. In this model, acute ischemia is initiated by inducing a coronary thrombosis by electrocoagulation in conscious dogs with previous myocardial infarction in another coronary zone. Using this model, Holland et al.[50] found that ventricular fibrillation occurred in 9 of 10 saline-treated animals but only 4 of 10 animals treated chronically with bretylium (10 mg/kg every 12 hours for 4 doses) (p < .03) (Fig. 5). Amiodarone and beta-blockers but not Class I agents also are effective in this model.

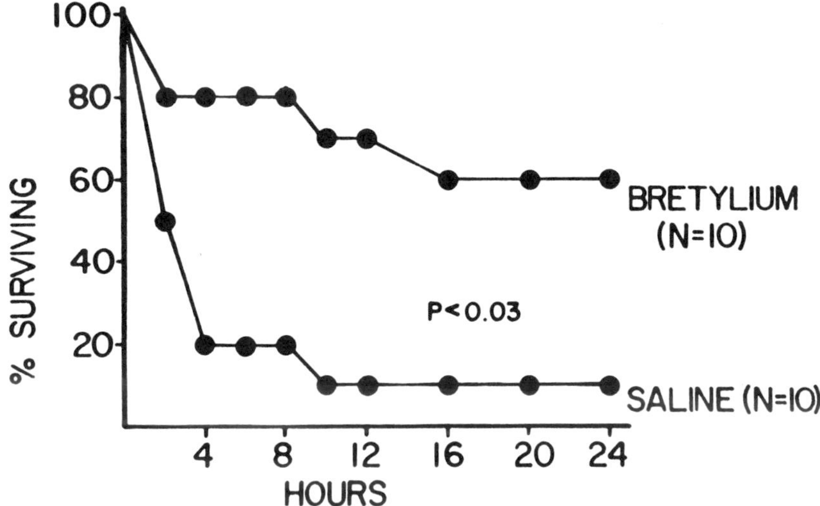


**Figure 5.**   Effect of bretylium on survival in a canine model of sudden coronary death (ischemic ventricular fibrillation). Cumulative survival is shown from time of initiation of thrombogenic electric current flow to intimal surface of left circumflex coronary artery for dogs treated with saline or bretylium (10 mg/kg every 12 hours: 4 prestudy doses). (From Holland K, Patterson E, Lucchesi BR: Prevention of ventricular fibrillation by bretylium in a conscious canine model of sudden coronary death. *Am J Cardiol* 105:711, 1983. By permission of the author and publisher.)

Wenger et al.[51] developed a method for quantitating antifibrillatory effects of drugs after coronary reperfusion in dogs using a logistic risk-regression analysis. Bretylium was shown to reduce the risk of VF during reperfusion estimated from the volume of ischemic mycardium.

The effect of bretylium on ventricular tachycardia induced by programmed electrical stimulation was investigated by Patterson et al.[52,53] in a chronic (3–14 day) infarction canine model (Fig. 6). In the control study, ventricular tachyarrhythmia (sustained or nonsustained) was consistently induced in all animals (14 of 14). Acute administration of bretylium led to little change or transient deterioration in spontaneous and electrically induced cardiac rhythms. Improvement in response was noted at 3 hours, however (7 of 12 animals protected), and response was augmented by propranolol administration (in 4 animals). Chronic bretylium infusions (3–4 days) consistently prevented VT induction (7 of 7). Vulnerability to arrhythmia recurred after bretylium washout (1–3 days). Thus, chronic but not acute therapy with bretylium was ef-

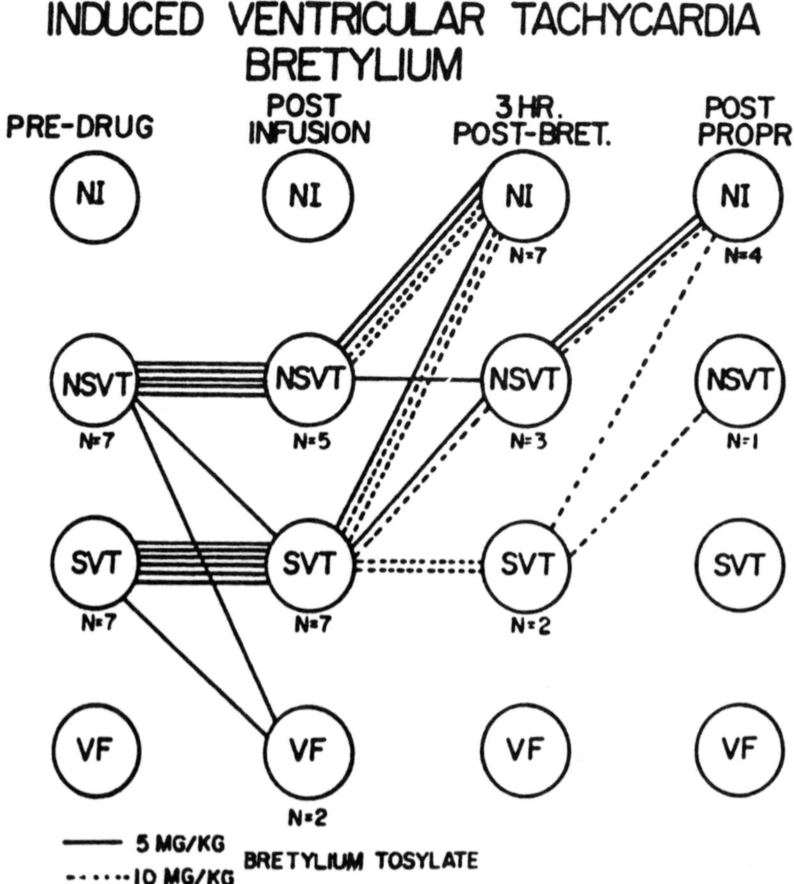



**Figure 6.** Incidence of induced ventricular arrhythmias by programmed electrical stimulation in postinfarction dogs treated with bretylium acutely and chronically. (From Patterson E, Gibson JK, Lucchesi BR: Post-myocardial infarction reentrant ventricular arrhythmias in conscious dogs: Suppression by bretylium tosylate. *J Pharmacol Exp Ther* 216:453, 1981. By permission of the author and publisher.)

fective for postinfarction VT. The slowly developing (direct) drug effect appeared to be beneficial, and the early, augmented sympathetic effect detrimental.

*Defibrillation Thresholds and Bretylium*

An early study suggested that bretylium, in contrast to standard antiarrhythmic agents, might lower rather than raise the energy requirement necessary for electrocardioversion from ventricular fibrillation.[54,55] However, subsequent studies have suggested little effect of bretylium on internal or external (transthoracic) defibrillation thresholds.[56-58]

## Bretylium Pharmacokinetics

The pharmacokinetics of bretylium have been relatively well studied only since its introduction into clinical therapeutics and after a sensitive gas chromatographic assay was developed.[59-61] However, plasma drug concentration measurements generally are not used in clinical practice.

## Canine Pharmacokinetics.

After intravenous injections of bretylium in open-chest and intact dogs, plasma or serum concentrations decrease rapidly in a biexponential fashion, whereas myocardial concentrations increase gradually, peaking between 1.5 and 6 hours[44] (Fig. 7). The ratio of myocardial to serum drug concentrations increases progressively, reaching about 12 by 6-12 hours. Thereafter, there is parallel elimination of drug from myocardial tissue and serum, with a terminal elimination half-life of 10.5 hours.

## Human Pharmacokinetics (also see Chapter 6)

Early studies of drug metabolism were limited by the absence of a sensitive drug assay.[62-64] However, they established that bretylium was eliminated primarily by urinary excretion of unchanged drug after intravenous administration and that oral drug was absorbed poorly. These early studies also suggested that plasma concentrations of about 1-1.5 mcg/ml were attained after intramuscular injections (4-5 mg/kg), and that elimination half-life was 5-10 hours or more.[63,64]

Using a sensitive gas chromatographic assay, Anderson et al.[65] determined the disposition of single intravenous and oral doses of bretylium in normal volunteers. Intravenous injection led to serum concentrations 10 times higher than oral administration (Fig. 8). Elimination kinetics followed a biexponential curve. Terminal elimination half-life was 13.6 hours after intravenous injections and 6 hours after oral dosing. Bretylium bound negligibly to

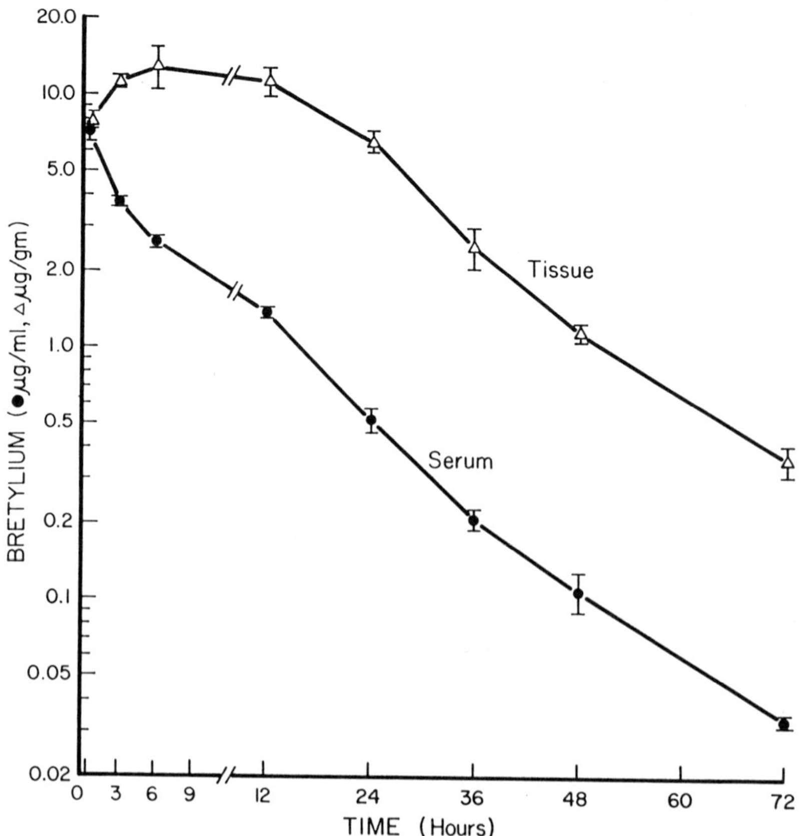


**Figure 7.** Accumulation of bretylium and its elimination kinetics in myocardial tissue and serum in intact dogs after bolus injection of 6 mg/kg. Myocardial tissue was obtained by pervenous endomyocardial biopsy. (From Anderson JL, Patterson E, Conlon M, et al: Kinetics of antifibrillatory effects of bretylium: Correlation with myocardial drug concentrations. *Am J Cardiol* 46:583, 1980. By permission of the author and publisher.)

plasma proteins and elimination was accounted for entirely by renal excretion.

Subsequently, bretylium disposition was determined in 7 cardiac patients with arrhythmia.[66] A comparison of results in patients and normal volunteers is presented in Table 2. Elimination half-life of a single intravenous dose was 13.5 hours, similar to that in normal subjects. Total body clearance was accounted for virtually completely by renal clearance, which averaged 397 ml/min.

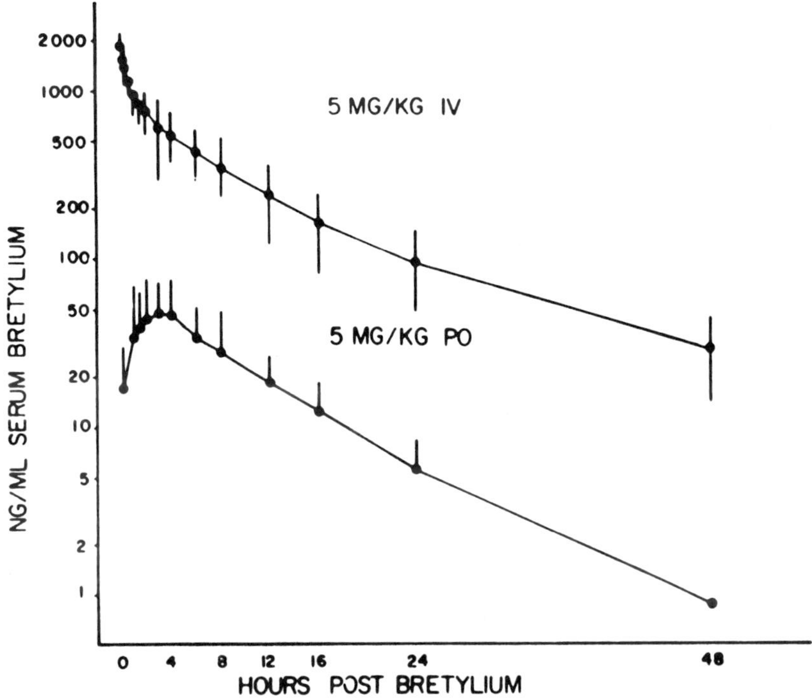


**Figure 8.** Serum concentration time curves for bretylium given intravenously and orally to normal subjects (means ± SD). From Anderson JL, Patterson E, Wagner JG, et al: Oral and intravenous bretylium disposition. *J Cardiovasc Pharmacol* 3:485, 1981. By permission of the author and publisher.)

## Table 2

### Pharmacokinetics of Single Intravenous Doses of Bretylium in Patients with Cardiac Arrhythmias (n = 7) and Normal Subjects (n = 10)

| Measurement | Patients | Normals |
|---|---|---|
| Area under curve, 0–24 hr | | |
| (mcg/ml × hr) | 5.69 (42.6) | 9.08 (34.5) |
| Amount excreted (mg), 0–24 hr | 128 (21.0) | 161 (12.0) |
| Renal clearance (ml/min) | 397 (41.7) | 300 (27.8) |
| Total body clearance (ml/min) | 428 (24.2) | 299 (31.9) |
| Creatinine clearance (ml/min) | 79.7 (13.3) | 112 (17.9) |
| Fraction of drug reaching | | |
| circulation | 0.98 (34.5) | 1.01 (8.7) |
| Elimination rate constant (hr$^{-1}$) | 0.052 (52.6) | 0.051 (12.8) |

Note: The data shown are means (coefficients of variation, in percentages) and are adapted from Anderson et al.[65,66]

Seven patients responding to intravenous drug were placed on oral bretylium in a mean dosage of 40 mg/kg/day. The mean steady state predose (trough) concentration of bretylium was 186 ng/ml during oral therapy, with a range of 72 to 461 ng/ml. Urinary bretylium excretion in 24 hours accounted for 18.3 percent (range, 9–31 percent) of administered drug, consistent with limited absorption. These findings demonstrate the difficulty by oral administration of achieving serum drug concentrations (i.e., about 1–2 mcg/ml or more) associated with therapeutic doses given intravenously. Investigational oral therapy with bretylium has generally been abandoned. The clinical pharmacology of bretylium is summarized in Table 3.

## Clinical Studies and Recommended Applications

## General Observations and Recommendations

Bretylium is considered to be a first-line agent for the treatment and prophylaxis of ventricular fibrillation,[7,8] especially after

Table 3
A Summary of Parameters of Clinical Pharmacology of Bretylium

| | |
|---|---|
| How supplied | 10 ml ampule, contains 500 mg bretylium tosylate in water (50 mg/ml) |
| Administration | Parenteral (IV preferred, or IM) |
| Therapeutic range of steady-state plasma concentrations | Uncertain (estimate: 0.5–3 mcg/ml) |
| Bioavailability (oral drug) | 20% (range, 10%–40%) |
| Total body clearance (ml/min/kg) | 4–6 (primarily renal clearance) |
| Volume of distribution at steady state (l/kg) | 2–5 |
| Elimination half-life mean, hours (range) | 13.5 (4–20) |
| Protein binding | <10% |
| Percent excreted unchanged in urine | 90–100% |
| Dosing (see text for details) | Loading: 5–10 mg/kg<br>Maintenance: 1–2 mg/min or 5–10 mg/kg every 6 hours |

Sources: Primarily from data in Anderson et al.[65,66]

myocardial infarction. It is also indicated for other life-threatening ventricular arrhythmias (i.e., ventricular tachycardia) that have not responded to lidocaine or other first-line agents. Bretylium cannot be recommended for the suppression of simple or frequent ventricular ectopy. It has not been tested or approved for use in acute supraventricular arrhythmias, although, like other drugs that prolong atrial refractoriness, it may slow the cycle length or terminate experimental atrial flutter.[67]

Bretylium has been subjected to clinical trials for serious ventricular arrhythmias associated with ischemic heart disease (both acute and chronic), valvular and primary myocardial heart disease, cardiac surgery, cardiopulmonary resuscitation, and delayed repolarization (prolonged QTU) syndromes. Bretylium has also been tested for prophylactic use in acute myocardial infarction.

Clinical reports on the use of bretylium span almost 20 years in several thousand patients, most with drug-refractory, life-threatening arrhythmia, and often as a last resort treatment for refractory ventricular fibrillation.[9,10] These essentially uncontrolled observations have suggested benefit in about 60–70 percent of patients,[10] but such studies lack parallel controls. The nature of malignant arrhythmias poses difficult practical and ethical problems to the design of scientifically controlled clinical studies.[10] As a result, the benefit of bretylium in the setting of cardiac arrest still lacks precise definition.

Clinical observations suggest that bretylium is much more effective against ventricular fibrillation (antifibrillatory effect) and acute prefibrillatory rhythms, such as runs of rapid (unstable) ventricular tachycardia, than against chronic (more stable) ventricular tachycardias or ventricular ectopy (antiarrhythmic effect).[68–82] In clinical practice, antifibrillatory effects occur quickly, but may require 10–15 minutes or more to develop fully.[69] Maximal antiarrhythmic effects may be delayed for several hours or more.[64,78]

## Early Studies in Postinfarction and Postoperative Arrhythmias

In his initial clinical study, Bacaner reported bretylium to be uniformly effective in 13 patients with ventricular fibrillation (VF, n = 9) or tachycardia (VT, n = 4).[6] Of note, in a subsequent study that included 37 patients with postinfarction arrhythmias, 7 patients experiencing 1–5 episodes of lidocaine-refractory ventricular fibrillation responded to bretylium.[79] Bretylium was effective in 7 of 10 patients with acute mycardial infarction with drug refractory VT or VF in the report of Terry et al.,[68] and 5 patients survived to discharge. Dhurandhar et al.[69] also treated refractory VF accompanying myocardial infarction with bretylium; 10 of 18 patients survived.

Bernstein and Koch-Weser[80] treated 30 patients with recurrent VF or VT (or both) refractory to standard therapy with bretylium. Ischemic heart disease was present in 28; 17 had acute myocardial infarction. Arrhythmias were successfully treated in 18 (60 percent) and partially suppressed in 5. Treatment with bretylium early after arrhythmia onset and without concomitant antiarrhythmic therapy favored a successful response.

Cohen et al.[81] used bretylium to treat 25 patients with resistant VT. Twenty had ischemic heart disease and 12, a recent infarction. Fourteen (56 percent) responded to bretylium and survived.

In the cardiac postoperative setting, Dhurandhar et al.[42] reported that bretylium allowed reversal of ventricular fibrillation in each of 9 patients coming off cardiopulmonary bypass. Six later died because of severe underlying cardiac dysfunction or cerebral ischemia. Castaneda and Bacaner[77] reported that bretylium appeared to prevent or suppress ventricular arrhythmias in 35 patients who underwent prosthetic valve surgery, but the significance of the results of such uncontrolled observations is uncertain.

## Studies of Bretylium for Cardiac Arrest (Ventricular Fibrillation)

Holder et al.[70] used bretylium in 27 consecutive cases of resistant ventricular fibrillation found in 330 consecutive cardiac arrests attended by the cardiac arrest team at a Canadian hospital. In each case, ventricular fibrillation had been sustained for at least 30 minutes and was resistant to multiple injections of lidocaine, electroversions, and injections of procainamide, propranolol, or phenytoin. Ventricular fibrillation could be terminated in 20 of the 27 patients by direct-current shock within 9–12 minutes of administration of bretylium. Twelve (44 percent) of these patients survived to discharge. These observations were dramatic but uncontrolled.

Nowak et al.[73] tested bretylium as first-line therapy for cardiopulmonary arrest in a randomized, double-blind study of 59 patients seen in the emergency ward. Among patients presenting with either ventricular fibrillation or asystole, survival was 35 percent in those treated initially with bretylium, compared with 6 percent in patients treated with conventional resuscitative measures (including lidocaine) plus placebo (p < 0.05).

In another report, Harrison and Amey[72] observed a signficant difference in outcome in those treated with bretylium earlier in the course of resuscitation using the American Heart Association Advanced Cardiac Life Support protocol (average, 14 min) than later (24 min) (p < 0.05).

In a Seattle Heartwatch study, Haynes et al.[71] compared clinical outcome of 146 patients experiencing ventricular fibrillation outside the hospital and treated initially with either bretylium or lidocaine in a randomized fashion. No significiant difference was observed between the two drugs in the percentage of patients converted to an organized rhythm (bretylium, 89 percent; lidocaine, 93 percent), the number of electrical defibrillations administered, and the time needed to establish an organized rhythm. The proportion of successfully resuscitated patients also was comparable (bretylium, 58 percent; lidocaine, 60 percent). Survival to hospital discharge was achieved in 35 percent (25 of 74) of bretylium-treated patients and 26 percent (19 of 72) of lidocaine patients (p = NS). Bretylium and lidocaine were concluded to be comparable as primary antiarrhythmic agents for the treatment of out-of-hospital ventricular fibrillation. Because the study of Haynes et al. did not have a placebo control group, it did not answer the question of net overall contribution of antiarrhythmic drug therapy to cardiopulmonary resuscitation of ventricular fibrillation.

Adult Advanced Cardiac Life Support recommendations have recently been revised (June 1986).[83] In this revision, lidocaine is now confirmed as the drug of choice in the management of ventricular fibrillation and tachycardia, based on studies (such as those mentioned) that indicate at least comparable efficacy and safety to other agents. Bretylium is recommended for ventricular fibrillation (and pulseless ventricular tachycardia) and for persistent arrhythmia despite lidocaine administration and repeated cardioversion.

Recent preliminary observations from the Seattle group raise questions about the role of antiarrhythmic drug therapy for persistent out-of-hospital ventricular fibrillation and emphasize repeated electrocardioversion.[84] Ventricular fibrillation that persisted after the first shock was encountered in 202 patients. These patients then were randomly selected to receive either lidocaine or epinephrine, and outcomes were compared. No significant advantages to lidocaine were observed, including proportions subsequently defibrillated, achieving an organized rhythm, successfully resuscitated (lidocaine group, 46 percent; epinephrine group, 49 percent), and eventually surviving (19 percent in each group). Moreover, higher survival rates were observed in a historical control group receiving only bicarbonate (29 percent) or no drugs between shocks (33 percent survival). Delay between shocks was the only detectable factor associated with a poorer outcome. Delays in initiating intravenous therapy were postulated to affect outcome adversely, and repeated shocks were considered to be the initial treatment of choice for persistent ventricular fibrillation.

## Bretylium and Suppression of VT at Programmed Electrical Stimulation

Suppression of the ability to induce chronically occurring ventricular tachycardia by programmed electrical stimulation during intracardiac electrophysiologic study has become an important prognostic test of the efficacy of antiarrhythmic agents.[85-87] In the canine chronic-infarct model, chronic but not acute administration of bretylium prevents induction of VT.[52,53] Reports of such tests of bretylium in humans are limited but are less positive.[37,88,89]

Bauernfeind et al.[88] repeated programmed stimulation early (30 min) after bretylium administration in 10 patients. Ventricular tachycardia could be reinduced in 9. Failure in part may have been due to an inadequate delay before retesting. However, Greene et al.[89] could reinduce VT (4 patients) or VF (1 patient) after bretylium had been infused continuously (average rate of 2.3 mg/min) for 4–9 days. Patients in both studies had failed to respond to multiple other agents (an average of 6.8 in the study of Greene et al.[89]).

This experience, although small, suggests that bretylium is not particularly effective in preventing induction by programmed stimulation of VT refractory to other agents. However, amiodarone, another Class III agent, has been reported to reduce the spontaneous development of VT and VF despite continued electrophysiologic inducibility of the arrhythmia.[90] Thus, the ideal test predictor for clinical effectiveness of antiarrhythmic drugs continues to be debated, especially for Class III agents.[87] Bretylium may be more antifibrillatory than antiarrhythmic.[91] Alternatively, it may display less direct electrophysiologic effect (prolongation of action potential and refractory period), which may be important in the treatment of induced VT in the clinical setting than the experimental setting.

## Torsades de Pointes Ventricular Tachycardia

This unusual ventricular arrhythmia is associated with heterogeneous, delayed repolarization and a prolonged QT interval and may be precipitated by quinidine or similar antiarrhythmic agents.[92,93] It may lead to syncope or sudden death. First-line treatment may include atrial or ventricular pacing, beta blockers, and lidocaine in addition to the discontinuation of the offending drug. Bretylium has also been tried in this setting[92,94,95] and has been successful in many but not all cases. Its potential efficacy in this setting may be related more to its propensity to release catecholamines than to its effect of prolonging the action potential duration. An electrophysiologic antagonism between quinidine and bretylium has been reported experimentally,[96] again related, in all probability, to the effect of bretylium-induced release of catecholamines.

Because bretylium protects the hypothermic ventricle with delayed repolarization from ventricular fibrillation experimentally, it may be worthy of a trial in clinical hypothermia.[97]

## Bretylium and Ventricular Ectopy

Bretylium generally is not indicated for suppression of isolated ventricular ectopic beats. Only a few studies, most older, with limited study design and methodology, have examined the antiectopic activity of the drug.[9,10] The limited data available indicates low ventricular antiectopic activity. In the study of Romhilt et al.,[64] the antiarrhythmic effects of bretylium were evaluated in 8 patients; a mean decrease in ectopy of at least 50 percent was observed in 5. Maximal ectopic suppression of approximately 60–70 percent occurred 9–12 hours after administration of 4 mg/kg intramuscular drug. No concurrent placebo controls were studied. Taylor et al.[74] observed no difference in ventricular ectopy in 38 patients receiving bretylium in the postinfarction period and in a similar number not so treated. Several other authors, though not presenting quantitative data, have reported no effects or only mild effects of bretylium on ventricular ectopic activity.

## Prophylactic Use in Myocardial Infarction

Loumanmäki et al.[98] compared prophylaxis with bretylium and lidocaine in 31 consecutive patients with acute infarction. Treatment groups did not differ in arrhythmia occurrence, although hypotension was a greater problem with bretylium. Taylor et al.[74] enrolled 101 patients with uncomplicated myocardial infarction in a controlled study of bretylium or no therapy. Differences in arrhythmia end-points were not significant. However, bretylium had to be withdrawn in 25 of 63 treated patients, primarily because of excessive hypotension.

Puddu et al.,[75] Torresani,[76] and others have reported a low mortality in a large but nonrandomized experience (1255 patients with acute infarctions). Among 412 patients treated with conventional antiarrhythmic drugs, there were 21 cases of primary VF (5 percent) versus only 11 cases (1.3 percent) in 843 patients who received low dose bretylium (10 mg/kg per 24 hours, infusioned for 5 days).

Unless results of much larger, randomized studies indicate otherwise, it is unlikely that bretylium will be accepted widely as prophylactic therapy in acute myocardial infarction, given the better tolerance of lidocaine.

## Adverse Effects and Contraindictions

The major adverse effects of bretylium are related to its modification of adrenergic function. Bretylium generally is free of other toxic effects. Initial catecholamine release may be associated with increases in heart rate and blood pressure, which are usually mild but variable.[14,60] A transient increase in ventricular ectopy may occur in 10–15 percent of patients,[80] and rarely, sustained ventricular tachycardia or fibrillation has appeared shortly after drug administration.[82] Other symptoms associated with catecholamine release include anxiety, excitement, flushing, substernal pressure, and headache. Angina pectoris occasionally may be precipitated. Concern has also been raised about the potential to extend ischemic damage.[19]

Hypotension often accompanies bretylium therapy and may begin within 15 minutes. Hypotension has required discontinuation of drug in about 10 percent of patients.[4,80,98] Because hypotension often is postural, patients should remain supine after administration of drug until blood pressure stabilizes. Supine hypotension is less pronounced but occurs to some degree in at least 50 percent of patients receiving bretylium. An asymptomatic fall in systolic pressure usually need not be treated unless it is severe (i.e., <80 mm Hg). In hypovolemic hypotensive patients, volume repletion is appropriate. Hypotension requiring treatment also may respond to vasopressors. Cautious dosing with pressors should be used because bretylium may induce catecholamine hypersensitivity. In patients with severely compromised cardiac function whose blood pressure is dependent on sympathetic stimulation for support, ominous hypotension may develop more frequently.[81,98] Bretylium probably should not be administered to patients with this degree of circulatory failure.

Protriptyline, a secondary amine antidepressant, may provide partial pharmacologic reversal of hypotension complicating bretylium therapy.[99] In patients with symptomatic hypotension requiring continued bretylium therapy, protriptyline has been given in dosages of 5–10 mg every 6–8 hours. The potential interaction of protriptyline with the antiarrhythmic action of bretylium should be studied further.[100]

Nausea or retching, which has been reported in about 10 percent of patients, usually is related to rapid intravenous injection (in < 8–10 min).

Diseases associated with a fixed cardiac output, such as severe aortic stenosis or pulmonary hypertension, may prevent compensation for the peripheral vasodilatation caused by bretylium.[8] In these conditions, bretylium should be avoided if possible and vasoconstrictor amines given, if needed, to support blood pressure.

Bretylium may accumulate in patients with renal failure, and appropriate modifications in dosage should be made. Intramuscular bretylium may cause irritation at injection sites. The safety of bretylium in children and during pregnancy has not been established.

In contrast to most antiarrhythmic agents, bretylium does not usually cause significant changes in electrocardiographic intervals[37] or precipitate of atrioventricular block.


## Drug Dosage and Administration

Bretylium is commercially supplied in 10 ml ampules containing 500 mg of bretylium tosylate in water for intravenous or intramuscular injection. On ampule thus contains a dose of 5–10 mg per kg weight for a typical patient.

## Initial Therapy

For ventricular fibrillation and hemodynamically unstable ventricular tachycardia, the minimum suggested initial dose is 5 mg/kg, which is given by rapid intravenous injection together with other usual resuscitative measure, including electrocardioversion before and after injection, if needed. If VF persists, the dose may be increased to 10 mg/kg and repeated, together with other resuscitative measures. There is comparatively little experience with total doses of more than 30 mg/kg, although higher doses have been used occasionally without apparent adverse effect.

For other ventricular, hemodynamically stable arrhythmias, bretylium is infused more gradually. One ampule of drug is diluted with a 5 percent dextrose or 0.9 percent sodium chloride solution to a volume ratio of at least 1:4, to a minimum of 50 ml. The diluted solution is infused to provide a total dose of 5−10 mg/kg of body weight over a period of a least 8 minutes, preferably 15 to 30 minutes, to prevent nausea and vomiting. The doses may be repeated at up to 1−2 hour intervals if arrhythmia persists.

## Maintenance therapy

After the initial dose of bretylium, a diluted solution (described earlier) may be administered as a constant infusion at a rate of 1−2 mg/min. Alternatively, a dose of 5−10 mg/kg may be infused slowly (over 15−30 min) every 6 hours.

## Intramuscular Therapy

Intravenous therapy is preferred whenever possible. If intramuscular therapy is necessary, an undiluted dose of 5−10 mg/kg may be given. Injection sites should be rotated and should avoid major nerve territories.

## **Related Investigational Antiarrhythmic Agents**

### Bethanidine

Bethanidine sulfate has a chemical structure (see Fig. 1) and pharmacologic properties that resemble those of bretylium but is better absorbed after oral administration, probably because it has an uncharged structure.[101] Bethanidine also is a potent sympathetic ganglionic blocker, causing prominent initial catecholamine release and subsequent hypotensive reactions. Bethanidine acutely elevates the ventricular fibrillation threshold in dogs. Its accumulation in myocardium after intravenous injection is rapid (within 15 min), in contrast to that of bretylium, resulting in tissue to plasma concentrations of about 50–100 to 1.[102]

Bacaner et al. awakened interest in the use of bethanidine as an orally effective analog of bretylium with a report of its antifibrillatory properties in dogs.[101] In a subsequent clinical study, 23 patients with ventricular arrhythmias refractory to standard agents (16 with VF) were treated with oral bethanidine.[103] Protriptyline (15–120 mg/d) was given concurrently to reduce hypotension caused by bethanidine. Ventricular arrhythmias were suppressed in 18 (78 percent) of the patients.

In an electrophysiologic study from the same group, Benditt et al.[104] treated 14 survivors of out of hospital cardiac arrest (primarily VF) not associated with myocardial infarction, who showed inducible arrhythmias at programmed electrical stimulation. Oral bethanidine was given in an initial dose of 16–20 mg/kg, with a supplemental dose of 10 mg/kg as needed. Inducible VT or VF was suppressed in 8 patients (57 percent), 6 of whom had presented with VF. Despite protriptyline, hypotension was often problematic. In another electrophysiologic study, Somberg et al.[105] and Wynn et al.[106] reported that intravenous bethanidine prevented VT induction in 8 (40 percent) of 20 patients.

Despite these early favorable reports, bethanidine generally was ineffective at programmed stimulation and was tolerated poorly in a recent multicenter trial in 56 patients with ventricular tachyarrhythmias.[107] In 59 trials of bethanidine administered acutely (20–30 mg/kg) or given for 24 hours, a successful result at programmed stimulation was observed in only 6 (11 percent) and a partial success in 3 (5 percent). Side effects were common, with symptomatic hypotension in 51 percent of trials, despite protriptyline. In another electrophysiologic study, bethanidine therapy was associated with little acute electrophysiologic activity, causing no significant changes in cardiac conduction or refractoriness.[108]

Recent experimental studies suggest differing electrophysiologic effects between bethanidine and bretylium. For example, Dangman and Miura[109] observed a decrease in the rate of membrane depolarization in canine ventricular and Purkinje fibers and a reduction in action potential duration in Purkinje fibers after bethanidine. An increase in Purkinje automaticity and abnormal automaticity was ascribed to catecholamine release. The effects of bethandine on the action potential resembled those of a Class I (lidocaine) rather than a Class III agent (bretylium). Unlike bretylium, bethanidine did not prevent sudden death in a conscious canine model of ischemic ventricular fibrillation in the study of Patterson et al.[110]

Because of these more recent experimental and clinical results, enthusiasm for developing bethanidine as an orally effective alternative to bretylium has waned.

## Meobentine

Meobentine sulfate is another compound related to bretylium.[111] Animal studies have led to differing conclusions regarding the degree of its antiarrhythmic/antifibrillatory activity.[111–113] In contrast to bretylium, meobentine is absorbed adequately when given orally and devoid of sympathetic ganglionic activity in animals.[111] Therefore, it was administered to 26 patients with serious ventricular arrhythmias (19 with sustained VT or VF) in a multicenter trial.[114] It was administered in two ways: by acute intravenous infusion (16 mg/kg over 90 min), and in multiple oral doses (400–1000 mg every 6 hours for at least 2 days). Meobentine was effective in 2 of 5 trials monitored by ambulatory recordings (>75 percent suppression of ectopy). Effectiveness was observed in 5 (22 percent) of 22 trials monitored by programmed electrical stimulation (suppression of induced VT). Partial efficacy was noted in 1, and 4 were not restudied because of recurrence of clinical arrhythmia or severe adverse effects. Meobentine caused increases in refractory periods of the right ventricle averaging 12 msec ($p < 0.05$), and right atrium of 33 msec ($p < 0.01$). Overall, only 3 patients (12 percent) were continued on drug for an extended period of time. Adverse experiences included hypotension in 50 percent (despite animal studies showing little antisympathetic activity) and gastrointestinal effects (nausea, vomiting, or diarrhea) in 56 percent (oral trials). These reactions often required dosage reduction (8 patients) or drug discontinuation (6 patients). Thus, clinical trials suggest modest efficacy of meobentine against chronic, severe ventricular arrhythmias in generally refractory patient groups and an unexpectedly high adverse effect potential.[114,115]

## Clofilium

Clofilium phosphate is a quaternary ammonium compound related to bretylium but devoid of sympathetic ganglionic effects.[116]

Initial experimental studies suggested it could prolong action potential duration and refractoriness without affecting conduction, characteristics of a Class III agent. Steinberg et al.[117] showed that in a canine 2-day myocardial infarct preparation, clofilium reduced the disparity in action potential duration between normal and infarcted Purkinje tissue (where it was prolonged) by lengthening action potential to a greater relative extent in normal tissue. Kowey et al.[118] compared the effects of clofilium and bretylium on dispersion of refractoriness and vulnerability to ventricular fibrillation in an ischemic feline cardiac model. Acute coronary occlusion reduced VF threshold by 73 percent, increased dispersion of refractoriness, and frequently resulted in spontaneous ventricular fibrillation. Bretylium increased refractory period and VF threshold and prevented occlusion-related dispersion in refractoriness. Spontaneous VF was prevented. Clofilium increased resting effective refractory period and VF threshold in low (0.5 mg/kg) and high (5 mg/kg) doses. High but not low-dose clofilium partially blunted the fall in VF threshold and increase in dispersion of refractoriness. Thus, Class III effects, consisting of increases in refractoriness and decreases in ischemia-related dispersion in refractoriness partially could explain reduced vulnerability to VF. However, sympathetic blockade (with bretylium) appeared requisite for full protection, since clofilium was less potent, even in high doses, than bretylium.

Limited data is available about the effects of clofilium in patients. Greene et al.[119] evaluated the effects of single doses of clofilium (60–300 mcg/kg) in 15 patients undergoing electrophysiologic testing for a variety of ventricular (n = 10) and supraventricular (n = 5) arrhythmias. No changes in blood pressure or heart rate were observed after clofilium, and no side effects occurred. Conduction times were not altered in atrium, AV node, His-Purkinje tissue, and ventricle. Class III effect was evidenced by lengthening of QT interval and atrial and ventricular effective refractory periods. Inducible supraventricular arrhythmias were improved in 4 of 4 patients, and ventricular arrhythmias in 5 of 9 patients.

Thus, clofilium appears to be less active than bretylium for reducing vulnerability to ischemia-related VF but shows promise in treating chronic, reentrant atrial and ventricular arrhythmias. Clinical experience, however, is extremely limited. Nonetheless, clofilium appears to be well tolerated and devoid of the sympathetic ganglionic side effects of bretylium. Unfortunately, quaternary ammonium compounds generally are absorbed poorly, which may limit clofilium's utility.

## Conclusion

Bretylium tosylate, the first clinically approved Class III antiarrhythmic agent, is a unique quaternary ammonium compound with prominent ventricular antifibrillatory activity. Proportionate lengthening of Purkinje fiber and ventricular muscle action potential and refractory period are the electrophysiologic hallmarks of its Class III effect. Intravenous administration of bretylium leads to a biphasic hemodynamic response resulting from initial norepinephrine release from adrenergic nerve terminals followed by sympathetic ganglionic blockade. Initial electrophysiologic effects also reflect (indirect) sympathetic interactions, whereas those related to direct activity may develop more gradually. Electrocardiographic intervals usually are unchanged after bretylium, and cardiac conduction is unchanged. Bretylium is eliminated unchanged by renal excretion, with a terminal half-life of about 13 hours. In several animal models and clinical circumstances, it shows substantial activity against ventricular fibrillation, including instances where therapy with standard (Class I) agents has failed. Bretylium has only weak activity against isolated ventricular ectopy. The exact mechanisms of bretylium's clinical actions, whether indirect (sympathetic neuronal) or direct (Class III), continue to be debated. Indirect actions may be more prominent with initial, and direct actions with delayed, effects. Bretylium has been approved as a first-line agent for prophylaxis and treatment of ventricular fibrillation, and as a second-line agent for other life-threatening ventricular tachyarrhythmias. Hemodynamic changes (e.g., hypotension) are the most commonly observed adverse reactions. Nausea may result from rapid administration. Bethanidine, meobentine, and clofilium are related compounds that have undergone testing. The role of these related agents in future arrhythmia management is uncertain, but bretylium will continue to serve as a prototype for future drug development.

## References

1. Lucchesi BR, Patterson ES: Antiarrhythmic drugs. In M Antonaccio (ed): *Cardiovascular Pharmacology* 2d ed. New York, Raven Press, 1984, p. 329.

2. Patterson E, Lucchesi BR: Bretylium: A prototype for future development of antidysrhythmic agents. *Am Heart J* 106:426, 1983.
3. Boura ALA, Green AF, McCoubrey A, et al: Darenthin: Hypotensive agent of a new type. *Lancet* 1:17, 1959.
4. Dollery CT, Emslie-Smith D, McMichael J: Bretylium tosylate in the treatment of hypertension. *Lancet* 2:296, 1960.
5. Bacaner MB: Bretylium tosylate for suppression of induced ventricular fibrillation. *Am J Cardiol* 17:528, 1966.
6. Bacaner MB: Treatment of ventricular fibrillation and other acute arrhythmias with bretylium tosylate. *Am J Cardiol* 21:530, 1968.
7. Bretylium (Bretylol) for ventricular arrhythmias. (editorial review). *Med Lett* 20:105, 1978.
8. Product information: Bretylol® (bretylium tosylate) injection. McGaw Park, Ill.: American Critical Care, 1980.
9. Heissenbuttel RH, Bigger JT: Bretylium tosylate: A newly available antiarrhythmic drug for ventricular arrhythmias. *Ann Intern Med* 91:229, 1979.
10. Koch-Weser J: Drug therapy. Bretylium. *N Eng J Med* 300:473, 1979.
11. Anderson JL: Bretylium: An update on pharmacologic studies and clinical uses. In E Rapaport (ed): *Cardiology Update. Reviews for Physicians, 1983.* New York, Elsevier Biomedical, 1983, p 241.
12. Anderson JL: Bretylium tosylate: Profile of the only available Class III antiarrhythmic agent. *Clin Ther* 7:205, 1985.
13. Boura ALA, Green AF: The actions of bretylium: Adrenergic neurone blocking and other effects. *Br J Pharmacol* 14:536, 1959.
14. Gokhale SD, Gulati OD, Kelkar VV: Mechanism of the initial adrenergic effects of bretylium and guanethidine. *Br. J Pharmacol* 20:362, 1963.
15. Chatterjee K, Mandel WJ, Vyden JK, et al: Cardiovascular effects of bretylium tosylate in acute myocardial infarction. *JAMA* 223:757, 1973.
16. Schreiber G, Sokolovsky M: Competitive inhibition of acetylcholinesterase by bretylium: possible mechanism for its induction of norepinephrine release. *J Cardiovasc Pharmacol* 7:1065, 1985.
17. Hammermeister KE, Boerth RC, Warbasse JR: The comparative inotropic effects of six clinically used antiarrhythmic agents. *Am Heart J* 84:643, 1972.
18. Markis JE, Koch-Weser J: Characteristics and mechanism of inotropic and chronotropic actions of bretylium tosylate. *J Pharmacol Exp Ther* 178:94, 1971.
19. Maroko PR, Kjekshus JK, Sobel BE, et al: Factors influencing infarct size following experimental coronary artery occlusions. *Circulation* 43:67, 1971.
20. Euler DE, Zeman TW, Wallock ME, et al: Deleterious effects of bretylium on hemodynamic recovery from ventricular fibrillation. *Am Heart J* 112:25, 1986.
21. Vaughan Williams EM: A classification of antiarrhythmic actions reassessed after a decade of new drugs. *J Clin Pharmacol* 24:129, 1984.
22. Papp, JG, Vaughan Williams EM: The effect on intracellular atrial

potentials of bretylium in relation to its local anaesthetic potency. *Br J Pharmacol* 35:352P, 1969.

23. Bigger JT Jr, Jaffe CC: The effect of bretylium tosylate on the electrophysiologic properties of ventricular muscle and Purkinje fibers. *Am J Cardiol* 27:82, 1971.

24. Wit AL, Steiner C, Damato AN: Electrophysiologic effects of bretylium tosylate on single fibers of the canine specialized conducting system and ventricle. *J Pharmacol Exp Ther* 173:344, 1970.

25. Mirro MJ, Webel RR, Kelly DJ, et al: Electrophysiologic properties of bretylium tosylate on atrial myocardium. *J Cardiovasc Pharmacol* 3:1312, 1981.

26. Namm DH, Wang CM, Sayad S, et al. Effects of bretylium on rat cardiac muscle: The electrophysiological effects and its uptake binding in normal and immunosympathectomized rat hearts. *J Pharmacol Exp Ther* 193:194, 1974.

27. Bacaner MB, Clay JR, Shrier A, et al: Potassium channel blockade: A mechanism for suppressing ventricular fibrillation. *Proc Natl Acad Sci USA* 83:2223, 1986.

28. Varro A, Nakaya Y, Elharrar V, et al: Effect of antiarrhythmic drugs on the cycle length-dependent action potential duration in dog Purkinje and ventricular muscle fibers. *J Cardiovasc Pharmacol* 8:178, 1986.

29. Goldberger AL, Curtis GP: An "automatic" classification of antiarrhythmic drugs. *J Electrocardiol* 15:397, 1982.

30. Cardinal R, Sasyniuk BI: Electrophysiological effects of bretylium tosylate on subendocardial Purkinje fibers from infarcted canine hearts. *J Pharmacol Exp Ther* 204:159, 1978.

31. Nishimura M, Watanabe Y: Membrane action and catecholamine release action of bretylium tosylate in normoxic and hypoxic canine Purkinje fibers. *J Am Coll Cardiol* 2:287, 1983.

32. Gibson JK, Steward JR, Li Y-P, et al: Electrophysiologic effects of bretylium tosylate on the canine heart during coronary artery occlusion and reperfusion. *J Cardiovasc Pharmacol* 5:517, 1983.

33. Inoue H, Toda I, Nozaki A, et al: Effects of bretylium tosylate on inhomogeneity of refractoriness and ventricular fibrillation threshold in canine heart with quinidine-induced long QT interval. *Cardiovasc Res* 19:655, 1985.

34. Cervoni P, Ellis CH, Maxwell RA: The antiarrhythmic action of bretylium in normal, reserpine-pretreated and chronically denervated dog hearts. *Arch Int Pharmacodyn Ther* 190:91, 1971.

35. Waxman MB, Wallace AG: Electrophysiologic mechanisms of bretylium tosylate on the heart. *J Pharmacol Exp Ther* 183:264, 1972.

36. Fujimoto T, Hamamoto H, Peter T, et al: Electrophysiologic effects of bretylium on canine ventricular muscle during acute ischemia and reperfusion. *Am Heart J* 105:966, 1983.

37. Anderson JL, Brodine WN, Patterson E, et al: Electrophysiologic effects of bretylium in man. Correlation with plasma bretylium concentrations. *J Cardiolvasc Pharmacol* 4:871, 1982.

38. Touboul P, Porte J, Huerta F, et al: Etude des proprietes electrophysiologiques du tosylate de bretylium chez l'homme. *Arch Mal Coeur Vaiss* 69:503, 1976.

39. Bacaner MB: Quantitative comparison of bretylium with other anti-fibrillatory drugs. *Am J Cardiol* 21:504, 1968.
40. Bacaner MB, Schrienemachers D: Bretylium tosylate for suppression of ventricular fibrillation after experimental myocardial infarction. *Nature* 220:494, 1968.
41. Kniffen FJ, Lomas TE, Counsell RE, et al: The antiarrhythmic and antifibrillatory actions of bretylium and its o-iodobenzyl trimethyl ammonium analog, UM 360. *J Pharmacol Exp Ther* 192:120, 1975.
42. Dhurandhar RW, Teasdale SJ, Mahon WA: Bretylium tosylate in the management of refractory ventricular fibrillation. *Can Med Assoc J* 105:161, 1971.
43. Sanna G, Archidiacono R: Chemical ventricular defibrillation of the human heart with bretylium tosylate. *Am J Cardiol* 32:982, 1973.
44. Anderson JL, Patterson E, Conlon M, et al: Kinetics of antifibrilla-tory effects of bretylium: Correlation with myocardial drug concentra-tions. *Am J Cardiol* 46:583, 1980.
45. Euler DE, Scanlon PJ: Mechanism of the effect of bretylium on the ventricular fibrillation threshold in dogs. *Am J Cardiol* 55:1396, 1985.
46. Chow MS, Kluger J, DiPersio DM, et al: Antifibrillatory effects of lidocaine and bretylium immediately postcardiopulmonary resuscita-tion. *Am Heart J* 110:938, 1985.
47. Frame VB, Wang HH: Importance of interaction with adrenergic neurons for antifibrillatory action of bretylium in the dog. *J Cardiov-asc Pharmacol* 8:336, 1986.
48. Anderson JL, Rodier HE, Green LS: Comparative effects of beta-adrenergic blocking drugs on experimental ventricular fibrillation threshold *Am J Cardiol* 51:1196, 1983.
49. Patterson E, Holland K, Eller BT, et al: Ventricular fibrillation re-sulting from ischemia at a site remote from previous myocardial in-farction. A conscious canine model of sudden coronary death. *Am J Cardiol* 50:1414, 1982.
50. Holland K, Patterson E, Lucchesi BR: Prevention of ventricular fi-brillation by bretylium in a conscious canine model of sudden coro-nary death. *Am Heart J* 105:711, 1983.
51. Wenger TL, Lederman L, Starmer CF, et al: A method for quantitat-ing antifibrillatory effects of drugs after coronary reperfusion in dogs: Improved outcome with bretylium. *Circulation* 69:142, 1984.
52. Patterson E, Gibson JK, Lucchesi BR: Prevention of chronic canine ventricular tachyarrhythmias with bretylium tosylate. *Circulation* 64:1045, 1981.
53. Patterson E, Gibson JK, Lucchesi BR: Postmyocardial infarction re-entrant ventricular arrhythmias in conscious dogs: Suppression by bretylium tosylate. *J Pharmacol Exp Ther* 216:453, 1981.
54. Babbs DF, Yim GKW, Whistler SJ, et al: Elevation of ventricular defibrillation threshold in dogs by antiarrhythmic drugs. *Am Heart J* 98:345, 1979.
55. Tacker WA, Niebauer MJ, Babbs CF, et al: The effect of newer anti-arrhythmic drugs on defibrillation threshold *Crit Care Med* 8:177, 1980.
56. Koo CC, Allen JD, Pantridge JF: Lack of effect of bretylium tosylate

on electrical ventricular defibrillation in a controlled study. *Cardiovasc Res* 18:762, 1984.

57. Kerber RE, Pandian NG, Jensen SR, et al: Effect of lidocaine and bretylium on energy requirements for transthoracic defibrillation: Experimental studies. *J Am Coll Cardiol* 7:397, 1986.

58. Dorian P, Fain ES, Davy JM, et al: Effect of quinidine and bretylium on defibrillation energy requirements. *Am Heart J* 112:19, 1986.

59. Patterson E, Stetson P, Lucchesi BR: Sensitive gas chromatographic assay for the quantitation of bretylium in plasma, urine, and myocardial tissue. *J Chromatog* 181:33, 1980.

60. Lai CM, Kamath BL, Carter JE, et al: GLC determination of bretylium in biological fluids. *J Pharm Sci* 69:681, 1980.

61. Narang PK, Adir J, Josselson J, et al: Pharmacokinetics of bretylium in man after intravenous administration. *J Pharmacokinet Biopharm* 8:363, 1980.

62. Duncombe WG, McCoubrey A: The excretion and stability to metabolism of bretylium. *Br J Pharmacol* 15:260, 1960.

63. Kuntzman R, Tsai I, Chang R, et al: Disposition of bretylium in man and rat. *Clin Pharmacol Ther* 5:829, 1970.

64. Romhilt DW, Bloomfield SS, Lipicky RJ, et al: Evaluation of bretylium tosylate for the treatment of premature ventricular contractions. *Circulation* 45:800, 1972.

65. Anderson JL, Patterson E, Wagner JG, et al: Oral and intravenous bretylium disposition. *Clin Pharmacol Ther* 28:468, 1980.

66. Anderson JL, Patterson E, Wagner JG, et al: Clinical pharmacokinetics of intravenous and oral bretylium tosylate in survivors of ventricular tachycardia or fibrillation. *J Cardiovasc Pharmacol* 3:485, 1981.

67. Boyden PA: Effects of pharmacologic agents on induced atrial flutter in dogs with right atrial enlargement. *J Cardiovasc Pharmacol* 8:170, 1986.

68. Terry G, Vellani CW, Higgins MR, et al: Bretylium tosylate in the treatment of refractory ventricular arrhythmias complicating myocardial infarction. *Br Heart J* 32:21, 1970.

69. Dhurandhar RW, Pickron J, Goldman AM: Bretylium tosylate in the management of recurrent ventricular fibrillation complicating acute myocardial infarction. *Heart Lung* 9:265, 1980.

70. Holder DA, Sniderman AD, Fraser G, et al: Experience with bretylium tosylate by a hospital cardiac arrest team. *Circulation* 55:541, 1966.

71. Haynes RE, Chinn RL, Copass MK, et al: Comparison of bretylium tosylate and lidocaine in management of out-of-hospital ventricular fibrillation. A randomized clinical trial. *Am J Cardiol* 48:353, 1981.

72. Harrison BE, Amey BD: The use of bretylium in prehospital ventricular fibrillation. *Am J Emerg Med* 1:1, 1983.

73. Nowak, RM, Bodnar TJ, Dronen S, et al: Bretylium tosylate as initial treatment for cardiopulmonary arrest: Randomized comparison with placebo. *Ann Emerg Med* 10:8, 1981.

74. Taylor SH, Saxton C, Davies PS, et al: Bretylium tosylate in prevention of cardiac dysrhythmias after myocardial infarction. *Br Heart J* 32:326, 1970.

75. Puddu PE, Jouve R, Torresani J, et al: Letter to the editor. *Heart Lung* 9:910, 1980.
76. Torresani J: Bretylium tosylate in patients with acute myocardial infarction. *Am J Cardiol* 54:20A, 1984.
77. Castaneda AR, Bacaner MB: Effect of bretylium tosylate on the prevention and treatment of postoperative arrhythmias. *Am J Cardiol* 25:464, 1970.
78. Duff HJ, Roden DM, Yacobi A, et al: Bretylium: Relations between plasma concentrations and pharmacologic actions in high-frequency ventricular arrhythmias. *Am J Cardiol* 55:395, 1985.
79. Day HW, Bacaner MB: Use of bretylium tosylate in the management of acute myocardial infarction. *Am J Cardiol* 21:530, 1968.
80. Bernstein JG, Koch-Weser J: Effectiveness of bretylium tosylate against refractory ventricular arrhythmias. *Circulation* 45:1024, 1972.
81. Cohen HC, Gozo EG, Langendorf R, et al: Response of resistant ventricular tachycardia to bretylium: Relation to site of ectopic focus and location of myocardial disease. *Circulation* 47:331, 1973.
82. Anderson JL, Popat K, Pitt B: Paradoxical ventricular tachycardia and fibrillation after intravenous bretylium therapy. *Arch Intern Med* 141:801, 1981.
83. Adult Advanced Cardiac Life Support. Part III. *JAMA* 255:2933, 1986.
84. Weaver WD, Fahrenbruch CE, Dennis D, et al: Efficacy of epinephrine and lidocaine for persistent ventricular fibrillation. (abstract) *Circulation* 72:III-8, 1985.
85. Mason JW, Winkle RA: Ability of induced ventricular tachycardia to predict long-term efficacy of antiarrhythmic drugs. *N Eng J Med* 303:1073, 1980.
86. Anderson JL, Mason JW: Criteria for selection of patients for programmed electrical stimulation. *Circulation* 73 (Suppl 2):II-50, 1986.
87. Anderson JL, Mason JW: Testing the efficacy of antiarrhythmic drugs. (editorial) *N Eng J Med* 315:391, 1986.
88. Bauernfeind RH, Hoff JV, Swiryn S, et al: Electrophysiologic testing of bretylium tosylate in sustained ventricular tachycardia. *Am Heart J* 105:973, 1983.
89. Greene HL, Werner JA, Gross BW, et al: Failure of bretylium to suppress inducible ventricular tachycarida. *Am Heart J* 105:717, 1983.
90. Hamer AW, Finerman WB, Peter T, et al: Disparity between the clinical and electrophysiologic effects of amiodarone in the treatment of recurrent ventricular tachyarrhythmias. *Am Heart J* 102:992, 1981.
91. Anderson JL: Antifibrillatory versus antiectopic therapy. *Am J Cardiol* 54:7A, 1984.
92. Reynolds EW, Vander Ark CR: Quinidine syncope and the delayed repolarization syndromes. *Mod Concepts Cardiovasc Dis* 45:117, 1976.
93. Smith WM, Gallagher JJ: "Les torsades de pointes": An unusual ventricular arrhythmia. *Ann Intern Med* 93:578, 1980.
94. Koster KW, Wellens HJJ: Quinidine induced ventricular flutter and fibrillation without digitalis therapy. *Am J Cardiol* 38:519, 1976.

95. Redleaf PD, Lerner IJ: Thiazide-induced hypokalemia with associated major ventricular arrhythmias: Report of a case and comment on therapeutic use of bretylium. *JAMA* 206:1302, 1958.

96. Deazevedo IM, Watanabe Y, Dreifus LS: Electrophysiologic antagonism of quinidine and bretylium tosylate. *Am J Cardiol* 33:633, 1974.

97. Nielson KC, Owman C: Control of ventricular fibrillation during induced hypothermia in cats after blocking the adrenergic neurons with bretylium. *Life Sci* 7:159, 1958.

98. Luomanmäki K, Heikkilä J, Härtel G: Bretylium tosylate: Adverse effects in acute myocardial infarction. *Arch Intern Med* 135:515, 1975.

99. Woosley RL, Reele SB, Roden DM, et al: Pharmacologic reversal of the hypotensive effect that complicates antiarrythmic therapy with bretylium. *Clin Pharmacol Ther* 32:313, 1982.

100. Wilkerson RD: Antiarrhythmic effects of tricyclic antidepressant drugs in ouabain-induced arrhythmias in the dog. *J Pharmacol Exp Ther* 205:666, 1978.

101. Bacaner MB, Hoey MP, Macres MG: Suppression of ventricular fibrillation and positive inotropic action of bethanidine sulfate, a chemical analog of bretylium tosylate that is well absorbed orally. *Am J Cardiol* 49:45, 1982.

102. Anderson JL, Anastasiou-Nana M, Dayton VD, et al: Myocardial bethanidine kinetics after single-dose intravenous infusion: Correlation with plasma kinetics in closed-chest dogs. *J Cardiovasc Pharmacol* 7:609, 1985.

103. Bacaner MB, Benditt DB: Antiarrhythmic, antifibrillatory, and hemodynamic actions of bethanidine sulfate: An orally effective analog of bretylium for suppression of ventricular tacharrhythmias. *Am J Cardiol* 50:728, 1982.

104. Benditt DB, Benson DW, Dunnigan A, et al: Antiarrhythmic and electrophysiologic actions of bethanidine sulfate in primary ventricular fibrillation or life-threatening ventricular tachycardia. *Am J Cardiol* 53:1268, 1984.

105. Somberg JC, Butler B, Torres V, et al: Antiarrhythmic action of bethanidine. *Am J Cardiol* 54:343, 1984.

106. Wynn J, Torres V, Tepper D, et al: New therapy focus: bethanidine. *Cardiovasc Rev Rep* 5:199, 1984.

107. Teichman SL, Waspe LE, Matos JA, et al: Bethanidine sulfate: Efficacy in prevention of ventricular tachyarrhythmias during programmed stimulation. Report of a multicenter study of 56 patients. *J Am Coll Cardiol* 6:510, 1985.

108. DiMarco JP, Sellers TD, Shipe JR, et al: Acute electrophysiologic effects of bethanidine sulfate in patients with ventricular tachycardia or fibrillation. *Am Heart J* 108:1244, 1984.

109. Dangman KH, Miura DS: Electrophysiological effects of bethanidine sulfate on canine cardiac Purkinje fibers and ventricular muscle cells. *J Cardiovasc Pharmacol* 7:50, 1985.

110. Patterson E, Amalfitano DJ, Lucchesi BR: Development of ventricular tachyarrhythmias in the conscious canine during the recovery

phase of experimental ischemic injury: Effect of bethanidine administration. *J Cardiovasc Pharmacol* 6:470, 1984.
111. Wastila WB, Copp BC, Walton E, et al: Meobentine sulfate: A new antidysrhythmic agent. *J Pharm Pharmacol* 33:594, 1981.
112. Michelson EL, Naito M, David D, et al: Meobentine sulfate: Antiarrhythmic efficacy and mechanism of action in a chronic canine model of myocardial infarction susceptible to ventricular tachyarrhythmias. (abstract) *(Am J Cardiol* 47:392, 1981.
113. Zimmerman JM, Patterson E, Pitt B, et al: Antidysrhythmic actions of meobentine sulfate. *Am Heart J* 107:1117, 1984.
114. Anderson JL, Reid PR, Platia EV, et al: Meobentine sulfate: Antiarrhythmic and electrophysiologic effects assessed by programmed electrical stimulation and ambulatory monitoring in patients with complex ventricular tachyarrhythmia. *Am Heart J* 110:774, 1985.
115. Duff HJ, Oates JA, Roden DM, et al: The antiarrhythmic activity of meobentine sulfate in man. *J Cardiovasc Pharmacol* 6:650, 1984.
116. Steinberg MI, Molloy BB: Clofilium—a new antifibrillatory agent that selectively increases cellular refractoriness. *Life Sci* 25:1397, 1979.
117. Steinberg M, Sullivan M, Wiest S, et al: Cellular electrophysiology of clofilium, a new antifibrillatory agent, in normal and ischemic canine Purkinje fibers. *J Cardiovasc Pharmacol* 3:881, 1981.
118. Kowey PR, Friehling TD, O'Connor KM, et al: The effect of bretylium and clofilium on dispersion of refractoriness and vulnerability to ventricular fibrillation in the ischemic feline heart. *Am Heart J* 110:363, 1985.
119. Greene HL, Werner JA, Gross BW, et al: Prolongation of cardiac refractory times in man by clofilium phosphate, a new antiarrhythmic agent. *Am Heart J* 106:492, 1983.

Chapter 13

# Antiarrhythmic Properties of Melperone, a Neuroleptic Agent that Lengthens Cardiac Repolarization

Helge Refsum and Eivind S. Platou

Melperone is classified as a Class III antiarrhythmic drug.[1-6] Its antiarrhythmic activity has been demonstrated in several studies.[7-17] But, as for the other Class III antiarrhythmic drugs, the discovery of melperone's antiarrhythmic activity was a secondary event. Melperone is a butyrophenone derivative, and it has been in clinical use as a neuroleptic drug for 20 years.[18,19] Reported side-effects of melperone are few,[18] even in intensive care patients.[20] Melperone does not cause cardiorespiratory depression. On the other hand, suggestions of antiarrhythmic effects of melperone initiated several electrophysiologic studies.

## Electrophysiologic Effects

In isolated rat atria, Refsum et al.[1] found that melperone significantly prolonged refractoriness without affecting excitability, and that the drug had a significant bradycardic effect. As a consequence of these results, a series of electrophysiologic studies were undertaken in dogs with monophasic action potential recordings, His bundle recordings, programmed electrical stimulation, and experimentally induced atrial fibrillation and flutter. From these

From: *Control of Cardiac Arrhythmias by Lengthening Repolarization*, edited by Bramah N. Singh, MD, Futura Publishing Company Inc., Mount Kisco, NY, © 1988.

studies it could be concluded that melperone prolongs homogeneously monophasic action potential duration (Fig. 1)[21,22] and causes a concentration-dependent increase in atrial, AV nodal, and ventricular refractoriness (Fig. 2).[3,23,24] These effects of melperone are direct effects of the drug, and they are present regardless of autonomic nervous blockade.[25-27]

In the (clinically relevant) doses used in these studies, there are no indications of Class I antiarrhythmic effects, and the increases in refractoriness seem to be accounted for by increases in action potential duration (Class III antiarrhythmic effect).

Melperone has direct negative chronotropic effect on the sinus node,[1] probably due to prolongation of the sinus node action potential duration.[4] In low doses, we observed in our dog studies an increase in heart rate due to activation of the sympathetic nervous system secondary to peripheral vasodilation.[3] This effect could be prevented by β-adrenoceptor blockade.[25,27]

Melperone does not change atrial or His-Purkinje conduction times or QRS width,[3,5,25] but in low and median doses the drug reduces AV nodal conduction time. This effect seems to be a direct effect of the drug and is present irrespective of various interventions on the autonomic nervous system.[25,27]

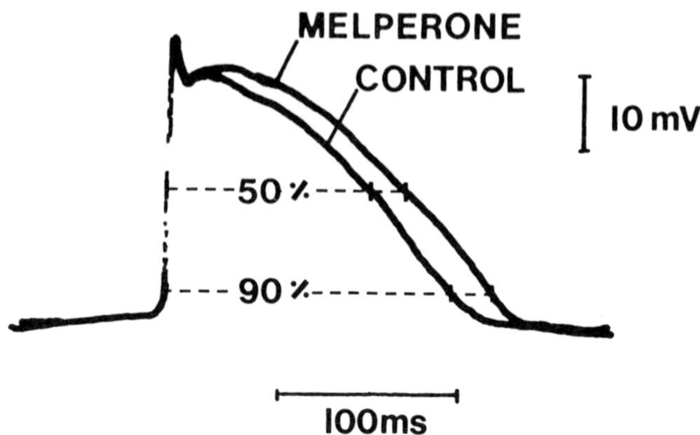


**Figure 1.** Monophasic action potentials recorded with suction electrode technique from the right ventricle of a pentobarbital anesthetized dog. Superposed are control recording and the effect of melperone 2.5 mg/kg. (From Platou ES, Myhre ESP, Smiseth OA, et al: Melperone: α-Adrenoceptor blocker with Class III antiarrhythmic action. In H Refsum, OD Mjøs (eds): α-Adrenoceptor Blockers in Cardiovascular Disease. Edinburgh, Churchill Livinstone, 1985, p. 311.)

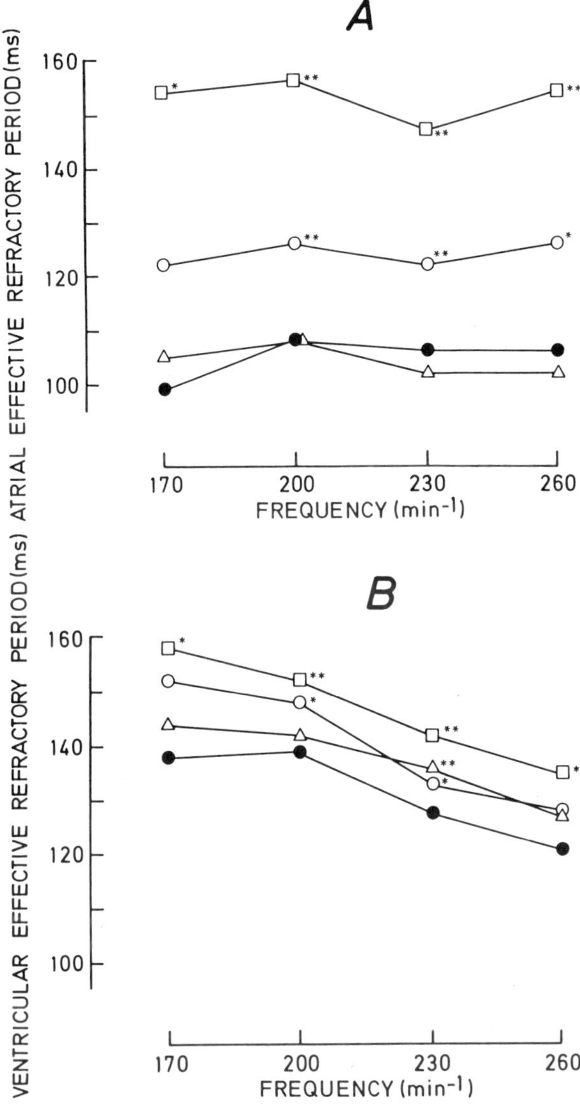



**Figure 2.** Effect of melperone on median atrial (A) and ventricular (B) effective refractory period at increasing frequencies of stimulation. Control = ●; effect of melperone 0.5 mg/kg = △; effect of melperone 2.5 mg/kg = ○; and effect of melperone 12.5 mg/kg = □. Asterisks indicate those values that are significantly different from the control value, **p $<$ 0.025, *p $<$ 0.05. (From Refsum H, Amlie JP, Platou ES, et al: Electrophysiological effects in the dog heart in situ—A new antiarrhythmic drug. *Cardiovasc Res* 15:131, 1981.)

## Antiarrhythmic Effects

We have found that melperone effectively converts electrically induced self-perpetuating atrial fibrillation and flutter in intact dogs (Fig. 3).[12] The potency of melperone in this study was comparable to that of amiodarone and was most probably due to its Class III antiarrhythmic effect. Antiarrhythmic effect also has been shown experimentally in rabbits and guinea pigs using ouabain and aconitine induced arrhythmias.[8]

It is interesting to note that melperone even prolongs action potential duration of hypoxic myocardium.[4] Melperone-induced increase in fibrillation threshold of normal as well as ischemic rat hearts has been demonstrated.[14] Melperone has been shown further to effectively prevent early postinfarction ventricular arrhythmias in rats.[11]

Melperone also is effective in reperfusion arrhythmias,[15] an effect that partly may be due to the $\alpha_1$-adrenoceptor blocking action of the drug. Thus, the combination of Class III antiarrhythmic action and $\alpha$-blockade might be particularly useful in the management of arrhythmias associated with acute myocardial ischemia and reperfusion.

## Hemodynamic Effects

Most antiarrhythmic drugs in clinical use today have negative inotropic effects, which may be detrimental in patients with heart failure. However, the positive inotropic effect of melperone as well as some other Class III antiarrhythmic drugs, for example, bretylium[29] and sotalol,[30] has been shown. A correlation between action potential duration and the force of contraction has been demonstrated,[31] and Class III antiarrhythmic action and positive inotropy may be linked.[32]

We have shown that melperone has a positive inotropic effect in isolated heart muscle preparations of rat[1] (Fig. 4) and cat,[33] in the intact dog heart[27,33] and in dogs with acute left ventricular heart failure.[34] The positive inotropic property also has been demonstrated by others.[2,4]

Hemodynamic observations in intact dogs demonstrated a decrease in blood pressure together with a reflex activation of the sympathetic nervous system after intravenous injections of mel-

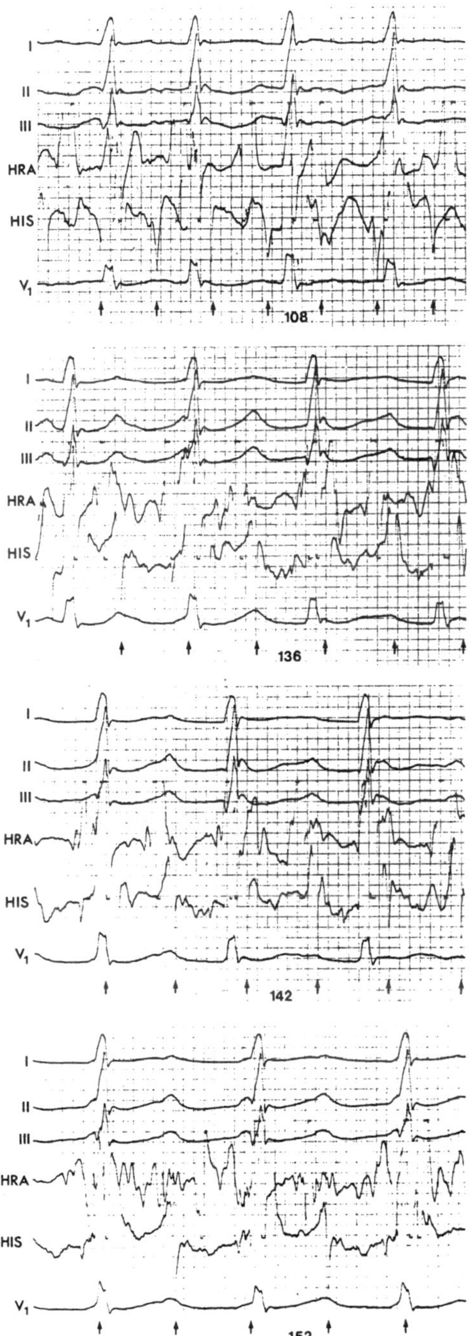

**Figure 3.** Tracings of experimentally induced atrial flutter in a dog and the effect of melperone. The arrows indicate the flutter waves. The top tracing shows atrial flutter before intravenous injection of melperone, flutter cycle is 108 msec. The following tracings show that melperone 2.5, 5.0, and 7.5 mg/kg (cumulative doses) increase the duration of the flutter cyclus to 136, 142, and 152 msec. Paper speed 250 mm/sec. Abbreviations: I, II, III, $V_1$, represent ECG leads; HRA and HIS represent high right atrial and His-bundle electrograms. (From Refsum H, Platou ES: Class III antiarrhythmic drugs in experimental atrial fibrillation and flutter. In S Levi, R Gerard (eds): *Recent Advances in Cardiac Arrhythmias. I. Antiarrhythmic Agents and Cardiac Pacing*. London, John Libbey, 1983, p 311.)

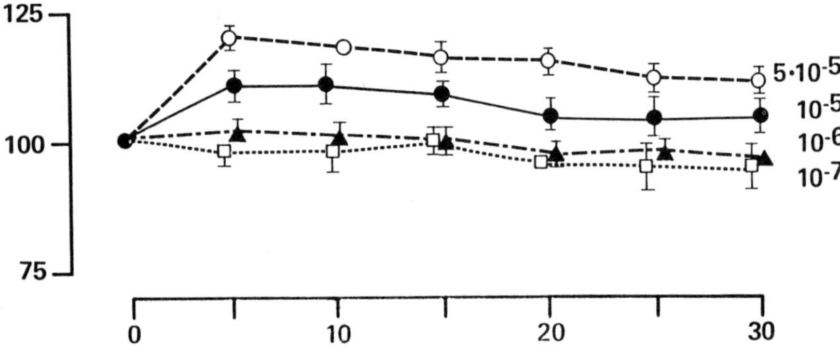


**Figure 4.** Time course of the contractile force of electrically stimulated, isolated rat atria after addition of melperone in concentrations from $10^{-7}$ to $5 \times 10^{-5}$ M. The values were calculated as a percentage of the values recorded immediately before addition of drug (time 0). The rate of contractions was kept constant (180 beats/min). Mean ± SEM of 3 to 5 recordings. Ordinate: Contractile force (Percent of control values), Abscissa: time (min). (From Refsum H, Passwal M, Olsson S-O: Comparison of the electrophysiologic effects of two neuroleptics, melperone and thioridazine, on isolated rat atria. *Eur J Pharmacol* 49:285, 1978.)

perone.[3,25,27] The vasodilating effect was present already after low doses of melperone[33] (Fig. 5) with a decrease in total peripheral resistance and an increase in heart rate. Despite these changes and the increase in maximum rise of left ventricular pressure, cardiac output did not increase. A reduced venous return to the right atrium can explain these findings, and a significant decrease of right ventricular end-diastolic pressure supports this notion.[33]

On the basis of these observations, we studied the effect of melperone in dogs with acute ischemic left ventricular failure.[34] In the failing heart, melperone significantly decreased left ventricular end-diastolic pressure (Fig. 6) and total peripheral resistance and increased stroke volume. There was a moderate fall in mean aortic blood pressure but no reflex increase in heart rate, which may be explained by reduced baroreceptor response during cardiac failure.[35] Hence, cadiac output was maintained at markedly reduced preload and moderately reduced oxygen consumption.

The vasodilating effect of melperone is due to $\alpha_1$-adrenoceptor blocking effect of the drug.[6,27,35] After $\alpha$-blocker (phenoxybenzamine) pretreatment, melperone has no or only minor hemodynamic effects even after high doses.[6,27]

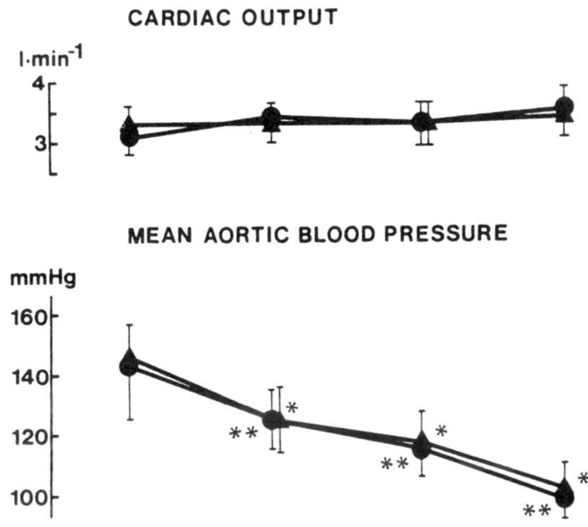


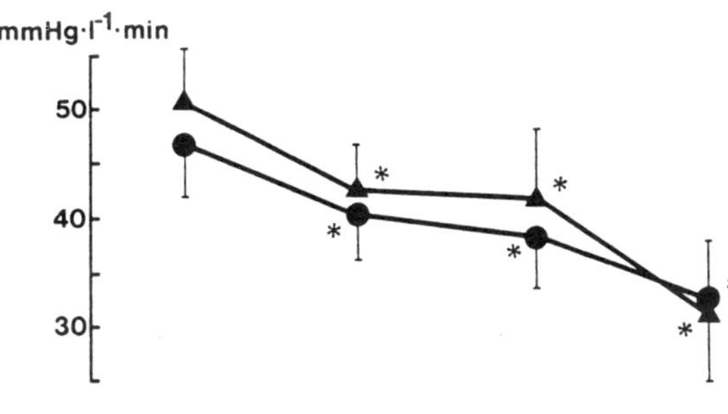


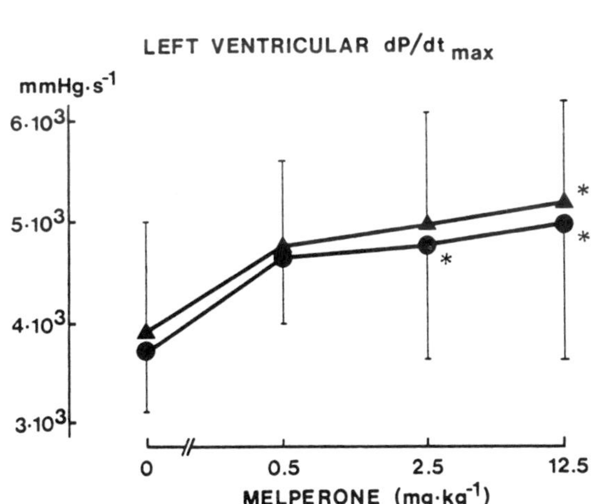


**Figure 5.** Effects of melperone in cumulative doses of 0.5, 2.5, and 12.5 mg/kg (log scale) on cardiac output, mean aortic blood pressure, total peripheral resistance, and left ventricular $dP/dt_{max}$ in 8 pentobarbital-anesthetized dogs at spontaneous heart rate (dots) and when paced at 200/min (triangles). Median values ± 95 percent confidence interval of the median, $**p < 0.001$, $*p < 0.05$. (From Platou ES, Smiseth OA, Refsum H, et al: Vasodilator and inotropic effects of the antiarrhythmic drug melperone. *J Cardiovasc Pharmacol* 4:645, 1982.)

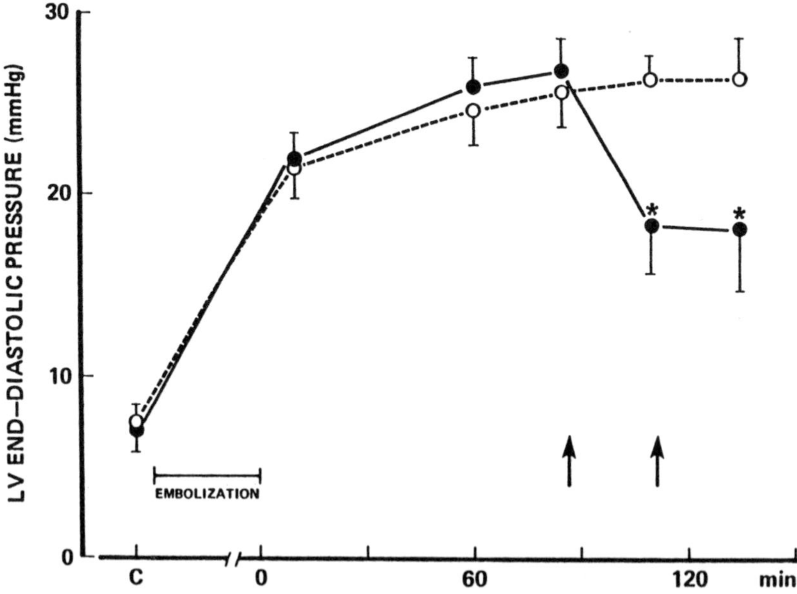


**Figure 6.** Effects of melperone on left ventricular end-diastolic pressure during acute ischemic left ventricular failure in close-chest, pentobarbital-anesthetized dogs. Acute ischemic failure was induced by embolization of the left main coronary artery with 50μm plastic microspheres. Open circles: 6 dogs that received no treatment; closed circles: 6 dogs that received melperone 1.0 mg/kg at 90 min (arrow) plus 1.5 mg/kg at 115 min (arrow) after coronary embolization. C = control values before embolization. Mean values ± SEM, *p < 0.01. (From Smiseth OA, Platou ES, Refsum H, et al: Haemodynamic and metabolic effects of the antiarrhythmic drug melperone during acute left ventricular failure in dogs. *Cardiovasc Res* 15:724, 1981.)

## Clinical Studies

When melperone was tested as a sedative in an intensive care unit,[20] it was observed that arrhythmias were reduced in patients with cardiac arrhythmias. The effect of melperone 50 mg IV, therefore, was tested double-blind in 26 patients hospitalized with acute myocardial infarction and ventricular arrhythmias.[10] Continuous EKG monitoring was done for 3 hours. Melperone was superior to a placebo in reducing the total number of ventricular ectopic beats as well as the number of minutes with either frequent, multifocal, R-on-T-type, or runs of ventricular beats. Mild sedation and slight blood pressure reduction were noted.

Edvardsson and Olsson[36] showed that a small IV dose of 10 mg melperone significantly prolonged right atrial monophasic action potential duration in humans. No sedative effect was noted after this dose.

Duff et al.[17] gave melperone to 15 patients with coronary heart disease with ejection fraction of 35 ± 13 percent and inducible sustained ventricular tachycardia. The patients were tested electrophysiologically before and after 3 days on melperone 30–120 mg/day orally. Ventricular effective refractory period increased significantly with increasing dose. Even though these patients had experienced failure of 4 ± 2 antiarrhythmic drugs, 4 patients had partial and 1 complete response to melperone. Postural hypotension in 4 patients was the only reported side effect.

Platou et al.[16] gave melperone IV to 8 patients with recurrent, life-threatening, drug-resistant ventricular tachycardia (VT) and fibrillation (VF), where one to four conventional antiarrhythmic drugs (including amiodarone in 3 patients) had failed to control the arrhythmias: One post-myocardial infarction patient had incessant VT and VF and was defibrillated 225 times. Immediate control of the arrhythmias was obtained by melperone 50 mg IV. Another patient was in cardiogenic shock, ventilated on respirator, and had recurrent VT and VF. Her arrhythmias were controlled by melperone. In 2 other patients with acute myocardial infarction with VT and VF, the arrhythmias could be controlled by melperone. One patient with hypertrophic cardiomyopathy and 1 patient with frequent VT after aneurysmectomy, received melperone as a result of electrophysiological drug testing. In 2 other patients, amiodarone produced intolerable side effects and was successfully substituted by melperone.

Two of these 8 patients experienced hypotension, 1 severe hypotension, that, however, could be corrected with saline infusion. Three patients experienced an acute sense of fear, a "bad trip" that was attenuated by slower IV infusion. Melperone was discontinued in 2 patients due to sedation, but it had to be reinstituted in 1 of them.

The promising results in the small groups of cardiac patients studied so far encourage further clinical studies. As melperone has been used widely as a neuroleptic, its pharmacology including side effects is well known. Apart from mild sedation, the incidence of side effects is low, particularly those arising from the extrapyramidal system.[18,37] Melperone has no significant peripheral anticholinergic or β-adrenoceptor blocking activity.[25,38]

## Pharmacokinetics

Melperone, γ-(4-methyl-piperidino)-p-fluorobutyrophenone hydrochloride, Buronil[R] (Ferrosan, Malmö, Sweden) is a colorless powder, soluble in polar liquids such as water, alcohol, and chloroform. Given as tablets, the absorption is complete and the bioavailability is 60−70 percent when compared to parenteral administration.[39] Melperone is metabolized mainly in the liver, hence, the reason for the significant first-pass effect. The distribution halftime is short, 0.11 hours. The elimination half-life after a single oral or parenteral dose is 3−4 hours, and about 6 hours after intramuscular injection. The pharmacokinetics are partly dose dependent. The hepatic metabolism probably is saturable, which makes more unchanged melperone available to the systemic circulation at higher doses.[39] With chronic dosage the elimination half-life, therefore, is somewhat longer, about 8 hours.[40] Protein binding is about 50 percent. Seven inactive metabolites have been found.

## Conclusions

Melperone has Class III antiarrhythmic action, and the effectiveness of this action has been demonstrated in various experimental situations as well as in patients. Melperone has direct bradycardic effect due to prolongation of the sinus node action potential. Melperone also has a direct enhancing effect on AV nodal conduction.

Melperone has slight positive inotropic effect, and we suggest that the positive inotropic effect is due to the same basic mechanism as the Class III antiarrhythmic effect. This may be a common feature of several Class III antiarrhythmic drugs. Melperone has vasodilating effects due to $\alpha_1$-adrenoceptor blocking action. The $\alpha_1$-adrenoceptor blocking action may add to the Class III antiarrhythmic action in reperfusion arrhythmias.

Melperone thus combines the properties of Class III antiarrhythmic action, slight positive inotropy, and $\alpha_1$-adrenoceptor blockade. Theoretically, this combination should be advantageous, particularly in patients with myocardial failure and ischemia, and melperone therefore may be a valuable addition to the antiarrhythmic armamentarium.

# References


1. Refsum H, Passwal M, Olsson S-O: Comparison of the electrophysiological effects of two neuroleptics, melperone and thioridazine, on isolated rat atria. *Eur J Pharmacol* 49:285, 1978.
2. Arlock P, Gullberg B, Olsson S-O: Cardiac electrophysiology of four neuroleptics: Melperone, haloperidol, thioridazine and chlorpromazine. *Naunyn Schmiedebergs Arch Pharmacol* 304:27, 1978.
3. Refsum H, Amlie JP, Platou ES, et al: Electrophysiological effects of melperone in the dog heart in situ—A new antiarrhythmic drug. *Cardiovasc Res* 15:131, 1981.
4. Millar JS, Vaughan Williams EM: Differential actions on rabbit nodal, atrial Purkinje cell and ventricular potentials of melperone, a bradycardic agent delaying repolarization: effect of hypoxia. *Br J Pharmacol* 75:109, 1982.
5. Millar JS, Vaughan Williams EM: Pharmacological mapping of regional effects in the rabbit heart of some new antiarrhythmic drugs. *Br J Pharmacol* 79:701, 1983.
6. Platou ES, Myhre ESP, Smiseth OA, et al: Melperone: $\alpha$-Adrenoceptor blocker with class III antiarrhythmic action. In H Refsum, OD Mjøs (eds): *α-Adrenoceptor Blockers in Cardiovascular Disease*. Edinburgh, Churchill Livingstone, 1985, p 311.
7. Olsson S-O, Duker G, Refsum H: Melperone—A new antiarrhythmic drug. In *7th International Congress of Pharmacology, Paris 1978*. Oxford, Pergamon Press, 1978, p 437.
8. Petersen EN: Experimental antiarrhythmic properties of melperone, a neuroleptic butyrophenone. *Acta Pharmacol Toxicol* 42:388, 1978.
9. Platou ES, Refsum H, Amlie JP, et al: Anti-arrhythmic action of melperone in the dog heart in situ. *Acta Pharmacol Toxicol* 44: 185, 1979.
10. Møgelvang JC, Petersen EN, Folke PE, et al: Antiarrhythmic properties of a neuroleptic butyrophenone, melperone, in acute myocardial infarction. A double blind trial. *Acta Med Scand* 208:61, 1980.
11. Kane KA, McDonald FM, Parratt JR: What pharmacological properties are necessary for the prevention of early post-infarction ventricular dysrhythmias? *Br J Pharmacol* 72:512P, 1981.
12. Platou ES, Refsum H: Class III antiarrhythmic action in experimental artrial fibrillation and flutter in dogs. *J Cardiovasc Pharmacol* 4:838, 1982.
13. Refsum H, Platou ES: Class III antiarrhythmic drugs in experimental atrial fibrillation and flutter. In S Levi, R Gerard (eds): *Recent Advances in Cardiac Arrhythmias. I. Antiarrhythmic Agents and Cardiac Pacing*. London, John Libbey, 1983, p 311.
14. Marshall RJ, Muir AW, Winslow E: Effects of antiarrhythmic drugs on ventricular fibrillation thresholds of normal and ischaemic myocardium in the anaesthetized rat. *Br J Pharmacol* 78:165, 1983.
15. Kane KA, Parratt JR, Williams FM: An investigation into the characteristics of reperfusion-induced arrhythmias in the anaesthetized rat and their susceptibility to antiarrhythmic agents. *Br J Pharmacol* 82:349, 1984.

16. Platou ES, Gjesdal K, Sivertssen E: Effect of melperone in patients with life-threatening, drug-resistant ventricular tachycardia. *III World Conference on Clinical Pharmacology and Therapeutics 1986. Acta Pharmacol Toxicol* 58 (Suppl V):286, 1986.
17. Duff HJ, Mitchell LB, Kavanagh KM, et al: Melperone: Antiarrhythmic and electrophysiologic activity in man. *Circulation* 74 (Suppl II):99, 1986.
18. Kirkegaard, AA, Kirkegaard G, Geismar L, et al: Additional studies on side effects of melperone in long term therapy for 1–5 years in psychiatric patients. *Drug Res* 31:737, 1981.
19. Olsson S-O, Refsum H: Melperones effekter på hjärtat. *Observ Med* 8:136, 1981.
20. Mark A, Feldt-Rasmussen M, Wikhjelm B, et al: Erfahrungen mit Methylperon (NFN) auf einer Intensivstation. *Therapowoche* 26:6823, 1976.
21. Landmark K, Amlie JP, Refsum H: Classification of cardioactive drugs in vivo by using programmed electrical stimulation in combination with monophasic action potential recordings at different pacing rates. *Acta Med Scand* (Suppl) 645:37, 1981.
22. Platou ES, Steinnes K, Refsum H: A method of simultaneous epicardial monophasic action potential recordings from the dog heart in situ. *Acta Pharmacol Toxicol* 54:94, 1984.
23. Landmark K, Amlie JP, Refsum H, et al: Correlation between melperone plasma concentrations and changes in the effective refractory period of the right atrium and ventricle of the dog. *Acta Pharmacol Toxicol* 45:166, 1979.
24. Platou ES, Refsum H, Amlie JP, et al: Plasma levels and cardiac electrophysiological effects of melperone in the dog. *Eur J Pharmacol* 82:1, 1982.
25. Platou ES, Refsum H, Amlie JP, et al: Influence of β-Adrenergic and cholinergic blockade on the electrophysiological effects of melperone in the dog heart in situ. *Cardiovasc Res* 15:137, 1981.
26. Platou ES, Refsum H, Myhre ESP, et al: The mode of antiarrhythmic action of melperone. *Acta Pharmacol Toxical* 50:108, 1982.
27. Platou ES, Myhre ESP, Refsum H: *A*-Adrenoceptor blockade and class III antiarrhythmic activity combined: Hemodynamic and electrophysiological effects of melperone in the dog. *Can J Physiol Pharmacol* 64:1286, 1986.
28. Platou ES, Refsum H: Class III antiarrhythmic drugs: Effects of amiodarone and melperone in experimentally induced atrial fibrillation and flutter in dogs. In G Breithardt, F Loogen (eds): *New Aspects in the Medical Treatment of Tachyarrhythmias. Role of Amiodarone.* München, Urban and Schwarzenberg, 1983, p 92.
29. Amsterdam EA, Spann JF Jr, Mason DT, et al: Characterization of the positive inotropic effects of bretylium tosylate: A unique property of antiarrhythmic agent. *Am J Cardiol* 25:81, 1970.
30. Kaumann AJ, Olson CB: Temporal relation between long-lasting aftercontractions and action potentials in cat papillary muscles. *Science* 161:293, 1968.
31. Morad M, Trautwein W: The effect of the duration of the action poten-

tial on contraction in the mammalian heart muscle. *Pfluegers Arch* 299:66, 1968.

32. Platou ES, Refsum H, Hotvedt R: Class III antiarrhythmic action linked with positive inotropy: Antiarrhythmic, electrophysiological, and hemodynamic effects of the sea anemone polypeptide $ATX_{II}$ in the dog heart in situ. *J Cardiovasc Pharmacol* 8:459, 1986.

33. Platou ES, Smiseth OA, Refsum H, et al: Vasodilator and inotropic effects of the antiarrhythmic drug melperone. *J Cardiovasc Pharmacol* 4:645, 1982.

34. Smiseth OA, Platou ES, Refsum H, et al: Haemodynamic and metabolic effects of the antiarrhythmic drug melperone during acute left ventricular failure in dogs. *Cardiovasc Res* 15:724, 1981.

35. Higgins CB, Vatner SF, Eckberg DL, et al: Alterations in the baroreceptor reflex in conscious dogs with heart failure. *J Clin Invest* 51:715, 1972.

36. Edvardsson N, Olsson SB: Effect of intravenous melperone on atrial repolarization in man. *Scand J Clin Lab Invest* 41:87, 1981.

37. Gunne L-M, Bàràni S: A monitoring test for the liability of neuroleptic drugs to induce tardive dyskinesia. *Psychopharmacol* 63:195, 1979.

38. Olsson S-O, Passwal M, Refsum H: In vitro autonomic effects of four neuroleptics: chlorpromazine, haloperidol, melperone and thioridazine. *Acta Pharmacol Toxicol* 41 (Suppl IV): 66, 1977.

39. Borgström L, Larson H, Molander L: Pharmacokinetics of parenteral and oral melperone in man. *Eur J Clin Pharmacol* 23:173, 1982.

40. Bjerkenstedt L, Härnryd C, Grimm V, et al: A double blind comparison of melperone and thiothixene in psychotic women using a new rating scale, the CPRS. *Arch Psychiatr Nervenkr* 226:157, 1978.

Chapter 14

# Electropharmacologic Properties of Amiodarone

Bramah N. Singh

---

Although developed specifically as a coronary vasodilator and an antianginal compound, amiodarone hydrochloride (Fig. 1) recently has attracted considerable experimental and clinical interest as an antiarrhythmic agent. Indeed, few, if any, other antidysrhythmic compounds have stimulated as much interest as has amiodarone over the last 10 years. Its extreme potency in the prophylactic control of most supraventricular and ventricular arrhythmias is now well established.[1-10] However, the fundamental mechanism whereby amiodarone induces its salutary effects for the most part remains uncertain. For this reason, the effects of the compound on cardiac electrophysiology relative to its associated pharmacologic properties are of much theoretical as well as practical importance. As in the case of numerous antiarrhythmic agents, the overall effects of amiodarone on the cardiac action potentials may result from its direct as well as indirect actions. Barring its intrinsic effects, the compound has the propensity to noncompetitively antagonize alpha- and beta-adrenergic receptors[11,12] with a poorly understood and complex interrelationship with thyroid hormone metabolism.[13,14] The purpose of this chapter is to discuss the overall pharmacodynamic actions of the drug with a particular reference to its electrophysiologic properties.

---

From: *Control of Cardiac Arrhythmias by Lengtening Repolarization*, edited by Bramah N. Singh, MD, Futura Publishing Company Inc., Mount Kisco, NY, © 1988.

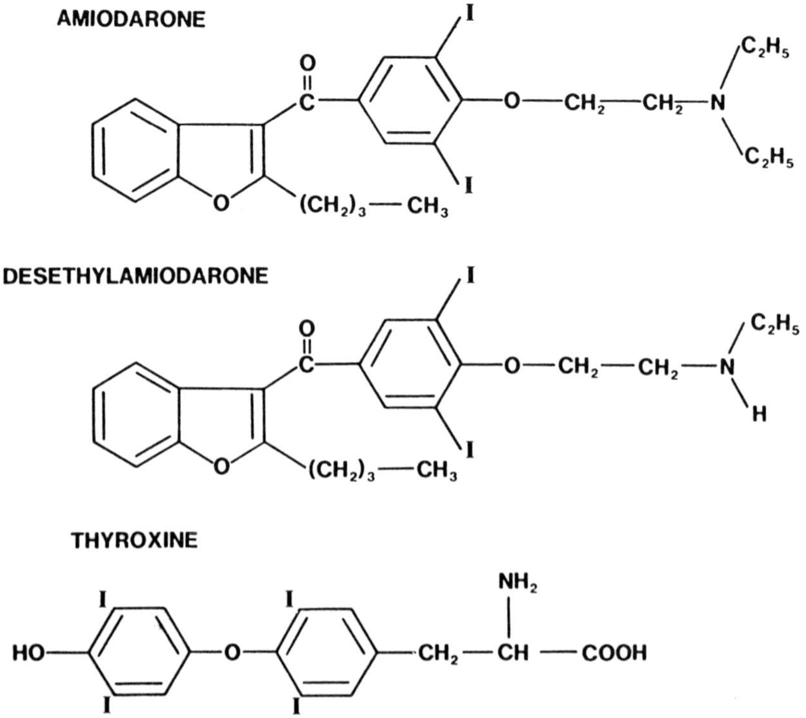

Figure 1. Structural formulas of amiodarone, desethylamiodarone, and thyroxine. Note the presence of iodine in amiodarone and desethylamiodarone.

## Development of Amiodarone

Amiodarone was synthesized by Labaz laboratories in Belgium as an antianginal agent during a systematic search for potent coronary vasodilators.[15] Amiodarone was one of a series of derivatives that were synthesized on the basis of the benzofuran moiety of the khellin molecule and its natural congeners, all of which were reasonably potent coronary vasodilators. The very first compound was benziodarone, in which the presence of two iodine atoms was believed to augment the overall pharmacologic properties compared to those of its precursor, benzarone. Benziodarone had but a short-lived clinical evaluation, as it was found to induce jaundice and hepatotoxicity in humans. It was soon superseded by amiodarone, which was found to be a more potent coronary vasodilator. In a series of comprehensive pharmacologic studies, Charlier et al.,[12] in a variety of isolated tissue preparations and in intact unconscious dogs, clearly demonstrated somewhat unusual properties of the compound. The studies indicated a slow onset and offset of action of amiodarone. For example, when it was given orally to instrumented dogs, the fall in heart rate, tension–time index, and systemic pressure were gradual and did not appear to reach a steady state at a constant daily dose for about 5–6 weeks. Similarly, the regression of the observed changes was not complete even after 5 weeks of drug withdrawal.

When intravenous amiodarone was given, there was an increase in coronary blood flow and reduced myocardial oxygen consumption. Intravenous amiodarone also tended to attenuate the tachycardia and enhanced contractility produced by isoproterenol suggesting an interaction with the autonomic nervous system. Although the differences between the effects of the parenterally and orally administered amiodarone were not emphasized by Charlier et al.[12] the overall effects noted in their studies were construed as representing a "new biologic profile" for an anti-anginal compound. The first report documenting the clinical antianginal actions of the compound appeared in 1967.[16]

The antiarrhythmic effects of amiodarone in experimental animals were first reported in 1969.[17] The earliest attempt to delineate the fundamental mechanism of action in cardiac muscle was reported in 1970[18] and again in 1971 as an integral part of a doctoral dissertation.[19] In common with the drug sotalol,[20] it was suggested that amiodarone might be a potent antiarrhythmic compound. The first clinical report with the drug as an antiarrhythmic agent was with the *intravenous* amiodarone in 1970[21] and after oral therapy in 1974.[22] The effects of the compound now have been studied in a variety of animal and clinical arrhythmias. The emergence of amiodarone has been a major landmark in the development of antiarrhythmic therapy,[23] but the precise cellular mode of action of the compound remains incompletely understood. In the section that follows, the relevant data that bear on this issue are discussed within a brief compass. The discussion of the electrophysiologic actions of the compound will be preceded by a brief description of the compound's interaction with the autonomic nervous system. The thesis will be developed that the precise understanding of the action of this unusually potent compound may provide further ideas about the development of similar but safer compounds, while leading to newer insights into the fundamental mechanisms of arrhythmias themselves.

## Amiodarone and Antiadrenergic Antagonism

The acute antiadrenergic actions of amiodarone have previously been established both in vitro[11] and in vivo[24-25,26] experimental models. Polster and Broekhuysen[11] compared the effects of the competitive beta-antagonist, propranolol, in isolated rabbit atria to those of amiodarone. The $pA_2$ value for propranolol was 8.33. Amiodarone acted as a noncompetitive beta antagonist with a $pD_2$ value of 4.17 with isoproterenol as an agonist. The effects of amiodarone on alpha-receptor blockade were investigated in isolated rat-aortic strips induced to contract by norepinephrine. The $pA_2$ value for phentolamine was found to be 8.69, whereas the $pD_2$ value for amiodarone was 4.06, the drug having no effect on calcium permeability in this preparation. Subsequently, Charlier[24] found that in anesthetized dogs, amiodarone produced bradycardia independently of beta-receptor blockade, as the effect persisted after the administration of propranolol. It is of interest that, although amiodarone has been found to decrease cholinergic receptors in the rat heart and brain,[27] some studies have failed to demonstrate a significant interaction with the cholinergic component of the autonomic nervous system.[18,26]

It is known that bradycardia develops in a stepwise manner as a function of time on a constant dose of amiodarone[12,19] raising the possibility of progressive decrease in myocardial beta adrenoceptors. This possibility recently has drawn increasing attention.[28,29] It is now confirmed that amiodarone does antagonize beta receptors in a noncompetitive fashion (Fig. 2) and exerts a significant effect on beta-receptor density following acute as well as chronic administration. For example, Vankatesh et al.[30] have shown that, when amiodarone and its principal metabolite desethylamiodarone were given acutely and chronically to rabbits, there was a significant reduction in myocardial beta-receptor density ($B_{max}$) without an effect on receptor affinity ($K_D$). The effect of chronic amiodarone administration over 6 weeks (Fig. 3) was more pronounced (-44 percent) than that (-23 percent) following acute intravenous drug injection. However this difference was unrelated to dose since the effects of 20 mg/kg and 40 mg/kg chronic dosing regimens on $B_{max}$ were statistically indistinguishable. Nor was the greater effect after chronic therapy attributable to serum and tissue levels after chronic dose drug administration, since both the serum and myocardial levels 15 minutes after acute intravenous amiodarone administration were considerably higher than the corresponding levels after 6 weeks of chronic drug dosing.

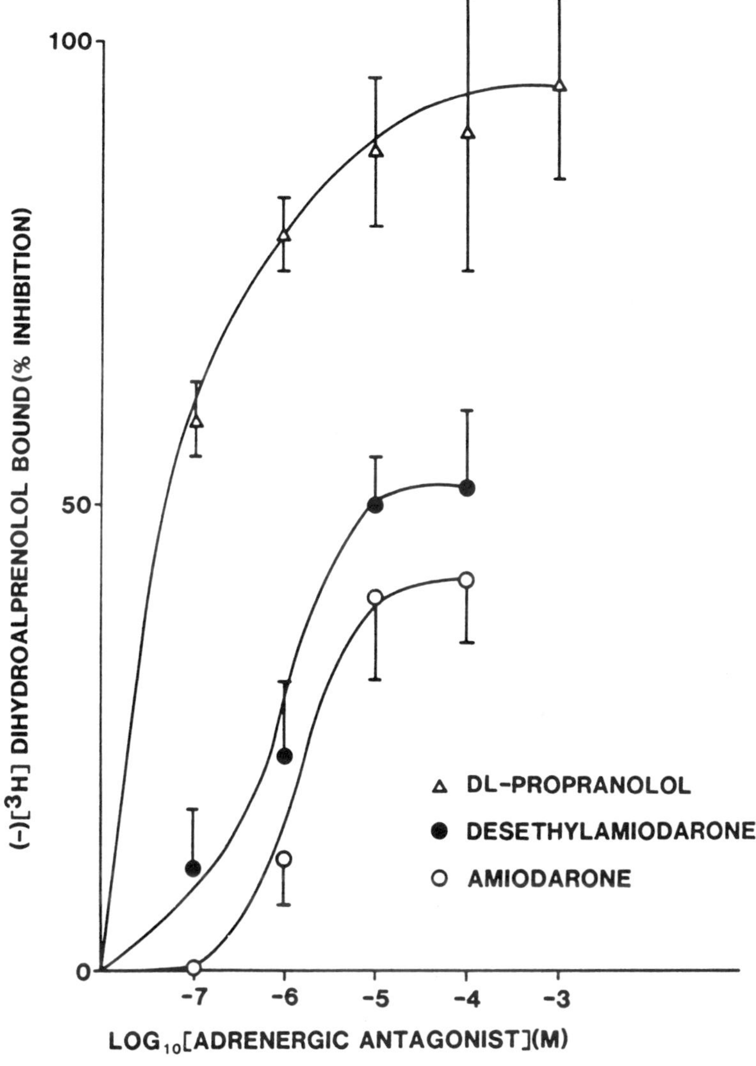



**Figure 2.** Differences between amiodarone, desethylamiodarone, and propranolol in their ability to inhibit ³H-DHA binding to beta-receptors. Note differences in the curves: the competitive nature for propranolol and noncompetitive for the benzofuran derivatives. (Based on data from Vankatesh et al.[30].)

The data confirm and extend the results of Nokin et al.,[28] who also performed direct ligand-binding assays on rat myocardial beta-adrenoceptors, but differ in providing evidence for a greater effect following chronic drug administration than after acute. The

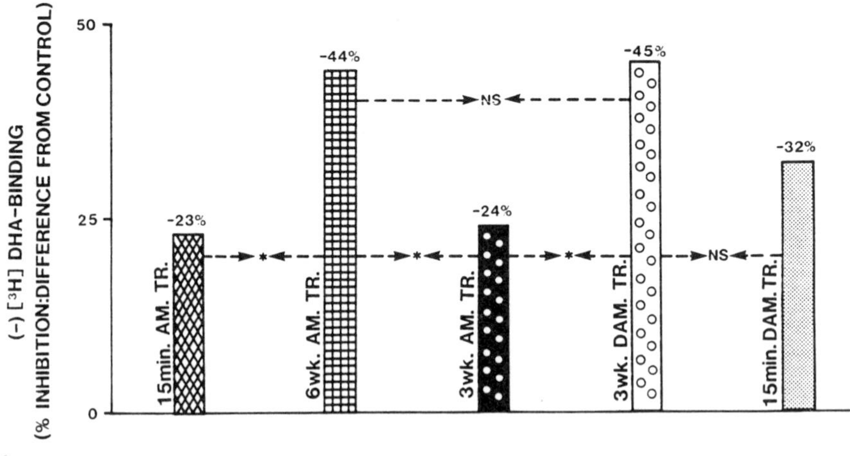


**Figure 3.** Effects of acute and chronic treatment with amiodarone (AM) and desethylamiodarone (DAM) on beta-receptor density ($B_{max}$) in the rabbit ventricular myocardium. Both agents depress $B_{max}$ with amiodarone exhibiting the trend to produce a greater reduction following chronic than after acute drug administration (TR-treatment). The data raise the possibility that the chronic effect may be due to the summated effects of the parent compound and those of the metabolite. The greater chronic effect also may result from an added effect of selective hypothyroidism (discussed in the text). (From Vankatesh N, Padbury JF, Singh BN:Effects of amiodarone and desethylamiodarone on rabbit myocardial beta-adrenorecptors and serum thyroid hormones— Absence of relationship to serum and myocardial drug concentrations. *J Cardiovasc Pharmacol* 8:989, 1986.)

observations of Nokin et al.[28] also are of interest in that they showed that both pretreatment with propranolol as well as with amiodarone abolished the increases in beta-receptor density induced by myocardial ischemia following coronary artery ligation. The effects of amiodarone on adrenergic receptors are similar in different animal species. For example, Sharma et al.,[29] who studied the effects of chronic (6 weeks) oral amiodarone administration to cats on beta- and alpha-receptor density in ventricular muscle, found no effect on alpha-receptor density but the drug produced a significant reduction in beta-receptor density without a change in receptor affinity. The reason for the dissociated effect of amiodarone on alpha and beta receptors as determined by radio-ligand binding is unclear at present especially in light of the fact that in in vitro systems noncompetitive effects against alpha- and beta-adrenergic receptors have been demonstrated.[11] Gagnol et al.[31]

also have found that, in rat heart membrane preparations, amiodarone noncompetitively antagonized the activation of adenylate cyclase by isoproterenol, glucagon, and secretin but not by sodium fluoride. The authors suggested that the noncompetitive beta-antagonistic properties of amiodarone might be due to the inhibition of the coupling of beta receptors with the regulatory unit of the adenylate cyclase complex and /or to a decrease in the number of functional beta receptors at the surface of the myocardial cell. The net result in vivo is the attenuation of the positive chronotropic actions of catecholamines,[31] a property of obvious significance in mediating the antiarrhythmic and antiischemic effects of the compound.

The fact that bradycardia during chronic amiodarone therapy develops as a function of time is consistent with the data of Vankatesh et al.,[30] indicating a gradual decrease in the number of beta receptors. In part, this may be due to the additive effect of the metabolite during chronic drug administration. This also may be explained on the basis of a secondary consequence of selective hypothyroidism induced by amiodarone.[13,14,30] It is known that a significant decrease in the density of myocardial beta-andrenoceptors occurs in hypothyroidism, and the converse in hyperthyroidism.[32] The changes in cardiac rate and rhythm during altered thyroid state therefore in part may be due to the associated alteration in the adrenergic state.[30,32] Thus, if the principal mechanism of action of amiodarone were a selective inhibition of $T_3$ action on cardiac muscle, the marked reduction in beta-receptor density in cardiac muscle following chronic amiodarone treatment in part may be due to the drug-induced myocardial hypothyroid state (discussed later). The observations of Bacq et al.,[33] on the effects of amiodarone on neurotransmitter overflow from the spleen induced by electrical stimulation of the splenic nerve, suggest that the drug also might exert a significant adrenergic blocking action at high drug concentrations. However, at present, the significance of such an effect on the net pharmacologic action of the drug is unclear.

## Electrophysiologic Effects of Amiodarone

When the action of amiodarone on cardiac muscle is considered, a number of features of its pharmacology appears to be of importance. First, the drug is not soluble in the usual physiologic media; thus, superfusion studies in isolated cardiac tissues can be undertaken only in homologous plasma or blood or in an especially modified extracellular environment.[34,35] Second,when the drug is given intravenously to experimental animals and to humans, the electrophysiologic effects are much less striking than those noted after the chronic administration at a constant dose over long periods of time.[36-37,38] An explanation for the delayed onset of the action of the drug thus appears crucial to a better understanding of its actions in the control of cardiac arrhythmias. Third, the elimination half-life of amiodarone is extremely long and variable[39-40,41] and the steady-state effect of the compound can not be predicted simply on the basis of the plasma and tissue drug levels of the parent compound or its active metabolite, desethylamiodarone.[42,43] For these reasons, the acute and the chronic effects of amiodarone and its metabolite need to be differentiated. Fourth, the interpretation of its effects need to allow for the fact that the compound is an iodinated molecule with a complex interrelationship with the metabolism of the thyroid hormone to which it bears a structural resemblance (Fig. 1). There are features of the drug's electrophysiologic actions that closely resemble those of hypothyroid cardiac muscle and are prevented by the administration of relatively small amounts of thyroxine. Finally, amiodarone is a coronary vasodilator[44] exhibiting a significant interaction with the autonomic nervous system, which may be of importance in mediating the overall pharmacologic and electrophysiologic effects of the compound in controlling cardiac arrhythmias. These various aspects of drug action will be considered further in this chapter. The coronary and systemic hemodynamic and the pharmacokinetic effects will not be discussed as they have been presented elsewhere in this book.

## Early Electrophysiologic Observations

In the first reported studies,[18] amiodarone was given 20 mg/kg intraperitoneally (as a 5 percent aqueous solution) for 1–6 weeks to rabbits from which atria and ventricular tissues were removed and cellular electrophysiology studied by the standard microelectrode technique. The drug had no significant effect on the resting membrane potential or the action potential amplitude in either tissue; it produced about a 10 percent reduction in the $V_{max}$ at a stimulus frequency 10 percent above the spontaneous frequency of the sinus node in the case of the atria and at 1 Hz in the case of the ventricular fibers. The major effect was a considerable prolongation of the action potential duration in both atrial and ventricular tissue (Fig. 4). Thus, by inference, the voltage-dependent effective refractory period was also prolonged. As far as the effects of amiodarone in the atrial muscle were concerned, they bore a striking resemblance to those induced by thyroid gland ablation in the rabbit.[45] Two other features of importance were noted. First, the effect of the drug on the action potential duration was slow in onset and continued to increase in a stepwise manner as a function of time on a *constant* daily dose. For example, at a daily intraperitoneal dose of 20 mg/kg of amiodarone in the rabbit, it

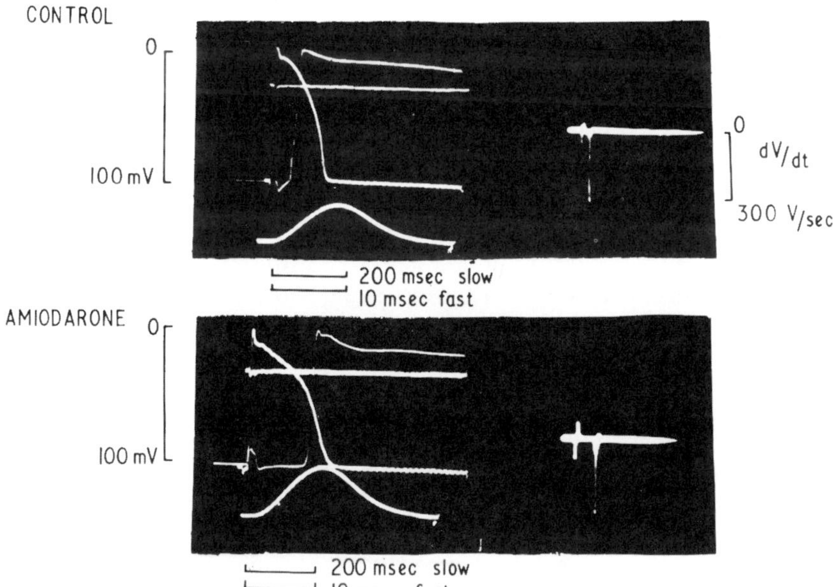



**Figure 4.** The effects of chronic amiodarone administration on the characteristics of transmembrane potentials in rabbit ventricular myocardium. The upper panel shows a typical recording from the ventricular muscle of a control rabbit, the lower from one treated with amiodarone 20 mg/kg intraperitoneally for 6 weeks. In each panel, the upper trace represents zero potential; the middle trace, the transmembrane potential at slow and fast sweep speeds. In the right upper trace is shown the extracellular electrogram and in the lower trace, the differentiated signal of the rate of rise of phase 0 of the action potential. Note that the major effect of the drug was to increase the time course of repolarization (and, by inference, the effective refractory period) with a minimal effect on the upstroke velocity of phase 0. (From Singh BN, Vaughan Williams EM: The effect of amiodarone, a new antianginal drug, on cardiac muscle. *Br J Pharmacol* 39:657, 1970. By permission of the journal.)

was found that the ventricular action potential increased by 11 percent after 1 week, 23 percent after 3 weeks, and 30 percent after 6 weeks of drug administration. Second, 5 μg of thyroxine given daily at the same time as amiodarone for the last 3 weeks of the 6-week drug administration period precluded the expected development of the action potential lengthening effected by the drug alone. Moreover, the administration of iodine as potassium iodide in amounts equivalent to those contained in the daily amiodarone dose used in these experiments did not produce changes similar to those induced by the drug. It therefore was postulated that the actions of chronically administered amiodarone may have been mediated through a depressant effect on thyroxine-dependent pathways.

## Subsequent Electrophysiologic Observations: Significance of Acute Superfusion and Allied Studies

A number of studies[35,46–49] in recent years have further enlarged our understanding of the actions of amiodarone in various cardiac tissues. The salient findings are discussed.

### Amiodarone and Slow Channel Potentials

In the sinus node preparations of the isolated rabbit atria superfused with amiodarone, Goupil and Lenfant[50] reported significant drug-induced decreases in the action potential amplitude, the maximal diastolic potential, and the slope of phase 4 of pacemaker potentials. That amiodarone does decrease phase 4 depolarization in the SA node and reduce the amplitude of the pacemaker potentials in the rabbit sinoatrial node (Fig. 5) was recently confirmed by Yabek et al.[35] In their study, the sinus cycle length was lenghtened significantly by amiodarone as well as desethylamiodarone.

A recent study[49] in which amiodarone was injected directly into the sinus and AV nodal arteries has raised the possibility that the drug also might act by inhibiting the slow-channel in nodal tissues. It is thus conceivable that the drug's acute effects[36] to a significant extent may be mediated via its antiadrenergic (discussed later) and calcium antagonistic actions in the SA and AV nodes. These effects are consistent with the marked decreases in sinus cycle length by the depression of phase 4 depolarization noted in the studies reported by Yabek et al.[35] as well as in those

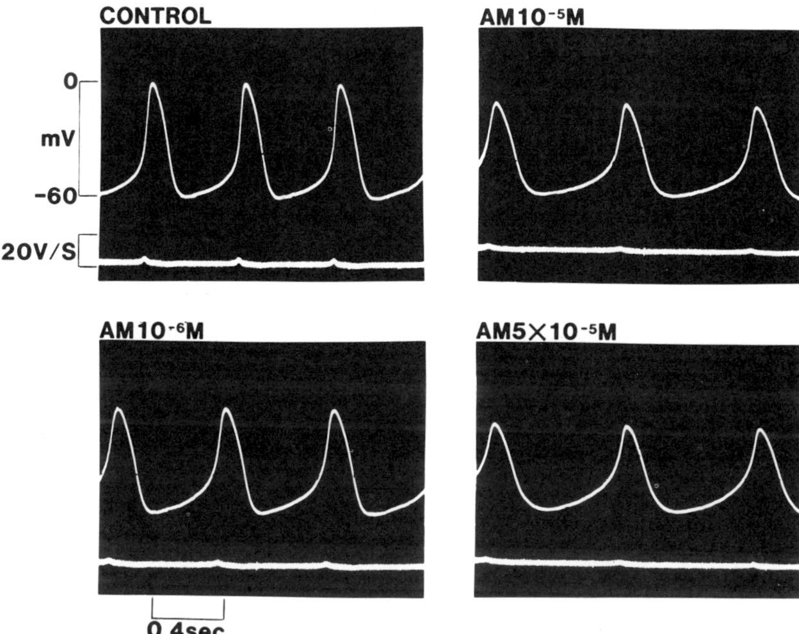



**Figure 5.** The effects of increasing amiodarone concentrations on a single dominant sinus node pacemaker cell action potential. The preparation is discharging spontaneously. In this and all subsequent illustrations of intracellular recordings the lower trace shows the phase 0 (upstroke) $V_{max}$. Voltage and time calibrations are the same for each illustration in the figure. (From Yabek S, Kato R, Singh BN: Acute electrophysiologic effects of amiodarone and desethylamiodarone in isolated cardiac muscle. *J Cardiovasc Pharmacol* 8:197, 1986. By permission of the authors and of the journal.)

of Goupil and Lenfant.[50] It also is conceivable that the slow channel blocking action may be the basis for impaired myocardial contractility evident with the intravenous drug in high doses (see Chapter 5).

*Amiodarone Effects on Fast Channel Potentials*

The studies of Yabek et al.[35] also have focused on defining the effects of amiodarone and its metabolite on the electrophysiologic parameters of other cardiac tissues during acute superfusion studies. Over a range of concentrations, $10^{-6}$ to $5 \times 10^{-5}$M (0.68–34 μg/ml), both amiodarone and desethylamiodarone dissolved in appropriate superfusion media exerted distinct but quantitatively and qualitatively similar electrophysiologic actions in isolated canine and rabbit cardiac muscle. At 1.0 Hz stimulus frequency, neither drug had a significant effect on action potential amplitude, overshoot, upstroke velocity of phase 0 or the resting membrane potential of rabbit atria, canine ventricular muscle, or Purkinje fibers even at the highest drug concentration (34 μg/ml). Modest increases in the action potential durations at 50 percent and 90 percent repolarization times ($APD_{50}$) and ($APD_{90}$) and in the effective refractory period (ERP), however, occurred in the ventricle (Fig. 6); in the atria these changes were less marked. A lack of change in the ratio of $APD_{90}$/ERP indicated that the change in the ERP essentially was due to a voltage-dependent mechanism. An unexpected finding reported by Yabek et al.[35] was that both amiodarone and its metabolite significantly *decreased* $APD_{90}$ and *shortened* the ERP, especially at the higher concentrations (Fig. 7). In the case of amiodarone, similar observations have previously been made by Aomine et al.[48] It is noteworthy that the shortening of the Purkinje fiber ERP was accompanied by a lengthening of the ERP in ventricular muscle. The ERP in the Purkinje fiber normally is longer than that in the ventricular muscle. Therefore, the observed differential effect of amiodarone and its metabolite on the voltage-dependent changes in the ERP may contribute to an overall electrical stability in the heart and constitute an antiarrhythmic mechanism.[35] The possibility must be considered that such an effect might mediate, at least in part, the acute antiarrhythmic actions of the compound. However, it must be emphasized that it is not known whether such a differential effect on repolarization also is induced by the drug during chronic administration.

*Effects on Fast Sodium Channel Kinetics and Use Dependency*

Singh and Vaughan Williams[18] reported that in rabbits treated chronically with amiodarone $V_{max}$ was reduced only by about 10 percent. Although such an effect was not felt to be significant, recent data have suggested that the overall mignitude of the effect may vary with animal species used, the concentrations of the drug and its metabolite that are tested, and the route of drug administration. The depressant effect of amiodarone has been most striking as a function of stimulation frequency[46] and in depolarized myocardial fibers.[47] During superfusion studies involving the left atrial free wall, amiodarone produced a slow development of concentration-dependent prolongation of the action potential duration; this was accompanied by a significant decrease in $V_{max}$ re-

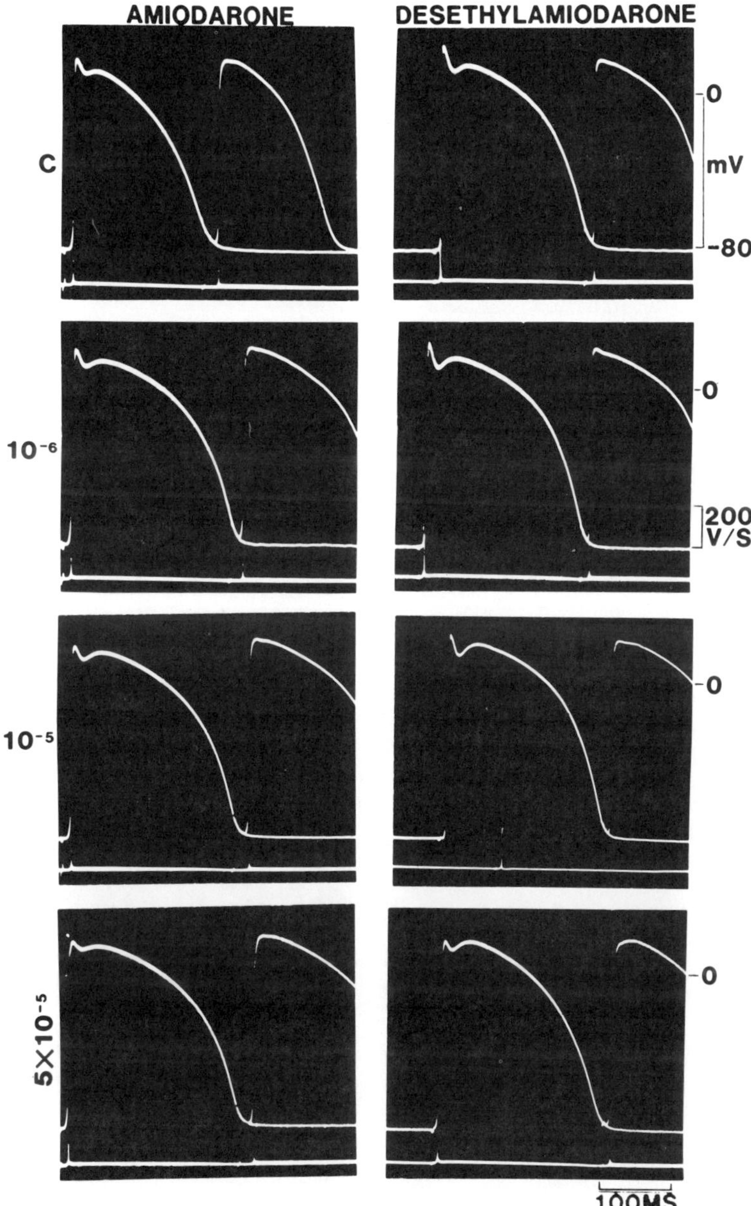



**Figure 6**. Effects of increasing concentrations of amiodarone and desethyl-amiodarone on ventricular myocardial action potentials. For each drug, the various action potentials were obtained from a single myocardial cell. Voltage and time calibrations are the same for each illustration. (From Yabek S, Kato R, Singh BN: Acute electrophysiologic effects of amiodarone and desethylamiodarone in isolated cardiac muscle. *J Cardiovasc Pharmacol* 8:197, 1986. By permission of the authors and of the journal.)

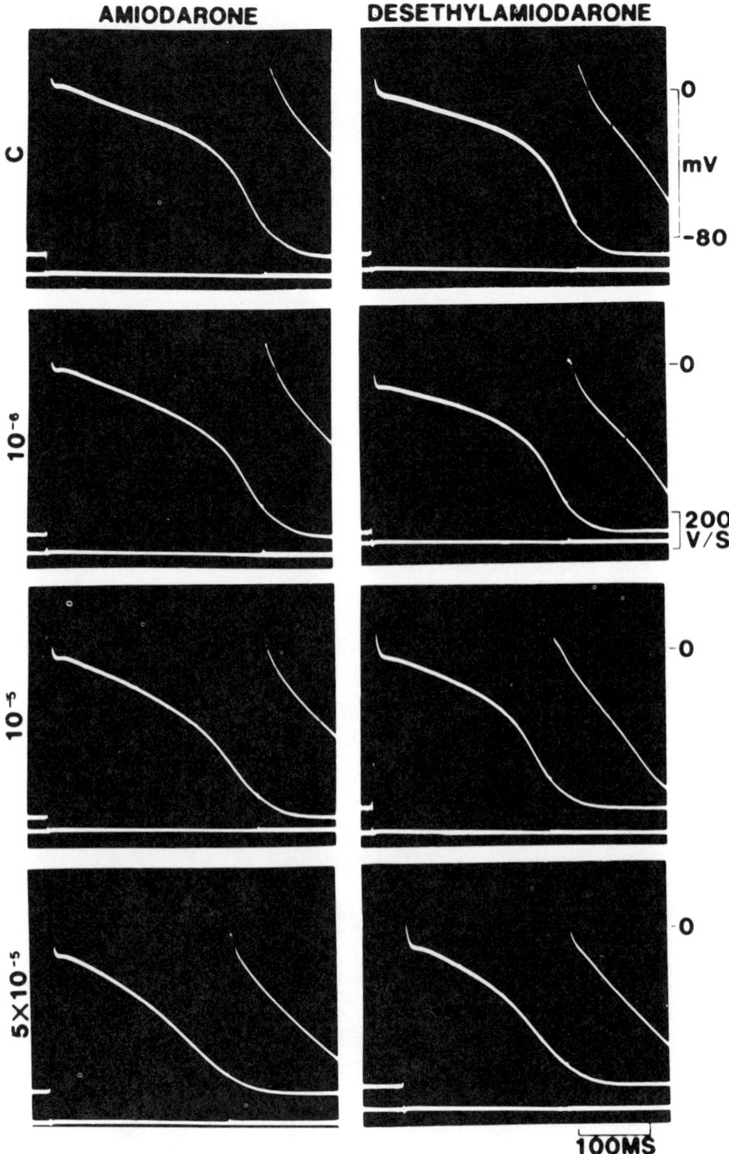



**Figure 7.** Results from a typical experiment showing the effects of increasing amiodarone and desethylamiodarone concentrations on Purkinje fiber action potentials. For each drug, the four action potentials were obtained from a single Purkinje fiber cell. Voltage and time calibrations are the same for each panel. The onset of the second action potential marks the end of the effective refractory period. (From Yabek S, Kato R, Singh BN: Acute electrophysiologic effects of amiodarone and desethylamiodarone in isolated cardiac muscle. *J Cardiovasc Pharmacol* 8:197, 1986. By permission of the authors and of the journal.)

flecting an inhibitory effect on the fast sodium channel as has been reported in the case of nerve fibers.[51] Yabek et al.[35] found a significant rate-dependent block of $V_{max}$ in canine Purkinje fibers and ventricular muscle at a concentration of 34 μg/ml of amiodarone and desethylamiodarone.

Of particular interest are the findings of Mason et al.[46,47] who, during voltage clamp studies, showed that high concentrations of amiodarone (over 50 μg/ml) exerted a rate-dependent depressant effect on the inactivated fast Na channels both in guinea pig myocardial fibers acutely superfused with amiodarone and in similar fibers removed from animals chronically treated with the drug over a period of 28 days. Amiodarone had a particular affinity for inactivated sodium channels and had a marked effect on the recovery kinetics of inactivation. For example, under drug-free conditions and at normal resting membrane potentials, recovery from inactivation was usually complete in 10 milliseconds.[47] Under the influence of amiodarone,the partial recovery of $V_{max}$ occurred rapidly, but a considerable fraction tended to recover slowly. This slow component of recovery at -80 to -90mV, had a time constant of about 163 milliseconds. Thus, their data indicated that the use-dependent block of $V_{max}$ induced by amiodarone developed during inactivation and recovered during rest. The data from Mason et al.[47] also are of interest in so far as they showed that the drug lengthened the action potential duration both acutely and after chronic drug administration; it also reduced or prevented the occurrence of depolarization-induced automaticity.

## Ionic Correlates of the Electrophysiologic Effects of Amiodarone

Although the effects of amiodarone on the gross parameters of cardiac action potential now are delineated reasonably well in acute superfusion studies and after chronic drug administration, there remains a paucity of data on the ionic correlates of these changes. Using the double sucrose gap technique in the frog and the ferret ventricular fibers, Neliat[52] provided further confirmation of the drug's effect in lengthening the action potential duration, in reducing the slope of diastolic depolarization in the atrium and in inhibiting the pacemaker activity in the Purkinje fibers and of the repetitive activity in the atrium. In a further study, Neliat[53] demonstrated that amiodarone had the dominant action in decreasing the delayed outward potassium current consistent with the prolongation of the action potential duration. He also found that high concentrations of the drug depressed inward currents retarding the kinetics of reactivation of the fast sodium and the slow calcium currents. Further data however are needed to define the significance of these changes in altering conduction and refractoriness in cardiac muscle relative to the mechanisms of control of cardiac arrhythmias. The delineation of the ionic mechanisms mediating the acute and the chronic repolarization changes relative to those in refractoriness are likely to be of crucial importance in providing further insights into the nature of amiodarone action.

### Electrophysiologic Effects of Amiodarone Following Chronic Administration

The acute superfusion effects with amiodarone and its metabolite, although modest with respect to repolarization, have been found to be no greater at the higher drug concentrations than at the lower ones. It appears that despite very high concentrations of amiodarone, a finite duration of exposure of the myocardium to the drug on a chronic basis is necessary for the full expression of the electrophysiologic effects. The most striking and consistent electrophysiologic effects of amiodarone occur when the drug is administered chronically, as originally reported.[18] These effects have now been shown[38] to occur in atria, sinus node fibers, AV nodal fibers, and in ventricular tissues (Fig. 8). The chronic effects in Purkinje fibers have not been defined clearly. The nature of the stepwise increase in the intensity of the effect as a function of time remains uncertain. Investigations have been undertaken to determine whether the phenomenon of the delayed onset of drug action is due to the formation of the active metabolite or to the slow build-up of amiodarone in the tissues or the myocardial membranes. Neither possibility is well supported by experimental data.

### Significance of the Activity of Desethylamiodarone

It has been found that although the metabolite (desethylamiodarone) is active, having qualitatively the same pharmacodynamic profile, its action is not immediate (discussed later). The drug has the propensity to reduce beta adrenoceptors after acute as well as chronic administration,[28] to alter thyroid hormone metabolism after chronic administration,[54] and to interact pharmacokinetically with cardiac glycosides.[55] As in the case of the parent compound, the metabolite appears to influence electrophysiologic parameters as a function of time and its elimination half-life

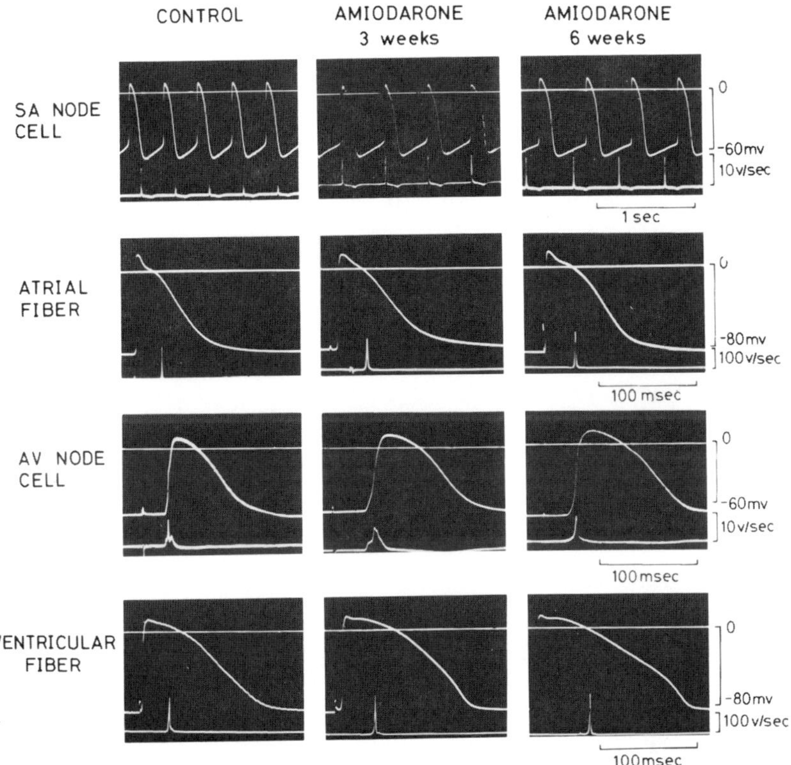



**Figure 8.** Effects of chronic administration of amiodarone on various types of cardiac action potentials in the rabbit heart compared to representative control recordings. Note the stepwise increase in repolarization time as a function of time on a constant daily dose. (From Ikeda N, Nademanee K, Kannan R, et al: Electrophysiologic effects of amiodarone: Experimental and clinical observations relative to serum and tissue concentrations. *Am Heart J* 108:890, 1984. By permission of the authors and of the American Heart Association.)

is longer than that of amiodarone.[56] Thus, whereas the activity of the metabolite will be additive to that of the parent compound during chronic administration, the delay in the onset of amiodarone action cannot be attributed solely to the effects of desethylamiodarone.

*Significance of Myocardial and Sarcolemmal Amiodarone Concentrations*

The more pronounced pharmacologic efficacy of amiodarone following chronic administration, despite low plasma drug concentrations and the lesser effects of the drug after acute intravenous administration, when drug levels are maximum has not been explained on the basis of the pharmacokinetic behavior of the drug. The recent studies of Vankatesh et al.[57] have shown that the stepwise increase in cardiac repolarization as a function of time is not related to the rate of accumulation of amiodarone in myocardial tisues or in the sarcolemmal preparations (Fig. 9). Data obtained from the transmembrane action potential recordings from rabbit ventricular myocardium were correlated with drug concentrations in the serum, myocardium, and myocardial sarcolemma following acute intravenous drug administration and after 4 weeks oral administration of 20 mg/kg/day amiodarone. Following the 15 minutes of acute drug administration when amiodarone concentrations were maximal in the serum ($4.72 \pm 1.23$ μg/ml), cardiac mus-

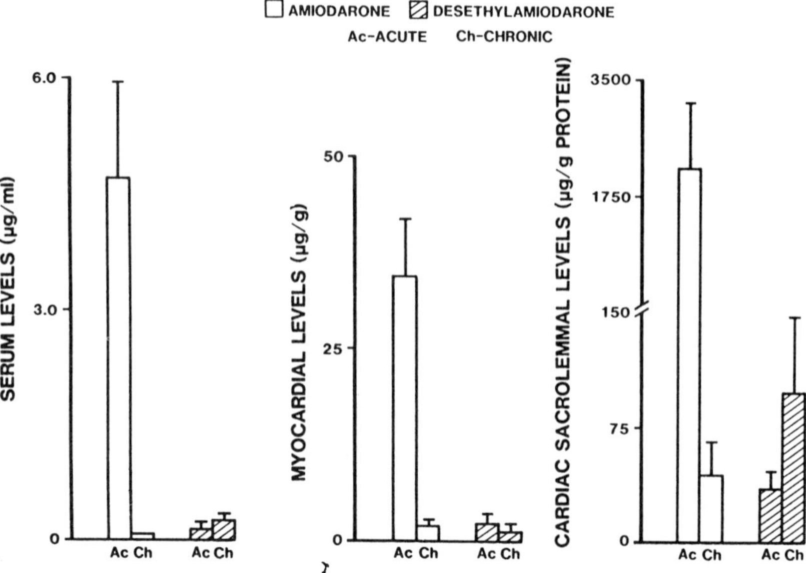


**Figure 9.** Concentrations of amiodarone and desethylamiodarone in the serum, myocardium, and ventricular sarcolemmal preparations. Note the significant reduction in the concentrations of amiodarone following chronic (Ch) treatment in all of the tissues analyzed and the levels of desethylamiodarone in the serum and sarcolemma following chronic therapyy; p<0.0001. Ac-acute. (From Vankatesh N, Somani P, Berhson M, et al: Electropharmacology of amiodarone: Absence of relationship to serum myocardial and cardiac sarcolemmal membrane drug concentrations. *Am Heart J* 112:916, 1986. By permission of the authors and of American Heart Association.)

cle (34.5±7.6 μg/g) and sarcolemma (1.94 mg/g protein), the electrophysiologic changes were insignificant. However, following chronic treatment when the levels of amiodarone were low in the serum (0.05±0.01 μg/ml amiodarone, 0.25±0.08 μg/ml of desethylamiodarone), cardiac muscle (1.91±0.9 μg/g amiodarone, 1.35±1.33 μg/g of desethylamiodarone,) and the myocardial membranes (0.043 mg/g protein of amiodarone, 0.097 mg/g protein of amiodarone, 0.097 mg/g protein of desethylamiodarone), there was a 54.3 percent increase in action potential duration at 90 percent repolarization (p<0.01) and 65 percent increase in the effective refractory period (p<0.01) of rabbit ventricular myocardium. These data are further supported by the observations of Lambert et al.,[42] who found that the increases in the ventricular effective refractory period as a function of time were dissociated from the tissue or serum concentrations of amiodarone as well as from the myocardial disposition of the metabolite. It is also noteworthy that Patterson et al.[58] recently showed (Figs. 10 and 11) that such differences between the acute and chronic dosing of amiodarone in their experimental canine model of sudden death could not be accounted for by lower serum and tissue levels of amiodarone following acute drug administration. Thus, the magnitude of the electrophysiologic and antiarrhythmic effects induced by amiodarone are not explained by the pharmacokinetics of the drug, but probably are related to the drug-induced changes in cellular metabolism. A finite duration of exposure of the myocardium to the drug on a chronic basis appears necessary for the maximal steady state electrophysiologic effects to become established.

## Amiodarone Action and Metabolism of Thyroid Hormones

Aspects of this issue have been discussed elsewhere in this book. See Chapter 15. Here, only the electrophysiologic interactions in the myocardium are presented. It has been emphasized repeatedly that the electrophysiologic changes induced by amiodarone following chronic drug administration closely resemble those produced by thyroid gland ablation.[44,59−61] Such an effect is not due to the iodine contained in the amiodarone molecule, since the administration of iodine alone in doses equivalent to those contained in the effective dose of amiodarone had no significant effect on the time course of atrial action potentials.[18] On the other hand, the concomitant administration of amiodarone and thyroid hormone

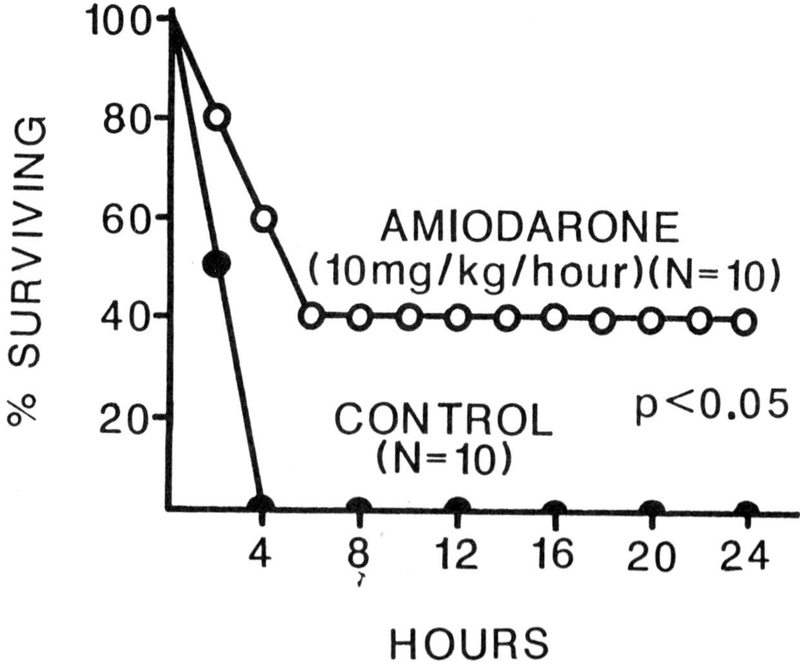


**Figure 10.** Survival in conscious canine preparation of sudden coronary death after short-term intravenous amiodarone administration. Cumulative survival curves are shown for control and intravenous amiodarone groups. Survival was by intravenous amiodarone significantly increased (pp<0.05). (From Patterson E, Eller BT, Abrams GD, et al: Ventricular fibrillation in conscious canine preparations of sudden coronary death. Prevention by short- and long-term amiodarone administration. *Circulation* 68:85, 1983. By permission of the authors and of the American Heart Association.)

prevented the development of repolarization changes evident after amiodarone alone.[18] These observations raised the possibility that the fundamental electrophysiologic effect of amiodarone at least in part may be mediated by the selective blockade of $T_3$ action on cardiac muscle[62-65] as the inhibition of the peripheral conversion of $T_4$ and $T_3$ resulting in a decrease of $T_3$, an increase in $rT_3$, and a minimal increase in $T_4$ in the plasma[54] due to the blockade of 5'-monodeiodinase[66] could account for the observed elctrophysiologic changes. Thus, a direct inhibition of $T_3$ nuclear binding by amiodarone or its metabolite desethylamiodarone[67,68] has been postulated to result in a hypothyroid state at a cellular level.[69,70] Since the electrophysiologic effects of hypothyroidism[44,59-61] on repolarization are nearly identical to those observed after long-

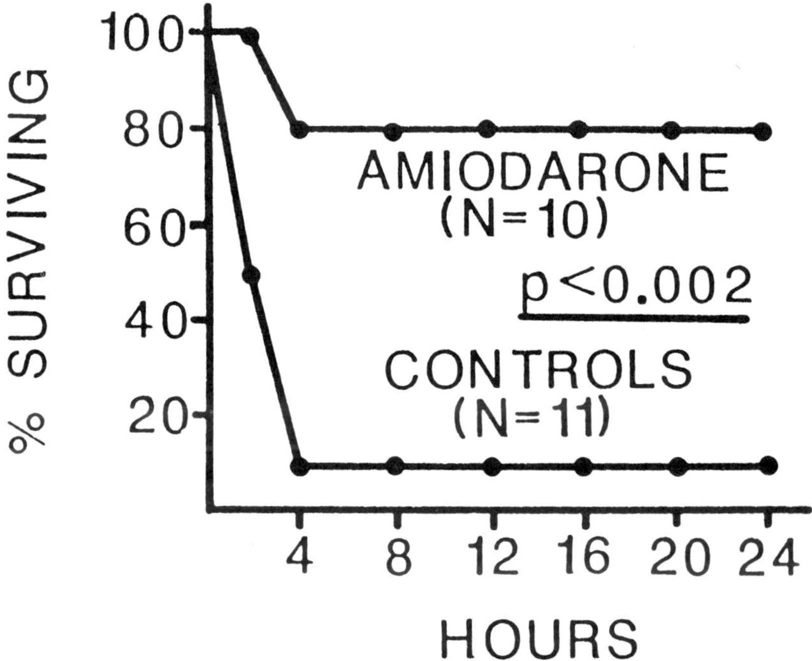


**Figure 11.** Survival curves for conscious canine preparation of sudden coronary death after long-term amiodarone. Cumulative survival curves for control and amiodarone-treated animals are shown. Amiodarone-treated animals received 10 mg/kg/day oral drug for 24 days before intimal stimulation of the left circumflex coronary artery on day 28 after anterior myocardial infarction. Survival was increased significantly (p<0.002) by amiodarone treatment. (From Patterson E, Eller BT, Abram GD, et al: Ventricular fibrillation in conscious canine preparation of sudden coronary death. Prevention by short- and long-term amiodarone administration. *Circulation* 68:857, 1983. By permission of the authors and of the American Heart Association.)

term amiodarone treatment, this phenomenon has been thought to exhibit some cardiospecificity.[18,69,70] Currently available data indicate that such a possibility remains a tenable hypothesis that, if vindicated, may have far-reaching theoretical and practical implications.

## Amiodarone–Membrane Lipid Interactions and Effects on Membrane Fluidity

Amioadrone is a complex molecule with a large, nonpolar hydrophobic moiety and a small hydrophilic side chain. This amphiphilic nature confers on the drug the propensity to alter lipid metabolism of the myocardium. For example, Gross and Somani[71] have shown that amiodarone alters the lipid metabolism of the cardiac cell as evidenced by the development of lysosomal and myelinoid inclusion bodies. From the standpoint of the drug's electropharmacologic actions, its effects on the membrane lipid dynamics are of more direct relevance, however. Chatelain[72] determined the in vitro effects of amiodarone on lipid dynamics using the fluorescent probe DPH in the erythrocyte ghost,[72] the brain synaptic membrane,[73] and the multilamellar vesicles synthesized from neutral phospholipids.[74] In both preparations, incubation with an increasing concentration of amodarone led to a significant decrease in membrane fluidity. Whether this is the basis for the known electrophysiologic actions of amiodarone remains to be determined. It clearly will be of interest to determine whether a decrease in membrane fluidity occurs in hypothyroid tissues.

It also should be emphasized that experimental data indicate the effects of amiodarone at the level of membrane proteins. For example, it has been found that the drug selectively inhibits the $Na^+/K^+$ ATPase of the guinea-pig myocardial particulate fraction;[75] its interaction with beta-adrenergic receptors has been well defined, as has its inhibitory effects on the adenylate cyclase activity.[29] However, the available data on the alterations produced by amiodarone in biological membranes must be regarded as preliminary, and further work is necessary to delineate the significance of the observed effects in mediating the compound's electrophysiologic and antiarrhythmic actions.

## In Vivo Electrophysiologic Effects of Amiodarone

### Experimental Observations

Chronic therapy with excellent control of arrhythmias[5,76] in humans has been associated with plasma amiodarone levels of $1-3$ µg/ml with slightly lower levels of desethylamiodarone. As indicated earlier, in acute in vitro experiments, concentrations up to 34 µg/ml of amiodarone and of the metabolite had considerably less effect on repolarization or refractoriness than when the drug was administered on a chronic basis.[8] This is consistent with little or no effect on ventricular refractoriness in unanesthetized patients following acute intravenous drug (5 mg/kg) administration[36,38,77,78] despite plasma levels often exceeding 10 µg/ml.[38]

There now are increasing data that suggest that the overall effects in anesthetized animals and in humans may differ as the extracardiac or other associated pharmacologic actions of the compound may influence the net effects under these circumstances. For example, in *anesthetized* animals, intravenous amiodarone in doses up to 10 mg/kg has been reported to increase the ventricular effective refractory period by 30 percent[79] in the absence of a significant increase in the $QT_c$ interval, as noted in another study.[44] Jaillon et al.[80] showed that in pentobarbital-anesthetized animals, intravenous amiodarone (1.25–10 mg/kg) produced a dose-related decrease in heart rate and prolonged the sinus node recovery time while having no effect on His-Purkinje conduction time. There were modest increases in the atrial and ventricular effective refractory periods with a marked decrease in the atrioventricular nodal conduction. Similar results have been reported by others[79,81] in adult as well as neonatal dogs. In the latter, the effects of amiodarone have been found to be less striking, consistent with the findings of Yabek et al.[82] in acute superfusion studies. The overall observations suggest that the reported variable and modest antiarrhythmic actions of acutely administered amiodarone[77,78] in part may be due to the noncompetitive alpha- and beta-adrenergic receptor antagonism.[11,12] The inhibitory actions on alpha-and beta-receptors are known to be associated with distinct electrophysiologic effects,[83,84] which may contribute to the observed effects of amiodarone during intravenous injections. Such effects thus are likely to be most pronounced in anesthetized animals or man.

## Clinical Electrophysiologic Effects

The experimental and clinical data emphasize that the maximal or steady-state effects with amiodarone in cardiac muscle do not become apparent acutely, despite extremely high drug concentrations. This is reflected in the marked differences found between the effects of acute intravenous versus chronic oral drug therapy. For example, following intravenous amiodarone administration the electrophysiologic effects are much less striking.[36–38] The main acute effect is the lengthening of AV nodal refractoriness and intranodal conduction (AH interval) time[36–38,78,79] with minimal effect on the effective refractory periods of the atrial, the ventricular, the bypass tract or the His-Purkinje tissue when the drug is administered in a dose of 5 mg/kg body weight. There is no significant effect on the HV or QRS intervals nor the $QT_c$ duration.

The acute effect on the atrioventricular node may be due to the blockade of the slow channels[49] and/or the noncompetitive adrenergic antagonism exerted by the drug.[11,12,28] At somewhat higher doses (10 mg/kg) intravenous amiodarone has been shown to increase the ventricular effective refractory period by 20–30 milliseconds and some lengthening of the QRS duration at fast stimulus frequencies consistent with a use-dependent effect on fast sodium channels.[36] Despite the well-documented in vitro depressant effects of amiodarone on sinus node automaticity, intravenous amiodarone in conscious humans does not produce the expected reduction in heart rate,[36–38] presumably due to the opposing effects of sympathetic activation resulting from the peripheral vasodilator actions of the drug.[13,14]

In contrast, when administered chronically, amiodarone predictably lengthens repolarization ($QT_c$) and refractoriness in most cardiac tissues as a function of time with little or no change in the QRS duration and a modest increase in the HV interval with a significant prolongation of the AH interval.[5,85–87] As far as the effects on repolarization are concerned, they are consistent with those previously noted with studies in rabbits chronically treated with amiodarone. For example, 20 mg/kg of amiodarone[18] increased the ventricular action potential by 11 percent at 1 week, 23 percent at 3 weeks, and 30 percent after 6 weeks of drug administration. This is consistent with the prolongation of the monophasic action potentials in experimental animals.[88] In humans[89] after 6 weeks of oral treatment with amiodarone, the duration of the monophasic action potentials recorded by suction electrodes in atria also was increased by about 30 percent (Fig. 12). These observations are concordant with the observation that the $QT_c$ interval in humans increased in a stepwise fashion on a constant dose of amiodarone, reaching what appeared to be a steady-state effect after 6 weeks.[62]

After chronic treatment in humans, there is a marked increase in the effective and the functional refractory periods in most cardiac tissues (atria, ventricles, AV node, His-Purkinje system, accessory tracts of the heart) as a function of time with little or no change in the QRS duration and a modest increase in the HV interval.[36,37] An increase in the QRS duration however does occur[36] as do increases in the infranodal conduction (anterograde or retrograde) following fast stimulation frequencies, again reflecting effects on the fast sodium channel.[90] It is clear that the overall electrophysiologic changes, which are accompanied by a stepwise

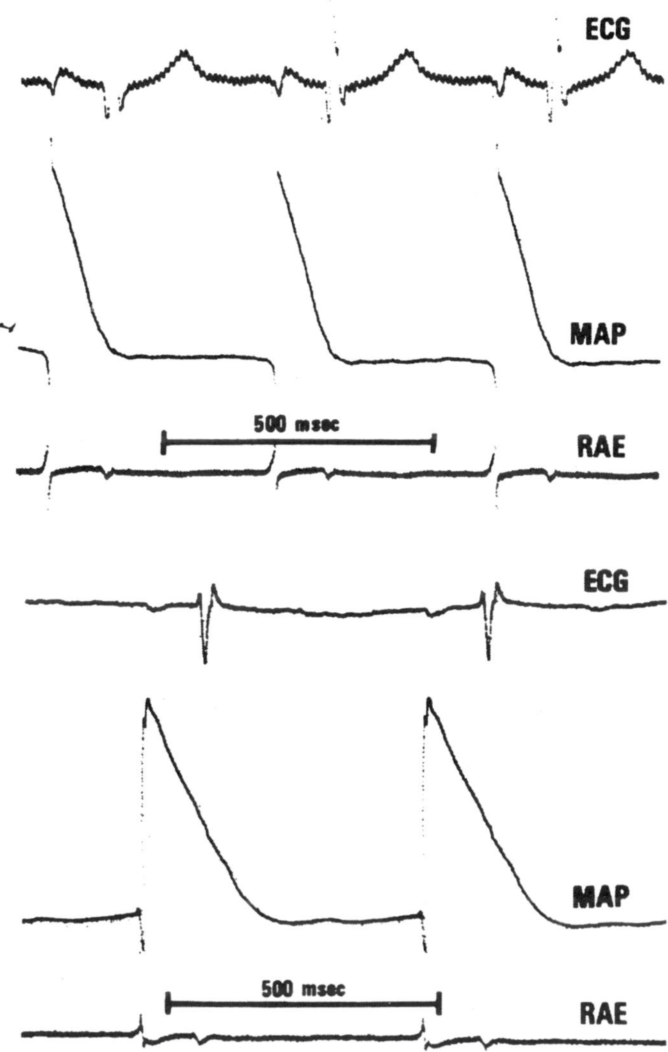


**Figure 12.** Monophasic action potentials recorded by the suction electrode technique in patients before and after 6 weeks of treatment with amiodarone (600 mg/day). The tracings were obtained from the catheter placed in the right atrium and simultaneous recordings of the surface EKG were taken. Note that amiodarone slowed the heart rate and lengthened the $QT_c$ interval of the surface EKG coincident with the lengthening of the monophasic action potential duration. (From Olson B, Brorson L, Varnauskas E: Class III antiarrhythmic action in man: Observations from monophasic action potential recordings and amiodarone treatment. *Br Heart J* 35:1255, 1973. By permission of the authors and of the journal.)

decrease in heart rate, are significantly greater during chronic therapy than after acute intravenous administration. There is now substantial evidence that such a difference, also noted in animals, is not accountable in terms of differences in serum drug concentrations.

These compounds exert significant but quantitatively and qualitatively similar acute electrophysiologic effects in isolated cardiac muscle. However, unlike the effects during chronic therapy, which are dominated by a marked lengthening of the action potential duration, those after acute superfusion with these drugs are associated with less striking alterations in repolarization and refractoriness despite extremely high drug concentrations. These differences are consistent with the observations that the overall electrophysiologic effects of intravenously administered amiodarone in humans differ from those found after long-term chronic drug administration. On the other hand, the potency of desethylamiodarone was no greater than that of amiodarone in terms of the electrophysiologic effects, which indicates that the known latency of the onset of the antiarrhythmic actions of amiodarone is unlikely to be due solely to the formation of the metabolite. The depressant effect of amiodarone on the characteristics of the sinus node potentials suggest that the drug might exert an acute calcium antagonistic and antiadrenergic effect, the summation of which might be of particular significance in the AV node. Finally, the fact that amiodarone exerted a marked use-dependent effect on $V_{max}$ in isolated cardiac muscle suggests the possiblity of a significant beneficial acute effect on conduction and refractoriness during rapid tacharrhythmias. However, whatever might be the clinical significance of these overall direct and indirect electrophysiologic effects of amiodarone, they require a careful comparison of the antiarrhythmic actions of the intravenously and chronically administered drug.

## Effects of Amiodarone in Experimental Arrhythmias

The antiarrhythmic effects of amiodarone now has been demonstrated in a wide variety of eperimentally induced cardiac arrhythmias. As might be predicted from the electrophysiologic actions, the antiarrhythmic effects of acute intravenous doses versus chronic oral dosing of amiodarone differ significantly. For example, in ventricular fibrillation produced by chloroform inhalation or calcium chloride administration in mice or rats, the effects of intravenous amiodarone were found to be weak.[17] However, high doses of the drug were found to be effective in suppressing ventricular tachyarrhythmias produced by aconitine hydrochloride in the rat and dog.[17,18] It also has been reported that the intravenous drug may be effective in the suppression of multifocal premature ventricular ectopic beats produced by the injections of epinephrine and barium chloride in the anesthetized dogs and rabbits. Pretreatment with amiodarone of anesthetized guinea-pigs also has been reported to increase the dose of intravenous infusion of ouabain required to produce ventricular fibrillation due to glycoside intoxication.[18]

A number of studies have emphasized the antifibrillatory effects of acutely and chronically administered amiodarone in a variety of experimental models of arrhythmia. For instance, Lubbe et al.[91] reported that pretreatment of rats with amiodarone for 2 minutes to 3 weeks before the hearts were removed and studied as a Langendorff preparation induced a dose-related decrease in the spontaneous heart rate with an increase in the ventricular fibrillation threshold both before and after coronary artery ligation. The drug also reduced the numbers of premature ventricular ectopic beats as well as ventricular tachycardia and fribrillation following coronary artery ligation and reperfusion. The study provided convincing evidence for the protective effects of the compound against the increases in ventricular vulnerability in the early phases following coronary artery occlusion and against reperfusion-induced ventricular fibrillation. These data are consistent with those reported by Schoenfeld,[92] who found 25–50 mg/kg of orally administered amiodarone had a markedly protective effect against both early and late fatal ventricular fibrillation following coronary artery ligation in rats.

The antifibrillatory effects of amiodarone also have been established in a number of experimentally induced models of ischemic arrhythmias in conscious as well as anesthetized animals.[9,58,93] Following coronary ligation in the dog, Rosenbaum et al.[9] found that amiodarone prevented the occurrence of ventricular fibrillation in all 10 pretreated animals given 40 mg/kg oral amiodarone for 1–4 weeks. In contrast, ventricular fibrillation occurred in 7 of 8 untreated animals. The drug also exerted a potent effect on the occurrence of premature ventricular contractions. Chew et al.[93] found that chronic pretreatment with amiodarone for a period of 4 weeks also markedly attenuated the frequency of ventricular arrhythmias following coronary artery ligation in conscious instrumented dogs.

Particularly noteworthy are the data reported by Patterson et al.[58] in a sudden death canine model produced by sequential ligation of coronary arteries. In this model, both short-term and long-term administration of amiodarone reduced the incidence of ventricular fibrillation. In the control series, there was a 91–100 percent (two series) incidence of ventricular fibrillation, 60 percent following short-term intravenous drug administration and only 20 percent following chronic drug administration. The significant differences between the effects of acute and chronic administration of the drug were not accounted for on the basis of differences in the plasma or myocardial tissue levels of amiodarone. The data emphasize the greater efficacy of chronically administered amiodarone as an antifibrillatory agent and indicate its particular role in the prevention of sudden death especially in patients with ischemic heart disease (see Chapter 20). The role in this setting is further supported by the animal data which have suggested a significant cardioprotective action following coronary artery ligation.

## Conclusions on the Potential Antiarrhythmic Mechanisms of Action of Amiodarone

As will be discussed in the other sections of this book, there is little doubt about the potency of amiodarone as a broad-spectrum antiarrhythmic agent for the prophylactic control of most supraventricular and ventricular tachyarrhythmias. Although the most readily measurable correlate of its antiarrhythmic action appears to be its propensity to lengthen the action potential duration in most cardiac tissues (the so-called Class III action), this alone is unlikely to be the sole basis of the drug's extraordinary potency as an antiarrhythmic compound. There are numerous compounds which produce a comparable degree of lengthening of the action potential duration[94,95] but are considerably less potent than amiodarone in the control of arrhythmias. Thus, the question arises as to which of the various electrophysiologic properties discussed in this chapter are the major determinants of the drug's antiarrhythmic potency. For the present, this remains essentially conjectural. It has been indicated that there are major differences between the actions of the acutely administered drug and those following protracted oral administration, the differences not being accountable in terms of serum, tissue, or membrane concentrations of the compound or its active metabolite. The dominant action of the drug is its ability to prolong the cardiac action potential duration, which probably forms the basis of its antifibrillatory effects, undoubtedly modulated by the complex array of its associated pharmacologic properties and its antiischemic potential. The relative significance of the drug's associated effects on the slow channel, the fast channel, alpha- and beta-adrenergic receptors, cholinergic receptors, and adrenergic neurone-blocking actions remain to be determined. The intriguing possibility that the so-called Class III antiarrhythmic action is mediated by the selective interference with the effects of the drug on the cardiac $T_3$ nuclear receptors still constitutes a challenge for experimental verification at the level of cellular and membrane electrophsyiology.

*Acknowledgment:* the research behind this chapter was supported by grants from the Medical Research Service of the Veterans Administration and the American Heart Association, the Greater Los Angeles Affiliate, Los Angeles, California.

# References


1. Rosenbaum MB, Chiale PA, Haedo A, et al: Ten years of experience with amiodarone. *Am Heart J* 106:957, 1983.
2. Heger JJ, Prystowky EN, Jackman WN, et al: Amiodarone: Clinical efficacy and electrophysiology during long term therapy for recurrent ventricular tachycardia or ventricular fibrillation. *N Eng J Med* 305:539, 1981.
3. Nademanee K, Hendrickson J, Kannan R, et al: Antiarrhythmic efficacy and electrophysiologic actions of amiodarone in patients with life-threatening arrhythmias. *Am Heart J* 103:950, 1982.
4. Nademanee K, Hendrickson JA, Cannom DS, et al: Control of refractory life-threatening ventricular arrhythmias by amiodarone. *Am Heart J* 101:759, 1981.
5. Heger JJ, Prystowsky EN, Miles WM, et al: Clinical use and pharmacology of amiodarone. *Med Clin North Am* 68(5):1339, 1984.
6. Nademanee K, Singh BN, Hendrickson JA, et al: Amiodarone in refractory life-threatening ventricular arrhythmias. *Ann Intern Med* 98:577, 1983.
7. Graboys TB, Podrid PJ, Lown B: Efficacy of amiodarone for refractory supraventricular tachyarrhythmias *Am Heart J* 106:870, 1983.
8. Zipes DP, Prystowsky EN, Heger JJ: Amiodarone: Electrophysiologic actions, pharmacokinetics and clinical effects. *J Am Coll Cardiol* 3:1059, 1984.
9. Rosenbaum MB, Chiale PA, Halpern MS, et al: Clinical efficacy of amiodarone as an antiarrhythmic agent. *Am J Cardiol* 38:934, 1976.
10. Singh BN, Collett JT, Chew CYC: New perspectives in the pharmacologic therapy of cardiac arrhythmias. *Prog Cardiovasc Dis* 22:243, 1980.

11. Polster P, Broekhuysen J: The adrenergic antagonism of amiodarone. *Biochem Pharmacol* 25:131, 1976.
12. Charlier R, Deltour G, Baudine A, et al: Pharmacology of amiodarone, an antianginal drug with a new biological profile. *Arzneim Forsch* 18:1408, 1968.
14. Singh BN: Amiodarone: Historical development and pharmacologic profile. *Am Heart J* 106:788, 1983.
15. Charlier R, Deltour G, Tondeur R, et al: Recherche dans la serie des benzofurannes. VII. Etude pharmacologique preliminaire du butyl-2(diiodo 3'5'-beta-N-diethylamino-ethoxy-4'benzoyl)-3 benzofurannes. *Arch Int Pharmacodyn* 139:255, 1962.
16. Vastesaeger M, Gillot P, Rasson G: Etude clinique d'une nouvelle medication ant-angoreuse. *Acta Cardiol*(Brussels) 22:483, 1967.
17. Charlier R, Delaunois G, Bauthier J, et al: Recherche dans la serie des benzofurannes. XL. Propriete anti-arrhythmiques de l'amiodarone. *Cardiologia* 54:83, 1969.
18. Singh BN, Vaughan Williams EM: The effect of amiodarone, a new anti-anginal drug, on cardiac muscle. *Br J Pharmacol* 39:657, 1970.
19. Singh BN: A study of the pharmacological actions of certain drugs and hormones with a particular reference to cardiac muscle. D. Phil. thesis, University of Oxford, England,1971.
20. Singh BN, Vaughan Williams EM: A third class of antiarrhythmic action. Effects on atrial and ventricular intracellular potentials and other pharmacologic actions on cardiac muscle of MJ1999 and AH3474. *Br J Pharmacol* 39:675, 1970.
21. Van Schepdael J, Solvay H: Etude clinique de l'amiodarone dans les troubles du rhythme cardiaque. *Presse Med* 78:1849, 1970.
22. Rosenbaum MB, Chiale PA, Ryba D, et al: Control of tachyarrhythmias associated with Wolff-Parkinson-White syndrome by amiodarone hydrochloride. *Am J Cardiol* 34:215, 1974.
23. Singh BN, Zipes DP (eds): Amiodarone: Basic concepts and clinical applications. *Am Heart J* 106:787, 1983.
24. Charlier R: Cardiac actions in the dog of a new antagonist of adrenergic excitation which does not produce competitive blockade of adrenoceptors. *Br J Pharmacol* 39:668, 1970.
25. Charlier R, Delaunois G, Bauthier J: Opposite effects of amiodarone and beta-blocking agents on cardiac functions under adrenergic stimulation. *Arzneimitt Forschung* 22:545, 1972.
26. Kobayashi M, Godin D, Naudeau R: Acute effects of amiodarone in the isolated dog heart. *Can J Physiol Pharmacol* 61:308, 1983.
27. Cohen-Armon M, Schreiber G, Sokolovsky M: Interaction of the anti-arrhythmic drug amiodarone with the muscarinic receptor in rat heart and brain. *J Cardiovasc Pharmacol* 6:1148, 1984.
28. Nokin P, Clinet M, Shoenfeld P: Cardiac beta-adrenoceptor modulation by amiodarone. *Biochem Pharmacol* 32(17)2473, 1983.
29. Sharma AD, Corr PB, Sobel BE: Modulation by amiodarone of cardiac adrenergic receptors and their electrophysiologic responsiveness of catecholamines. (abstract) *Circulation* 68 (II):393, 1983.
30. Vankatesh N, Padbury JF, Singh BN: Effects of amiodarone and de-sethylamiodarone on rabbit myocardial beta-adrenoceptors and serum thyroid hormones—absence of relationship to serum and myocardial

drug concentrations. *J Cardiovasc Pharmacol* 8:989, 1986.
31. Gagnol JP, Devos C, Clinet M, et al: Amiodarone: Biochemical aspects and hemodynamic effects. *Drugs* 29(Suppl 3):1, 1985.
32. Williams LT, Lefkowitz RJ, Hathaway DR, et al: Thyroid hormone regulation of beta-adrenergic receptor number. *J Biol Chem* 252:2787, 1977.
33. Bacq ZM, Blakeley AGN, Summers RJ: The effects of amiodarone, alpha and beta receptor antagonist, on adrenergic transmission in the cat spleen. *Biochem Pharmacol* 25:1195, 1976.
34. Hauswirth O, Singh BN: Ionic mechanisms in heart muscle in relation to the genesis and the pharmacologic therapy of cardiac arrhythmias. *Pharmacol Rev* 30:5, 1978.
35. Yabek S, Kato R, Singh BN: Acute electrophysiologic effects of amiodarone and desethylamiodarone in isolated cardiac muscle. *J Cardiovasc Pharmacol* 8:197, 1986.
36. Wellens HJJ, Brugada P, Abdollah H, et al: A comparison of the electrophysiologic effects in intravenous and oral amiodarone in the same patient. *Circulation* 69:120, 1984.
37. Morady F, Dicarlo LA, Krol RB, et al: Acute and chronic effects of amiodarone on ventricular refractoriness, intraventricular conduction and ventricular tachycardia induction. *J Am Coll Cardiol* 7(1):148, 1986.
38. Ikeda N, Nademanee K, Kannan R, et al: Electrophysiologic effects of amiodarone: Experimental and clinical observations relative to serum and tissue concentrations. *Am Heart J* 108:890, 1984.
39. Holt DW, Tucker GT, Jackson PR, et al: Amiodarone pharmacokinetics. *Am Heart J* 106:840, 1983.
40. Storey GCA, Adams PC, Campbell RWF, et al: High performance liquid chromatographic measurement of amiodarone and desethylamiodarone in small tissue samples after enzymatic digetion. *J Clin Pathol* 36:785, 1983.
41. Kannan R, Nademanee K, Hendrickson JA, et al: Amiodarone kinetics after oral doses. *Clin Pharmacol Ther* 31:438, 1982.
42. Lambert C, Vermeulen M, Cardinal R, et al: Effect of induction of amiodarone biotransformation on ventricular refractory periods in rats. *J Pharmacol Exper Therap* 238:307, 1986.
43. Kato R, Vankatesh N, Yabek S, et al: The comparative electrophysiologic effects of desethylamiodarone and amiodarone after chronic dosing in rabbits. Unpublished.
44. Singh BN, Jewitt DE, Downey JM, et al: Effects of amiodarone and L8040, novel antianginal and antiarrhythmic drugs, on cardiac and coronary hemodynamics and on cardiac intracellular potentials. *Clin Exp Pharmacol Physiol* 3:426, 1976.
45. Freeberg, AS, Papp GJ, Vaughan Williams EM: The effects of altered thyroid state on atrial intracellular potentials. *J Physiol* 207:357, 1970.
46. Mason JW, Hondeghem LM, Katzung BG: Amiodarone blocks inactivated cardiac sodium channels. *Pflueg Arch* 396:79, 1983.
47. Mason JW, Hondeghem LM, Katzung BG: Block of inactivated sodium channels and of depolarization-induced automaticity in guinea-pig papillary muscle by amiodarone. *Circ Res* 55:277, 1984.

48. Aomine M, McCullough J, Mayuga R, et al: Cellular electrophysiologic effects of acute exposure to amiodarone on guinea pig heart. *Fed Proc* 43:961, 1984.
49. Gloor HO, Urthaler F, James TN: Acute effects of amiodarone upon the canine sinus node and atrioventricular junctional region. *J Clin Invest* 71:1457, 1983.
50. Goupil N, Lenfant J: The effects of amiodarone on the sinus node activity of the rabbit heart. *Eur J Pharm* 39:23, 1976.
51. Courtney KR: Mechanism of frequency-dependent inhibition of sodium currents in myelinated nerve by the quarternary lidocaine derivative GEA 968. *J Pharmacol Exp Therap* 195:225, 1975.
52. Neliat G: Electrophysiologic effects of butoprozine on isolated heart preparations. Comparison with amiodarone and verapamil. *Arch Int Pharmacodyn* 255:220, 1982.
53. Neliat G: Effects of butoprozine on ionic currents in frog atrial and ferret ventricular fibers. Comparison with amiodarone and verapamil. *Arch Int Pharmacodyn* 255:237, 1982.
54. Vankatesh N, Al-Sarraf L, Hershman JM, et al: Effects of desethylamiodarone on thyroid hormone metabolism in rats: Comparison with the effects of amiodarone. *Proc Soc Exp Biol Med* 181:233, 1986.
55. Vankatesh N, Al-Sarraf L, Singh BN: Digoxin-desethylamiodarone interaction in rats. Comparison with that of amiodarone. *J Cardiovasc Pharmacol* 8:309, 1986.
56. Kannan R, Ikeda N, Drachenberg M, et al: Serum and myocardial kinetics of amiodarone and its major metabolite desethylamiodarone in rabbits. *J Pharm Sci* 73:1208, 1984.
57. Vankatesh N, Somani P, Bersohn M, et al: Electropharmacology of amiodarone: Absence of relationship to serum myocardial and cardiac sarcolemmal membrane drug concentrations. *Am Heart J* 112:916, 1986.
58. Patterson E, Eller BT, Abrams GD, et al: Ventricular fibrillation in conscious canine preparation of sudden coronary death. Prevention by short- and long-term amiodarone administration. *Circulation* 68:857, 1983.
59. Johnson PN, Freedberg AS, Marshall JM: Action of thyroid hormone on the transmembrane potentials from sino atrial nodal cells and atrial muscle cells in isolated atria of rabbits. *Cardiology* 58:273, 1973.
60. Gavrilescu S, Luca C, Streian C, et al: Monophasic action potential of right atrium and electrophysiologic properties of AV conducting system in patients with hypothyroidism. *Br Heart J* 38:1350, 1976.
61. Sharp NA, Neel DS, Parsons RL: Influence of thyroid hormone levels on the electrical and mechanical properties of rabbit papillary muscle. *J Mol Cell Cardiol* 17:119, 1985.
62. Pritchard DA, Singh BN, Hurley PJ: Effects of amiodarone on thyroid function in patients with ischemic heart disease. *Br Heart J* 37:856, 1975.
63. Burger A, Dinichert C, Nicod P, et al: Effect of amiodarone on serum triiodothyronine, thyroxine and thyrotropin: A drug influencing peripheral metabolism of thyroid hormones. *J Clin Invest* 58:255, 1976.
64. Melmed S, Nademanee K, Reed AW, et al: Hyperthyroxinemia with

bradycardia and normal thyrotropin secretion after chronic amiodarone administration. *J Clin Endocrin Met* 53:997, 1981.

65. Hershman JW, Nademanee K, Masahiro S, et al: Thyroxine and triiodothyronine kinetics in cardiac patients taking amiodarone. *Acta Endocrinologica* 111:193, 1986.

66. Sogol PB, Hershman JM, Reed AW: The effects of amiodarone on serum thyroid hormones and hepatic thyroxine 5'-monodeiodination in rats. *Endocrinology* 113;1464, 1983.

67. Wiersinga WM, Broenik MM: In vitro inhibition of nuclear thyroid hormone binding by amiodarone and desethylamiodarone in rat liver and cardiac muscle. (abstract) 59th American Thyroid Association, New Orleans, Oct. 5–8, 1983.

68. Latham KR, Sellittie DF, Goldstein RE: Interaction of amiodarone and desethylamiodarone with nuclear thyroid hormone receptors. (abstract) *J Am Coll Cardiol* 5:466, 1985.

69. Singh BN, Nademanee K: Amiodarone and thyroid function: Clinical implications during antiarrhythmic therapy. *Am Heart J* 106(4):857, 1983.

70. Nademanee K, Singh BN, Hendrickson JA, et al: Pharmacokinetic significance of reverse $T_3$ levels during amiodarone treatment: A potential method of monitoring chronic drug therapy. *Circulation* 66:202, 1982.

71. Gross SA, Somani P: Amiodarone-induced ultrastructural changes in the canine myocardial fibers. *Am Heart J* 112:771, 1986.

72. Chatelain P: Effects of amiodarone on lipid dynamics in erythrocyte membrane in vitro and after chronic treatment. *Arch Int Pharmacodyn* 276:327, 1985.

73. Chatelain P: Modulation by amiodarone of membrane fluidity and $Na^+$-$K^+$-ATPase activity in rat brain synaptosomes. *Biochem Biophys Res Commun* 129:148, 1985.

74. Chatelain P, Ferriera J, Laruel R, et al: Amiodarone-induced modifications of the phospholipid physical state. A fluorescence polarization study. *Biochem Pharmacol* 35(18):3007, 1986.

75. Broekhuysen J, Charlier R, Ghislain J: Action of amiodarone on guinea-pig heart sodium and potassium activated adenosine triphosphatase. *Biochem Pharmacol* 21:2951, 1972.

76. Mostow ND, Rakita L, Vrobel TR, et al: Amiodarone: Correlation of serum concentration with suppression of complex ventricular ectropic activity. *Am J Cardoiol* 54:569, 1984.

77. Gomes JAC, Kang PS, Hariman RJ, et al: Electrophysiologic effects and mechanisms of termination of supraventricular tachycardia by intravenous amiodarone. *Am Heart J* 107:214, 1984.

78. Hariman RJ, Gomes AC, Kang KS, et al: Effects of intravenous amiodarone in patients with inducible repetitive ventricular responses and ventricular tachycardia. *Am Heart J* 107:1109, 1984.

79. Platou ES, Refsum H: Class III antiarrhythmic action in experimental atrial fibrillation and flutter in dogs. *J Cardiovasc Pharmacol* 4:839, 1982.

80. Jaillon P, Heckle J, Jais J-M, et al: Acute effects of intravenous prifuroline and amiodarone on canine automaticity, conduction and refractoriness. *J Cardiovasc Pharmacol* 4:486, 1982.

81. Pickoff AS, Singh S, Flinn CJ, et al: Dose-dependent electrophysiologic effects of amiodarone in the immature canine heart. *Am J Cardiol* 52:621, 1983.
82. Yabek S, Kato R, Singh BN: Electrophysiologic effects of amiodarone in canine adult and neonatal myocardial and Purkinje fibers. *J Amer Coll Cardiol* 5(5):1109, 1985.
83. Rosen MR, Gelband H, Hoffman BR: Effects of phentolamine on electrophysiologic properites of isolated canine Purkinje fibers. *J Pharmacol Exp Ther* 179:586, 1971.
84. Giotti A, Ledda F, Mannaioni DF: Effects of noradrenaline and isoprenaline, in combination with alpha- and beta-receptor blocking substances on the action potential of cardiac Purkinje fibers. *Physiology* 2229:99P, 1973.
85. Nademanee K, Hendrickson J, Kannan R, et al: Antiarrhythmic efficacy and electrophysiologic actions of amiodarone in patients with life-threatening arrhythmias. *Am Heart J* 103:950, 1982.
86. Waxman HL, Groh WC, Marchlinski FE, et al: Amiodarone for control of sustained ventricular tachyarrhythmias: Clinical and electrophysiological effects in 51 patients. *Am J Cardiol* 50:1066, 1982.
87. Finerman WR Jr, Hamer A, Peter T: Electrophysiologic effects of chronic amiodarone therapy in patients with ventricular arrhythmias. *Am Heart J* 104:987, 1982.
88. Cabasson J: Analysis of the electrophysiologic effects of amiodarone, perhexiline and bepridil on the cardiac rhythms of the unanesthetized dog in chronic heart block. *Arch Int Pharmacodyn* 233:65, 1978.
89. Olson B, Brorson L, Varnauskas E: Class III antiarrhythmic action in man: Observations from monophasic action potential recordings and amiodarone treatment. *Br Heart J* 35:1255, 1973.
90. Shenasa M, Denker S, Mahmud R, et al: Effect of amiodarone on conduction and refractoriness of the His-Purkinje system in the human heart. *J Amer Coll Cardiol* 4:105, 1984.
91. Lubbe WF, McFadyen ML, Muller CA, et al: Protective action of amiodarone against ventricular fibrillation in the isolated perfused rat heart. *Am J Cardiol* 43:533, 1978.
92. Schoenfeld P: Comparison des effets de l'amiodarone et du propranolol sur l'incidence et al severité des arrhythmies ventriculaires après ligature de l'artère coronarien chez le rat anesthesié. *J Cardiol* 11:499, 1982.
93. Chew CYC, Collet JT, Campbell C, et al: Beneficial effects of amiodarone pretreatment on early ischemic ventricular arrhythmias relative to infarct size and regional myocardial blood flow in the conscious dog. *J Cardiovasc Pharmacol* 4:1028, 1982.
94. Singh BN, Hauswirth O: Comparative mechanisms of action of antiarrhythmic drugs. *Am Heart J* 87:367, 1974.
95. Singh BN, Nademanee K: Control of cardiac arrhythmias by selective lengthening of repolarization: Theoretic considerations and clinical observations. *Am Heart J* 109:421, 1985.

# Chapter 15

# Thyroid Hormone Metabolism and Amiodarone

## Jerome M. Hershman

In 1968, Charlier et al.[1] showed that when amiodarone was given at a constant daily dose to conscious instrumented dogs, progressive bradycardia developed over a period of weeks. When the drug was discontinued, the return to normal heart rate was equally slow. Subsequent studies in experimental animals[2] indicated that although the cardiac electrophysiologic changes induced by the drug closely resembled those found with hypothyroidism in animals and humans[3–6] generalized hypothyroidism did not occur. Pritchard et al.[7] administered 600 mg/day of amiodarone to patients with ischemic heart disease for 6 weeks. They found significant increases in serum thyroxine ($T_4$) levels with minor decreases in levels of triiodothyronine ($T_3$). There was a decrease in heart rate and a lengthening of the $QT_c$ interval of the surface electrocardiogram. These changes were not associated with altered thyroid state. The suggestion was made that the drug acted by inhibiting the peripheral conversion of $T_4$ to $T_3$. A year later Burger et al.[8] reported similar findings during the course of a study in which 400 mg/day of amiodarone was given for 28 days and thyroid function tests were undertaken serially. In addition to the reported effects of $T_4$ and $T_3$, they found significant increases in reverse $T_3$ ($rT_3$); these effects were not produced by iodine in amounts equivalent to those contained in 400 mg/day of amiodarone. Their data indicated that the effects of amiodarone on thyroid hormone indices could not be attributed to iodine contained in the drug molecule. Burger et al.[8] also found no effect of amiodarone on

From: *Control of Cardiac Arrhythmias by Lengthening Repolarization*, edited by Bramah N. Singh, MD, Futura Publishing Company Inc., Mount Kisco, NY, © 1988.

thyroxine-bound globulin (TBG), but the drug increased the response of thyroid-stimulating-hormone (TSH) to thyrotropin-releasing-hormone (TRH). Very similar data were reported by Jonckheer et al.[9] but unlike the data from the relatively short-term studies of Pritchard et al.[7] and Burger et al.,[8] a number of patients in this series developed hyperthyroidism and hypothyroidism. Some of the cases of altered thyroid state developed after the drug had been withdrawn for many months.

As indicated elsewhere in this book, in recent years, amiodarone has attracted considerable attention as a potent antiarrhythmic agent.[10-15] Clinical observations during its increasing use in the control of arrhythmias have raised a number of questions in relation to thyroid hormone metabolism.[16] This chapter deals with the significance of iodine present in the amiodarone molecule and its role in the development of altered thyroid state and with the effect of the drug on thyroid hormone metabolism with a particular reference to the biochemical changes that accompany its short-term and long-term administration. Data is provided to enable the clinician to evaluate the clinical significance of such changes in relation to altered thyroid state. The complex interaction between thyroid hormone effects and electrophysiologic actions of amiodarone during chronic administration was discussed in Chapter 14.

## Amiodarone and Iodine Metabolism

There now is substantial evidence that the altered thyroid state (discussed later) that occurs in a small number of patients during chronic therapy with amiodarone is not an intrinsic property of amiodarone.[16,17] It appears to be related to the iodine contained in the molecule, which amounts to 37 percent iodine by weight. It is estimated that its metabolism results in the release of 3 mg of inorganic iodine per 100 mg amiodarone each day.[18] Because the normal daily dietary intake of iodine is 200 to 800 $\mu$g, the iodine load of 12 mg from a daily dose of 400 mg of amiodarone is very substantial.

In a study of 15 patients taking 300 mg amiodarone per day, urinary inorganic iodide excretion rose from control value of 270 mcg/day to 10,800 mcg/day.[19] Plasma inorganic iodide rose fortyfold, thyroid iodide uptake was reduced by 75 percent, and thyroid clearance of iodide fell from 6 ml/min to 0.5 ml/min. The absolute thyroid uptake of iodide (iodide clearance $\times$ plasma concentration) was increased twofold to threefold. The fall in thyroid clearance of iodide (iodide trapping) in response to a large iodide load is an adaptive mechanism to prevent the accumulation of excessive amounts of iodine in the thyroid gland. Large doses of iodide inhibit the biosynthesis of thyroid hormone (the Wolff-Chaikoff effect).[20] Inhibition of iodide transport so that intrathyroid iodide concentrations fall below the critical level needed to sustain the Wolff-Chaikoff effect is an adaptive mechanism to avoid hypothyroidism.[21] It is likely that such a mechanism operates to prevent the development of hypothyroidism in most patients given amiodarone long term.

## Changes in Thyroid Function Tests Induced by Amiodarone

The biochemical changes that accompany the chronic administration of amiodarone now are well defined. In euthyroid patients, amiodarone causes an increase in serum thyroxin ($T_4$) and reverse triiodothyronine ($rT_3$) levels and a reduction of serum triiodothyronine ($T_3$) levels.[8,22] The free $T_4$ levels also are increased in proportion to the increase of total serum $T_4$ concentration (see Fig. 1). Thse data in adults are similar to those reported by Attuel[23] in children.

The basis for the changes in thyroid hormone levels has been carefully investigated. Kinetic studies in humans show a reduction in $T_4$ clearance rate while the daily production rate remains the same or increases.[24,25] Similar data have been reported in a rabbit model.[9] In euthyroid man, the principal source of $T_3$ production is extrathyroidal conversion of $T_4$ to $T_3$ by 5'- monodeiodination; this accounts for about three-fourths of daily $T_3$ production. In patients taking amiodarone, conversion of $T_4$ to $T_3$ is reduced by 60 percent and the $T_3$ production rate falls by nearly 50 percent.[25] On the average, serum $T_3$ levels are reduced by about 20 percent, but there is considerable variability of the response among individuals. Jonckheer et al[9] were the first to report a "low $T_3$ syndrome" in patients taking amiodarone. Systemic illness, aging, and several drugs in addition to amiodarone (propranolol, corticosteroids) also reduce serum $T_3$ levels and could influence the level in a given patient.[26] Baseline serum TSH levels rise slightly during the first few weeks of treatment and then return to normal in several months.[22] In some patients, serum TSH levels become subnormal

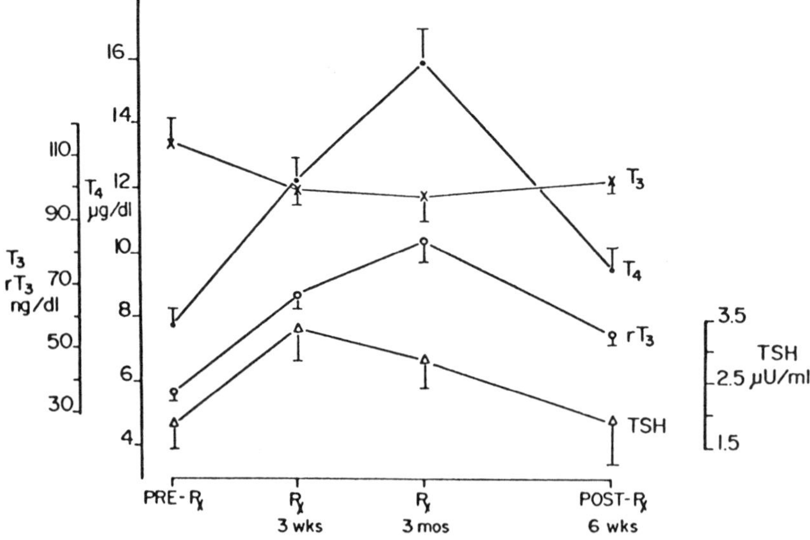


**Figure 1.** Summary of changes in thyroid function in 15 patients before, during, and after amiodarone treatment (means ± SE). $T_4$ (p < 0.005), $T_3$ (p < 0.01), and $rT_3$ (p < 0.001) were all different from the pretreatment baseline levels. TSH (p < 0.05) was increased only after 3 weeks. (From Melmed S, Nademanee K, Reed AW, et al: Hyperthyroxemia with brady-cardia and normal thyrotropin secretion after amiodarone administration *J Clin Endo Metab* 53:997, 1981. By permission of the authors and the journal.)

during chronic therapy. In others, the serum TSH levels are elevated modestly above the normal range but without the development of clinical hypothyroidism (discussed later).

## Mechanisms of Changes in Thyroid Hormone Levels

Amiodarone appears to act by inhibiting the outer ring mono-deiodination of thyroxine.[5,7,22,25] For example, studies in rats have shown that amiodarone reduces conversion of $T_4$ to $T_3$ in the liver, a major site of this process.[27] Amiodarone inhibits 5'-deiodinase activity. This would account for the elevation of serum $T_4$ and $rT_3$ levels (because both of these hormones are metabolized by this enzymatic pathway), as well as the reduction of serum $T_3$ levels. In addition, amiodarone may block binding of $T_3$ to nuclear receptors and thus block the action of thyroid hormone. However, this action needs to be distinguished from the drug's effect in inhibiting the peripheral conversion of $T_4$ to $T_3$. The latter effect is exhibited by a large number of pharmacologic compounds that do not produce the same electrophysiologic effects of chronically administered amiodarone.

In isolated pituitary nuclei, amiodarone blocked binding of $T_3$ by the nuclei,[28] but this was not found using isolated hepatic nuclei.[27] The difficulty of maintaining amiodarone in solution as well as the effects of various vehicles for solubilizing it may account for some of the discrepant findings of in vitro studies.

Rats treated with amiodarone had a reduction of pituitary 5'-deiodinase activity in one report[29] but not in another.[30] In the pituitary gland, the major source of $T_3$ is that generated locally by 5'-deiodination of $T_4$. Inhibition of intrapituitary production of $T_3$ as well as inhibition of the binding of $T_3$ to nuclear receptors would block the inhibitory action of $T_3$ on TSH secretion and result in enhanced secretion of TSH. This could explain the rise in TSH in patients taking amiodarone during the first few weeks of therapy. Amiodarone stimulated TSH release in cultured pituitary cells.[28]

Studies of deiodination or nuclear binding of $T_3$ in cardiac tissue are difficult technically. In a recent report, acute administration of amiodarone reduced cardiac 5'-deiodinase activity.[31] In rats treated with amiodarone, there was a reduction of cardiac $Ca^{++}$ myosin ATPase, an enzyme induced by thyroid hormone.[28] Two hepatic enzymes induced by thyroid hormone, alpha-glycerophosphate dehydrogenase and malic enzyme, are reduced in rats treated with amiodarone, but the cardiac levels of these enzymes are unchanged.[32] Reduced intracardiac generation of $T_3$ caused by amiodarone could account for the reduced action of $T_3$ on the heart. The effects of amiodarone on the heart, reduced cardiac $Ca^{++}$ myosin ATPase, and lengthening of repolarization could be attributed to "cardiac hypothyroidism," as postulated by Singh and Nademanee[16] (also see Chapter 14).

## Significance of Changes in $rT_3$

Nademanee et al.[17] showed that the increases in serum reverse $T_3$ levels induced by amiodarone occurred as a function of dose and duration of therapy. It also was found that, since many of the side effects as well as the suppressant effects of amiodarone varied as a function of dose and duration of drug therapy, efficacy and toxicity of amiodarone could be monitored by the serial measurements of serum $rT_3$. The utility of this approach has not been investigated extensively.[17,33] However, it has been found that increase in the level of serum $rT_3$ threefold to fivefold above the baseline usually is associated with an adequate antiarrhythmic response and side effects are likely to occur when such a limit is exceeded, as when the level of the hormone continues to increase at a constant dose once an apparent steady-state "amiodaronization" has been attained. There has been a report [33] indicating that exceedingly high levels of $rT_3$ may be associated with sudden death. However, this study was a limited one and further data are needed to confirm or deny such a possibility.

It should be emphasized that in the use of $rT_3$ levels in monitoring toxicity and efficacy of amiodarone, a number of limitations should be appreciated. First, there is considerable variability in the measurement of the hormone from laboratory to laboratory; each center needs to establish its own normal and so-called therapeutic range. Second, increases in serum $rT_3$ levels may occur during the course of systemic illnesses, fasting, and surgery, situations in which the use of $rT_3$ in monitoring efficacy and toxicity of amiodarone clearly is limited. The concomitant use of drugs such as corticosteroids or beta-adrenergic blocking drugs that also alter the levels of $rT_3$ is likely to confound the use of the technique in monitoring amiodarone therapy by the serial determinations of the hormone. Finally, the expected increases in $rT_3$ do not occur in the event hypothyroidism develops, and higher than expected levels may develop if hyperthyroidism supervenes. Preliminary data at our institution, however, suggest that the serial measurements of $rT_3$ may be of great clinical utility in avoiding the development of certain potentially serious complications, such as pulmonary toxicity induced by amiodarone.

## Significance of Altered Hormone Indices During Chronic Amiodarone Therapy

In recent years, data have suggested that the effects of amiodarone on thyroid hormone indices constitute a spectrum of abnormality. This has been demonstrated most clearly by Nademanee et al.[34] Serial thyroid hormone indices were determined serially in 76 patients given amiodarone for 6–32 months, means 16 ± (SD), for control of arrhythmias. The mean data are presented in Table 1. Over this period, 68 (89 percent) remained euthryroid, 6 (8 percent) developed hypothyroidism, and 2 (3 percent) developed hyperthyroidism. In patients who remained euthyroid, thyroid hormone

## Table 1
### Changes in Thyroid Hormone Indices as a Function of Duration and of Cumulative Dose of Amiodarone Therapy in Patients with Cardiac Arrhythmias

| | Control | 1 Month | 3 Months | 6 Months | 12 Months | 18 Months | 24 Months |
|---|---|---|---|---|---|---|---|
| $T_4$ (μg/dl) (normal) | 8 ± 2 (n = 72) (4−12) | 11 ± 3 (44) | 12 ± 3** (59) | 12 ± 3** (50) | 12 ± 3** (40) | 12 ± 2** (37) | 12 ± 3** (30) |
| $T_3$ (ng/dl) (normal) | 108 ± 32 (n = 72) (66−170) | 102 ± 30 (42) | 91 ± 25* (58) | 90 ± 24* (52) | 90 ± 27* (37) | 98 ± 27* (37) | 98 ± 23** (29) |
| $rT_3$ (ng/dl) (normal) | 29 ± 10 (n = 70) (15−50) | 65 ± 31 (53) | 79 ± 27** (64) | 77 ± 27** (55) | 68 ± 23** (39) | 69 ± 17 (43) | 67 ± 17** (28) |
| TSH (μU/ml) (normal) | 3 ± 2 (n = 70) (1−60) | 5 ± 4 (33) | 4 ± 3 (48) | 4 ± 4 (37) | 5 ± 4 (36) | 5 ± 3 (34) | 3 ± 2 (28) |
| CM (g) | 0 | 29 | 64 | 117 | 168 | 200 | 310 |

The data shown are means ± standard deviations from *n* observations. The statistical significance of differences shown are from control.

*p < 0.05

**p < 0.01

CM = Cumulative dose

The range of values in parenthesis under control column are "laboratory normals" for euthyroid patients not given amiodarone or other drugs.

Source: Nademanee K, Singh BN, Callahan B, et al: Amiodarone, thyroid hormone indices, and altered thyroid function: Long-term serial effects in patients with cardiac arrhythmias. *Am J Cardiol* (in press). By permission of the authors and the journal.

alterations attained steady-state values at 3 months: $T_4$ increased 42 percent ($p < 0.01$), $rT_3$ increased by 172 percent ($p < 0.01$), $T_3$ decreased 16 percent ($p < 0.05$) without significant effect on thyroid-stimulating-hormone.

These serial data acquired over the long term, relative to clinically altered thyroid state, permitted the authors to determine the 90 percent tolerance limits for the various hormones in patients remaining euthyroid on amiodarone. For these patients, the 90 percent tolerance limits (95 percent confidence) over the follow-up period for $T_4$ was 5–19 μg/dl (range in normal subjects, 4–12), for $T_3$ 36–163 ng/dl (range for normals, 60–160), for $rT_3$ 22–131 ng/dl (range for normals, 15–50), and for thyroid stimulating hormone 0–14 μU/ml (range for normals, 1–6). The data are illustrated graphically in Figure 2. The changes in hormone indices in hyperthyroid (see Table 2) or hypothyroid (see Table 3) patients were not related to the cumulative dose or duration of drug therapy. The most reliable diagnostic indices for amiodarone-induced altered thyroid state were thyroid-stimulating-hormone level over 20 μU for hypothyroidism, and $T_4$ over 20 ng/dl and/or high $T_3$ over 200 ng/dl for hyperthyroidism. All the levels were within the 90 percent tolerance limits derived for these hormones from patients remaining euthyroid on amiodarone long term. The data provide the basis for the diagnosis of abnormal thyroid function in patients with drug-induced changes in thyroid function tests due to amiodarone and suggest the need for baseline and periodic determinations of thyroid function tests during chronic amiodarone therapy (discussed later). This approach, when related to the clinical states of the patients, was found to be of much diagnostic utility in the recognition of hyperthyroidism and hypothyroidism developing during amiodarone therapy. For example, a serum $T_4$ level of 15 μg/dl normally is consistent with thyrotoxicosis in patients not on amiodarone. The data on tolerance limits indicate that a $T_4$ level up to 19 μg/dl during amiodarone therapy is compatible with euthyroidism. Conversely, a serum $T_4$ level of 5 μg/dl (normally within the euthyroid range) is strongly suggestive of hypothyroidism. None of the euthyroid patients had thyroid-stimulating-hormone levels $\geq 20$ μU/ml.


## Amiodarone as a Cause of Subclinical Hypothyroidism

A finding of theoretical importance was that a subset of patients reported by Nademanee et al.[34] developed TSH levels be-

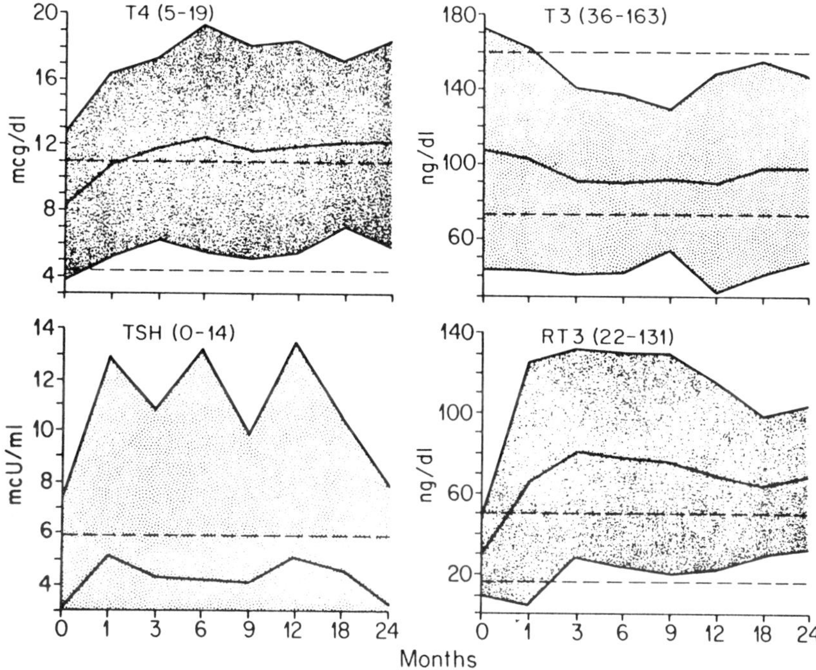



**Figure 2.** The delineation of the tolerance limits for various thyroid hormone indices in patients treated chronically with amiodarone. The ordinate in each panel shows the hormone values and the abscissa the time course of drug treatment. The shaded areas indicate the 90 percent tolerance limits of the hormone indices in patients who remained euthyroid on amiodarone during the period of treatment. The areas delimited by broken horizontal lines for $T_4$, $T_3$, and $rT_3$ indicate the range of values for the hormones in euthyroid subjects not taking amiodarone; in the case of TSH (thyroid-stimulating-hormone) only the upper limit is indicated since the lower limit may be zero in some subjects (From Nademanee K, Singh BN, Callahan B, et al: Amiodarone, thyroid hormone indices, and altered thyroid function: Long-term serial effects in patients with cardiac arrhythmias. *Am J Cardiol* 58:981, 1986. By permission of the authors and the journal.)

tween 10 and 20 $\mu$U/ml without clinical or other biochemical evidence of hypothyroidism (see Table 4). This occurred in 13 of the patients in the series. None of these patients subsequently developed further increases in TSH levels or clinical hypothyroidism. The mechanism for such increases in the TSH levels in these patients is uncertain. It may represent a stable nonprogressive subclinical hypothyroidism. Alternatively, it may be due to hypothyroidism limited to certain organs, since tissue selectivity of

Table 2

Patterns of Changes in Thyroid Hormone Indices in Patients Developing
Hypothyroidism During Amiodarone Therapy Relative to Tolerance in
Patients Remaining Euthyroid.

| Parameters (90% tolerance limits) | $T_3$ 36–163 ng/dl | $rT_3$ 22–131 ng/dl | $T_4$ 5–19 µg/dl | TSH 0–14 µU/ml | Cumulative Dose (g) | Duration of Therapy (months) |
|---|---|---|---|---|---|---|
| Patient 1 | 92 | 39 | 6 | 25 | 294 | 24 |
| Patient 2 | 54 | 32 | 5 | 80 | 44 | 3 |
| Patient 3 | 84 | 84 | 5 | 66 | 150 | 11 |
| Patient 4 | 88 | 21 | 4 | 40 | 17.8 | 0.5 |
| Patient 5 | 109 | 33 | 6 | 35 | 144 | 10 |
| Patient 6 | 40 | 14 | 4 | 137 | 24 | 4 |
| Means ± SD | 78 ± 23 | 37 ± 23 | 5 ± 1 | 64 ± 38 | 112 ± 107 | 9 ± 9 |

TSH = thyroid stimulating hormone.
Source: Nademanee K, Singh BN, Callahan B, et al: Amiodarone, thyroid hormone indices, and altered thyroid function: Long-term serial effects in patients with cardiac arrhythmias. *Am J Cardiol* 58:981, 1986. By permission of the authors and the journal.

amiodarone action has been reported by Polster and Broekhuys-en.[35] Moreover, electrophysiologic studies have shown that the effects of chronically administered amiodarone[2] on cardiac repolarization are very similar to those of experimental hypothyroidism[3] and are prevented by the concomitant administration of thyroid hormones[2] in doses less than those produced daily endogenously.

## Clinically Detectable Altered Thyroid State

Patients taking amiodarone develop a significant but variable incidence of thyroid dysfunction.[36–42] Table 5 summarizes the data from various series that have been selected from the literature. The incidence of hypothyroidism varies from 5 to 22 percent, and that of hyperthyroidism from 2 to 10 percent. Although both conditions are relatively common, especially hypothyroidism in the older population,[43] the incidence of these disorders is much greater in patients taking amiodarone than in the general population. The series cited in Table 5 were prospective evaluations of cardiac patients and excluded those with overt preexisting thyroid disease.

### Table 3
### Thyroid Hormone Indices in Patients Developing Hyperthyroidism During Amiodarone Therapy

|  | Patient 1 | Patient 2 | Patient 3 | Patient 4 |
|---|---|---|---|---|
| Indication for amiodarone | VT/VF | Recurrent AF | VT/VF | VT |
| Duration of treatment (months) | 30 | 14 | 39 | 9 |
| Cumulative dose (grams) | 301 | 188 | 432 | 117 |
| $T_4$ ($\mu$g/dl) | 29 | 20 | 22 | 21 |
| $T_3$ (ng/dl) | 490 | 157 | 225 | 205 |
| TSH ($\mu$U/ml) | 0 | 0 | NA | NA |
| $rT_3$ (ng/dl) | 110 | 122 | 113 | 105 |

VT/VF = Ventricular tachycardia/ventricular fibrillation.

AF = Atrial fibrillation

NA = Not available

Source: Nademanee K, Singh BN, Callahan B, et al: Amiodarone, thyroid hormone indices, and altered thyroid function: Long-term serial effects in patients with cardiac arrhythmias. *Am J Cardiol* 58:981, 1986. By permission of the authors and the journal.

### Table 4
### Changes in Thyroid Hormone Indices Relative to Those in Thyroid-Stimulating-Hormone Levels in Patients Treated Chronically with Amiodarone

| Subgroups by TSH Levels | $T_3$ (ng/dl) | $rT_3$ (ng/dl) | $T_4$ ($\mu$g/dl) |
|---|---|---|---|
| Group 1 (n = 287) < 10 $\mu$U/ml | 95 ± 25 | 64 ± 28 | 11 ± 3 |
| Group 2 (n = 28) 10–20 $\mu$U/ml | 95 ± 28 | 65 ± 30 | 9 ± 3 |
| Group 3 (n = 14) > 20 $\mu$U/ml | 78 ± 28* | 34 ± 21** | 6 ± 3** |

The data represent means ± SD; n = the number of patient determinations. Since the total number of patients was 76, more than one determination was made in nearly all patients during maintenance amiodarone therapy. Significances of differences shown by asterisks are those for Group 3 versus Group 1 or Group 2: *$p < 0.05$; **$p < 0.01$. All p values were adjusted to a level of $p < 0.05$ for multiple tests using Bonferroni correction. There was no significant difference between any of the values in Group 1 versus the corresponding ones in Group 2.

Source: Nademanee K, Singh BN, Callahan B, et al: Amiodarone, thyroid hormone indices, and altered thyroid function: Long-term serial effects in patients with cardiac arrhythmias. *Am J Cardiol* 58:981, 1986. By permission of the authors and the journal.

Table 5
Reported Incidence of Amiodarone-Induced Thyroid Dysfunction

| Study | Year | N | % Hypothyroidism | % Hyperthyroidism |
|---|---|---|---|---|
| Chevigne-Brancart & Vandalem[36] | 1982 | 174 | 8 | 12 |
| Amico et al.[37] | 1984 | 26 | 19 | 0 |
| Martino et al.[38] | 1984 | 188 | 5 | 10 |
|  |  | 41 | 22 | 2 |
| Posner et al.[39] | 1984 | 92 | 12 | 2 |
| Sanmarti et al.[40] | 1984 | 45 | 9 | 4 |
| Borowski et al.[41] | 1985 | 45 | 9 | 4 |
| Valenzuela et al.[42] | 1985 | 30 | 3 | 3 |
| Nademanee et al.[34] | 1986 | 76 | 8 | 3 |

N = refers to the numbers of patients in the series.

Martino et al.[38] found that there was a difference in the frequency of thyroid dysfunction in relation to dietary iodine intake: In west Tuscany, Italy, where dietary iodine is low, there was a preponderance of hyperthyroidism compared with hypothyroidism. In Massachusetts, where iodine intake is much higher, there was a preponderance of hypothyroidism, and hyperthyroidism was relatively rare. Other reports from the United States confirm a preponderance of hypothyroidism and suggest that its frequency increases with long-term therapy.[44]

The overall data suggest that the iodine content of amiodarone is the main factor responsible for the thyroid dysfunction; underlying thyroid disease also predisposes to both hypothyroidism and hyperthyroidism.

## Hypothyroidism

The clinical presentation of hypothyroidism may be typical with cold intolerance, sluggishness, mental apathy, constipation, bradycardia, and edema. Even myxedema coma has been reported as a consequence of amiodarone therapy.[45] However, hypothyroidism is often relatively asymptomatic (subclinical) and detected by thyroid function tests in patients with minimal symptoms.[44] In others, bradycardia in excess of what usually is expected during amiodarone therapy should alert the possibility of hypothyroidism.

The diagnosis of hypothyroidism is established by a serum

TSH >20 $\mu$U/ml and $T_4$ <6 $\mu$g/dl. Because amiodarone raises serum $T_4$ and free $T_4$ levels, these measurements may remain within the usual normal range. As discussed earlier, some patients, who have no symptoms of hypothyroidism while taking amiodarone, have modestly elevated serum TSH levels of 10 to 20 $\mu$U/ml (upper limit of normal 5 $\mu$U/ml); their serum $T_4$ and $T_3$ levels are clearly normal.[34] In our experience, the elevated serum TSH in this range does not indicate impending thyroid failure. Although one can classify such patients as showing subclinical hypothyroidism, in the absence of symptoms, there is no reason to treat these patients with thyroid hormone nor discontinue amiodarone therapy.

Studies of hypothyroid patients taking amiodarone showed that they had higher thyroid radioiodine uptake than euthyroid patients while taking the drug.[46] The hypothyroid patients also had abnormal iodide perchlorate discharge tests, which indicates a block in the organic binding of iodine. The increased TSH secretion in the hypothyroid patients enhanced iodide transport and increased intrathyroidal iodide, and the defect in organic binding of iodide prevented the escape from the Wolff-Chaikoff inhibition of biosynthesis.

The possibility must be considered that amiodarone or its iodine content has a direct toxic effect on the thyroid. In a prospective study of patients recovering from myocardial infarction, 13 were given amiodarone and 22 were given a placebo for 30 days.[47] Antithyroid microsomal antibodies were not present in all patients before the study. After 30 days, 55 percent of those receiving amiodarone had antimicrosomal antibodies, while none of those in the placebo group developed the antibodies. After withdrawal of the amiodarone, the antibodies disappeared.

Treatment of the hypothyroidism complicating amiodarone therapy is straightforward. Thyroxine is given in a dose sufficient to relieve symptoms of hypothyroidism. Because of the underlying cardiac disease, therapy should be initiated with a dose of 25–50 $\mu$g of thyroxine daily, and gradually increased at intervals of 4 to 6 weeks while amiodarone is continued. The serum $T_4$ level will increase in proportion to the dose of $T_4$ and stabilize after 2 weeks, but it may take 6 weeks for the serum TSH to fall to a stable level reflecting the equilibrium response to the dose of thyroxine. Normalization of serum TSH levels may not be a reasonable goal for many patients, because a dose sufficient to accomplish this may precipitate cardiac decompensation or an arrhythmia.

## Hyperthyroidism

The clinical presentation of hyperthyroidism often is dramatic with recurrence of the arrhythmia while the patient is taking amiodarone. This is particularly so in the case of atrial arrhythmias. Similarly, the initial bradycardiac response that invariably develops on amiodarone disappears, being replaced by an increase in heart rate. Other findings may include muscle weakness, weight loss, anorexia, nervousness, restlessness, tremor, diffuse or nodular goiter, and congestive heart failure.

A mild increase of serum $T_4$ and free $T_4$ levels by itself is not sufficient to make the diagnosis of hyperthyroidism, because this occurs in euthyroid patients taking amiodarone.[22] The range of euthyroid serum $T_4$ levels in euthyroid patients taking amiodarone was found to be 5–19 μg/dl.[34] An increased serum $T_3$ level and free $T_3$ level supports the diagnosis of hyperthyroidism. The thyroid uptake of radioiodine is usually reduced in hyperthyroid patients taking amiodarone because of the large iodine load;[46,48] however, in one report, 24-hour thyroid uptake was elevated in most amiodarone-treated hyperthyroid patients with diffuse or nodular goiter.[49]

In many euthyroid patients on chronic amiodarone therapy, the TSH response to thyrotropin-releasing-hormone (TRH) is suppressed.[38] In one study the conversion of the TSH response to TRH from a normal to a suppressed response was found to be a harbinger of hyperthyroidism.[50] However, many of the patients in this report had preexisting nodular goiter and many have been predisposed to iodine-induced hyperthyroidism.

Amiodarone-treated hyperthyroid patients have an increased thyroid iodine content measured by X-ray fluorescence,[48] but this also may be found in euthyroid patients taking amiodarone. After withdrawal of the drug, the thyroid iodine content falls into the normal range.

In regard to the pathogenesis of the hyperthyroidism, there are two mechanisms.[51,52] Many of the patients have multinodular or uninodular goiter; these nodules are autonomous in their biosynthesis of thyroid hormone. The excess iodine load provided by amiodarone is a large amount of substrate for production of thyroid hormone by the autonomous hyperfunctioning nodules. Most patients with amiodarone-induced toxic diffuse goiter have detectable thyroid-stimulating immunoglobulins, which are found in hyperthyroid patients with Graves' disease.[53] In these patients, the stimulated gland takes up the iodine and secretes excessive amounts of thyroid hormone. Perhaps those with undetectable thyroid-stimulating immunoglobulin have low levels of this stimulator and become hyperthyroid only with the availability of excess iodine.

Treatment of amiodarone-induced hyperthyroidism involves two considerations: first, discontinuation of the amiodarone; and second, use of antithyroid drugs. The condition usually is self-limited and will respond well to discontinuation of the amiodarone with disappearance of clinical findings and normalization of thyroid function tests within a few months. However, if the amiodarone is regarded as life-saving and irreplaceable, it can be continued. Treatment with the usual doses of propylthiouracil or methimazole also causes improvement despite continuation of the amiodarone. We prefer to use propylthiouracil rather than methimazole because propylthiouracil blocks peripheral conversion of $T_4$ to $T_3$, whereas methimazole does not. A beta-adrenergic blocking agent, such as propranolol, also may be useful to control the symptoms and tachycardia of hyperthyroidism.

## Summary

Amiodarone blocks peripheral 5'-deiodination of $T_4$ and $rT_3$, resulting in increased serum $T_4$, free $T_4$, and $rT_3$ levels and in reduced serum $T_3$ concentration without a change in thyroxine-binding globulin. Amiodarone blocks the action of thyroid hormone by the inhibition of 5'-deiodinase, which reduces production of $T_3$ in peripheral tissues and possibly by blocking nuclear binding of $T_3$. The significant incidence of thyroid dysfunction caused by the drug is attributable mainly to chronic iodine overload in susceptible patients. The diagnosis of altered thyroid state can be established by considering the overall clinical picture and the tolerance limits of hormone indices established in patients remaining euthyroid on amiodarone therapy. To screen for thyroid disease, thyroid function should be assessed before initiating therapy and semiannually during therapy or when clinical features of thyroid dysfunction occur. Subclinical hypothyroidism as denoted by modest increases in TSH levels do not require treatment or the discontinuation of amiodarone therapy. An appreciation of the mechanism of the interaction between amiodarone and thyroid hormone metabolism permits an early recognition and appropriate treatment of thyroid dysfunction that occurs in susceptible patients during chronic therapy with the drug.

## References


1. Charlier R, Deltour G, Baudine A, et al: Pharmacology of amiodarone, an antianginal drug with a new biological profile. *Arzeimittelforsch* 18:1408, 1968.
2. Singh BN, Vaughan Williams EM: The effect of amiodarone, a new anti-anginal drug, on cardiac muscle. *Br J Pharmacol* 39:657, 1970.
3. Freedberg AS, Papp JG, Vaughan Williams EM: The effects of altered thyroid state on atrial intracellular potentials. *J Physiol* (London) 207:357, 1970.
4. Cotoi S, Conspanpinescu L, Gavrilescu S: The effect of thyroid state on monophasic action potentials in the human heart. *Experientia* 28:797, 1972.
5. Jaeger JM, Houser SR, Freeman AR, et al: Effect of thyroid hormone on canine cardiac Purkinje fiber action potential. *J Physiol* 240:H934, 1981.
6. Sharp NA, Neel DS, Parsons RL: Influence of thyroid hormone levels on the electrical and mechanical properties of rabbit papillary muscle. *J Cell Molec Cardiol* 17:119, 1985.
7. Pritchard DA, Singh BN, Hurley PJ: Effects of amiodarone on thyroid function in patients with ischemic heart disease. *Br Heart J* 37:856, 1975.
8. Burger A, Dinichert D, Nicod P, et al: Effect of amiodarone on serum triiodothyronine, reverse triiodothyronine, thyroxin and thyrotropin. *J Clin Invest* 58:255, 1976.
9. Jonckheer MH, Blockx P, Broechaert I, et al: 'Low $T_3$ syndrome' in patients chronically treated with an iodine-containing drug, amiodarone. *Clin Endocrinol* 9:27, 1978.
10. Rosenbaum MB, Chiale PA, Ryba D, et al: Control of tachyarrhythmias associated with the Wolf-Parkinson-White syndrome by amiodarone hydrochloride. *Am J Cardiol* 34:215, 1974.
11. Rosenbaum MB, Chiale PA, Halpern MS, et al: Clinical efficacy of amiodarone as an antiarrhythmic agent. *Am J Cardiol* 38:934, 1976.
12. Marcus FI, Fontaine GH, Frank R, et al: Clinical pharmacology and therapeutic applications of the antiarrhythmic drug, amiodarone. *Am Heart J* 101:480, 1981.
13. Nademanee K, Hendrickson JA, Cannom DS, et al: Control of refractory life-threatening ventricular arrhythmias by amiodarone. *Am Heart J* 101:759, 1981.
14. Nademanee K, Singh BN, Hendrickson JA, et al: Amiodarone in refractory life-threatening ventricular arrhythmias. *Ann Int Med* 98:577, 1983.
15. Heger JJ, Prystowsky E, Jackman WM, et al: Amiodarone: Clinical efficacy and electrophysiology during long-term therapy for recurrent ventricular tachycardia or ventricular fibrillation. *N Eng J Med* 305:538, 1981.
16. Singh BN, Nademanee K: Amiodarone and thyroid function: Clinical implications during antiarrhythmic therapy. *Am Heart J* 106:857, 1983.
17. Nademanee K, Singh BN, Hendrickson JA, et al: Pharmacokinetic significance of serum reverse $T_3$ levels during amiodarone treatment:

A potential method for monitoring chronic drug therapy. *Circulation* 66:202, 1982.

18. Andreasen F, Agerbaek H, Bjerregaard P, et al: Pharmacokinetics of amiodarone after intravenous or oral administration. *Eur J Clin Pharmacol* 19:293, 1981.

19. Rao RH, McCready VR, Spathis GS: Iodine kinetic studies during amiodarone treatment. *J Clin Endocrinol Metab* 62:563, 1986.

20. Wolff J: Iodide goiter and the pharmacologic effects of excess iodide. *Am J Med* 47:101, 1969.

21. Braverman LE, Ingbar SH: Changes in thyroidal function during adaptation to large doses of iodine. *J Clin Invest* 42:1216, 1983.

22. Melmed S, Nademanee K, Reed AW, et al: Hyperthyroxinemia with bradycardia and normal thyrotropin secretion after chronic amiodarone administration. *J Clin Endocrinol Metab* 53:997, 1981.

23. Attuel P: Amiodarone in cardiac arrhythmias. *Royal Society of Medicine International Congress and Symposium.* Series 6. The Royal Society of Medicine, p 39, 1979.

24. Lambert MJ, Burger AJ, Galeazzi RL, et al: Are selective increases in serum thyroxine ($T_4$) due to iodinated inhibitors to $T_4$ monodeiodination indicative of hyperthyroidism? *J Clin Endocrinol Metab* 55:1058, 1982.

25. Hershman JM, Nademanee K, Sugawara M, et al: Thyroxine and triiodothyronine kinetics in cardiac patients taking amiodarone. *Acta Endocrinol* 111:193, 1986.

26. Brent GA, Hershman JM: Effects of nonthyroidal illness on thyroid function tests. In L Van Middlesworth *The Thyroid Gland.* Chicago, Year Book Medical Publishers, p 83, 1986.

27. Sogol PB, Hershman JM, Reed AW, et al: The effects of amiodarone on serum thyroid hormones and hepatic thyroxine 5'-monodeiodination in rats. *Endocrinology* 113:1464, 1983.

28. Franklyn JA, Davis JR, Gammage MD, et al: Amiodarone and thyroid hormone action. *Clin Endocrinol* 22:257, 1985.

29. Safran M, Frang S-L, Bambini G, et al: Effects of amiodarone and desethylamiodarone on pituitary deiodinase activity and thyrotropin secretion in the rat. *Am J Med Sci* 292:136, 1986.

30. Valenzuela M, Pineda G: Amiodarona no inhibe la actividad de al 5'dyodasa hipofisaria en ratas hipotiroideas. *Rev Med Chile* 115:103, 1987.

31. Bambini G, Fang SL, Roti E, et al: Effect of amiodarone and desethylamiodarone on cardiac reverse $T_3$ 5'-monodeiodination. Program of the 61st Meeting of the American Thyroid Assoc., Sept. 10–13, 1986, T-22.

32. Pekary AE, Hershman JM, Reed AW, et al: Amiodarone inhibits $T_4$ to $T_3$ conversion and alpha-glycerophosphate dehydrogenase and malic enzyme levels in rat liver. *Horm Metab Res* 18:114, 1986.

33. Kerin NZ, Blevins RD, Benaderet D, et al: Relation of serum reverse $T_3$ to amiodarone antiarrhythmic efficacy and toxicity. *Am J Cardiol* 57:128, 1986.

34. Nademanee K, Singh BN, Callahan B, et al: Amiodarone, thyroid hormone indices, and altered thyroid function: Long-term serial effects in patients with cardiac arrhythmias. *Am J Cardiol* 58:981, 1986.

35. Polster P, Broekhuysen J: The adrenergic antagonism of amiodarone. *Biochem Pharmacol* 26:131, 1976.
36. Chevigne-Brancart M, Vandalem JL: Thyroid function during and after amiodarone therapy. Abstract N. Prog 64th Annual Meeting of the Endocrine Society, 128, 1982.
37. Amico JA, Richardson V, Alpert B, et al: Clinical and chemical assessment of thyroid function during therapy with amiodarone. *Arch Intern Med* 144:487, 1984.
38. Martino E, Safran M, Aghini-Lombardi F, et al: Environmental iodine intake and thyroid dysfunction during chronic amiodarone therapy. *Ann Intern Med* 101:28, 1984.
39. Posner J, Sobel RJ, Glick S: Effect of amiodarone on thyroid hormone economy. Isr J Med Sci 20:113, 1984.
40. Sanmarti A, Permanyer-Miralda, Catellanos JM, et al. Chronic administration of amiodarone and thyroid function: A follow-up study. *Am Heart J* 180:1262, 1984.
41. Borowski GD, Garofano CD, Rose LI, et al. Effect of long-term amiodarone therapy on thyroid hormone levels and thyroid function. *Am J Med* 78:443, 1985.
42. Valenzuela M, Cristian BC, Pineda G, et al: Incidencia de disfunction tiroidea en pacientes en tratamiento cronico con amiodarona. *Rev Med Chile* 113:1072, 1985.
43. Sawin CT, Castelli WP, Hershman JM: The aging thyroid; thyroid deficiency in the Framingham Study. *Arch Intern Med* 145:1386, 1985.
44. Hawthorne GC, Campbell NPS, Geddes JS, et al: Amiodarone-induced hypothyroidism. A common complication of prolonged therapy: A report of eight cases. *Arch Intern Med* 145:1016, 1985.
45. Mazonson PD, Williams ML, Cantley LK, et al: Myxedema coma during long-term amiodarone therapy. *Am J Med* 77:751, 1984.
46. Wiersinga WM, Touber JL, Trip M, et al: Uninhibited thyroidal uptake of radioiodine despite iodine excess in amiodarone-induced hypothyroidism. *J Clin Endocrinol Metab* 63:485, 1986.
47. Monteiro E, Galvae-Teles A, Santos ML, et al: Antithyroid antibodies as an early marker for thyroid disease induced by amiodarone. *Br Med J* 292:227, 1986.
48. Leger AF, Fragu P, Rougier P, et al: Thyroid iodine content measured by x-ray fluorescence in amiodarone-induced thyrotoxicosis: Concise communication. *J Nucl Med* 24:582, 1983.
49. Martino E, Aghini-Lombardi A, Lippi F, et al: Twenty-four hour radioactive iodine uptake in 35 patients with amiodarone associated thyrotoxicosis. *J Nucl Med* 26:1402, 1985.
50. Staubli M, Studer H: Amiodarone-treated patients with suppressed TSH test are at risk of thyrotoxicosis. Klin Wocheschr 63:168, 1985.
51. Fradkin JE, Wolff J: Iodide-induced thyrotoxicosis. *Medicine* 62:1, 1983.
52. Klein I, Levey GS: Iodide excess and thyroid function. *Ann Intern Med* 98:406, 1983.
53. Martino E, Macchia E, Aghini-Lombardi F, et al: Is humoral thyroid autoimmunity relevative in amiodarone iodine-induced thyrotoxicosis (AHT)? *Clin Endocrinol* 24:627, 1986.

# Chapter 16

# Amiodarone in the Management of Supraventricular Tachycardias

William G. Stevenson, Daniel Rieders,
Koonlawee Nademanee, James Weiss,
and Bramah N. Singh

In 1976, Rosenbaum et al.[1] reported on the efficacy of amiodarone in the prophylactic control of a variety of supraventricular tachyarrhythmias. Subsequently, numerous reports have drawn attention to the potency of the drug in the treatment of atrial flutter and fibrillation and in reentrant supraventricular tachycardias both with and without preexcitation,[2] although the largest clinical experience, particularly in the United States as reported elsewhere in this book, has been in the control of life-threatening ventricular arrhythmias. However, in recent years, there has been an increasing use of the drug in recalcitrant supraventricular tachyarrhythmias. In this chapter, the salient available experience with the intravenous and the oral formulation of the drug in the management of various supraventricular arrhythmias is discussed in light of the known electrophysiologic actions of the drug. It is emphasized that the bulk of the reported experience is of an uncontrolled nature and dogmatic conclusions cannot be made regarding the precise role of the drug in the treatment of various supraventricular arrhythmias, although the evidence for the efficacy of the compound in most recalcitrant arrhythmias is reasonably secure. The discussion does not include the effects of the compound in patients with preexcitation syndromes, which is discussed in Chapter 18.

---

From: *Control of Cardiac Arrhythmias by Lengthening Repolarization*, edited by
Bramah N. Singh, MD, Futura Publishing Company Inc., Mount Kisco, NY,
© 1988.

## Electropharmacologic Considerations

Amiodarone is the first Class III antiarrhythmic drug to be used in the treatment of supraventricular arrhythmias and it has several desirable effects that contribute to its efficacy in this regard.[3,4] In attempting to delineate its antiarrhythmic profile in patients with various supraventricular arrhythmias, it clearly is relevant to appreciate that the net electrophysiologic effects of the drug differ somewhat quantitatively when it is administered intravenously and when it is taken orally over long periods of time.[35] As indicated in Chapter 14, the acute effects are dominated by those on the atrioventricular node, probably resulting from the drug's antiadrenergic and calcium antagonistic properties. These effects lead to a significant lengthening of the intranodal conduction time (the AH interval) and the prolongation of the effective and the functional refractory periods of the AV node. Thus, these changes will produce a slowing of the ventricular response in atrial flutter and fibrillation and occasionally may result in the conversion to sinus rhythm. This is unlikely to be a common occurrence however, as the effective refractory period is prolonged but slightly with only a minor increase in the time course of repolarization. The slowing of the intranodal conduction often reaches a critical level that, in reentrant paroxysmal supraventricular tachycardias, may lead to a sudden termination at the antegrade limb of the tachycardia circuit.

Following chronic therapy with amiodarone, the electrophysiologic picture in the atria is dominated by a marked lengthening of the atrial action potential duration, an effect that was reported by Olsson et al.[6] in 1973 (Fig. 1). They found that after 6 weeks of amiodarone (600 mg/day) administration, the atrial monophasic action potential duration measured by the suction electrode technique was prolonged 30 percent above the baseline. It also was found that, in untreated patients converted from atrial fibrillation to sinus rhythm, the atrial monophasic action potential duration was substantially longer in those who remained in sinus rhythm than in those who relapsed.[7] The data emphasized the antifibrillatory effects of prolonged atrial repolarization and refractoriness. Thus, it appears that, during chronic amiodarone administration, one might expect a greater antifibrillatory effect in atrial flutter and fibrillation than during acute drug administration. The lengthening of the atrial refractory period may suppress intraatrial reentry. Finally, it is known that following chronic oral therapy with amiodarone there is a greater effect on the AV nodal ef-

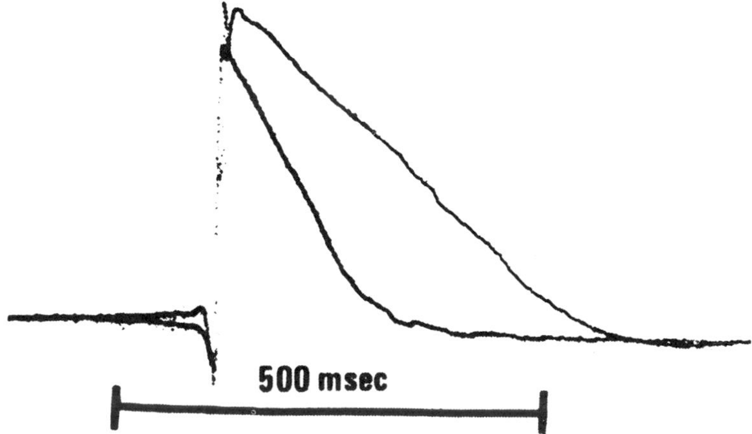



**Figure 1.** Superimposed traces of monophasic action potentials from the atria recorded by the suction electrode technique before and after 6 weeks of treatment with oral amiodarone. Note the lengthening of the action potential duration induced by amiodarone. By inference, the effective refractory period also is prolonged. (From Olsson JB, Brorson L, Varnauskas E: Antiarrhythmic action in man: Observations from monophasic action potential recordings and amiodarone treatment. *Br Heart J* 35:1255, 1973. By permission of the authors and the journal.)

fective and functional refractory periods than after acute drug administration.[3,5,8] Such a difference is relevant to the effects of the drug in attenuating the exercise-induced increments in ventricular response in atrial flutter and fibrillation and in preventing the recurrences of paroxysmal supraventricular tachycardia utilizing antegrade conduction at the AV node. It also should be emphasized that amiodarone is a potent suppressant of atrial premature contractions,[1] which may serve as the triggering mechanism for supraventricular tachyarrhythmias.

Amiodarone also suppresses sinus node automaticity and therefore can precipitate bradyarrhythmias in susceptible patients.[9] These overall considerations are pertinent to the understanding of the mechanism of the salutary effects of amiodarone in various atrial arrhythmias to be discussed in this chapter.

## Intravenous Amiodarone in Supraventricular Arrhythmias

As already indicated, the electrophysiologic effects of the intravenous drug indicate its potential value in slowing the ventricular response in atrial flutter and fibrillation and in termination of paroxysmal reentrant supraventricular tachycardias (PSVT). The available clinical experience is in line with these theoretical considerations.

## Paroxysmal Supraventricular Tachycardias

As expected from its acute effect on the atrioventricular node, intravenous amiodarone has been effective in terminating PSVT in 36 to 88 percent[10-17] of cases (see Table 1). Curry[17] gave an infusion of 5 mg/kg of intravenous amiodarone over 10 minutes via a central vein to 7 patients with PSVT. Amiodarone terminated 5 of the cases with PSVT to sinus rhythm within 6 minutes, the termination occurring because of the block in the antegrade AV limb of the tachycardia circuit. Programmed electrical stimulation failed to initiate the tachycardia 30 minutes after the termination of the tachycardia. In 1 patient, there was slowing of the tachycardia and an easier programmed termination after amiodarone. In contrast, the United Kingdom clinical experience survey conducted by Gosling et al.,[18] while providing further evidence for the efficacy of intravenous amiodarone in PSVT, revealed a somewhat lower rate of conversion. However, the majority of the patients had failed to respond to at least two other antiarrhythmic agents. It should be

### Table 1
#### Intravenous Amiodarone for Acute Termination of Supraventricular Arrhythmias

| Study | Atrial Fibrillation* | | Atrial Tachycardia | | PSVT | |
|---|---|---|---|---|---|---|
| | N | Success | N | Success | N | Success |
| Benaim & Uzan[10] (1978) | 45 | 38% | 19 | 47% | 11 | 36% |
| Storelli et al.[11] (1985) | 17 | 24% | — | — | 33 | 88% |
| Strasberg et al.[12] (1985) | 26 | 46% | — | — | — | — |
| Installe et al.[13] (1981) | 18 | 33% | — | — | — | — |
| Blandford et al.[14] (1981) | 3 | 33% | — | — | — | — |
| Faniel & Schoenfield[15] (1983) | 26 | 81% | — | — | — | — |
| Holt et al.[16] (1985) | 7 | 14% | 1 | 100% | — | — |
| Curry[17] (1986) | 7 | 14% | — | — | 7 | 71% |

*New onset or recent recurrences

emphasized that further data are needed to define the comparative efficacy and safety of intravenous amiodarone versus other agents (e.g., beta blockers, but especially verapamil, diltiazem, or adenosine) in the acute conversion of PSVT.

## Atrial Flutter and Fibrillation

Curry[17] and Gosling et al.[18] noted that, although intravenous amiodarone was uniformly effective in slowing the ventricular response in these arrhythmias, rarely did it produce a conversion to sinus rhythm (Fig. 2). In this regard, the effects of acutely administered amiodarone resembles those of beta blockers or calcium channel blockers such as verapamil or diltiazem. Amiodarone has been administered intravenously in an attempt to rapidly convert recent onset atrial fibrillation (Table 1). The rapid effect of amiodarone on the AV node generally results in a prompt slowing of the ventricular response. Sinus rhythm was restored over 1 to 24 hours in 14–81 percent of patients. However, these are uncontrolled observational trials and it is likely that some patients would have converted spontaneously during this time. Hence, the role of amiodarone in this setting requires further evaluation. A recent small trial[19] compared the effects of IV amiodarone (7 mg/kg) followed by infusion of IV digoxin (0.5 mg over 30 minutes) in patients with atrial fibrillation complicating acute myocardial infarction. Eigh-

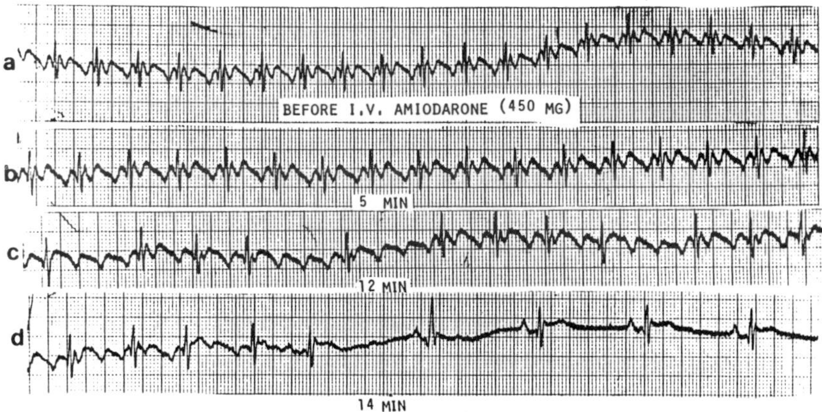


**Figure 2.**   Effects of intravenous amiodarone in the conversion of a recent onset atrial flutter. Note the progressive increase in the degree of AV block and the slowing of the flutter rate before the restoration of sinus rhythm. From Koonlawee Nademanee, unpublished observations.

teen patients were selected randomly to receive amiodarone and 16 to receive digoxin. The two groups were very similar; 3 patients selected for amiodarone and 1 for digoxin converted to sinus rhythm before the initiation of treatment. During the 24 hours, the conversion rate on amiodarone was 83 percent versus 75 percent in the digoxin group, with reversion occurring slightly earlier in the amiodarone group. This data establishes the safety of IV therapy but appears to offer no significant advantages over digoxin. In this setting, the comparative effects of beta blockers or calcium antagonists versus IV amiodarone will be of practical importance in the setting of acute infarction as well as in the post operative phase of patients undergoing open heart surgery.[15]

Perhaps it should be indicated that the value of amiodarone for the slowing of the ventricular response in these cases or for the conversion to sinus rhythm appears to be limited since it produces thrombophlebitis when given in a peripheral vein and hypotension, although transient, may develop during rapid infusions. The data indicate that the major role of amiodarone in supraventricular tachyarrhythmias is in the form of oral therapy for chronic prophylaxis. This will be discussed later.

## Orally Administered Amiodarone in the Treatment of Supraventricular Tachyarrhythmias

Although used for many years in Europe for the treament of supraventricular arrhythmias, only recently has amiodarone emerged as an important agent for the prophylactic control of refractory cases. The drug now is used increasingly for the treatment of refractory cases of atrial flutter and fibrillation.[20,21] However, although used widely in paroxysmal supraventricular tachycardias in the past, its role in this arrhythmia is undergoing redefinition with the increasing availability of other, somewhat simpler compounds, such as encainide and sotalol.

### Atrial Fibrillation and Flutter

In this setting, the utility of amiodarone is in (1) slowing the ventricular response at rest, and with exercise (2) converting the arrhythmia to sinus rhythm and (3) maintaining the stability of sinus rhythm during chronic oral therapy. However, it should be indicated that the conversion rate that occurs with the drug during chronic therapy is unpredictable, it may occur after a long period of therapy, and the precise efficacy in this regard is uncertain.

Amiodarone often will maintain sinus rhythm in patients who have chronic or paroxysmal atrial fibrillation refractory to several Class I antiarrhythmic compounds. In this context, amiodarone may be effective when most other agents have failed. Recently, we analyzed our data in 59 patients with chronic or paroxysmal atrial fibrillation that had not been controlled successfully with Class 1 antiarrhythmic agents. The clinical characteristics and previous antiarrhythmic therapies of these patients are shown in Tables 2 and 3.

Table 2
Amiodarone for Atrial Fibrillation/Flutter Clinical Characteristics

| | |
|---|---|
| Number | 59 |
| Age (years) | 63 ± 10 |
| Men | 40 |
| Heart Disease | |
|     Coronary | 14 |
|     Valvular | 14 |
|     Hypertension | 10 |
|     Dilated cardiomyopathy | 9 |
|     Other | 4 |
|     No structural abnormalities | 10 |
| Congestive failure | 21 |
| Paroxysmal AF | 35 |
| Chronic AF | 24 |
| Symptoms < 1 yr | 14 |
| Symptoms > 1 yr | 45 |

AF = Atrial fibrillation/flutter.

Table 3
Previous Drug Therapy

| Antiarrhythmic Agents | % of Patients |
|---|---|
| Any Class I drug | 92 |
| Disopyramide | 38 |
| Procainamide | 50 |
| Quinidine | 69 |
| Digoxin | 80 |
| Beta blockers | 52 |
| Calcium channel blockers | 31 |

Therapy was initiated with a loading dose of 600–1200 mg/day for 1 to 2 weeks, following which the dose was decreased to 400–800 mg/day for 2 to 8 weeks. The daily dose then was tapered slowly over several months to 200–400 mg as dictated by the clinical response.

Amiodarone was successful in restoring sinus rhythm in 10 of the 24 (42 percent) patients with chronic atrial fibrillation. In 4 additional patients, amiodarone maintained sinus rhythm following cardioversion for atrial fibrillation. Thus, amiodarone was effective in maintaining sinus rhythm in 59 percent of patients with chronic atrial fibrillation. In 35 patients with recurrent paroxysmal atrial fibrillation, amiodarone prevented arrhythmia recurrences in 94 percent of patients. Echocardiograms and LV ejection fractions were available in 39 and 44 patients, respectively. As shown in Table 4, patients with chronic atrial fibrillation, congestive heart failure, and significantly impaired left ventricular ejection fraction were less likely to remain in sinus rhythm than patients without these risk factors. Patients who had been in chronic atrial fibrillation for longer than 1 year also were less likely to be maintained in sinus rhythm, although this difference was of borderline significance.

It was of particular interest that left atrial size was not predictive of chronic antiarrhythmic efficacy of amiodarone. The relationship of these clinical features to amiodarone efficacy has been recently examined by others.[22–24] A duration of chronic atrial fibrillation for longer than 1 year, a left atrial diameter greater than 50 mm and a low left ventricular ejection fraction were related to drug failure in some, but not all studies. As in our study, efficacy was relatively good even in the high risk groups. Thus, the

Table 4

Determinants of Probability of Successful Treatment

| Characteristics | Present | Absent | P |
|---|---|---|---|
| Paroxysmal | 94 | — | <0.001 |
| Chronic | 58 | — | |
| Congestive Failure | 62 | 89 | <.05 |
| LA size >5 cm | 73 | 82 | NS |
| LV EF <.4 | 38 | 83 | <.01 |
| Symptoms >1 year | | | |
|    Paroxysmal | 92 | 100 | NS |
|    Chronic | 42 | 80 | NS |

presence of factors previously shown to predict recurrence of atrial fibrillation during therapy with Class 1A antiarrhythmic drugs does not preclude a good response to amiodarone.[25,26]

Amiodarone controlled atrial fibrillation but was discontinued due to side effects in 9 (15%) patients (Table 5). In 12 (20%) patients, amiodarone failed to maintain sinus rhythm although control of the ventricular rate was improved. Three of these patients also had adverse effects significant enough to warrant discontinuation of therapy (Table 5). As the daily dose of amiodarone was tapered to 200 mg or less, 16 of 28 (58%) patients suffered a recurrence of atrial fibrillation 17 ± 14.5 months after initiating therapy. However, control was almost invariably again achieved by increasing the dose. The minimum daily maintenance doses that prevented recurrences of atrial fibrillation are shown in Table 6. Life table analysis of the probability of successful therapy is shown in Figure 3. The probability of continued successful therapy with amiodarone was 76% at 1 year and 61% at 2 years.

Our results are similar to previous studies which have found

Table 5
Adverse Reactions to Amiodarone

| | | |
|---|---|---|
| Total Patients | 59 | |
| Minor | 28 | 47.5% |
| Severe Reactions | 12 | 20.3% |
|   Neurologic | 5 | 8.5% |
|   Myopathy | 1 | 1.7% |
|   Pneumonitis | 1 | 1.7% |
|   Skin Discoloration | 2 | 3.4% |
|   Gastrointestinal | 3 | 5.0% |

Table 6
Maintenance Dose of Amiodarone for
Prophylaxis of Atrial Fibrillation

| mg/day | % Patients Controlled |
|---|---|
| <200 | 4 |
| 200 | 29 |
| 300 | 13 |
| 400 | 47 |
| >400 | 7 |

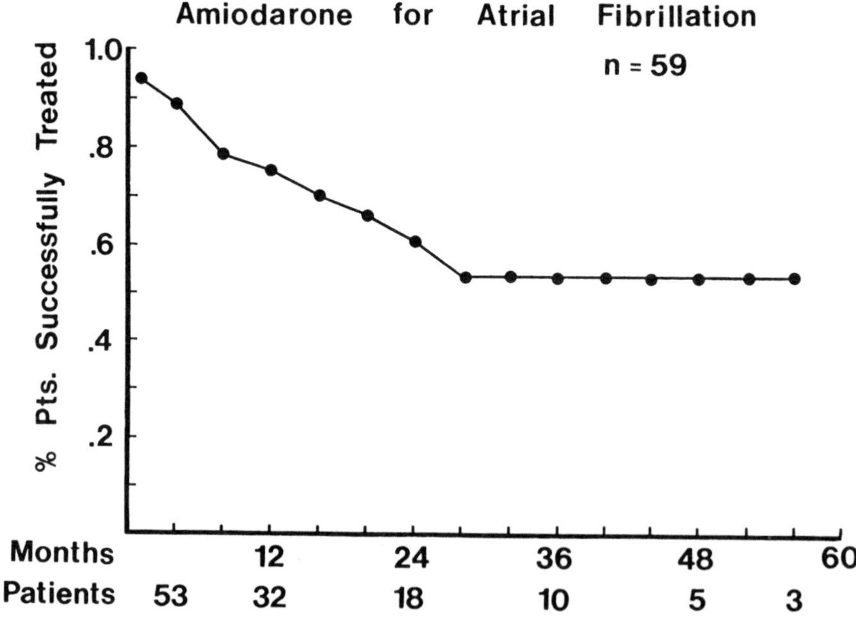


**Figure 3.** Cumulative probability of successful therapy with amiodarone for maintenance of sinus rhythm in patients with persistent or paroxysmal atrial fibrillation.

an efficacy of 29% to 77%[23,24,28−32] for maintaining sinus rhythm in patients with persistent atrial fibrillation and 50 to 97 percent for preventing paroxysmal atrial fibrillation (Table 7). The majority of these studies were conducted in patients with atrial fibrillation resistant to other antiarrhythmics. Vitolo et al. randomly chose patients successfully converted from atrial fibrillation to either quinidine (400 mg every 8 hours) or amiodarone 400 mg 5 days per week. Atrial fibrillation recurred within 6 months in 67 percent of the quinidine treated patients but in only 22 percent of the amiodarone treated patients.[27] Martin et al.[33] compared the effects of low dose amiodarone (200 mg/day maintenance) and disopyramide (400 mg/day) in patients with atrial fibrillation and flutter; amiodarone was effective in 55 percent. In cases of amiodarone failure, relapses to atrial fibrillation were associated with slower ventricular responses. Thus, amiodarone appears to be significantly more effective for the chronic prophylaxis of atrial fibrillation than available Class I antiarrhythmic drugs such as quinidine or disopyramide.

**Table 7**
**Chronic Amiodarone Therapy for Preventing Recurrences of Atrial Fibrillation**

| Study | Persistent AF | | Paroxysmal AF | |
|---|---|---|---|---|
|  | N | Success | N | Success |
| Rowland et al.[28] (1986) | 34 | 35% | — | — |
| McCarthy et al.[29] (1986) | 14 | 29% | — | — |
| Gold et al.[22] (1986) | 14 | 57% | 54 | 85% |
| Horowitz et al.[24] (1985) | 11 | 45% | 27 | 55% |
| Blomstrom et al[30] (1984) | 13 | 77% | 8 | 50% |
| Wheeler et al.[31] (1979) | 8 | 50% | 5 | 60% |
| Podrid & Lowin[32] (1981) | — | — | 20 | 80% |
| Martin et al.[33] (1986) | — | — | 43 | 88% |
| Ward et al.[37] (1980) | — | — | 15 | 53% |
| Rosenbaum et al.[1] (1976) | — | — | 30 | 97% |
| Naccarelli et al.[36] (1985) | (Duration not specified) | | 29 | 62% |
| Haffajee et al.[20] (1983) | (Duration not specified) | | 48 | 85% |
| Graboys et al.[21] (1983) | (Duration not specified) | | 95 | 78% |
| Vitolo et al.[27] (1981) | (Duration not specified) | | 28 | 79% |

When amiodarone is administered to patients already taking digoxin or warfarin, it is important to monitor closely for toxicity since amiodarone decreases the metabolism of these medications.[34,35] In general, we decrease the dose of warfarin by half at the time therapy with amiodarone is begun.

## Paroxysmal Supraventricular Tachycardia Without Preexcitation

Paroxysmal supraventricular tachycardia incorporating an accessory atrioventricular connection is discussed elsewhere in this book. In a small number of reported patients with PSVT without evidence of preexcitation or with documented intra-AV nodal re-entry, amiodarone has been found to be effective[1,31–33,36] in preventing tachycardia recurrences (Table 8). This is consistent with its effect on the atrioventricular node. The small number of cases reported is probably due to the relative ease in controlling PSVT with simpler medications. At present, it is not known whether the effect of acutely administered amiodarone on inducible PSVT is predictive of long-term response during chronic prophylaxis.

<table>
<tr><td colspan="3" align="center">Table 8<br>Chronic Amiodarone for Paroxysmal SVT in Patients<br>Without Preexcitation</td></tr>
<tr><td>Study</td><td>N</td><td>Success</td></tr>
<tr><td>Nacarelli et al.[37] (1985)</td><td>4</td><td>100%</td></tr>
<tr><td>Haffajee et al.[20] (1983)</td><td>6</td><td>67%</td></tr>
<tr><td>Podrid & Lowin[32] (1981)</td><td>6</td><td>100%</td></tr>
<tr><td>Wheeler et al.[31] (1979)</td><td>2</td><td>100%</td></tr>
<tr><td>Rosenbaum et al.[1] (1976)</td><td>39</td><td>95%</td></tr>
</table>

## Atrial Tachycardia

Chronic administration of amiodarone for the conversion and prophylaxis of ectopic atrial tachycardia has been reported in a small number of patients.[31,37–39] In general, it has been effective in approximately two-thirds of patients, regardless of the presumed mechanism of the tachycardia (automaticity or reentry). Intravenous amiodarone has been reported to acutely terminate atrial tachycardia in 47 percent of 19 patients in one series.[10]

## Summary

Amiodarone has displayed a broad spectrum of activity against supraventricular arrhythmias consistent with its effects on atrial and AV nodal refractoriness and AV nodal conduction. These effects represent a summation of direct and indirect electrophysiologic actions of the compound. It is extremely effective for maintaining sinus rhythm in most patients with paroxysmal atrial fibrillation and almost half of patients with persistent atrial fibrillation even if multiple other antiarrhythmic drugs have failed. It also is effective in preventing recurrences of atrioventricular nodal reentry and atrial tachycardias, although these arrhythmias commonly are controllable with simpler agents. However, side effects prevent long-term therapy in approximately 20 percent of patients. The role of intravenous amiodarone for the acute management of supraventricular arrhythmias requires further evaluation although preliminary data indicate that, in line with the known electrophysiologic effects of the drug, ventricular response in atrial flutter/ fibrillation is shown with a low rate of conversion to sinus rhythm, there being a higher rate of conversion in paroxysmal supraventricular tachycardia.

## References


1. Rosenbaum MB, Chiale PA, Halpern MS, et al: Clinical efficacy of amiodarone as an antiarrhythmic agent. *Am J Cardiol* 38:934, 1976.
2. Leak D, Eydt JN: Control of refractory cardiac arrhythmias with amiodarone. *Arch Int Med* 139:425, 1979.
3. Wellens HJJ, Brugada P, Abdollah H, et al: A comparison of the electrophysiologic effects of intravenous and oral amiodarone in the same patient. *Circulation* 69:120, 1983.
4. Finerman WB, Hamer A, Peter T, et al: Electrophysiologic effects of chronic amiodarone therapy in patients with ventricular arrhythmias. *Am Heart J* 104:987, 1982.
5. Ikeda N, Nademanee N, Kannan R, et al: Electrophysiologic effects of amiodarone: Experimental and clinical observation relative to serum and tissue drug concentration. *Am Heart J* 68:890, 1984.
6. Olsson JB, Brorson L, Varnauskas E: Antiarrhythmic action in man: Observations from monophasic action potential recordings and amiodarone treatment. *Br Heart J* 35:1255, 1973.
7. Olsson SB, Cotoi S, Varnauskas E: Monophasic action potential and sinus rhythm stability after conversion of atrial fibrillation. *Acta Med Scand* 190:381, 1971.
8. Singh BN: Amiodarone: Historical development and pharmacologic profile. *Am Heart J* 106:788, 1983.
9. McGovern B, Garan H, Ruskin JN. Sinus arrest during treatment with amiodarone. *Br Med J* 284:160, 1982.
10. Benaim R, Uzan C: Les effect antiarrhythmiques de l'amiodarone injectable (a propos de 153 cas). *Rev Med* 1959:19, 1978.
11. Storelli A, Andriulo C, Chisena A, et al: L'amiodarone endovena nella terapia della tachiaritmie parossistiche sopraventriolari. *Cr Ital Cardiol* 15:290, 1985.
12. Strasberg B, Arditti A, Sclarovsky S, et al: Efficacy of intravenous amiodarone in the management of new atrial fibrillation with fast ventricular response. *Int J Cardiol* 7:47, 1985.
13. Installe E, Schoevaerdts JC, Gadisseux P, et al: Intravenous amiodarone in the treatment of various arrhythmias following cardiac operations. *J Thorac Cardiovasc Surg* 81:302, 1981.
14. Blandford RL, Crampton J, Kudlac H. Intravenous amiodarone in atrial fibrillation complicating myocardial infarction. *Br Med J* 284:16, 1981.
15. Faniel R, Shoenfeld P: Efficacy of intravenous amiodarone in converting rapid atrial fibrillation and flutter to sinus rhythm: Intensive care patients. *Eur Heart J* 4:180, 1983.
16. Holt P, Crick JCP, Davies DW, et al: Intravenous amiodarone in the acute termination of supraventricular arrhythmias. *Int J Cardiol* 867, 1985.
17. Curry PVL: The efficacy of intravenous amiodarone. *Br J Clin Pharmacol* 40:152, 1986.
18. Gosling RH, Wildey W, Wirth MA: Intravenous amiodarone: UK clinical experience survey. *Br J Clin Pharmacol* 40:147, 1986.
19. Cowan JC, Gardiner P, Reid DS, et al: Amiodarone in the manage-

ment of atrial fibrillation complicating myocardial infarction. *Br J Clin Pract* 40:155, 1986.

20. Haffejee CL, Love JC, Candada AT, et al: Clinical pharmacokinetics and efficacy of amiodarone for refractory tachyarrhythmias. *Circulation* 67:1347, 1983.

21. Graboys TB, Podrid PJ, Lown B: Efficacy of amiodarone for refractory supraventricular tachyarrhythmias. *Am Heart J* 106:870, 1983.

22. Gold RC, Haffajee CL, Charos G, et al: Amiodarone for refractory atrial fibrillation. *Am J Cardiol* 57:124, 1986.

23. Yee KG, Heger JJ, Prystowsky EN, et al: Predictors of clinical efficacy for amiodarone in supraventricular tachyarrhythmias (abstract) *Circulation* 11:438, 1984.

24. Horowitz LN, Spielman SR, Greenspan AM, et al: Use of amiodarone in the treatment of persistent and paroxysmal atrial fibrillation resistant to quinidine therapy. *J Am Coll Cardiol* 6:1402, 1985.

25. Henry WL, Morganroth J, Pearlman AS, et al: Relation between echocardiographically documented left atrial size and atrial fibrillation. *Circulation* 53:273, 1976.

26. Hillstad L, Bjerkelund C, Dale J, et al: Quindine in maintenance of sinus rhythm after electroconversion of chronic atrial fibrillation. *Br Heart J* 33:518, 1971.

27. Vitolo E, Tronci M, Larovere MT, et al: Amidarone versus quinidine in the prophylaxis of atrial fibrillation. *Acta Cardiol* (Brussels) 6:431, 1981.

28. Rowland E, McKenna WJ, Krikler D: Amiodarone for the conversion of established atrial fibrillation and flutter. *Br J Clin Pract* 40 (Suppl 44):39, 1986.

29. McCarthy ST, McCarthy GL, John S, et al: Amiodarone as a treatment for atrial fibrillation refractory to digoxin therapy. *Br J Clin Pract* 40 (Suppl 44):49, 1986.

30. Blomstrom P, Edvardsson N, Olsson SB: Amiodarone in atrial fibrillation. *Acta Med Scand* 216:517, 1984.

31. Wheeler PH, Puritz R, Ingram DV, et al: Amiodarone in the treatment of refractory supraventricular and ventricular arrhythmias. *Postgrad Med J* 55:1, 1979.

32. Podrid PJ, Lowin B: Amiodarone therapy in symptomatic sustained refractory atrial and ventricular tachyarrhythmias. *Am Heart J* 101:374, 1981.

33. Martin A, Benbow LJ, Leach C, et al: Comparison of amiodarone and disopyramide in the control of paroxysmal atrial fibrillation and atrial flutter. *Br J Clin Pract* 40 (Suppl 44):52, 1986.

34. Hamer A, Peter T, Mandel WJ, et al: The potentiation of warfarin anticoagulation by amiodarone. *Circulation* 65:1025, 1982.

35. Nademanee K, Kannan R, Hendrickson JA, et al: Amiodarone–digoxin interaction: Clinical significance, time course of development, potential pharmacokinetic mechanisms and therapeutic implications. *J Amer Coll Cardiol* 4:111, 1984.

36. Ward DE, Camm AJ, Spurrelli RAJ: Clinical antiarrhythmic effects of amiodarone in patients with resistant paroxysmal tachycardias. *Br Heart J* 44:91, 1980.

37. Naccarelli G, Rinkenberger RL, Dougherty AH, et al: Amiodarone: Pharmacology and antiarrhythmic and adverse effects. *Pharmacotherapy* 5:298, 1985.
38. Wiener I, Lyons H. Amiodarone for refractory automatic atrial tachycardia: Observations on the electrophysiologic actions of amiodarone. *PACE* 7:707, 1984.
39. Tonet JL, Bernardeau C, Lechat P, et al: Comparison between the efficacy of amiodarone and quinidine in the treatment of atrial cardiac arrhythmias. *Br J Clin Pract* 40 (Suppl 44):42, 1986.

Chapter 17

# Amiodarone in the Wolff-Parkinson-White Syndrome

## Hein J. Wellens and Pedro Brugada

Amiodarone, although originally introduced as an antianginal agent, has been in use as an antiarrhythmic drug for more than 15 years.[1,2] Our own group has been especially interested in the use of amiodarone in the Wolff-Parkinson-White syndrome and has published many articles on the effects of the drug over a 10-year period.[3-12]

The purpose of this article is to review that experience with emphasis on the practical usage of amiodarone in the Wolff-Parkinson-White syndrome in light of the reported data from other investigative centers. A number of questions will be discussed: (1) What are the electrophysiological effects of amiodarone? (2) Has intravenous amiodarone the same effects as oral amiodarone? (3) What is the value of programmed electrical stimulation of the heart in predicting efficacy of the drug? (4) Why does amiodarone work? (5) Can the effect of amiodarone be antagonized by sympathetic stimulation? (6) Can the effect of amiodarone be predicted from the results of noninvasive tests? (7) How does one select the appropriate dose of amiodarone in an individual patient?

## The Arrhythmias in the Wolff-Parkinson-White Syndrome

In the Wolff-Parkinson-White syndrome, apart from the AV node-His pathway, an accessory pathway is present between the atrium and ventricle. The common indication for antiarrhythmic

From: *Control of Cardiac Arrhythmias by Lengthening Repolarization*, edited by Bramah N. Singh, MD, Futura Publishing Company Inc., Mount Kisco, NY, © 1988.

treatment in the WPW syndrome is the occurrence of circus movement tachycardia, atrial fibrillation, or both. The *circus movement tachycardia* usually is the result of sustained circulation of an impulse in a circuit consisting of atrium-AV node-His bundle-bundle branch-ventricle-accessory atrioventricular connection (orthodromic tachycardia). Uncommonly, the passage of the impulse is reversed, and the ventricular excitation occurs via anterograde conduction over the bypass tract and retrograde via the AV node. This is an example of antidromic type of circus movement tachycardia. Rarely a circuit is used with two accessory pathways, one for atrioventricular and one for ventriculoatrial conduction. To initiate a circus movement tachycardia, unidirectional block must occur in one of the two connections between the atrium and ventricle. Thereafter, the electrophysiologic properties (conduction velocity and refractory period duration) in the tachycardia circuit must be such that the impulse can reenter its chamber of origin and continue to circulate. A more detailed description of the many ways in which a circus movement tachycardia can be initiated has been given elsewhere.[9] It should be stressed that a delicate balance between conduction velocity and duration of the refractory period in the circuit is required to sustain the circus movement tachycardia. Antiarrhythmic drugs can prevent the initiating mechanism such as the premature beat or a change in heart rate or can change conduction velocity and/or the duration of the refractory period in one or more components of the circuit.

In atrial fibrillation, the presence of an accessory AV pathway may lead to life-threatening ventricular rates (300/min or faster), if the duration of the refractory period of the accessory pathway in the anterograde direction is short. The purpose of antiarrhythmic drug administration is to prevent the occurence of atrial fibrillation and to lengthen the anterograde refractory period of the accessory pathway to such an extent that high ventricular rates during atrial fibrillation or flutter no longer are possible. This will preclude the development of ventricular fibrillation and prevent sudden death.


## The Electrophysiological Effects of Amiodarone in the WPW Syndrome

In 1976, programmed electrical stimulation of the heart was performed in 15 patients suffering from circus movement tachycardia.[3] Seven of the patients also had atrial fibrillation. The stimulation study was repeated after 14 days of oral amiodarone. The dose utilized in this study was 600 mg/day of amiodarone for 7 days followed by 300 mg/day for the next 7 days, at which time electrophysiologic evaluation was repeated. In general, the anterograde refractory periods of the accessory pathway, the right atrium, and the right ventricle lengthened (mean increases of 109, 41, and 23 msec, respectively). There also was slowing in the rate of the circus movement tachycardia (a mean increase in tachycardia cycle length of 80 msec). It also was found that only in a limited number of patients amiodarone prevented the initiation of circus movement tachycardia by programmed stimulation of the heart. It is of interest that, as in the case of other antiarrhythmic drugs, the degree of lengthening of the anterograde refractory period of the accessory pathway was related to the initial predrug value.[4] This finding was confirmed in a more recent study (Fig. 1). It should be emphasized however, that the effects of amiodarone on the electrophysiologic characteristics of the bypass tracts and on the inducibility of the orthodromic tachycardia may vary with drug dosage. For example, Feld et al.[13] and Rasmussen and Berning[14] found larger increases in the effective refractory period (anterograde and retrograde) of the bypass tracts following larger loading doses of amiodarone. They also found a greater success rate in preventing the reinduction of circus movement tachycardia, there being a less consistent relationship between the magnitude of increase in the effective refractory period relative to the predrug value.

## A Comparison of Intravenous and Oral Amiodarone

Nine patients with the WPW syndrome were studied by programmed electrical stimulation of the heart before, after intravenous (5 mg/kg body weight in 1 min) and after oral (total dose 9800 to 11,200 mg) amiodarone.[10] While both intravenous and oral amiodarone produced a lengthening of the anterograde refractory period of the accessory atrioventricular pathway, the increase was more marked after oral amiodarone administration. Only oral amiodarone significantly prolonged the refractory period of atrium and ventricle and the HV interval. In contrast, only intravenous amiodarone prolonged the AH interval. In the 5 patients in whom the refractory period of the AV node could be measured after both intravenous and oral amiodarone, there was the same degree of

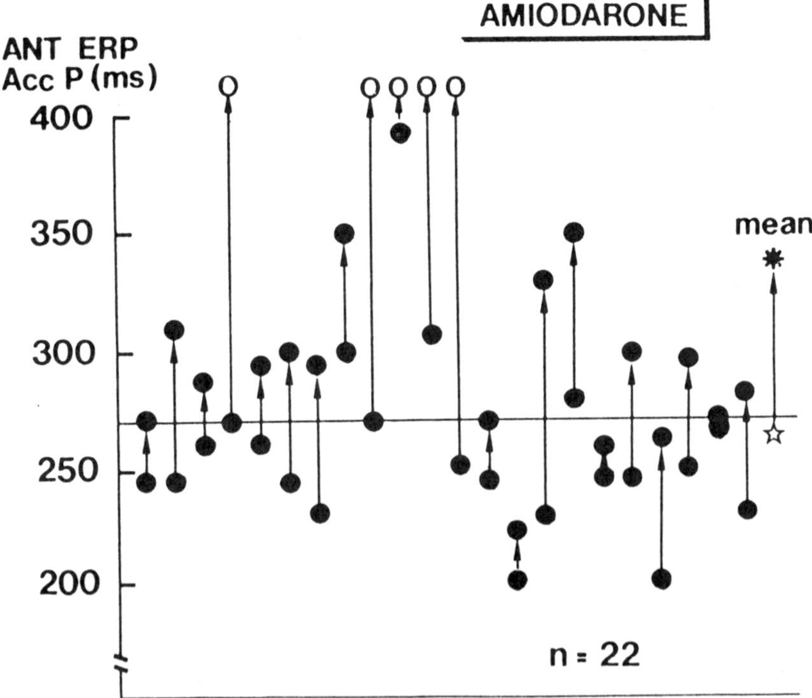


**Figure 1.** Effect of chronic oral amiodarone administration on the anterograde refractory period of the accessory pathway in relation to the initial (predrug) value of the anterograde refractory period of the accessory pathway. Open circles indicate patients in whom complete anterograde block in the accessory pathway developed following amiodarone. Note the importance of the initial value on the lengthening effects of amiodarone.

prolongation of the refractory period. Both intravenous and oral amiodarone slowed the rate of the circus movement tachycardia. Interestingly, while intravenous amiodarone led to a mean increase in tachycardia cycle length of 90 msec, an additional lengthening of the tachycardia cycle by 50 msec was seen after oral amiodarone. In all 9 patients, amiodarone was given intravenously during circus movement tachycardia. In 3 patients, this resulted in the termination of tachycardia by block in the AV node. In 2 of these 3 patients, tachycardia could not be reinitiated by programmed stimulation of the heart during oral amiodarone administration. In the remaining 7 patients, the circus movement tachycardia could still be provoked during the stimulation study on oral amiodarone. We concluded that test data indicated that intravenous and oral amiodarone do not have the same electrophysiologic effects. It is not clear whether cumulative effects, active metabolites, or both are responsible for these differences. The potential mechanisms that might account for the differences in the electrophysiologic effects of intravenous and oral amiodarone were discussed in Chapter 14. Table 1 gives a comparison of the electrophysiological effects of oral and intravenous amiodarone. The data are in line with the findings of Ikeda et al.[15] and those of Morady et al.[16] It is noteworthy that, in the case of Morady et al.,[16] the dose was 10 mg/kg. Despite the higher dose, the increases in right ventricular effective refractory period were modest, significantly less than those after protracted oral amiodarone administration.

Figure 2 schematically indicates the electrophysiologic effects of the different antiarrhythmic drugs on the different parts of the heart. As shown, chronically administered amiodarone affects all the different components of the heart involved in either a circus movement tachycardia or atrial fibrillation and flutter.

## The Value of Programmed Stimulation to Predict Clinical Efficacy of Amiodarone

Programmed stimulation before and after amiodarone administration will give information about its electrophysiological effects on the refractory period of the accessory pathway and the other components of the tachycardia circuit. Documentation of the changes in anterograde refractory period of the accessory pathway is of particular importance in the patients suffering from atrial fibrillation or flutter. From the preceding section, it has already become clear that in patients with circus movement tachycardia the arrhythmia may be variably reinitiated during programmed stimulation of the heart.

To obtain information about the predictive significance of this finding for clinical management of these patients, we decided to follow the patients during continued oral administration of amiodarone.[8] In 9 of 30 patients with circus movement tachycardia, the arrhythmia no longer could be reinitiated by programmed stimulation of the heart during oral amiodarone, indicating that in 70 percent of patients the tachycardia could still be initiated. However, during clinical follow-up with a mean of 40 months, only 4 patients had a spontaneous recurrence of tachycardia (13 percent). These data indicate that amiodarone frequently is successful clinically in

## Table 1

### Effect of Intravenous and Oral Amiodarone on Electrophysiologic Parameters (all measurements in msec)

| | No. of pts | Before Amiodarone A | | Intravenous Amiodarone B | | Oral Amiodarone C | | p Values | | |
|---|---|---|---|---|---|---|---|---|---|---|
| | | Range | Mean | Range | Mean | Range | Mean | A vs B | B vs C | A vs C |
| Sinus cycle length | 12 | 700−1090 | 799 ± 42 | 620−1000 | 792 ± 48 | 720−1300 | 940 ± 65 | NS | <.05 | <.05 |
| ERP RA | 12 | 160−320 | 232 ± 41 | 220−350 | 256 ± 42 | 200−370 | 268 ± 50 | NS | NS | <.05 |
| ERP RV | 12 | 200−240 | 229 ± 7 | 210−260 | 231 ± 10 | 210−300 | 247 ± 16 | NS | <.05 | <.05 |
| ERP AVN | 8 | 220−360 | 287 ± 31 | 260−350 | 326 ± 35 | 270−380 | 323 ± 37 | <.05 | NS | <.05 |
| ERP Ant AP | 9 | 230−300 | 265 ± 14 | 260−350 | 305 ± 21 | 275−>600 | 354 ± 32 | <.05 | <.05 | <.001 |
| AH interval | 11 | 55−90 | 76 ± 10 | 65−120 | 93 ± 16 | 60−120 | 83 ± 12 | <.05 | NS | NS |
| HV interval | 10 | 35−50 | 41 ± 6 | 35−50 | 43 ± 6 | 40−80 | 52 ± 10 | NS | <.05 | <.05 |

ERP = effective refractory period; RA = right atrium; RV = right ventricle; AVN = atrioventricular node; Ant AP = anterograde accessory pathway.

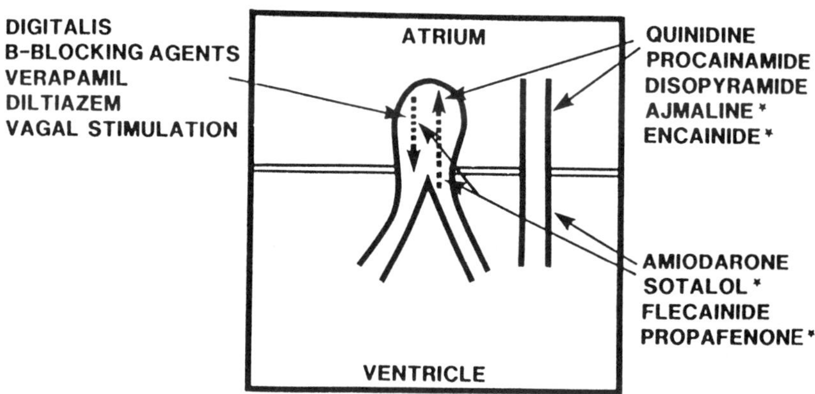


**Figure 2.** Illustration of the site of prolongation of the refractory period in the AV nodal–His pathway and the accessory atrioventricular pathway by different drugs. In general, drugs that prolong the refractory period of the accessory pathway also lengthen the refractory period of the atrium, His-Purkinje system, and ventricular muscle. Amiodarone affects all these components. Drugs marked by an asterisk are investigational in the U.S.A.

spite of the ability to reinitiate circus movement tachycardia by programmed stimulation during oral administration of amiodarone. Although there is some controversy, our data in the WPW syndrome in this regard resemble those reported for sustained monomorphic ventricular tachycardia, in which the failure to prevent reinduction by amiodarone does not preclude an excellent clinical outcome long term.

## Mechanism of Antiarrhythmic Action of Amiodarone

Programmed electrical stimulation of the heart allows partial insight into the mechanism of antiarrhythmic activity of amiodarone. Arrhythmias in the WPW syndrome require an initiating mechanism, usually a premature beat, and the correct balance in electrophysiologic properties within the circuit to be sustained. Programmed stimulation obviously will not provide us with information on the effect of amiodarone on the initiating premature beat, because that premature beat is given by the stimulation. Holter recordings are much better suited to provide an idea about the significance of the antiectopic actions of amiodarone. Programmed stimulation, however, can identify why the drug might interrupt conduction in the reentry circuit. As pointed out elsewhere,[8] this can be caused by a complete block in the accessory pathway or a prolongation of the refractory period in the accessory pathway, the AV node, or the bundle of His. We also found[11] that in some patients the rate-related shortening of the refractory period of the accessory pathway is prevented by amiodarone. This effect may lead to inability to sustain circus movement tachycardia. As already indicated, in many patients with circus movement tachycardia, the arrhythmia still can be initiated during programmed stimulation. Inability to initiate the circus movement tachycardia during amiodarone therapy predicts clinical success. However, many patients, in whom the arrhythmia can still be initiated by programmed stimulation have no recurrence during oral drug administration suggesting that in these patients the prevention of the tachycardia-initiating mechanism might be the reason for observed clinical success.

## Reversibility of Amiodarone-Induced Changes by Isoproterenol

It is clearly of practical importance to determine whether isoproterenol counteracts the amiodarone-induced changes in electrophysiologic properties of the heart. We have studied patients in whom electrophysiologic data were available before amiodarone administration, during oral amiodarone, and when isoproterenol was given while the patient was receiving oral amiodarone.[6,12] We found that the amiodarone-induced lengthening of the refractory period of the accessory pathway, the AV node, atrium and ventricle, the AH interval, and the slowing in tachycardia rate were completely reversed by isoproterenol administration.[6] Isoproterenol was administered at an initial dose of 0.25 to 1 µg/min and doubled every 3–5 minutes until an increase in sinus rate of at least 20 percent was attained. These observations suggest that sympathetic stimulation during exercise and anxiety may reverse amiodarone-induced changes in the electrophysiological properties of the heart. The converse also was found to hold. The facilitating effect of isoproterenol on the initiation of circus movement tachycardia could not be prevented by treatment with oral amiodarone.[12] This information is important not only for the patient with circus movement tachycardia but seems to be particularly relevant to the patient receiving amiodarone, because of atrial fibrillation in the presence of a short anterograde refractory period of the accessory AV-pathway. In these patients, beta blockade should accompany amiodarone administration to prevent further sympathetically mediated shortening of the anterograde refractory period of the accessory AV pathway following the onset of atrial fibrillation.

## Prediction of the Effect of Amiodarone from Results of Noninvasive Tests

We have demonstrated that both ajmaline[5] and procainamide[7] can be used to identify patients with a short anterograde refractory period of the accessory atrioventricular pathway. Failure to block anterograde conduction over the accessory pathway after the intravenous administration of these drugs was found to be highly suggestive of a short anterograde refractory period of that pathway.[5,7] We also showed that the amount of lengthening of the anterograde refractory period of the accessory pathway was related to its initial predrug value, lengthening being most marked in patients having a relatively long anterograde refractory period of their accessory pathway.[4] Not surprisingly, therefore, the effect of amiodarone on the anterograde refractory period of the accessory AV pathway may be predicted from the results of the ajmaline or procainamide test.[9] As shown in Table 2, block in the anterograde conduction over the accessory AV pathway following ajmaline or procainamide indicates a marked lengthening of the anterograde refractory period of the accessory AV pathway during oral amiodarone therapy.

The information that appropriate lengthening of the anterograde refractory period of the accessory pathway cannot be accom-

### Table 2
### Value of Ajmaline or Procainamide Test to Predict Effect of Long-Term Oral Amiodarone on Anterograde Effective Refractory Period of Accessory Pathway

| | Ant $ERP_{ap}$ (msec) | | |
|---|---|---|---|
| Aj/P test | $Am^-$ | $Am^+$ | Increase (msec) |
| + (12 patients) | 284 ± 25 | 384 ± 94 | 100 ± 85 |
| − (24 patients) | 237 ± 24 | 290 ± 37 | 53 ± 35 |

Ant $ERP_{ap}$ = anterograde effective refractory period of the accessory pathway; Aj = ajmaline; P = procainamide; $Am^-$ = before amiodarone; $Am^+$ = after amiodarone.

plished by drug administration, of course, is extremely important for the patient having atrial fibrillation in the presence of the WPW syndrome. Results of the ajmaline/procainamide test therefore are useful in selecting patients more likely to benefit from surgical interruption of their accessory pathway.

## How to Select the Appropriate Dose of Amiodarone?

Amiodarone is an extremely useful drug for the prophylactic treatment of cardiac arrhythmis in the WPW syndrome,[13,14,17,18] but since the drug may have potentially serious side effects during long-term drug administration the patient should be selected carefully and clinically monitored continually.

### Circus Movement Tachycardia

When tachycardia episodes are rare and well tolerated or tachycardia episodes can be terminated easily by vagal maneuvers, amiodarone therapy is not indicated. Only when tachycardias occur frequently, are rapid and poorly tolerated, and unresponsive to simpler treatment is amiodarone therapy started with a daily dose of 600 mg for a week, with a daily dose of 200 mg thereafter. It is of interest that in several patients after a few months of a daily dose of 200 mg the dose can be reduced to 100 mg daily. In reviewing a series of 76 patients (follow-up 10 to 102, mean 67, months) with circus movement tachycardia, we found that 11 patients had a weekly maintenance dose of amiodarone of 500 mg. Sixty-one and 4 patients had maintenance doses of 700 to 1400 mg and above 1400 mg, respectively. Since side effects of amiodarone usually are related to the dose given, it is not surprising that in patients with circus movement tachycardia side effects did not necessitate termination of amiodarone administration. The overall response of circus movement tachycardia to prophylactically administered amiodarone generally is excellent.[13] However, further comparative data derived from controlled studies involving newer agents such as sotalol or encainide will be of interest.

### Atrial Fibrillation

In patients with the WPW syndrome and atrial fibrillation, the severity of the arrhythmia primarily relates to the duration of the anterograde refractory period of the accessory pathway. As discussed earlier,[4] the extent of lengthening of the duration of the anterograde refractory period of the accessory pathway after amiodarone is related to the initial length of that refractory period. Unfortunately, in the presence of a short anterograde refractory period of the accessory pathway, the lengthening following amiodarone administration is disappointingly small in many cases. In the patient with documented atrial fibrillation and a short anterograde refractory period of the accessory pathway, therefore, we as do others favor[19] surgical interruption of the accessory pathway over drug therapy. It should be emphasized that in centers in which surgical approaches[20] to the bypass tracts are well developed, younger patients with atrial fibrillation complicating the WPW syndrome increasingly are offered surgical ablation in preference to a life-long commitment to drug therapy.

Amiodarone was given to 29 patients with electrocardiographically documented attacks of atrial fibrillation. During follow-up (11 to 110, mean 60, months) recurrences were prevented in 23 patients. The amiodarone dose was higher as compared to patients suffering from circus movement tachycardia. The majority of the patients are taking a maintenance dose of 300 or 400 mg daily. The value of amiodarone in patients with WPW and atrial fibrillation is based not only on the drug's effect on the duration of the anterograde refractory period but primarily on the resultant marked reduction in the number of episodes of paroxysmal atrial fibrillation.[17] This may be the result of the elimination of the premature beat initiating atrial fibrillation or due to the lengthening of the atrial refractory period after amiodarone administration.


## Conclusions

In recent years it has become clear that amiodarone is an effective drug in the prevention of circus movement tachycardia and atrial fibrillation in patients with the WPW syndrome, with generally acceptable side effects. Apart from its effects on the different components of the circuit in circus movement tachycardia and the anterograde refractory period of the accessory pathway in patients with atrial fibrillation or flutter, the chronically administered drug has important protective effects against mechanisms initiating these arrhythmias. Especially in circus movement tachycardia, arrhythmia control usually can be accomplished with relatively small dosages of amiodarone, with minimal side effects. The use of amiodarone in arrhythmias complicating the WPW syndrome is a major advance but the drug's clinical efficacy and utility in this setting needs to be balanced against its potential side effects. The intravenously administered drug has minimal effects on the electrophysiologic properties of the bypass tract; it is unlikely to be of value in the acute control of the ventricular response in atrial flutter and fibrillation complicating the WPW syndrome.

## References


1. Van Schepdael J, Solvay H: Étude clinique de l'amiodarone dans les troubles du rhythme cardiaque. *Presse Med* 78:1849, 1970.
2. Singh BN, Vaughan Williams EM: The effect of amiodarone, a new anti-anginal drug on cardiac muscle. *Br J Pharmacol* 39:657, 1970.
3. Wellens HJJ, Lie KI, Bar FW, et al: Effect of amiodarone in the Wolff-Parkinson-White syndrome. *Am J Cardiol* 46:665, 1980.
4. Wellens HJJ, Bar FW, Dassen W, et al: Effects of drugs in the Wolff-Parkinson-White syndrome. *Am J Cardiol* 46:665, 1980.
5. Wellens HJJ, Bar FW, Gorgels AP, et al: Use of ajmaline in patients with the Wolff-Parkinson-White syndrome to disclose a short refractory period of the accessory pathway. *Am J Cardiol* 45:130, 1980.
6. Wellens HJJ, Brugada P, Roy D, et al: Effect of isoproterenol on the anterograde refractory period of the accessory pathway with circus movement tachycardia. *Am J Cardiol* 50:180, 1982.
7. Wellens HJJ, Braat S, Brugada P, et al: Use of procainamide in patients with the Wolff-Parkinson-White syndrome to disclose a short refractory period of the accessory pathway. *Am J Cardiol* 50:1087, 1982.
8. Wellens HJJ, Brugada P, Abdollah H: Effect of amiodarone in paroxysmal supraventricular tachycardia with or without Wolff-Parkinson-White syndrome. *Am Heart J* 106:876, 1983.
9. Brugada P, Dassen WR, Braat S, et al: Value of the ajmaline-procainamide test to preduct the effect of long-term oral amiodarone on the anterograde effective refractory period of the accessory pathway in the Wolff-Parkinson-White syndrome. *Am J Cardiol* 52:70, 1983.
10. Wellens HJJ, Brugada P, Abdollah H, et al: A comparison of the electrophysiologic effects of intravenous and oral amiodarone in the same patient. *Circulation* 69:120, 1984.
11. Brugada P, Wellens HJJ: Effects of oral amiodarone on rate-dependent changes in refractoriness in patients with Wolff-Parkinson-White syndrome. *Am J Cardiol* 56:863, 1985.
12. Brugada P, Faccini M, Wellens HJJ: Effects of isoproterenol and amiodarone and the role of exercise in the initiation of circus movement tachycardia in the accessory atrioventricular pathway. *Am J Cardiol* 57:146, 1986.

13. Feld GK, Nademanee K, Weiss J, et al: Electrophysiologic basis for the suppression by amiodarone of orthodromic supraventricular tachycardias complicating pre-excitation syndromes. *J Am Coll Cardiol* 3:1298, 1984.
14. Rasmussen V, Berning J: Effects of amiodarone in the Wolff-Parkinson-White syndrome. *Acta Med Scand* 205:31, 1979.
15. Ikeda N, Nademanee K, Kannan R, et al: Electrophysiologic effects of amiodarone: experimental and clinical observations relative to serum and tissue concentrations. *Am Heart J* 108:890, 1984.
16. Morady F, Lorenzo LA, Kool RB, et al: Acute and chronic effects of amiodarone on ventricular refractoriness intraventricular conduction and ventricular tachycardia induction. *J Am Coll Cardiol* 7:148, 1986.
17. Rosenbaum MB, Chiale PA, Ryba D, et al: Control of tachyarrhythmias associated with Wolff-Parkinson-White syndrome by amiodarone hydrochloride. *Am J Cardiol* 34:215, 1974.
18. Rowland E, Kirkler DM: Electrophysiological assessment of amiodarone in treatment of resistent supraventricular arrhythmias. *Br Heart J* 44:82, 1980.
19. Kappenberger LJ, Fromer MA, Steinbrunn W, et al: Efficacy of amiodarone in the Wolff-Parkinson-White syndrome: Incidence after surgical ablation of the accessory pathway. *Circulation* 72:161, 1985.
20. Sharma RD, Klein GJ, Guiradon GM, et al: Atrial fibrillation in patients with Wolff-Parkinson-White syndrome: Incidence after surgical ablation of the accessory pathway. *Circulation* 72:161, 1985.

Chapter 18

# Relative Efficacy of Amiodarone and Propafenone in Patients with Recurrent Ventricular Tachycardia and Ventricular Fibrillation

James J. Heger, Eric N. Prystowsky, William M. Miles, Lawrence S. Klein, and Douglas P. Zipes

Clinical use of amiodarone dates to its introduction as an antianginal agent nearly two decades ago, whereas widespread recognition of amiodarone as an antiarrhythmic agent was fostered by the reports of Rosenbaum et al. beginning in 1974.[1,2] Since that time, there has been a large worldwide experience with amiodarone as an agent for treatment of recurrent ventricular arrhythmias. In a recent summary of published reports that included over 1000 patients treated for recurrent ventricular tachycardia or ventricular fibrillation, amiodarone was judged as an effective agent in 70 percent of patients with efficacy rates in individual studies ranging from 46 to 100 percent of treated patients.[3] Amiodarone usually was employed after one or several other available antiarrhythmic agents had been ineffective, so a direct comparison of amiodarone with other agents was not performed. Likewise, other new antiarrhythmic agents, such as propafenone, usually are employed in a similar manner. Previous experience with propafenone suggests it

From: *Control of Cardiac Arrhythmias by Lengthening Repolarization*, edited by Bramah N. Singh, MD, Futura Publishing Company Inc., Mount Kisco, NY, © 1988.

is an effective antiarrhythmic agent in patient populations similar
to those treated with amiodarone and also similar to the experience with amiodarone is that propafenone may prevent recurrence
of spontaneous ventricular arrhythmias despite continued inducibility of ventricular arrhythmias during propafenone treatment.[4]
Although either agent may be effective antiarrhythmic therapy, no
trials have compared directly the efficacy of amiodarone and propafenone. Such trials are difficult to accomplish utilizing a patient
population with life-threatening arrhythmias because of the necessity to provide adequate arrhythmia management and because the
pharmacologic features of amiodarone make a controlled, comparative trial relatively difficult. Since, in our experience, either amiodarone or propafenone may be employed to treat patients who
have recurrent ventricular arrhythmias unresponsive to multiple
previous antiarrhythmic drug trials, thus defining a population
with relatively resistant arrhythmias, we have retrospectively analyzed subgroups of patients treated with amiodarone and propafenone in an attempt to compare their antiarrhythmic efficacy.

## Methods

The study population was strictly defined in order to provide
homogeneous patient groups for comparison. Patients were included for analysis in this study only if they had experienced recurrent sustained ventricular tachycardia or ventricular fibrillation,
had failed multiple previous antiarrhythmic drug trials, underwent serial electrophysiologic testing, and were treated either with
amiodarone or propafenone as a single antiarrhythmic agent. From
a retrospective review of 230 consecutive patients treated with amiodarone and 86 consecutive patients treated with propafenone,
there were 68 amiodarone-treated patients and 16 propafenone-
treated patients who met all study criteria.

The treatment protocol was standard for each of the patients
evaluated. A control evaluation was performed after discontinuation of all prior antiarrhythmic agents for at least five half-lives of
the particular agent. During this antiarrhythmic drug-free state,
continuous electrocardiographic monitoring for at least 48 hours
was performed as well as a control electrophysiologic study. Drug
therapy with amiodarone was initiated at a dose of 800–1600 mg a
day for up to 2 weeks of in-hospital treatment. Propafenone was
administered at a dose of 600–900 mg a day in three divided doses

for up to 4 days of in-hospital monitoring. Continuous electrocardiographic monitoring was performed during all phases of in-hospital evaluation and at the end of initial in-hospital drug treatment phase, repeat electrophysiologic study was performed.

Electrophysiologic testing was performed using our standard, previously described protocol.[5] Programmed ventricular stimulation employed up to three ventricular extrastimuli from two right ventricular endocardial sites. Sustained ventricular tachycardia that occurred spontaneously or was induced by programmed ventricular stimulation was defined as that which lasted for 30 seconds or longer or required termination by electrical cardioversion or pacing due to hemodynamic collapse.

Antiarrhythmic drug therapy with either amiodarone or propafenone was considered a success during in-hospital therapy if the drug prevented spontaneous ventricular tachycardia or ventricular fibrillation, produced no intolerable side effects, and during electrophysiologic testing, either prevented induction of ventricular tachycardia or the induced ventricular tachycardia had a cycle length greater than 350 msec and was well tolerated hemodynamically, defined as maintenance of a systolic blood pressure of 90 mm Hg or greater while supine. Outpatient follow-up was conducted at 3-month intervals in the arrhythmia clinic at the Krannert Institute of Cardiology. The dose of propafenone during follow-up was either 600 or 900 mg a day, similar to that administered during hospital monitoring. Amiodarone dose was progressively reduced with 800 mg a day administered for the first month of follow-up and then an average of 400 mg a day administered for chronic maintenance therapy. During follow-up evaluation, patients were monitored for the occurrence of one of two end-points, either sustained symptomatic ventricular tachycardia or ventricular fibrillation or the occurrence of sudden cardiac death.

Statistical analysis of long-term follow-up data was performed using Kaplan-Meier life table analysis. Clinical and demographic variables, used to compare various subgroups of patients were analyzed either by chi-square analysis for noncontinuous variables or unpaired $t$ tests for continuous variables.

## Results

The study population of 84 patients (68 amiodarone-treated and 16 propafenone-treated) was composed of 66 men and 18 women whose mean age was 58 ± 9 years. The underlying heart disease was ischemic heart disease in 60 patients; dilated cardiomyopathy in 15 patients; and mitral valve prolapse, other valvular heart disease, and no identifiable heart disease in 3 patients each. The presenting clinical arrhythmia was recurrent ventricular fibrillation in 27 patients and recurrent sustained ventricular tachycardia in 57 patients and the mean left ventricular ejection fraction for the group was 0.33 ± 0.14.

Each of the 84 patients underwent electrophysiologic testing during drug therapy. Overall, 14 of 84 patients (17 percent) had no inducible ventricular tachycardia during drug therapy. The outcome of electrophysiologic testing for each drug treatment group is presented in Table 1. At repeat electrophysiologic study during drug therapy, ventricular tachycardia was no longer inducible in 11 of 68 (16 percent) amiodarone-treated patients and 3 of 16 (19 percent) propafenone-treated patients. This difference was not statistically significant. Each of the 14 patients whose arrhythmia became noninducible during drug therapy has continued amiodarone or propafenone without recurrence of symptomatic ventricular arrhythmia during follow-up. Of the remaining 57 amiodarone-treated patients, 27 had nonsustained ventricular tachycardia induced, and 30 patients continued to have sustained ventricular tachycardia induced during amiodarone treatment. Of the other 13 propafenone-treated patients, 2 had nonsustained ventricular tachycardia induced, and 11 continued to have sustained ventricular tachycardia induced. The patients who had nonsustained ventricular tachycardia induced were not analyzed further because the marked asymmetry between the two drug-treatment groups precluded statistical analysis.

Comparison of clinical features among the 14 patients in whom either drug prevented ventricular tachycardia induction and

### Table 1
### Results of Electrophysiologic Testing

| Number of Patients | Amiodarone | Propafenone | Total |
|---|---|---|---|
| Total | 68 | 16 | 84 |
| Electrophysiologic study result | | | |
|     Sustained VT | 30 | 11 | 41 |
|     Nonsustained VT | 27 | 2 | 29 |
|     VT not inducible | 11 | 3 | 14 |

VT = Ventricular Tachycardia

the 41 patients in whom sustained ventricular tachycardia could still be induced yielded no significant difference in the age, left ventricular ejection fraction, New York Heart Association classification for congestive heart failure, or number of prior antiarrhythmic drug trials (Table 2). Ischemic heart disease was more prevalent in those patients in whom sustained ventricular tachycardia remained inducible, 32 of 41 patients (78 percent), versus those patients in whom drug therapy prevented ventricular tachycardia induction, 6 of 14 patients (43 percent), (p < .01).

Each of the 41 patients who had inducible sustained ventricular tachycardia during drug therapy continued long-term antiarrhythmic therapy with amiodarone or propafenone as a single agent. Actuarial analysis of the proportion of these patients remaining free of recurrent ventricular tachycardia or ventricular fibrillation during follow-up is presented in Figure 1. From this analysis, the amiodarone and propafenone life table curves are significantly different (p = 0.02) indicating that amiodarone-treated patients had a lower risk of recurrent ventricular tachycardia or ventricular fibrillation than did propafenone-treated patients. At 11 months of follow-up, 44 percent of propafenone-treated patients remained free of recurrent ventricular tachycardia or ventricular fibrillation as compared to a recurrence-free rate during amiodarone treatment of 80 percent at 10 months and 63 percent at 30 months.

Comparisons of clinical parameters were performed between 30 amiodarone-treated patients and the 11 propafenone-treated pa-

Table 2

Electrophysiologic Study Subgroup Comparison

| | Subgroup | | |
|---|---|---|---|
| Parameter | No VT Induced | VT-S Induced | P |
| Number | 14 | 41 | NS |
| Sex Male/Female | 10/4 | 34/7 | NS |
| Disease category | | | |
|   Percent IHD | 43% (6/14) | 78% (32/41) | p < .01 |
|   LVEF | .41 ± .13 | .34 ± .15 | NS |
|   NYHA class I | 6 | 7 | |
|     II | 7 | 19 | NS |
|     III | 1 | 15 | |
| Prior drug trials | 3.7 ± 0.8 | 3.7 ± 1.7 | NS |

VT = Ventricular Tachycardia; S = Sustained; IHD = Ischemic Heart Disease; LVEF = Left Ventricular Ejection Fraction.

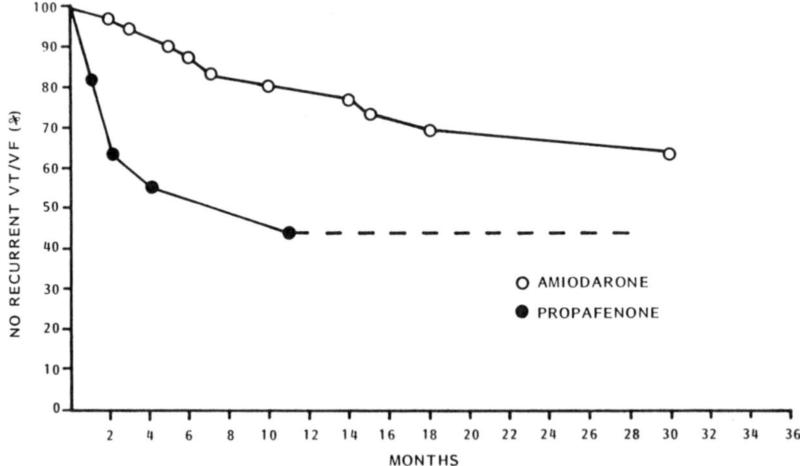


**Figure 1.** Life table analysis of the proportion of patients treated with amiodarone or propafenone who remained free of recurrent ventricular tachycardia or ventricular fibrillation during follow-up. The life table curves are significantly different with p = 0.02.

tients who had inducible sustained ventricular tachycardia and between the 15 patients who experienced recurrent ventricular arrhythmias and the 26 patients who remained free of recurrent arrhythmias (Tables 3 and 4). There were no significant differences in age, sex distribution, disease category, left ventricular ejection fraction, New York Heart Association classification for heart failure, or number of prior drug trials between these groups. The only significant difference was in comparing the patients with or without clinical recurrence of ventricular arrhythmias, where a significantly higher proportion of amiodarone-treated patients were in the group with no recurrence of arrhythmia, 22 of 26 (85 percent), than were in the group with arrhythmia recurrence, 8 of 15 (53 percent), (p < .05).

## Discussion

In this study, the antiarrhythmic efficacy of amiodarone and propafenone was compared in similar study populations. All patients had experienced recurrent sustained ventricular tachycardia or ventricular fibrillation, had failed multiple prior antiarrhythmic drugs, and underwent serial electrophysiologic testing with either

Table 3
Drug Subgroup Comparisons

| Parameter | Amiodarone | Propafenone | p |
|---|---|---|---|
| Number | 30 | 11 | — |
| Age (years) | 58 ± 12 | 58 ± 6 | NS |
| Sex | | | |
|   Men | 24 | 10 | NS |
|   Women | 6 | 1 | |
| Disease Category: | | | |
|   IHD (%) | 23 (77) | 9 (82) | NS |
|   LVEF | .35 ± .19 | .34 ± .10 | NS |
|   NYHA class | | | |
|     I | 4 | 3 | |
|     II | 15 | 5 | NS |
|     III | 11 | 3 | |
| Prior drug trials | 3.6 ± 1.5 | 3.4 ± 1.4 | NS |

VT = Ventricular Tachycardia; S = Sustained; IHD = Ischemic Heart Disease; LVEF = Left Ventricular Ejection Fraction.

Table 4
Subgroup Characteristics of Patients with VT-S at Drug EP Study

| Parameter | Follow-up Results | | p |
| | Recurrent VT-VF | No Recurrent VT-VF | |
|---|---|---|---|
| Number | 15 | 26 | — |
| Age | 57 ± 7 | 58 ± 8 | NS |
| Sex: | | | |
|   Men | 11 | 23 | NS |
|   Women | 4 | 3 | |
| Disease category: | | | |
|   IHD (%) | 12 (80%) | 20 (77%) | NS |
|   LVEF | .37 ± .13 | .18 ± .12 | NS |
|   NHYA class | | | |
|     I | 3 | 4 | |
|     II | 7 | 12 | NS |
|     III | 5 | 10 | |
| Prior drug trials | 3.8 ± 2.0 | 3.6 ± 1.5 | NS |
| Drug treatment: | | | |
|   Amiodarone | 8 | 22 | p < .05 |
|   Propafenone | 7 | 4 | |

VT = Ventricular Tachycardia; S = Sustained; IHD = Ischemic Heart Disease; LVEF = Left Ventricular Ejection Fraction.

amiodarone or propafenone as a single agent. One finding of this study was that amiodarone and propafenone were similarly effective in preventing induction of ventricular tachycardia by programmed ventricular stimulation. The proportion of patients in whom drug therapy prevented induction of ventricular tachycardia was low (17 percent), but this is consistent with our overall experience in patients who have sustained ventricular arrhythmias.[6] Moreover, the low response rate probably reflects that the population studied had arrhythmias that were relatively resistant to antiarrhythmic drugs, since both amiodarone- and propafenone-treated patients had failed more than three prior antiarrhythmic drug trials.

While amiodarone and propafenone had similar rates of efficacy in preventing induction of sustained ventricular arrhythmias, amiodarone appeared significantly more effective in preventing spontaneous recurrence of arrhythmia. In previous reports, we had noted that failure to prevent induction of ventricular tachycardia at electrophysiologic study did not preclude a successful long-term clinical response to amiodarone.[7] In patients who had either nonsustained or sustained ventricular tachycardia induced during amiodarone therapy, there was approximately a 25 percent probability of recurrent ventricular tachycardia or ventricular fibrillation at 24 months of follow-up and approximately 40 percent recurrence rate at 48 months of follow-up in these patients.[8] Likewise, we had noted that a substantial proportion of propafenone-treated patients remained free of clinical recurrence of their arrhythmia despite continued inducibility of ventricular arrhythmia during electrophysiologic testing.[4] With this information, the present study compared drug efficacy in a subset of patients who had sustained ventricular tachycardia induced by programmed ventricular stimulation during drug therapy and were similar for other clinical variables, such as type of heart disease and extent of left ventricular dysfunction. Therefore, in a study population that was relatively homogeneous in terms of clinical parameters, hemodynamic parameters, clinical arrhythmia, and electrophysiologic study results, a comparison of two antiarrhythmic drug regimens indicated amiodarone was more effective than propafenone.

Analysis of other clinical criteria indicated that patients who had ischemic heart disease were less likely to have noninducible ventricular tachycardia during amiodarone or propafenone therapy. Other variables analyzed did not discriminate between success of drug therapy in preventing induction of ventricular tachycardia or success of long-term drug therapy in preventing spontaneous recurrence of ventricular tachycardia or ventricular fibrillation. Previous analyses also have indicated that antiarrhythmic drug success was not predicted by clinical variables but that variables from electrophysiologic study, namely mode of ventricular tachycardia induction, was predictive of drug efficacy in patients treated with amiodarone or propafenone.[9,10]

Although the patient populations treated either with amiodarone or propafenone appeared comparable in regard to multiple clinical variables and both series were collected concurrently, this study did not employ a random allocation of patients to either drug therapy. Therefore, there may be an unintended selection bias favoring the amiodarone-treated patients that accounts for the improved efficacy noted. However, from the clinical variables identified and analyzed, no such bias appears evident. Moreover, while amiodarone appeared more effective in long-term follow-up, none of the clinical variables tested were reliable predictors of which drug would be effective either in preventing induction of ventricular tachycardia at electrophysiologic testing or in preventing spontaneous recurrence. In addition, since this study was not a crossover design, it is not known whether the efficacy of either drug tested predicts efficacy of the other. Finally, while amiodarone appeared more effective in prevention of recurrent ventricular arrhythmias in this select population, the choice of antiarrhythmic therapy includes factors, such as relative safety and side effects, which were not addressed in this study.

*The research behind this chapter was supported in part by the Herman C. Krannert Fund, Indianapolis, Indiana; by Grants HL-06308, and HL-07182 from the National Heart, Lung and Blood Institute of the National Institutes of Health, Bethesda, Maryland; and by the Attorney General of Indiana Public Health Trust and by the Roudebush Veterans Administration Medical Center, Indianapolis, Indiana; and by a Grant-In-Aid from the American Heart Association, Indiana Affiliate, Inc., Indianapolis, Indiana.*

## References

1. Rosenbaum MB, Chiale PA, Halpern MS, et al: Clinical efficacy of amiodarone as an antiarrhythmic agent. *Am J Cardiol* 38:934, 1976.
2. Rosenbaum MB, Chiale PA, Ryba D, et al: Control of tachyarrhythmias associated with Wolff-Parkinson-White syndrome by amiodarone hydrochloride. *Am J Cardiol* 34:215, 1974.

3. Heger JJ, Prystowsky EN, Miles WM, et al: Clinical use and pharmacology of amiodarone. In Zipes DP (ed): *Medical Clinics of North America*. Philadelphia, W.B. Saunders, 1984, 1339.
4. Chilson DA, Heger JJ, Zipes DP, et al: Electrophysiologic effects and clinical efficacy of oral propafenone therapy in patients with ventricular tachycardia. *J Am Coll Cardiol* 5:1407, 1985.
5. Prystowsky EN, Miles WM, Evans JJ, et al: Induction of ventricular tachycardia during programmed electrical stimulation: Analysis of pacing methods. *Circulation,* 73:II-33, 1986.
6. Prystowsky EN, Heger JJ, Lloyd EA, et al: Clinical electrophysiology of ventricular tachycardia. In Zipes DP (ed): *Cardiac Arrhythmias: Cardiology Clinics*. Philadelphia, W.B. Saunders, 1983, 253.
7. Heger JJ, Prystowsky EN, Jackman WM, et al: Amiodarone: Clinical efficacy and electrophysiology during long-term therapy for recurrent ventricular tachycardia or ventricular fibrillation. *N Eng J Med* 305:539, 1981.
8. Heger JJ, Prystowsky EN, Miles WM, et al: Clinical experience with amiodarone for treatment of recurrent ventricular tachycardia and ventricular fibrillation. *Br J Clin Prac* 40:1, 1986.
9. Klein LS, Fineberg N, Heger JJ, et al: Amiodarone: Prospective evaluation of a discriminant function to predict recurrence of ventricular arrhythmias. *Circulation* 72:III, 1985.
10. Minardo JD, Miles WM, Heger JJ, et al: Propafenone therapy for ventricular arrhythmias—Role of electrophysiologic testing. *Circulation* 74:II-312, 1986.

# Chapter 19

# Predictors of Long-Term Response to Amiodarone in Patients with Sustained Ventricular Tachyarrhythmias: Comparative Value of Ambulatory Monitoring and Programmed Electrical Stimulation Responses

Richard Kehoe, Terry Zheutlin,
Charles Davidson, Joseph Sarmiento,
Thomas Mattioni, Michelle Parker,
Catherine Dunnington, and Michael Lesch

The effectiveness of amiodarone for the therapy of a wide spectrum of cardiac arrhythmias has been well documented in numerous prior studies.[1-6] Despite the widely held view that amiodarone is a potent antiarrhythmic agent, considerable controversy exists as to which parameters are the best predictors of long-term arrhythmic outcome in patients receiving this agent for sustained ventricular tachyarrhythmias.[7,8] Certainly, the ability to accurately predict the recurrence of potentially lethal ventricular arrhythmias in such patients would be of great practical value since alternative

From: *Control of Cardiac Arrhythmias by Lengthening Repolarization,* edited by Bramah N. Singh, MD, Futura Publishing Company Inc., Mount Kisco, NY, © 1988.

antiarrhythmic drug therapy, ablative surgical techniques, or implantable automatically functioning cardioversion/defibrillation devices could be employed in those felt to remain at high arrhythmic risk.

To date, the techniques that have proved the most useful in assessing antiarrhythmic drug responses and in predicting arrhythmic outcome for patients with ventricular tachyarrhythmias have been programmed electrical stimulation (PES) and continuous ambulatory monitoring (AM). Either the suppression of ventricular tachycardia (VT) induction at PES[9] or the abolition of spontaneous VT runs during 24-hour AM[10] have been reported to predict a favorable response to amiodarone. However, it is difficult to determine which of these techniques offers the greater predictive accuracy since in the majority of prior studies, the assessment has been limited to either PES or AM and little data are available comparing the two methods within the same patient population. Accordingly, the relative value of AM and PES responses as predictors of amiodarone efficacy remains largely undetermined.

While it generally is felt that the abolition of inducible VT at PES in patients receiving amiodarone indicates a low risk of arrhythmic recurrence, the outcome of those with persistence of inducible VT despite therapy remains controversial.[7,8] Some investigators have reported arrhythmic recurrence rates as high as 60–70 percent at 2 years for such patients.[11] In contrast, others have reported a far better outcome for patients with persistent inducibility, citing recurrence rates of only 15–30 percent at similar lengths of follow-up.[1,2,12,13] The reasons for these reported differences in arrhythmic outcome are unclear, but may be related to differences in the study populations with respect to clinical and angiographic characteristics known to significantly influence arrhythmic risk.[14] Such characteristics include the type of underlying heart disease, nature of the presenting arrhythmia (VT or VF), the presence or absence of prior cardiac arrests, the extent of left ventricular dysfunction, and NYHA functional class.

In order to determine which clinical features and arrhythmia assessment techniques are the most useful in predicting long-term response to amiodarone, the clinical characteristics, PES and AM responses of 91 patients receiving amiodarone for recurrent sustained VT or documented ventricular fibrillation (VF) were determined prior to hospital discharge. These findings in turn were related to arrhythmic outcome as these patients were followed prospectively in our outpatient arrhythmia clinic.

## Methods

### Patient Selection

Between January 1982 and September 1986, 91 patients evaluated by the Clinical Cardiac Electrophysiology Service were discharged on long-term amiodarone therapy for the treatment of symptomatic sustained ventricular tachyarrhythmias. The presenting arrhythmia was sustained VT in 67 patients and documented VF in 24. Patients were excluded from this study if the presenting episode of VT/VF was secondary to acute myocardial infarction, electrolyte disturbance, drug intoxication, or a spontaneous or drug-induced prolonged QT syndrome.

The clinical, arrhythmic and angiographic characteristics of the study population are summarized in Tables 1 and 2. In all 91 patients, the presenting arrhythmia was associated with either cardiovascular collapse or hemodynamic compromise defined as systolic pressure <80 mm Hg. Fifty-five of the 67 patients with sustained VT required urgent DC cardioversion, and 9 required ei-

|  |  |
|---|---|
| **Table 1** | |
| **Clinical and Angiographic Characteristic** | |
| **of the Patient Population** | |
| Total patients | 91 |
| Men/Women | 71/20 |
| Age (years) | 61 ± 13 |
| Type of heart disease: | |
|   Coronary disease | 64 |
|   Prior MI | 62 |
|   Cardiomyopathy | 17 |
|   Valvular | 5 |
|   PEHD | 4 |
|   Congenital | 1 |
| LV Aneurysm | 47 |
| LV ejection fraction (%) | 38 ± 13 |
| Prior CHF | 41 |
| NYHA Class | |
|   I or II | 48 |
|   III or IV | 43 |

CHF = Congestive Heart Failure; LV = Left Ventricular; MI = Myocardial Infarction; NYHA = New York Heart Association; PEHD = Primary Electrical Heart Disease.

|  |  |
| --- | --- |
| **Table 2** | |
| **Arrhythmic Features of the Patient Population** | |
| Total patients | 91 |
| Type of presenting arrhythmia: | |
|    Sustained VT | 67 (74%) |
|    VF | 24 (26%) |
| Site of presenting arrhythmia: | |
|    In-hospital | 15 (16%) |
|    Out-of-hospital | 76 (84%) |
| Number requiring DC cardioversion | 82 (90%) |
| Prior MAE | 63 (69%) |
| Prior drug failure: | |
|    Spontaneous | 63 (69%) |
|    During PES | 28 (31%) |
| Amiodarone Loading Dose (mg) | 1293 ± 291 |
| Amiodarone Maintenance dose (mg) | 514 ± 134 |

DC = Direct Current; MAE = Major Arrhythmic Episodes; PES = Programmed Electrical Stimulation; VF = Ventricular Fibrillation; VT = Ventricular Tachycardia.

ther intravenous lidocaine or procainamide to terminate VT. All 24 patients with ventricular fibrillation were found pulseless and unconscious by arriving paramedics and required emergency DC fibrillation. All 91 patients had failed to respond to at least one (mean = 3 ± 1/patient) conventional or investigational antiarrhythmic drug prior to therapy with amiodarone. Sixty-three of the 91 patients (69 percent) had experienced at least one (range 1−4 /patient) documented prior major arrhythmic episode (MAE) defined as either VF or sustained VT requiring DC cardioversion.

The initial evaluation of each patient included a thorough history and a review of all available medical records to determine the following clinical variables: (1) history of prior left ventricular failure defined as dyspnea at rest with radiographic evidence of pulmonary vascular congestion; (2) history of spontaneous or exertional chest pain compatible with angina pectoris; (3) history of previous myocardial infarction; (4) prior coronary artery bypass grafting; and (5) site of presenting arrhythmia, in-hospital or out-of-hospital. The nature and extent of underlying heart disease was determined by cardiac catheterization and left ventriculography in 69 patients and by noninvasive methods in 22. Left ventricular ejection fraction was determined angiographically in 69 patients and by radionuclide techniques in 22. Patients who exhibited one or more dyskinetic left ventricular segments were considered to have left ventricular aneurysms.

## Programmed Stimulation Techniques

Seventy-six of the 91 patients underwent control drug–free PES studies. In 13 patients, a drug-free study was precluded by the emergence of sustained, hemodynamically compromising VT during the period of antiarrhythmic drug withdrawal. All 13 of these patients exhibited inducible VT during subsequent serial drug trials before the institution of amiodarone therapy. Two patients refused baseline PES study.

Control PES was performed in the post absorptive, nonsedated state after all antiarrhythmic agents (except digoxin) had been discontinued for at least 48 hours. PES was performed using temporary transvenous pacing catheters with an interelectrode separation of 10 mm. All stimulation was bipolar and performed at a stimulus current twice the diastolic threshold for capture with a pulse width of 2 msec. The pacing protocol included single ($S_1$) and double ($S_2S_3$) ventricular extrastimuli initially coupled to spontaneous rhythm and, thereafter, coupled to ventricular pacing at cycle lengths of 600, 500, and 400 msec. Rapid burst ventricular pacing (5–7 consecutive captures) in increments of 10 beats/minute was performed at rates ranging from 160–250 beats/minute, if single or double extrastimulus technique failed to initiate VT. If right ventricular apical stimulation did not result in VT induction, repeat stimulation of the right ventricular outflow tract was performed according to the same stimulation protocol.

Control PES responses were defined as follows: (1) *Inducible VT* indicates the reproducible (at least twice) initiation of 7 or more repetitive ventricular responses excluding bundle branch reentry with the mean rate of the induced VT exceeding 120 beats/minute; (2) *sustained VT* indicates an induced VT with a rate exceeding 120 beats/minute that required urgent termination due to hemodynamic compromise or a VT that lasted greater than 30 seconds; (3) *nonsustained VT* indicates an induced VT of 7 or more beats duration with a mean rate exceeding 120 beats/minute that terminated spontaneously within 30 seconds.

Patients were considered inducible at either control and post-amiodarone PES studies if either sustained or nonsustained VT could be reproducibly initiated at either right ventricular site in response to the stimulation protocol described earlier.

## Ambulatory Monitoring and Treadmill Studies

An attempt was made to obtain baseline drug-free 24-hour Holter monitoring data on each patient prior to PES studies. This was accomplished in 81 patients using an Avionics dual channel recorder (Model #445). The 24-hour tapes were analyzed using a Marquette Series 8000 Holter Analysis System and the recordings subsequently reviewed by two of the investigators for accuracy. The total number of isolated VPBs per 24 hours and the presence of VT runs, defined as 3 or more consecutive VPBs with a mean rate $\geq$ 100 beats/minute, were determined. In 10 patients, the development of symptomatic VT/VF during the drug-free period precluded the completion of 24-hour ambulatory monitoring. These patients were classified as having spontaneous VT runs.

Baseline drug-free symptom limited exercise treadmill studies also were obtained using the modified Bruce protocol in the 52 patients capable of upright exercise. The duration of exercise, the development of angina pectoris, or the emergence of symptomatic VT during exercise were determined.

## Amiodarone Treatment Schedule

All 91 patients underwent amiodarone loading for 14 days with loading doses ranging from 800 to 1600 mg/day; the mean loading dose for the group was 1293 $\pm$ 291 mg. Occasional downward dose adjustments were required before the end of the 14-day period, usually due to GI or neurologic side effects. Subsequently, patients were discharged on 800 mg of amiodarone daily for another 2 weeks. Ultimately, an attempt was made to reduce chronic maintenance doses to 400–600 mg/day. The mean amiodarone dosage employed for chronic therapy was 514 $\pm$ 134 mg/day.

## Post-amiodarone Studies

After 8–14 (mean 9 $\pm$ 2) days of amiodarone loading, repeat PES, 24-hour ambulatory monitoring, and symptom-limited, modified Bruce protocol treadmill exercise testing were repeated. These studies were omitted only at the request of the patient or the referring physician. The same variables as outlined earlier for drug-free control studies were obtained after amiodarone loading. These findings are summarized in Table 3.

Table 3

Summary of Baseline and Predischarge 24-Hour AM and Treadmill Responses

| | Baseline | Predischarge |
|---|---|---|
| Ambulatory Monitoring: | n = 91 | n = 90 |
| VPB frequency/24 hours | | |
| Mean | 3060 ± 4111 | 1932 ± 9910 |
| Median | 1291 | 109 |
| Percent Suppression | | |
| Mean (%) | — | 20 ± 258 |
| Median (%) | — | 92 |
| VPB Complexity | | |
| Pairs or less (pts) | 19 (21%) | 60 (67%) |
| VT runs (pts) | 72 (79%) | 30 (33%) |
| VT runs suppressed (pts) | — | 47 |
| VT runs presistent VT (pts) | | 25 |
| VT runs of new onset (pts) | — | 5 |
| Treadmill Responses | n = 52 | n = 61 |
| Duration (sec) | 716 ± 336 | 645 ± 287 |
| Maximum HR (beats/min) | 147 ± 22 | 125 ± 27 |
| VT runs (pts) | 11 | 8 |
| Symptomatic VT runs (pts) | 3 | None |

AM = 24-Hour Ambulatory Monitoring; HR = Heart Rate; VPB = Ventricular Premature Beat; VT = Ventricular Tachycardia.

## Follow-up

Patients were seen in our outpatient arrhythmia clinic every 3 months, at which time a clinical assessment, physical examination, 12 lead EKG, routine clinical serum chemistries, and a 24-hour Holter monitor were obtained. Patients were evaluated specifically for the interim development of either congestive heart failure or angina pectoris as defined earlier.

Amiodarone was considered effective in a given patient if there was no occurence of major arrhythmic episodes during follow-up. A major arrhythmic episode (MAE) was defined as syncope without other apparent cause, sustained symptomatic VT, documented VF, or sudden unexpected death.

The patient population was then divided into two groups based upon their response to amiodarone therapy. Group 1 was composed of the 71 patients (78 percent) who remained free of MAE during follow-up, and Group 2 was composed of the 20 patients (22 percent) who sustained arrhythmic recurrence.

## Statistical Methods

Comparisons between patient groups were made using two sample $t$ tests for continuous variables and chi-square tests for discrete variables. The Mann-Whitney U test was used to compare total VPB counts during 24-hour ambulatory monitoring because the counts were not distributed normally.

The Kaplan-Meier method was used to generate major arrhythmic event curves and standard life table techniques were used to summarize results. The outcome variable was recurrence of a MAE. Patients who died suddenly were considered to have had a recurrence. Patients in whom amiodarone was discontinued due to side effects or who died from nonarrhythmic causes were considered censored as of the date of drug discontinuation or death. No patients were lost to follow-up. Comparisons between major arrhythmic event recurrence curves were tested using the log rank test. A p value of $<.05$ was considered statistically significant.

For the various ambulatory monitoring and PES testing variables, sensitivity, specificity, positive predictive value, negative predictive value, and predictive accuracy were defined as follows:

Sensitivity = True Positive/(True Positive + False Negative)
Specificity = True Negative/(True Negative + False Positive)
Positive Predictive Value = True Positive/(True Positive + False Positive)
Negative Predictive Value = True Negative/(True Negative + False Negative
Predictive Accuracy = True Positive + True Negative/Total Population

A true positive for 24-hour AM was defined as the presence of spontaneous VT during predischarge monitoring with the development of MAE during follow-up; and a true negative for 24-hour AM, the absence of VT during predischarge monitoring and freedom from MAE during follow-up. A true positive for PES was defined as the presence of inducible VT at predischarge PES and the development of MAE during follow-up; and a true negative for PES, the absence of VT at predischarge PES and freedom from MAE during follow-up.

The positive and negative predictive values and predictive accuracy for 24-hour AM and PES were determined at 12, 24, and 36 months follow-up and compared.

## Results

## Ambulatory Monitoring and Treadmill Responses

Baseline 24 hour AM was completed in 81 patients (Table 3) and precluded in 10 patients who developed spontaneous symptomatic VT or VF during the drug-free period. At baseline, the mean isolated ventricular premature beat frequency (VPB) was 3060 ± 4111 per 24 hours and the median frequency 1281 per 24 hours. After therapy with amiodarone, the predischarge mean and median VPB frequencies per 24 hours decreased to 1932 ± 9910 and 109, respectively. The mean and median percent VPB suppressions resulting from amiodarone therapy were 20 percent and 92 percent, respectively.

Seventy-two patients (79 percent) exhibited VT runs at baseline 24-hour AM, whereas 19 patients (21 percent) had only couplets or multiform isolated VPBs. Of the 90 patients undergoing predischarge 24-hour AM, 30 (33 percent) had VT runs and 60 (67 percent) exhibited only pairs or isolated VPBs. Of the 72 patients with VT runs at baseline AM, 47 patients (65 percent) had abolition of all VT runs during the predischarge 24-hour AM and 25 patients (35 percent) exhibited persistent VT runs despite therapy. In 4 patients, VT runs were absent at baseline and first documented at the time of discharge 24-hour recording.

Only 11 patients (12 percent) exhibited VT runs during baseline treadmill exercise. The exercise-provoked VT was symptomatic and sustained in 3. All 11 patients with VT runs during exercise also exhibited VT during baseline AM. During predischarge exercise testing, 8 of these 11 patients had persistence of VT runs, but none had symptomatic or sustained arrhythmia. No patient exhibited angina pectoris during either baseline or predischarge exercise testing. The mean treadmill durations at baseline and predischarge studies were 716 ± 336 and 645 ± 287 seconds, respectively. The mean maximum heart rates achieved were 147 ± 22 and 125 ± 27 at baseline and predischarge studies, respectively.

## PES Responses

Baseline PES studies were undertaken in 76 patients (Table 4) and deferred in 13 because of spontaneous sustained VT or VF

Table 4
Summary of Baseline and Predischarge PES Responses

| | Baseline (n = 89) | Predischarge (n = 73) |
|---|---|---|
| Inducible VT: | | |
| Yes (pts) | 73 (82%) | 55 (75%) |
| No (pts) | 16 (18%) | 18 (25%) |
| Sustained (pts) | 57 | 35 |
| Nonsustained (pts) | 16 | 20 |
| Mode of Induction: | | |
| $S_2S_3$ (pts) | 57 | 45 |
| IVP (pts) | 3 | 10 |
| Spontaneous (pts) | 13 | — |
| Rendered free of inducible VT (pts) | — | 12 |
| Persistence of inducible VT (pts) | — | 51 |
| New onset inducible VT (pts) | — | 4 |

IVP = Incremental Ventricular Pacing; $S_2S_3$ = Paired Extrastimulus Testing; VT = Ventricular Tachycardia

during the drug withdrawal period. All 13 of these patients exhibited inducible VT during subsequent serial drug testing and were classified as having inducible VT. Two patients refused baseline PES. Of the 76 patients undergoing baseline PES, 60 had inducible VT and 16 did not. Thus, of the 89 patients ultimately undergoing PES evaluations, 73 (82 percent) were classified as having inducible VT and 16 patients (18 percent) as noninducible. The induced or spontaneous VT at control study was sustained in 57 patients and nonsustained in 16. VT was initiated in response to $S_2S_3$ extrastimulus testing in 57 patients, incremental ventricular pacing in 3 and occurred spontaneously in 13.

Predischarge PES studies were undertaken in 73 patients and deferred in 18 at the request of either the patient or the managing physician. Of the 73 undergoing predischarge PES, 55 patients (75 percent) exhibited inducible VT and 18 (25 percent) were noninducible. At predischarge PES, VT induction occurred in response to $S_2S_3$ extrastimulus testing in 45 patients and incremental ventricular pacing in 10. The induced VT at predischarge PES was sustained in 35 patients and nonsustained in 20.

Of the 73 patients who exhibited inducible VT at baseline PES, 63 underwent repeat PES prior to hospital discharge. Twelve of these 63 patients (19 percent) were free of inducible VT after amiodarone therapy, whereas 51 patients (81 percent) exhibited persistence of inducible VT despite therapy.

## Clinical Outcome

The study population was followed for a mean of 19 ± 15 months. During follow-up, 71 patients (78 percent) remained free of major arrhythmic events (MAE) and were designated as Group 1. The 20 patients (22 percent) who had subsequent MAE were designated as Group 2. For the 20 Group 2 patients, MAE was manifest as sudden death in 9 patients, sustained VT in 8 patients, and documented fatal VF in the remaining 3. The mean time to MAE was 8.8 ± 6.8 months. In addition to the 12 patients with presumed or documented sudden arrhythmic death, 5 additional patients died of noncardiac causes, and 4 eventually succumbed to progressive heart failure. Figure 1 depicts the actuarial analysis of amiodarone efficacy for the entire study population. The estimated percentage of patients remaining free of arrhythmic recurrence at 12, 24, and 36 months was 80 percent, 72 percent, and 69 percent, respectively.

## Comparison of Groups 1 and 2

The clinical and angiographic features of Groups 1 and 2 are summarized in Table 5. The groups were similar with respect to

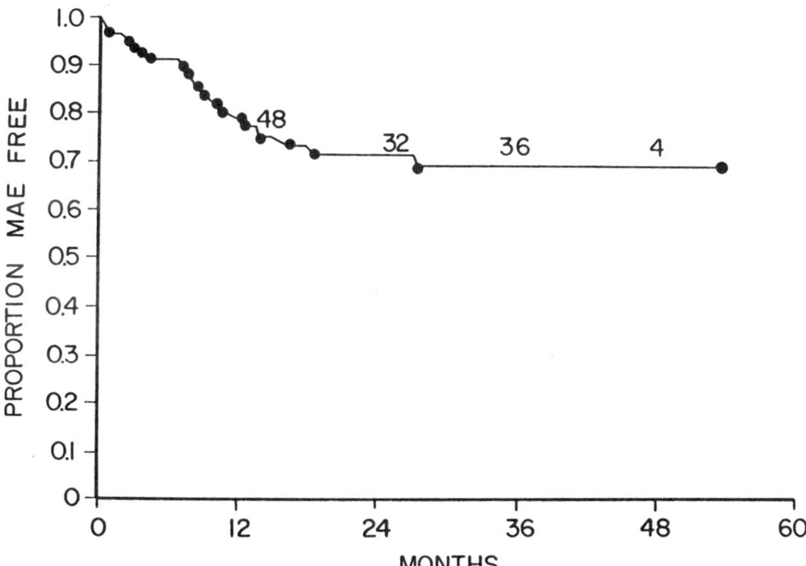


**Figure 1.** Life table analysis depicting the overall efficacy of amiodarone in 91 patients with sustained ventricular tachyarrhythmia. MAE = Major Arrhythmic Episodes during follow-up.

Table 5
Comparison of the Clinical and Angiographic Features of
Groups 1 and 2

| | Group 1 (n = 71) | Group 2 (n = 20) | p Value |
|---|---|---|---|
| Age (years) | 61 ± 13 | 62 ± 13 | NS |
| Prior MI (pts) | 50 (70%) | 12 (60%) | NS |
| Prior CHF (pts) | 32 (45%) | 9 (45%) | NS |
| NYHA Class III or IV (pts) | 31 (44%) | 12 (60%) | NS |
| Presenting MAE: | | | |
|   VF (pts) | 20 (28%) | 4 (25%) | NS |
|   VT (pts) | 51 (72%) | 16 (75%) | NS |
| Prior MAE (pts) | 44 (62%) | 19 (95%) | <.005 |
| Late CHF (pts) | 18 (25%) | 12 (60%) | <.004 |
| Late angina (pts) | 7 (10%) | 2 (10%) | NS |
| LV ejection fraction (%) | 37 ± 12 | 37 ± 15 | NS |
| LV aneurysm (pts) | 36 (51%) | 12 (60%) | NS |
| Amiodarone dose: | | | |
|   Loading (mg) | 1297 ± 300 | 1278 ± 258 | NS |
|   Maintenance (mg) | 514 ± 134 | 520 ± 136 | NS |

CHF = Congestive Heart Failure; LV = Left Ventricular; MAE = Major Arrhythmic Event; MI = Myocardial Infarction; NYHA = New York Heart Association; VF = Ventricular Fibrillation; VT = Ventricular Tachycardia.

age, sex, amiodarone loading and maintenance doses, presence of prior infarction, presenting MAE type (VT or VF), presence of LV aneurysm, new onset angina during follow-up, and mean LV ejection fraction. Although mean LV ejection fraction was similar for both groups, life table analysis revealed a trend towards a higher probability of arrhythmic recurrence for patients with LV ejection fractions less than 35 percent. For the 44 patients with ejection fractions of 35 percent or less, the percent sustaining arrhythmic recurrence was 18 percent at 12 months, 36 percent at 24 months, and 44 percent at 36 months. The percent sustaining arrhythmic recurrence for the 47 patients with ejection fractions greater than 35 percent was 20 percent, 23 percent, and 23 percent at 12, 24, and 36 months of follow-up, respectively. Although suggestive of enhanced arrhythmic risk for patients with lower ejection fraction, the observed difference in outcome failed to reach statistical significance (p < .06).

The groups did differ significantly with respect to history of prior MAE (44 of 71, Group 1 versus 19 of 20, Group 2; p < .005). The actuarial outcome of the 63 patients with a history of one or more prior MAEs is compared to the 28 patients presenting with their initial arrhythmic episode in Figure 2. The percentages remaining MAE free at 12, 24, and 36 months were 96 percent at all three points of follow-up for those free of prior MAE as compared to 74 percent, 65 percent, and 62 percent at the corresponding follow-up points for those with a history of prior MAE (p < .05).

Groups 1 and 2 also differed significantly with respect to the number of patients developing CHF during follow-up (18 of 71, Group 1 versus 12 of 20, Group 2 (p < .004). The outcome of the 30 patients who developed one or more episodes of congestive heart failure (CHF) during follow-up is compared to the 61 who remained free of CHF (Fig. 3). At 12, 24, and 36 months follow-up, the corresponding percentages remaining MAE free were 88 percent, 83 percent, and 83 percent for those without CHF and 68 percent, 52 percent, and 42 percent for those who developed CHF (p < .02).

## Comparison of 24-Hour AM Responses

The 24 hour AM and exercise treadmill characteristics of the two groups are summarized in Table 6. The groups were similar with respect to isolated VPB frequency at both baseline and predis-

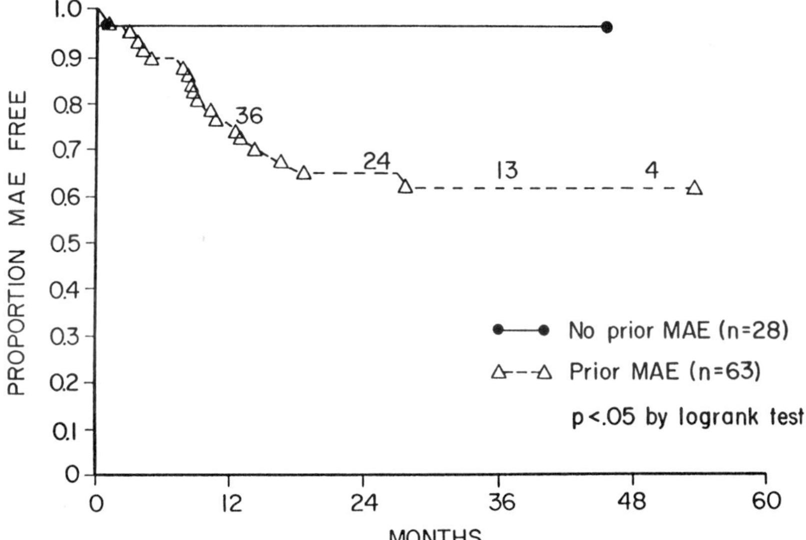


**Figure 2.**   Life table analysis comparing the efficacy of amiodarone for patients with and without a history of prior major arrhythmic episodes (MAE).

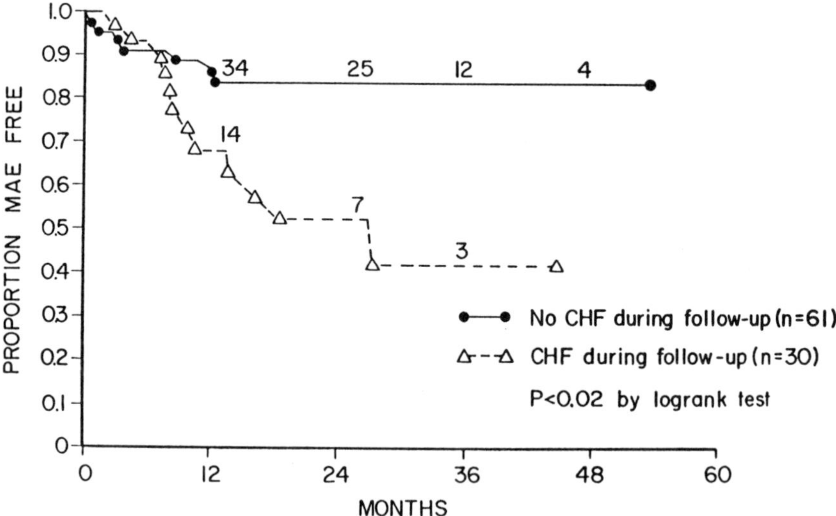



**Figure 3.** Life table analysis comparing the efficacy of amiodarone for patients with and without congestive heart failure (CHF) during follow-up.

Table 6

Comparison of 24-Hour AM and Exercise Treadmill Responses of Groups 1 and 2

| | Group 1 (n = 71) | Group 2 (n = 20) | p Value |
|---|---|---|---|
| VPB frequency/24%: | | | |
| Baseline (mean) | 2937 ± 4188 | 3628 ± 3866 | NS |
| Predischarge (mean) | 2368 ± 1224 | 416 ± 531 | NS |
| Percent VPB suppression: | | | |
| Mean (%) | 8 ± 285 | 70 ± 32 | NS |
| Median (%) | 93 | 82 | |
| VT runs baseline (pts) | 57 | 16 | |
| VT runs predischarge (pts) | 20 (28%) | 10 (50%) | NS |
| Suppression of VT runs (pts) | 39/56 (70%) | 8/16 (50%) | NS |
| Predischarge treadmill (time sec): | 662 ± 283 | 573 ± 305 | NS |
| VT runs (pts) | 7/49 (14%) | 1/12 (8%) | NS |

AM = 24-Hour Ambulatory Monitoring; VPB = Ventricular Premature Beats; VT = Ventricular Tachycardia.

charge 24-hour AM, mean and median percent VPB suppression, number with VT runs at baseline 24-hour AM, duration of treadmill exercise, and number with VT runs at predischarge treadmill study. Although just failing to achieve statistical significance, Group 2 patients had a higher incidence of spontaneous VT runs during predischarge AM with 10 of 20 Group 2 patients (50 percent) exhibiting this response as compared to only 20 of 71 patients (29 percent) for Group 1. (p < .06). Similarly, amiodarone therapy was more likely to have resulted in complete suppression of VT runs previously detected during baseline AM for Group 1 patients as compared to those in Group 2, although the number exhibiting complete suppression, 40 of 57 (70 percent) for Group 1 and 8 of 16 (50 percent) for Group 2 fell just short of statistical significance (p < .06).

The actuarial outcome of the 60 patients free of VT runs on predischarge AM is compared to the 30 who exhibited VT runs at discharge in Figure 4. The percentages remaining MAE-free for patients without VT runs at 12, 24, and 36 months were 87 percent, 76 percent, and 76 percent, respectively. The corresponding percentages remaining MAE-free were 67 percent, 63 percent, and 54 percent for patients with VT runs. Similarly, patients rendered

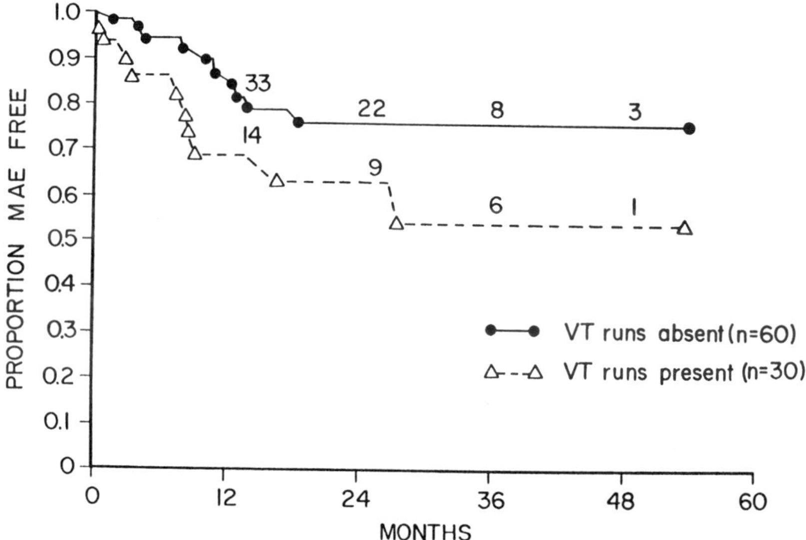


**Figure 4.** Life table analysis comparing the efficacy of amiodarone for patients with and without VT runs on predischarge 24-hour ambulatory monitoring.

free of VT runs initially present on baseline 24-hour AM had a lower incidence of arrhythmic recurrence as compared to those with persistent VT runs. Of the 47 patients rendered free of VT runs by amiodarone, 39 (83 percent) were MAE-free during follow-up as compared to only 17 of 25 patients (68 percent) for those with persistence of VT runs. Although suggestive of a more favorable outcome for patients rendered free of VT runs, this difference did not achieve statistical significance ($p < .07$).

## Comparison of PES Responses

The PES responses of the two groups are summarized in Table 7. No significant differences were observed between Groups 1 and 2 with respect to the presence or absence of inducible VT at predischarge PES, the number rendered noninducible by therapy, and the rate of the induced VT at predischarge study.

The actuarial outcome of the 18 patients free of inducible VT at predischarge PES is compared to the 55 exhibiting inducible VT at predischarge study in Figure 5. The percentage remaining MAE-free for patients with absence of inducible VT at predischarge PES was 66 percent at each of the 12, 24, and 36 month follow-up points and did not differ significantly from the corresponding 82 percent, 71 percent, and 67 percent MAE-free rates observed for patients with persistence of inducible VT. Similarly, there were no significant differences between the proportions remaining free of arrhythmic recurrence for the 12 patients rendered

Table 7

Comparison of PES Responses for Groups 1 and 2 in the 73 Patients Undergoing Predischarge Study

|  | Group 1 (n = 56) | Group 2 (n = 17) | p Value |
|---|---|---|---|
| Inducible VT: |  |  |  |
|   Present (pts) | 42 (75%) | 13 (76%) | NS |
|   Absent (pts) | 14 (25%) | 4 (24%) | NS |
| Rendered free of inducible VT | 8/47 (17%) | 4/16 (25%) | NS |
| Persistence of inducible VT | 39/47 (83%) | 12/16 (75%) | NS |
| Rate of inducible VT |  |  |  |
|   (beats/min) | 205 ± 42 | 185 ± 35 | NS |

PES = Programmed Electrical Stimulation; VT = Ventricular Tachycardia.

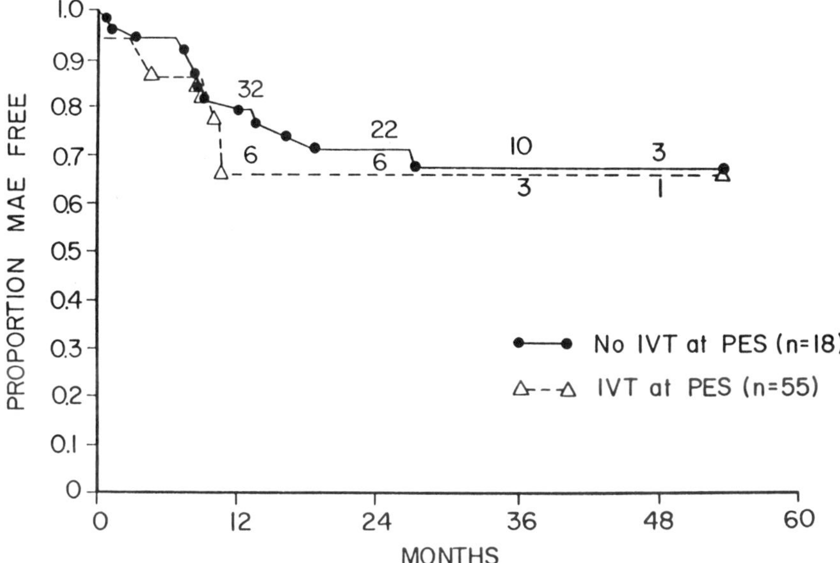


**Figure 5.** Life table analysis comparing the efficacy of amiodarone for patients with and without inducible ventricular tachycardia (IVT) at pre-discharge programmed electrical stimulation (PES).

free of inducible VT as compared to the 51 patients with its persistence. Four of the 12 patients (33 percent) rendered free of inducible VT by therapy with amiodarone sustained arrhythmic recurrence, an incidence not significantly different than that observed for the 51 patients with persistence of inducible VT, 12 of whom (24 percent) had recurrence.

## Comparison of Predictive Value for PES and AM

The positive and negative predictive values and predictive accuracies for PES and 24-hour AM at 12, 24, and 36 months of follow-up are summarized in Table 8. The positive and negative predictive values of 24-hour AM were greater at all points of follow-up than those of PES, but these differences did not achieve statistical significance. The overall predictive accuracy of 24-hour AM was significantly greater than that of PES with corresponding 12, 24, and 36 months values of 69 percent, 66 percent, and 67 percent for 24-hour AM versus 30 percent, 36 percent, and 37 percent for PES (p < .001).

Table 8

Comparison of Positive and Negative Predictive Values and Predictive Accuracy of PES (PES and AM responses in follow-up)

|  | 12 Months | 24 Months | 36 Months |
|---|---|---|---|
| Positive predictive value: |  |  |  |
| PES | 15% | 22% | 24% |
| AM | 27% | 30% | 33% |
| p | NS | NS | NS |
| Negative predictive value: |  |  |  |
| PES | 78% | 78% | 78% |
| AM | 90% | 83% | 83% |
| p | NS | NS | NS |
| Predictive accuracy: |  |  |  |
| PES | 30% | 36% | 37% |
| AM | 69% | 66% | 67% |
| p | <.001 | <.001 | <.001 |

AM = 24-Hour Ambulatory Monitoring; PES = Programmed Electrical Stimulation.

## Discussion

In this study, we examined the value of selected clinical, angiographic, and electrophysiologic variables as possible predictors of long-term arrhythmic outcome in patients being treated with amiodarone for sustained ventricular tachyarrhythmias. Importantly, the ability of PES and 24-hour AM responses were compared within the same patient population.

## Overall Efficacy of Amiodarone

Our findings confirm the results of several prior investigations that have indicated that amiodarone is an unusually effective antiarrhythmic agent in patients with life-threatening ventricular arrhythmias.[1-5,13] In our study population, all 91 patients had failed an average of three previously administered antiarrhythmic drugs and 63 patients had sustained at least one prior episode of sustained VT or VF in addition to the presenting event. Despite this unfavorable arrhythmic risk profile, only 20 of our 91 patients (22 percent) sustained arrhythmic recurrence at a mean follow-up of 19 ± 15 months. Actuarial analysis revealed that the percentages remaining free of recurrent MAE at 12, 24, and 36 months were 80 percent, 72 percent, and 69 percent, respectively. These efficacy rates correpond closely with those recently reported by Veltri et al.[15] and Kim et al.[16] in two separate studies, both of which examined amiodarone efficacy in patient populations similar to ours.

These findings also are in keeping with those of earlier investigators who reported the initial clinical experience with amiodarone. For example, Nademanee et al.[13] found amiodarone to be effective in preventing arrhythmic recurrence in 36 of 40 cardiac arrest survivors (90 percent) who were followed for a mean of 16 months. Similarly, Heger et al.[17] reported an overall efficacy rate of 79 percent at a mean follow-up of 16 months in 177 patients, the majority of whom presented with either sustained VT or VF. However, the majority of these earlier studies, while establishing the efficacy of amiodarone in a high-risk patient population, did not precisely define predictors of arrhythmic recurrence or express arrhythmic outcome as a function of both PES and AM responses. The relationship between the long-term response to amiodarone and these electrophysiologic variables, as well as selected clinical variables, will be described.

## Importance of Clinical and Angiographic Variables

One of the principal findings of our study was that the risk of arrhythmic recurrence on chronic amiodarone therapy is influenced strongly by a history of one or more prior major arrhythmic episodes (MAE). For example, of the 28 patients in our study in whom the presenting episode of VT/VF was the first manifestation of symptomatic ventricular arrhythmia, only 1 patient (4 percent) sustained arrhythmic recurrence during follow-up (Fig. 1). In contrast, 19 of the 63 patients (30 percent) with prior arrhythmic episodes recurred. The importance of prior MAE as a predictor of subsequent arrhythmic risk also was emphasized recently by DiCarlo et al.[18] in a study of 104 patients with sustained ventricular tachyarrhythmias who were treated with amiodarone. Patients with a history of prior cardiac arrest or syncope, essentially the same criteria we employed, were significantly more likely to sustain late arrhythmic recurrence than were those without such a history. Importantly, in their study the variable of prior MAE was an independent predictor of arrhythmic risk in a multiple regression analysis.

Another clinical variable found to be associated significantly with arrhythmic recurrence in our study was the development of congestive heart failure during the follow-up. Of the 30 patients exhibiting this finding, 12 (40 percent) subsequently sustained arrhythmic recurrence as compared to only 8 of the 61 patients (13 percent) who remained free of CHF after discharge. Using life table methods, the predicted arrhythmic recurrence rate for patients with late CHF was 48 percent at 2 years as compared to only 17 percent for patients free of late CHF (Fig. 3). These findings are in keeping with other studies, which have indicated that the extent of LV functional impairment is an important determinant of successful antiarrhythmic therapy.[14] Our findings further suggest that the emergence of even a transient deterioration in LV performance may indicate an alteration in electrophysiologic status, one that may herald the recurrence of potentially lethal ventricular tachyarrhythmia. Accordingly, the development of CHF during follow-up should be viewed as a potentially dangerous finding, one that may indicate the need to reassess the adequacy of antiarrhythmic protection.

Other clinical and angiographic features that could influence arrhythmic outcome were also examined in our study (Table 5). Importantly, neither the type of the presenting arrhythmia, sustained VT versus VF, nor the type of underlying heart disease was associated significantly with subsequent arrhythmic recurrence.

Somewhat surprisingly, the extent of left ventricular dysfunction, at least as assessed by mean LV ejection fraction, was similar for Group 1 and Group 2 patients, the mean ejection fraction being 37 percent for both groups. While mean LV ejection fraction was not significantly lower in our Group 2 patients, other investigators have found ejection fraction to be useful in assessing arrhythmic risk. In the study of DiCarlo et al.,[18] multivariate analysis revealed that an ejection fraction less than 40 percent was an independent predictor of subsequent cardiac arrest. Similarly, McGovern et al.[11] found that in patients with persistence of inducible VT, the probability of arrhythmic recurrence was directly related to the extent of LV functional impairment. In their series, for example, a patient with persistence of inducible VT and an LV ejection fraction of 25 percent was twice as likely to sustain arrhythmic recurrence, approximately 50 percent at 12 months, as a patient with similar PES responses and an ejection fraction of 50 percent.

One possible explanation for our observation that mean ejection fraction did not correlate with arrhythmic recurrence may be that the number of patients in our series with LV ejections greater than 50 percent, only 9 of 91 (10 percent), was quite small. Accordingly, a simple univariate analysis might not have detected any beneficial effect for patients with higher LV ejection fractions. However, when life table methods are used to examine amiodarone efficacy, a trend toward a more favorable arrhythmic outcome for patients with ejection fractions greater than 35 percent was observed. This trend, however, did not become apparent until after approximately 3 years of follow-up, at which time only 23 percent of patients with ejection fractions greater than 35 percent were predicted to have recurred as compared to 44 percent for those with ejection fractions less than 35 percent. Thus, in view of our findings and those reported by others,[11,18] it appears that the risk of arrhythmic recurrence in patients receiving amiodarone for sustained ventricular tachyarrhythmia is influenced by the extent of LV dysfunction, whether this finding is manifest as depression of LV ejection fraction or by the development of congestive heart failure during follow-up.

## Role of PES Responses

Some investigators have reported that PES responses are useful in further defining arrhythmic risk in patients receiving amiodarone.[9,11,19] In our study population, however, the long-term arrhythmic outcome of patients discharged with persistence of inducible VT, 67 percent MAE-free at 3 years, was virtually identical to the 66 percent MAE-free rate observed for patients discharged free of inducible VT (Fig. 5). Furthermore, of the 63 patients in our study who exhibited inducible VT at control PES, suppression of inducibility was achieved in 12 patients (19 percent), a response rate similar to that observed in other series.[9,17] However, the arrhythmic outcome of these 12 patients, 60 percent predicted to be MAE-free at 3 years, was not significantly different than the 68 percent MAE-free rate predicted for the 51 patients discharged with persistence of inducible VT.

These findings are in keeping with those of several previously published studies that have attempted to relate long-term efficacy of amiodarone to posttherapy PES responses. For example, in the study of Nademanee et al.,[13] the arrhythmic outcome of 40 cardiac arrest survivors treated with amiodarone appeared to be uninfluenced by the presence or absence of inducible VT at predischarge PES, only 5 percent of their study population sustaining arrhythmic recurrence despite the fact that 65 percent of their patients still exhibited inducible VT after therapy. In their study, the suppression of spontaneous VT during ambulatory monitoring appeared to be more predictive of outcome than were PES responses.

The relationship between PES responses and amiodarone efficacy also was examined by Heger et al.[17] in a large series of patients with either sustained VT or VF. Of the 101 patients in their study who exhibited persistence of inducible VT despite therapy, 80 patients (80 percent) remained free of arrhythmic recurrence at a mean follow-up of 14 months. This high efficacy rate, despite persistence of inducible VT at PES, also has been noted by several other investigators and suggests that programmed stimulation responses are not nearly as useful in predicting arrhythmic recurrence for patients receiving amiodarone as they have been for patients receiving other more conventional antiarrhythmic agents.[1-6,20,21]

The relatively benign outcome of patients with persistence of inducible VT despite amiodarone therapy, however, has been questioned in a few recent reports that have cited recurrence rates as high as 60–70 percent at 2 years for patients with unfavorable PES responses.[9,11,19] These findings, while not in keeping with the much larger body of data to the contrary, do raise valid questions as to the usefulness of PES in assessing subsequent arrhythmic risk in patients being treated with amiodarone. Potential explanations for the controversy regarding the ability PES responses to predict arrhythmic outcome in this setting will be explored later.

Since it is apparent that clinical and angiographic variables, such as the number of prior MAEs, the extent of LV dysfunction, and the emergence of congestive heart failure during follow-up, all significantly influence arrhythmic outcome, any analysis that does not consider these variables or attempt to control for their effects must be interpreted with caution. It is quite possible that the continuing confusion regarding the value of programmed stimulation responses as predictors of amiodarone efficacy could be resolved if such factors were taken into consideration.

For example, Horowitz et al.[9] assessed the prognostic significance of programmed stimulation responses in 100 consecutive patients treated with amiodarone for sustained ventricular tachyarrhythmias. They found that of the 20 patients rendered free of inducible VT by amiodarone therapy, no patient sustained arrhythmic recurrence at a mean follow-up of 18 months. In contrast, 38 of the 80 patients (48 percent) discharged with persistence of inducible VT experienced arrhythmic recurrence at mean follow-up of 12 months. However, the authors did not compare the clinical features of their inducible and noninducible groups and, thus, it is difficult to determine the extent to which arrhythmic outcome might have been influenced by differences in the clinical characteristics of their inducible and noninducible groups. It is conceivable that the more favorable outcome of the patients rendered free of inducible VT was determined as significantly by the beneficial effects of well-preserved LV ejection fraction or absence of congestive failure, as it was by their favorable PES responses. Accordingly, the true validity of PES responses as predictors of long-term response to amiodarone is difficult to determine from the study of Horowitz et al.

More recently, McGovern et al.[11] and Borggrefe and Breithardt[19] have reported that either the suppression of inducible VT or the rendering of VT more difficult to initiate by amiodarone therapy are predictive of freedom from arrhythmic recurrence. Potential limiting factors to both of these studies, however, are their short follow-up durations, relatively small patient populations, and limited clinical characterizations of the inducible and noninducible groups. Again, perhaps, the poorer outcome of their patients with persistence of inducible VT was related to the clinical and angiographic determinants of arrhythmic recurrence as discussed earlier.

To date, most attempts to relate PES responses to amiodarone efficacy have been limited to simple determinations of the presence or absence of inducible VT. However, it is possible that other invasive PES parameters might be useful in assessing arrhythmic risk. While limited data in this regard are available, some investigators have suggested that the end-points of either greater ease of inducibility or the induction of repetitive ventricular responses after single extrastimulus testing in sinus rhythm are predictive of arrhythmic recurrence.[22] Also, it has been reported that the rate and hemodynamic effects of the induced ventricular tachycardia after amiodarone therapy are predictive of the nature of subsequent recurrences.[9] For example, if the induced VT has been rendered slow and well-tolerated hemodynamically, it has been suggested that subsequent spontaneous VT episodes are likely to be of the same nature. At this time, however, these findings are probably best considered preliminary, since they have not been widely reproduced.

One last point with regard to programmed stimulation and amiodarone is worthy of mention. In view of the long elimination half-life of amiodarone and the extended period of time required to achieve peak effect, some of the confusion regarding the predictive value of PES responses could derive from differences in the timing of the posttherapy PES study. PES responses determined relatively early after the onset of therapy, for example at 7–10 days, might be more likely to reveal persistent inducibility and, thus, underestimate the value of PES, than would a posttreatment study undertaken later during therapy. The possibility that the discrepancy between PES responses and arrhythmic outcome might be related to the timing of the postamiodarone study was examined by Veltri et al. in 13 patients with sustained ventricular tachyarrhythmias.[20] All exhibited inducible VT at control study and 12 of the 13 patients still exhibited inducible arrhythmia at late PES studies undertaken after approximately 6 months of amiodarone administration. Thus, only 1 patient changed status from inducible to noninducible despite the fact that the late PES studies were performed at a time when amiodarone would have exerted its maximal electrophysiologic effect. Also noteworthy in Veltri's study, the persistence of inducibility at either early or late study did not appear to accurately predict outcome in that only 3 of the 11 patients (27 percent) with inducible sustained VT experienced arrhythmic recurrence at 24 months follow-up. These findings regarding the lack of change in PES responses at early versus late postamiodarone study are in keeping with observations from our own laboratory and suggest that the controversy regarding the ability of PES to predict amiodarone efficacy is not related to the timing of the posttherapy study.

## The Role of 24-Hour AM Responses

In contrast to the inability of PES responses to predict amiodarone efficacy in our study, 24-hour ambulatory monitoring (AM) responses did provide useful prognostic information. While amiodarone administration resulted in marked VPB suppression in both patient groups, the criterion that was the most useful in predicting outcome was the presence or absence of VT runs on predischarge 24-hour AM. For example, life-table analysis (Fig. 4) revealed that for patients free of VT runs at discharge AM, 76 percent were predicted to remain free of arrhythmic recurrence at 36 months as opposed to only 54 percent for patients who exhibited VT runs. It is of interest to note that other noninvasive electrocardiographic characteristics such as percent VPB suppression, treadmill exercise duration, and the presence or absence of asymptomatic VT runs on predischarge treadmill testing, were not of value in further assessing arrhythmic risk.

The utility of 24-hour AM responses in assessing amiodarone efficacy has been established by several prior investigations. In the study of DiCarlo et al.,[18] the presence of VT runs during predischarge AM was shown to be an independent predictor of arrhythmic recurrence in a prospective study of 104 cardiac arrest survivors receiving amiodarone. More recently, Veltri et al. also examined the role of AM responses as indicators of amiodarone efficacy.[15] Using the criterion of the presence or absence of VT runs during 72 hours of AM, they found a significantly higher arrhythmic recurrence rate for patients exhibiting VT runs, estimated to be 75 percent at 2 years, as compared to an estimated recurrence rate of only 12 percent at 2 years for patients free of VT runs. They were unable to demonstrate, however, that suppression of VT runs was an independent predictor of outcome since their patients who had recurrences had a significantly lower mean ejection fraction than those who remained free of recurrence. These observations again reenforce the importance of examining the relative merit of any predictive criterion, in this case 24-hour AM, in light of the extent of left ventricular dysfunction.

Kim et al.[16] examined the relative value of several ambulatory monitoring criteria in 80 patients undergoing amiodarone therapy for sustained ventricular tachyarrhythmias. They also found that the simple suppression of VT runs by amiodarone therapy predicted a significantly greater arrhythmia-free survival, 74 percent at 2 years for those without VT, as compared to only 48 percent at 2 years for patients with persistence of VT. These findings are quite similar to the 2-year arrhythmia-free survival rates predicted by similar 24-hour AM criteria in our own study population. It is important to note, however, that while the suppression of VT runs does predict a more favorable outcome, as many as 25 percent of patients exhibiting a favorable response can be expected to sustain arrhythmic recurrence over 2 years. These recurrence rates, felt by many to be unacceptably high, point out the need to develop better criteria for risk stratification.

Kim et al.[16] found that additional risk stratification could be achieved by combining the criterion of greater than 85 percent VPB suppression to that of abolition of VT runs. However, the additional benefit derived from use of these more stringent AM criteria was small. Based upon our findings and those of DiCarlo et al.,[18] ideally, the ability to predict the recurrence of life-threatening arrhythmias in patients receiving amiodarone can be enhanced if, in addition to 24-hour AM responses, selected clinical characteristics such as the development of heart failure, presence of multiple prior arrhythmic episodes, and left ventricular ejection fraction are incorporated into the overall risk assessment.

## Comparative Value of PES and AM Responses

When we compared the positive and negative predictive value of AM and PES responses, those of AM were always superior to PES, although these differences failed to reach statistical significance. The overall predictive accuracy of AM, however, was significantly better than that of PES (p < .001) at all points during follow-up. For example, the predictive accuracy of 24-hour AM was 69 percent, 66 percent, and 67 percent at 12, 24, and 36 months follow-up as compared to corresponding values of only 30 percent, 36 percent, and 37 percent for PES. Thus, in our own patient population, the criterion of absence of VT runs on predischarge 24-hour AM proved to be the most useful electrophysiologic variable for predicting long-term response to amiodarone and offered significantly greater overall predictive accuracy than did the criterion of absence of inducible VT at posttherapy PES. In view of these findings, it would appear that, when compared within the same patient population, AM responses provide prognostic information superior to that of PES.

Our findings raise questions as to the role of PES studies in patients receiving amiodarone. However, few long-term studies comparing the relative value of both PES and AM techniques thus far have been reported, and until further information is available, it would be reasonable to undertake posttreatment PES studies, if only because some investigators have reported an exceedingly low arrhythmic risk in patients rendered free of inducible VT by amiodarone.[9,11,19] Although this was not our observation, if a favorable PES response ultimately could be shown to predict virtual freedom from arrhythmic recurrence, a negative PES response could obviate the need to employ more aggressive and complicated forms of therapy, such as antitachycardia cardioversion/ defibrillation devices or ablative surgical techniques. Accordingly, it would be important to define more precisely the arrhythmic course of patients in whom inducible VT is suppressed by amiodarone therapy, particularly in the subset of patients with clinical characteristics indicative of high arrhythmic risk.[14]

## Summary

In summary, based on our findings and those reported by other investigators, amiodarone can be expected to provide effective anti-arrhythmic therapy for a significant proportion of patients with sustained, life-threatening ventricular tachyarrhythmia, even when multiple prior antiarrhythmic drug trials have been unsuccessful. Using life table methods, it generally can be expected that the empiric use of amiodarone will provide effective protection from arrhythmic recurrence in 80 percent of patients at 12 months, 72 percent at 24 months, and 69 percent at 36 months of follow-up.

In addition, it appears that arrhythmic recurrence despite amiodarone therapy is more accurately predicted by the persistence of VT runs during 24-hour AM than by the presence of inducible VT at posttherapy PES. The risk of arrhythmic recurrence, however, also is influenced heavily by certain clinical characteristics. Most notable amongst these are a history of prior major arrhythmic episodes, depression of LV ejection fraction to less than 35 percent, and the emergence of congestive failure during follow-up. Accurate risk assessment and the effective use of amiodarone require that not only electrophysiologic variables but also these important clinical characteristics be incorporated into the overall management strategy. In selected patients who exhibit unfavorable electrophysiologic or clinical characteristics, the use of alternative antiarrhythmic drugs or techniques, such as endocardial resection or the automatic implantable cardioverter/defibrillator may be indicated.

---

*We wish to thank Mary Mays for her invaluable secretarial assistance and also the nursing staff of the Intermediate Coronary Care Unit of Northwestern Memorial Hospital for the expert and humane care they delivered to the patients included in this study.*

## References

1. Heger JJ, Prystowsky EN, Jackman WM, et al: Amiodarone: Clinical efficacy and electrophysiology during long-term therapy for recurrent ventricular tachycardia or ventricular fibrillation. *N Eng J Med* 305:539, 1981.
2. Nademanee K, Singh BN, Hendrickson J, et al: Amiodarone in refractory life-threatening ventricular arrhythmias. *Ann Intern Med* 98:577, 1983.
3. Morady F, Sauve MJ, Malone P, et al: Long-term efficacy and toxicity

of high-dose amiodarone therapy for ventricular tachycardia or ventricular fibrillation. *Am J Cardiol* 52:975, 1983.

4. Rosenbaum MB, Chiale PA, Halpern MS, et al: Clinical efficacy of amiodarone as an antiarrhymic agent. *Am J Cardiol* 38:934, 1976.

5. Peter T, Hamer A, Mandel WJ, et al: Evaluation of amiodarone therapy in the treatment of drug-resistent cardiac arrhythmias: Long-term follow-up. *Am Heart J* 106:943, 1983.

6. Greene HL, Graham EL, Werner JA, et al: Toxic and therapeutic effects of amiodarone in the treatment of cardiac arrhythmias. *J Am Coll Cardiol* 2:1114, 1983.

7. McGovern B, Ruskin JN: The efficacy of amiodarone for ventricular arrhythmias can be predicted with clinical electrophysiologic studies. *Int J Cardiol* 3:71, 1983.

8. Waxman HL: The efficacy of amiodarone for ventricular arrhythmias cannot be predicted with clinical electrophysiological studies. *Int J Cardiol* 3:76, 1983.

9. Horowitz LN, Greenspan AM, Spielman SR, et al: Usefulness of electrophysiologic testing in evaluation of amiodarone therapy for sustained ventricular tachyarrhythmias associated with coronary heart disease. *Am J Cardiol* 55:367, 1985.

10. Podrid PJ, Lown B: Amiodarone therapy in symptomatic, sustained refractory atrial and ventricular tachyarrhythmias. *Am Heart J* 101:374, 1981.

11. McGovern B, Hasan G, Malacoff RF, et al: Long-term clinical outcome of ventricular tachycardia or fibrillation treated with amiodarone. *Am J Cardiol* 53:1558, 1984.

12. Morady F, Scheinman MM, Hess DS: Amiodarone in the management of patients with ventricular tachycardia and ventricular fibrillation. PACE 6:609, 1983.

13. Nademanee K, Hendrickson J, Kannar R, et al: Antiarrhythmic efficacy and electrophysiologic actions of amiodarone in patients with life-threatening ventricular arrhythmias: Potent suppression of spontaneous occurring tachyarrhythmia versus inconsistent abolition of induced ventricular tachycardia. *Am Heart J* 103:950, 1982.

14. Swerdlow CH, Winkle RA, Mason JA: Determinants of survival in patients with ventricular tachyarrhythmias. *N Eng J Med* 308:1436, 1983.

15. Veltri EP, Reid PR, Platia EV, et al: Amiodarone in the treatment of life-threatening ventricular tachycardia: Role of Holter monitoring in predicting long-term clinical efficacy. *J Am Coll Cardiol* 6:806, 1985.

16. Kim SG, Felder SD, Figura I, et al: Value of Holter monitoring in predicting long-term efficacy and in efficacy of amiodarone used alone and in combination with Class 1A antiarrhythmic agents in patients with ventricular tachycardia. *J Am Coll Cardiol* 9:169, 1987.

17. Heger JJ, Prystowsky EN, Zipes DP: Clinical efficacy of amiodarone in treatment of recurrent ventricular tachycardia and ventricular fibrillation. *Am Heart J* 106:887, 1983.

18. DiCarlo LA Jr, Morady F, Sauve MJ, et al: Cardiac arrest and sudden death in patients treated with amiodarone for sustained ventricular tachycardia or ventricular fibrillation: Risk stratification based on clinical variables. *Am J Cardiol* 55:372, 1985.

19. Borggrefe M, Breithardt G: Predictive value of electrophysiologic testing in the treatment of drug-refractory ventricular arrhythmias with amiodarone. *Eur Heart J* 7:735, 1986.
20. Veltri EP, Reid PR, Platia EV, et al: Results of late programmed electrical stimulation and long-term electrophysiologic effects of amiodarone therapy in patients with refractory ventricular tachycardia. *Am J Cardiol* 55:375, 1985.
21. Waxman HL, Groh WC, Marchlinski FE, et al: Amiodarone for control of sustained ventricular tachyarrhythmia: Clinical and electrophysiologic effects in 51 patients. *Am J Cardiol* 50:1066, 1982.
22. Naccarelli GV, Fineberg NS, Zipes DP, et al: Amiodarone: Risk factors for recurrence of symptomatic ventricular tachycardia identified at electrophysiologic study. *J Am Coll Cardiol* 6:814, 1985.
23. Marchlinski FE, Buxton AE, Flores BT, et al: Value of Holter monitoring in identifying risk for sustained ventricular arrhythmia recurrence on amiodarone. *Am J Cardiol* 55:709, 1985.

# Chapter 20

# The Role of Amiodarone in the Survivors of Sudden Arrhythmic Deaths

Koonlawee Nademanee,
William Stevenson, James Weiss, and
Bramah N. N. Singh

Sudden arrhythmic deaths represent a common mode of deaths in patients with cardiac disease.[1,2] In the United States alone, over 350,000 patients, mostly men, die suddenly every year.[3] In the last 10 years or so, a great deal has been learned about the mechanisms of sudden cardiac deaths in such patients and about the subsets of patients particularly prone to sudden arrhythmic deaths. Advances also have occurred in our knowledge of patients who are *not* at a high risk for sudden deaths despite the presence of significant ventricular arrhythmias.[4] Whether newer advances in therapy— pharmacologic, surgical, electrode catheter ablation, or the use of implantable devices—can make a significant inroad into the mortality figures of sudden arrhythmic deaths nevertheless remains uncertain and controversial.[5-7] An unequivocal reduction in mortality by the suppression of life-threatening ventricular arrhythmias in patients with heart disease remains to be demonstrated.

The purpose of this chapter is to critically discuss the subsets of patients particularly at risk for sudden cardiac deaths and to discuss the evolving role of amiodarone in the prevention of death from sudden, life-threatening arrhythmias with a particular reference to our own experience with the drug in 72 patients treated and followed for periods over 7 years.

From: *Control of Cardiac Arrhythmias by Lengthening Repolarization*, edited by Bramah N. Singh, MD, Futura Publishing Company Inc., Mount Kisco, NY, © 1988.

## Premature Ventricular Contractions as Markers of Sudden Cardiac Death

For many years it was considered that the frequency and the complexity of premature ventricular contractions (PVCs) constituted an important risk factor for the occurrence of sudden cardiac death.[4,8-12] With the advent of continuous ambulatory EKG monitoring in the 1970s, numerous studies were undertaken to determine the prevalence and the prognostic significance of premature ventricular contractions.[4,8-12] It is now clear that PVCs are common even in young healthy adults without apparent cardiac disease.[8] The prevalence of such ventricular arrhythmias tends to increase with age in subjects without clinically evident heart disease.[13] However, the occurrence of frequent and complex PVCs even with runs of nonsustained ventricular tachycardia does not appear to have much prognostic significance in subjects without cardiac disease at any age. The most important observation in this regard was reported by Kennedy et al.,[4] who followed 72 such patients for a decade (1973–1983). The data showed that the mortality rate in these subjects was not affected by the presence of ventricular ectopy, since the death rate in the group did not differ from that in a comparable group of subjects without ectopy. Thus, it is clear the use of antiarrhythmic therapy including the use of amiodarone in these patients is unlikely to make an impact on the incidence of sudden death. Such patients need suppressant treatment only in the case of disabling symptoms due to PVCs.

The issue of suppressant therapy however is less clear and more controversial in the case of PVCs associated with significant heart disease, especially scarring of the ventricular myocardium.[14] Numerous studies have indicated that patients with previous myocardial infarction, dilated cardiomyopathy, certain forms of valvular heart disease, and hypertrophic cardiomyopathy, among other cardiac problems are at a significantly increased risk of sudden cardiac death compared to otherwise identical subjects without complex ventricular ectopy.[14-17] The delineation of such a risk potential is particularly well documented in the case of survivors of acute myocardial infarction. The risk is further augmented by the presence of reduced ventricular function, particularly if the ejection fraction was below 40 percent.[18] However, it must be emphasized that although the risk of sudden death is increased a great deal by the severity of ventricular dysfunction, the presence of complex PVCs and runs of ventricular tachycardia on Holter recordings appear to contribute *independently* to mortality risk in the first year following acute myocardial infarction.[19]

While the evidence is compelling that the presence of complex PVCs and runs of ventricular tachycardia constitute a major risk factor for sudden death in the survivors of acute myocardial infarction, there still is no convincing data to suggest that suppressant antiarrhythmic therapy significantly reduces it.[20] The major studies that bear on this issue recently have been discussed critically by Furberg.[20] Neither short-term nor long-term trials involving Class I antiarrhythmic agents (such as quinidine, procainamide, disopyramide, lidocaine, mexiletine, aprindine, tocainide, and phenytoin sodium) produced evidence that these drugs exerted a significant effect on mortality. As suggested by Furberg,[20] the results of these trials can be interpreted in a number of ways. For example, it may be inferred that agents that act essentially by inhibiting fast channel function in the mycardium do not alter mortality, and they do not have a role in the treatment of patients with ventricular arrhythmias in the survivors of acute myocardial infarction. It also is possible that, since these agents exhibit a significant proarrhythmic action (perhaps up to $10-15$ percent), they exert an effect on mortality in certain subsets of patients, but such an effect is offset by their arrhythmogenic potential in others. Finally, the possibility still must be entertained that a suppression of ventricular arrhythmias in the survivors of acute myocardial infarction (and in patients with other forms of structural heart disease) may prolong survival but the effect has not been seen in the reported trials because of the limitations of the design and conduct of the studies. These limitations have indicated a sharper focus on the issues of methodology of trial design, such as selection of appropriate patient populations, pharmacologic agents and their dosing schedules, as well as larger sample sizes. Such an approach was embodied in the Cardiac Arrhythmia Pilot Study (CAPS),[21] which formed the basis for the definitive Cardiac Arrhythmias Sudden Death Trial (using several Class I agents), recently initiated under the auspices of the National Heart, Lung, and Blood Institute. It must be pointed out that this trial should be distinguished from the beta-blocker trials that examined the prophylactic effects of beta blockade on sudden death or reinfarction rate in the survivors of acute infarction.[20] These trials did show a reduction of sudden death by between 18 and 35 percent, but the beneficial effect could not be linked obligatorily to the suppression of ventricular arrhythmias. Indeed, none of the trials preselected the patients on the basis of the presence of arrhythmias. In one of the trials (involving propranolol), Holter recordings were obtained in 25 percent of the cases, and the data showed that the drug prevented the increase in the PVCs that occurs between the first few weeks to the sixth week of acute myocardial infarction. The degree of suppression of PVCs achieved in this study did not seem striking and appeared unlikely to account for the observed salutary effect on mortality.

The question also arises whether antiarrhythmic agents, which exert broader electrophysiologic actions than the available Class I agents, might be effective in the setting of patients with myocardial infarction or other forms of heart disease associated with complex PVCs. Little or no data currently are available in regard to Class III agents, especially amiodarone. The role of sotalol, N-acetylprocainamide, and other lesser known Class III agents has not been tested in this setting. However, it has been reported that in case of hypertrophic cardiomyopathy, verapamil and beta blockers were ineffective in suppressing complex PVCs and nonsustained ventricular tachycardia, whereas modest doses of amiodarone were not only a powerful suppressant but, by life-table methods of analysis, appeared to exert a beneficial effect on mortality.[16,22] The salutary effect appeared to be linked to the suppression of PVCs. These data are of much clinical significance, since they suggest that elimination of complex ectopic activity in patients with heart disease may prolong survival. Whether a similar effect may be obtained by the use of amiodarone in other forms of heart disease especially in the survivors of myocardial infarction remains unclear. The role of amiodarone in these subsets of patients requires delineation in terms of potency, efficacy, and the overall side effects profile relative to the roles of simpler conventional and experimental compounds. Ongoing clinical studies may provide definitive conclusions.


## Amiodarone in Patients with Ventricular Tachycardia

This is a group of patients whose prognosis is affected seriously by their ventricular arrhythmias. It has been found that if they have significant and complex ectopic activity, the elimination especially of the repetitive arrhythmias by Class I and Class II agents, alone or in combination, may prolong survival.[23] Similarly, if the drugs are effective in suppressing ventricular tachycardia reproducibly inducible by programmed electrical stimulation of the heart during acute drug testing, there is a long-term beneficial effect on recurrence of arrhythmia and, by inference, on mortality.[24-26] These observations have been based on uncontrolled observations but their validity generally is not questioned. It is noteworthy, however, that when conventional agents and most experimental agents fail to suppress symptomatic ventricular tachycardia in the setting of heart disease, amiodarone has been found to be effective in over 60 percent of the cases.[27-33] The subject has been discussed in Chapters 18 and 19 and will not be dealt further. The comparative efficacy of amiodarone and implantable antitachycardia devices or surgery has not been evaluated systematically but merits investigation.

## Pharmacologic Approaches to Patients with Out-of-Hospital Cardiac Arrest

The severest test of an antiarrhythmic drug is in the prevention of sudden death in the survivors of out-of-hospital cardiac arrest following cardiopulmonary resuscitation. As a group, these patients have now been well characterized and are known to have a recurrence rate of over 25–30 percent in the first year.[1,2,12,34] The attrition rates from one of the series of cases[12] are shown in Figure 1 and provide a basis for judging the effects of therapy, since it appears unethical to test the efficacy of a particular modality of therapy against a placebo control in this group of patients.

Patients who have been resuscitated from out-of-hospital cardiac arrests generally are men and over two-thirds have coronary artery disease, but usually without acute myocardial infarction as the basis for the sudden arrest. The remainder have cardiomyopathy (hypertrophic or dilated), valvular heart disease (including mitral valve prolapse), or their ventricular arrhythmias are caused by cardioactive or psychotropic drugs. The left ventricular ejection fraction in these patients generally is under 40 percent, a mean usually less than 30 percent. The commonest age group is between 40 to 60 years. The recent use of Holter monitoring has revealed that when these patients develop cardiac arrest while wearing a Holter recorder, the initial rhythm triggered by a ventricular ectopic beat often is a ventricular tachycardia that deteriorates into ventricular fibrillation as the terminal event.[15,35] Less commonly, during the course of resuscitation, asystolic arrest is found as the

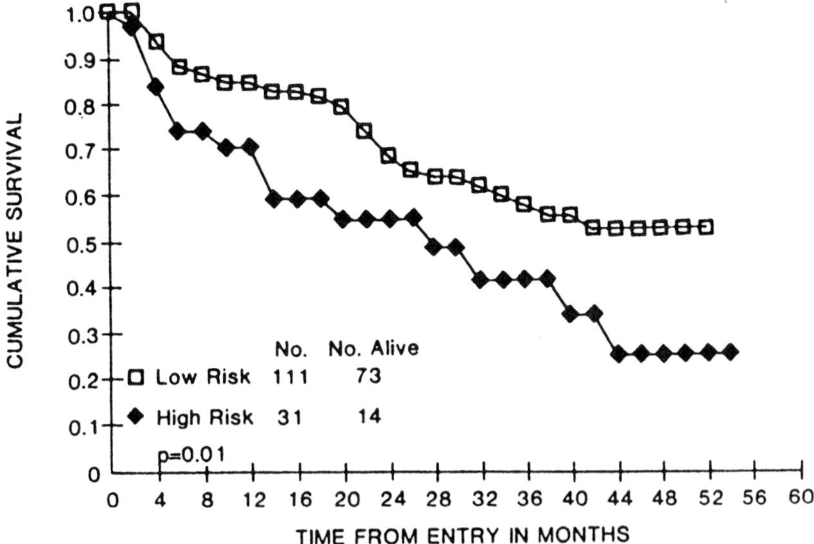


**Figure 1.** Life-table analysis for survivors of sudden cardiac arrests. high and low risk for death. In the low-risk group, cardiac arrest occurred as a result of an acute infarction; in the high risk group, the arrests were due to primary arrhythmic event. Note that in the latter, 70 percent patients had a recurrence within 44 months. (From Goldstein S, Landis JR, Leighton R, et al: Characteristics of the resuscitated out-of-hospital cardiac arrest victim with coronary heart disease. *Circulation* 64:977, 1981. By permission of the authors and of the American Heart Assocation.)

terminal event. Two other features of survivors of cardiac arrest need emphasis: two-thirds or more of these patients have complex or repetitive ventricular ectopic demonstrable on Holter recordings, and over 80 percent are found to have ventricular tachycardias or fibrillation reproducibly induced by programmed electrical stimulation of the heart.[26,36] These two features also are found in patients who present with symptomatic ventricular tachycardia but without the history of cardiac arrest. They provide the rationale for the use of Holter monitoring or electrophysiologic drug testing as the basis for the choice of drug therapy in both categories of patients with life-threatening ventricular tachyarrhythmias.[24–26,36] For example, Graboys et al[23] demonstrated that elimination of complex ventricular ectopy by antiarrhythmic agents in patients with previous cardiac arrests prevented recurrences. In the alternative approach, the suppression of inducible ventricular tachycardia/fibrillation during short-term drug testing in 31 patients with a history of cardiac arrests, Ruskin et al.[36] were able to find effective drug therapy in 19 patients who had predictably good outcome long term. The drugs used in these two studies utilizing different approaches were esentially Class I agents. However, it must be indicated that the numbers of these and most other studies involving Class I agents in patients with cardiac arrests have been small and durations of follow-up limited. It is difficult to draw firm conclusions from such studies regarding the role of Class I agents in the control of recurrent cardiac arrests. Larger, controlled studies with longer-term follow-up observations will be needed to define the precise efficacy of fast sodium channel blockers in the treatment of patients resuscitated from out-of-hospital cardiac arrests. Our own data documenting the efficacy of amiodarone in life-threatening ventricular arrhythmias refractory to Class I agents prompted us to examine the role of amiodarone in patients with sudden death resuscitated from out-of-hospital cardiac arrests. Our preliminary experience was reported in 1983[37] and is summarized in Figure 2. Our experience with a larger number of patients followed for a longer period of time forms the basis of this report, which highlights the evolving role of amiodarone in the survivors of cardiac arrest.

## Rationale for the Use of Amiodarone in Sudden Cardiac Arrest Survivors

As indicated in Chapter 14, amiodarone has a number of features that indicate the drug may have a significant antifibrillatory potential. For example, the compound has considerable potency for the suppression of premature ventricular contractions,[27,29,32] the trigger mechanism for ventricular tachycardia and fibrillation. The fact that the compound lengthens the action potential duration and the voltage dependent refractory period,[38] it prolongs the tachycardia cycle length, which may prevent the deterioration of ventricular tachycardia to ventricular fibrillation. The prolongation of the tachycardia cycle length also may occur as a result of the drug's Class I activity during fast rates (see Chapter 14). It also should be emphasized that the drug was developed as a coronary dilator; such an action coupled with its propensity to exert an anti-sympathetic activity[39] confers on the compound an important anti-ischemic potential, which may contribute to its beneficial antifibrillatory activity. In experimental animals, the compound has been found to elevate ventricular fibrillation threshold.[40]

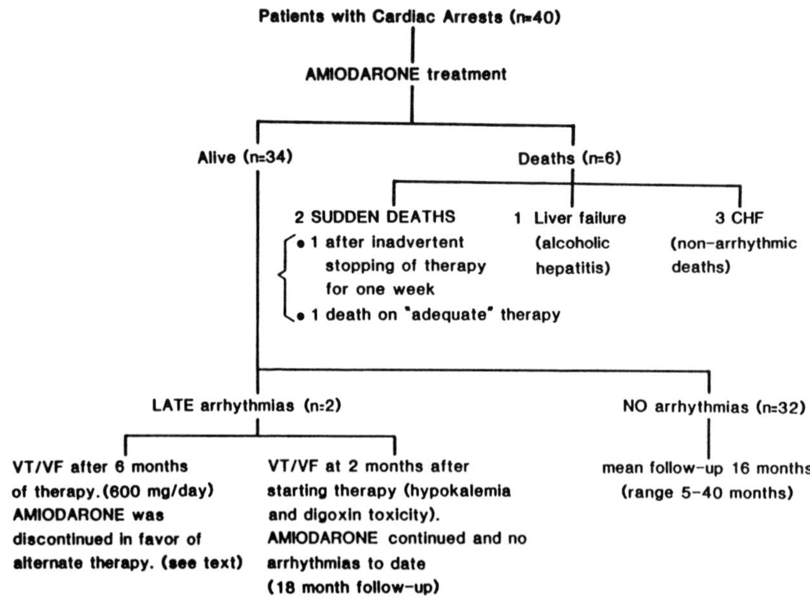


**Figure 2.** Flow diagram demonstrating the clinical outcome in 40 survivors of sudden cardiac arrest (36 out of hospital; 4 in hospital) treated prophylactically with amiodarone with intial loading doses and subsequent maintenance doses of the drug. Note the low recurrence rate of arrhythmia during long-term treatment. (From Nademanee K, Singh BN, Cannon DS, et al: Control of sudden recurrent arrhythmic deaths: Role of amiodarone. *Am Heart J* 106:895, 1983. By permission of the authors and of the American Heart Association.)

In terms of its overall use in the treatment of ventricular tachycardia and fibrillation in humans, two other features deserve mention. It is known that patients subject to recurrent cardiac arrests generally have reduced ventricular function and have a greater proclivity for proarrhythmic action in response to antiarrhythmic agents. As discussed in Chapter 7, amiodarone has a low or minimal negative inotropic effect and rarely has it been shown to aggravate cardiac failure, even in patients with markedly reduced ventricular ejection fraction. Furthermore, unlike most antiarrhythmic agents, there is increasing consensus that amiodarone has a very low arrhythmogenic potential.[41] Thus, the overall effect of amiodarone in patients with life-threatening arrhythmias is not confounded by its tendency to aggravate arrhythmias. For these reasons, the drug is of particular interest with respect to its potential role in the treatment of recurrent cardiac arrests.

## Experience in 72 Patients Resuscitated from Out-of-Hospital Cardiac Arrests

### Clinical Features

Seventy-two patients, 62 men, 10 women, mean age 62 years compose this series. Fifty-seven patients had coronary artery disease (47 with prior myocardial infarction), 11 had cardiomyopathy, and 4 valvular heart disease. The mean left ventricular ejection fraction (LVEF) was $29 \pm 11$ percent. Forty-three patients had history of 1 cardiac arrest, 19 had 2 arrests, and 10 had more than 2 cardiac arrests. The mean number of arrests was $1.60 \pm 0.89$ per patient. Most patients had failed on conventional therapy. The details of prior antiarrhythmic therapy are indicated in Table 1.

### Design of Study

Once the decision to treat the patient with amiodarone was made, other antiarrhythmic agents were stopped and amiodarone was started in a loading dose of 1200−1600 mg/day (usually in two equal doses) for 1−2 weeks; this was followed by an intermediate dose of 800 mg/day for 2−4 weeks, followed by a maintenance regimen of 200−400 mg/day; the actual dose was adjusted according to subsequent response. Whenever appropriate, serial Holter record-

Table 1

Antiarrhythmic Therapy in Survivors
of Sudden Cardiac Arrest Before
Treatment with Amiodarone

| Compound | Number of Patients |
|---|---|
| Quinidine | 50 |
| Procainamide | 55 |
| Disopyramide | 15 |
| Mexiletine | 6 |
| Tocainide | 1 |
| Beta blocker | 8 |
| Sotalol | 11 |
| Others | 5 |
| No drug | 0 |
| 1 drug | 17 |
| 2 drug | 33 |
| >2 drugs | 22 |

ings were obtained. Nearly all patients underwent electrophysiologic studies with programmed electrical stimulation under baseline conditions at a time they had been off all antiarrhythmic agents and before amiodarone therapy was initiated. In a proportion of patients, induction studies were performed at variable periods after the start of amiodarone therapy. The stimulation protocol used in these studies was identical to that reported previously from our laboratory.[30] However, the results of the induction studies were not used to make clinical decisions regarding the continued use of amiodarone in these patients.

When available, the results of the Holter recordings were used to make periodic adjustments of dose during the long-term follow-up of the patients, who were seen in the arrhythmia clinic at intervals of 3 to 6 months, once a steady-state therapy had been considered attained. Barring clinical parameters, appropriate laboratory tests (including liver function tests, thyroid function tests, and serum biochemistry) and 12-lead electrocardiograms were obtained during these outpatient evaluations.

## Clinical Outcome Relative to Mortality

The mean follow-up period for the 72 patients was 2.25 ± years (ranging from 1 month to 7 years). The overall survival with respect to sudden, cardiac, and total deaths analyzed by the life-table method is presented in Figure 3. There were 17 total deaths: 11 were sudden cardiac deaths, 4 congestive heart failure, 1 liver failure, and 1 malignancy. The cumulative second and third year cardiac-death rates were 15 percent and 18 percent, respectively. The cumulative sudden death rates were 8 percent, 12 percent, and 27 percent at 1, 2, and 4 years, respectively. After 4 years, there was no further instance of sudden death over the next 3½ years.

## Left Ventricular Ejection Fraction as a Determinant of Drug Efficacy

The effects of the left ventricular ejection fraction (LVEF) on the probability of recurrence of sudden death and of total cardiac deaths were analyzed by the life-table method using the 30 percent value of the LVEF as a cut-off point. The data are presented in Figures 4 and 5, respectively. Patients with ejection fractions greater than 30 percent had a more favorable outcome in both instances but the difference was significant only in the case of total

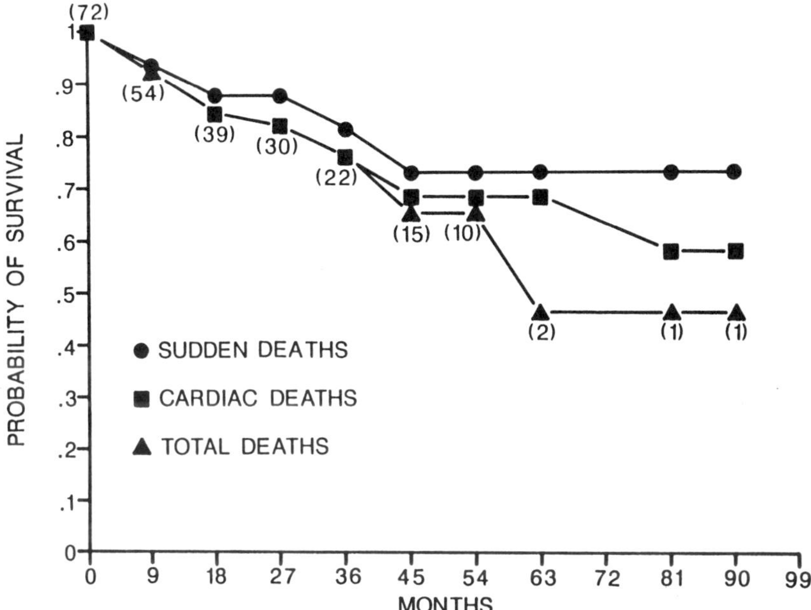


**Figure 3.** Effects of amiodarone on sudden death, cardiac deaths, and total deaths in survivors of out-of-hospital cardiac arrests. Note that nearly all cases of sudden deaths occurred in the first 45 months. The data in this figure and in subsequent figures were analyzed by the life-table analysis methods.

cardiac deaths (p = 0.03); that for sudden deaths was of borderline significance (p = 0.055). The trend however suggested that with a larger sample size the difference in the case of sudden deaths also may reach statistical significance.

## Predictive Significance of Electrophysiologic Drug Testing

Our current findings confirmed our previous data, as well as those of other investigators, regarding the effects of chronically administered amiodarone on inducible ventricular tachycardia cycle length and of the right ventricular effective refractory period. The mean data are shown in Table 2. The probability of survival as a function of the effects of amiodarone on the inducibility of ventricular tachycardia determined by the life-table analysis is shown in Figure 6. Although the numbers of patients in each group are relatively small, there was a clear trend for fewer recurrences of car-

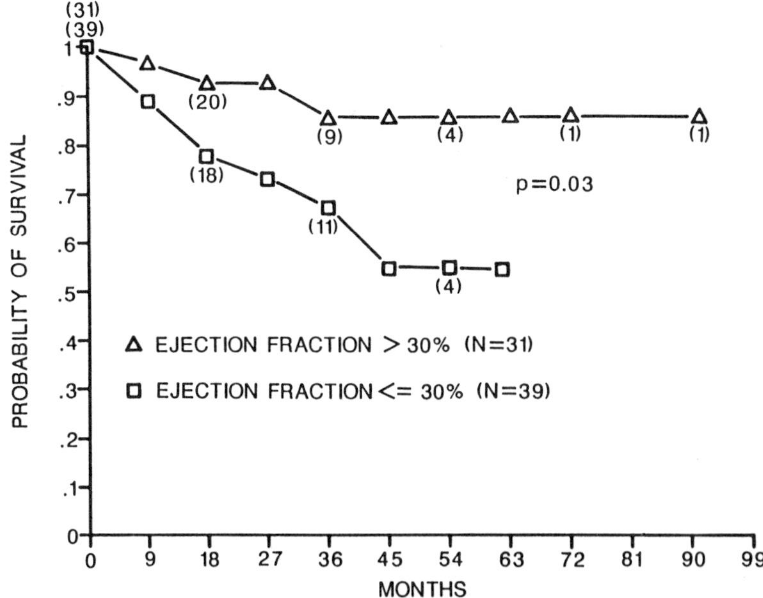


**Figure 4.** The occurrence of sudden death as a function of left ventricular ejection fraction (LVEF) in the survivors of cardiac arrests treated long term with amiodarone. The patients with LVEF exceeding 30 percent responded better to amiodarone than those with a lower LVEF.

diac arrest in patients in which the drug prevented reinduction of ventricular arrhythmia.

## Side Effects

The incidence of major and minor side effects that occurred in this series of patients treated long term with amiodarone is summarized in Table 3. The overall incidence of side effects was 53 percent: 38 percent minor and 15 percent major. The rate of development of corneal microdeposits has not been included in the overall analysis. Of particular interest, the total incidence of pulmonary toxicity was 6 percent, and there were no cases in which amiodarone could be incriminated as a cause of arrhythmia aggravation. There were no deaths directly attributable to the side effect of amiodarone. The incidence of major side effects tended to decrease as a function of duration of therapy, the converse for the minor side effects. The incidence of bluish-grey skin pigmentation

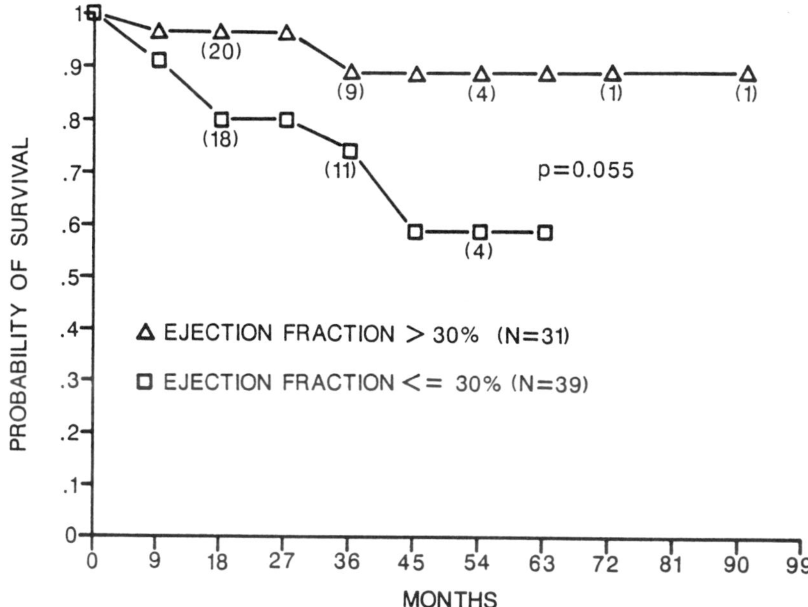


**Figure 5.** Effects of amiodarone on total cardiac deaths as a function of LVEF in survivors of out-of-hospital cardiac arrests. Note that those with LVEF lower than 30 percent had a significantly lower rate of survival.

over the face and other exposed areas of the body continued to increase in frequency and severity as a function of duration of therapy.

## Comments on the Role of Amiodarone in Survivors of Sudden Cardiac Arrest

The role of amiodarone in the prevention of recurrent cardiac arrests and in patients with recurrent symptomatic ventricular tachycardia remains controversial. However, the controversy appears to center less on the issue of efficacy and more on the toxicity profile of the drug during the chronic prophylactic treatment of life-threatening ventricular tachyarrhythmias. In 1983, we presented our experiences[37] in the first 40 survivors of out-of-hospital cardiac arrest; after a mean follow-up of 16 months, 32 patients were alive and well on the drug (Fig. 2) with late arrhythmic recurrence in 2. There was a low incidence of sudden cardiac death in

Table 2

Effects of Amiodarone on Tachycardia Cycle Length and
Right Ventricular Effective Refractory Period

|  | Control | Amiodarone | p Value |
|---|---|---|---|
| VT cycle length | 257 ± 48 | 409 ± 111 | < 0.01 |
| VERP | 247 ± 26 | 290 ± 26 | < 0.01 |

VT = Ventricular tachycardia; VERP = Ventricular effective refractory period

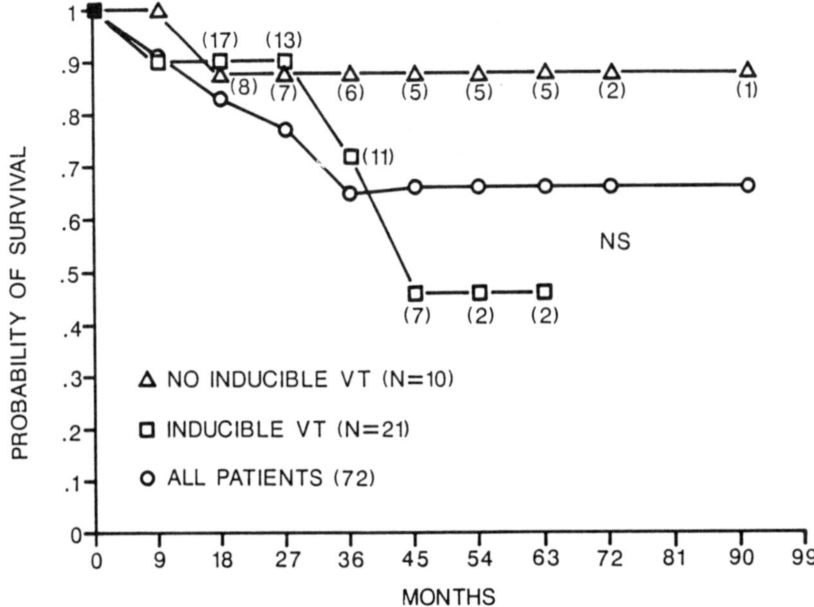


**Figure 6.** The probability of survival as a function of the effects of amiodarone on the inducibility of ventricular tachycardia determined by the life-table analysis. Although there was a difference in significance between those on amiodarone in whom the ventricular tachycardia was inducible versus those in whom it was not, there was a clear trend for a better survival in the groups in which the drug prevented reinduction of the tachycardia.

this series with the mortality rate at first year and second year less than 10 percent and 15 percent, respectively. Other studies in a similar subset of patients treated with amiodarone reported sud-

---

**Table 3**
**Side Effects Due to Amiodarone in 72 Patients Treated for
Sudden Cardiac Arrest**

---

Major side effects (11 of 72 patients: 15%):
    Pulmonary fibrosis = 4 (6%)
    Maximal muscle weakness = 1 (1.4%)
    Altered thyroid state = 3 (4.2%)
    Hepatotoxicity = 1 (1.4%)
    Peripheral neuropathy = 1 (1.4%)
    Bradyarrhythmias requiring Pacemaker insertion = 1 (1.4%)
Minor side effects (27 of 72 patients: 38%):
    Skin discoloration: Increased as a function of time (over 15%)
    GI disturbances
    CNS disturbances
    Photosensitivities
    Hepatic enzyme abnormalities
    Miscellaneous

---

Note: Total incidence 53% (38 of 72 patients).

den death recurrence of 9 percent[42] and 7.4 percent[43] during the first year of the follow-up period.

Our current data in a larger group of patients provide further confirmation of these findings; as far as we are aware, it is the first set of observations in which an antiarrhythmic agent has been used continuously for over 7 years in the survivors of primary arrhythmic arrests resuscitated out-of-hospital. The annual mortality in this long-term study was less than 5 percent. No comparable series of data are currently available for other antiarrhythmic agents nor for other modalities of treatment such as surgery or the use of implantable defibrillators. In the absence of a control series, it is difficult to evaluate the precise significance of the observed efficacy of the drug in this setting, especially in a group of patients in which it clearly would be unethical to perform a blind, placebo-controlled study. Nor would it have been possible to directly compare the effects of amiodarone to another agent, since all the patients had failed on conventional therapy. However, our treated group with sudden arrests may be compared to the previously reported series in which the survivors of cardiac arrest have been followed on either no therapy or nonstandardized therapy with antiarrhythmic regimens.[12] Of particular interest are the observations (see Fig. 1) of Goldstein et al.,[12] who followed three subsets of patients with cardiac arrests: those with acute myocardial infarction, those with ischemic events, and those with a primary arrhythmic event. The last group is comparable with the patients described in our series. After 44 months, in this group, over 70 percent of the patients were dead compared to 32 percent total deaths in our amiodarone treated patients over the same period. The results of the two series, of course, cannot be subjected to a valid statistical analysis but the data do suggest that amiodarone may have a significant potential for prolonging survival in patients with recurrent cardiac arrest.

It also is of interest that the drug appeared to be more effective in this regard in patients who had ventricular ejection fractions exceeding 30 percent compared to those with lower ones. This was particularly evident in the case of total deaths, although a beneficial trend also was apparent in the case of sudden deaths. Our data also indicated that the prevention by amiodarone of inducible ventricular tachycardia by programmed electrical stimulation also was highly predictive of a beneficial response as has been noted by numerous investigators. However, as also noted by many[28,31,44,45] and not by some,[46] a good clinical outcome on amiodarone in the survivors of cardiac arrest or those with life-threatening ventricular arrhythmias treated with amiodarone is not precluded by the failure of the drug to prevent reinduction of the arrhythmia by electrode catheter induction. The issue whether the effects on spontaneously occurring arrhythmias detected on ambulatory Holter recordings may constitute a more reliable guide in this context could not be addressed in the present study but has been discussed in Chapter 19.

Our data also emphasize that, during long-term theapy with amiodarone in patients with malignant arrhythmias, a careful surveillance of the impending development of toxicity can be obviated in most patients by simple clinical approaches, since serial chest x-rays and pulmonary function tests were performed routinely in these patients. The incidence of pulmonary fibrosis was 6 percent and deaths directly attributable to the toxicity of the drug did not occur. However, concern remains regarding the complex side effect profile particularly regarding the increasing incidence and intensity of skin pigmentation as a function of duration of drug therapy.

Although our data, considered in light of other studies in patients with cardiac arrests and in those with symptomatic sustained ventricular tachycardia occurring in patients with structural heart disease, are highly indicative of a beneficial effect of amiodarone on survival, the precise mechanism, or mechanisms, mediating such an effect remains unclear. To what extent the anti-ischemic potential of the drug or its antisympathetic actions modulate the drug's complex electrophysiologic effects on the myocardium to prevent ventricular fibrillation also remains to be determined.

## Conclusions

The most severe test of an antiarrhythmic regimen is in patients with recurrent cardiac arrests occurring in the community. Such patients have significant heart disease and often markedly impaired ventricular function, associated with frequent complex ventricular ectopic activity and a high incidence of electrical instability demonstrated by programmed stimulation of the heart. These features are associated with a high incidence of recurrence of cardiac arrests. There is no consistent evidence for a reduction in mortality by prophylactic therapy with conventional antiarrhythmic therapy. Experimental and increasing clinical experience support the use of amiodarone for the survivors of cardiac arrest, although long-term observations on the effects of the drug on mortality have been scant. We extended our initial observations in the use of the drug in this subset of patients when they had not responded to conventional compounds.

Seventy-two patients with cardiac arrests therefore were treated with amiodarone when other compounds had been found to be ineffective. During a period of follow-up exceeding 7 years, the annualized recurrence of sudden death was less than 5 percent and total mortality less than 15 percent. These figures are substantially lower than those reported in numerous historical controls. The life-table method of analysis indicated a beneficial effect of the drug on overall mortality, which was more striking in patients with a left ventricular ejection fraction exceeding 30 percent. Amiodarone prolonged the right ventricular effective refractory period and lengthened the cycle length of inducible tachycardia. When the drug prevented the inducible arrhythmia, the long-term beneficial effect was highly predictive but the converse was not found. There was a 53 percent incidence of overall toxicity with the drug, major ones in 15 percent (including 6 percent incidence of pulmonary fibrosis) and minor in 38 percent (excluding corneal microdeposits). Aggravation of heart failure, proarrhythmic effects, and fatal toxic reactions attributable to the drug were not encountered.

The results of this study, when considered in light of the previously reported shorter-term observations, suggest that amiodarone is a potent agent for the prevention of sudden arrhythmic deaths. It appears to have the potential to prolong survival. The precise mechanism of its beneficial effect remains to be established, but a balanced perspective needs to be developed in the case of a compound that has the property to prolong survival but has the proclivity to induce potentially serious side effects.

*Acknowledgement: We are much indebted to numerous colleagues who have assisted in the care of the patients the data from whom form the basis for the original observations reported in this chapter. In particular, we thank Jo Ann Hendrickson, BS, Vanida Intarachot, RN, Gregory Feld, MD, Daniel Rieders, MD, Clara Pruitt, RN, and other staff members of Clinical Electrophysiologic Laboratories at Wadsworth Veterans Administration Hospital and the Center for Health Sciences, UCLA School of Medicine.*

# References


1. Cobb LA, Werner JA, Trobaugh GB: Sudden cardiac death. I. A decade's experience of resuscitation, management and future directions. *Mod Conc Cardiovasc Dis* 49:31, 1980.
2. Cobb LA, Werner JA, Trobaugh GB: Sudden cardiac death. II. Outcome of resuscitation and future directions. *Mod Conc Cardiovasc Dis* 49:37, 1980.
3. Kannel WB, Adrienne Couples L, D'Aguestino RB: Sudden death risk in overt coronary heart disease: The Framingham study. *Am Heart J* 113:804, 1987.
4. Kennedy HL, Whitlock JA, Sprague MK: Long-term follow-up of asymptomatic healthy subjects with frequent and complex ventricular ectopy. *N Eng J Med* 312:193, 1985.
5. Singh BN: Effects of antiarrhythmic drugs on the cardiac action potential and in vitro cardiac electrophysiology. In PN Yu, JF Goodwin (eds): *Progress in Cardiology*, vol. 15. Philadelphia, Lea and Febiger, 1987, p 37.
6. Seger JJ, Griffin JC: Electrical treatment of cardiac arrhythmias. In PN Yu, JF Goodwin (eds): *Progress in Cardiology*, Vol. 15. Philadelphia, Lea and Febiger, 1987, p 113.
7. Fontaine G, Frank R, Tonet JL, et al: Electrode catheter ablation (fulguration) in the cardiac arrhythmias. In PN Yu, JF Goodwin (eds): *Progress in Cardiology*, vol. 15. Philadelphia, Lea and Febiger, 1987, p 123.
8. Brodsky M, Wu D, Denes P, et al: Arrhythmias documented by 24 hour continuous electrocardiographic monitoring in 50 male medical students without apparent heart disease. *Am J Cardiol* 39:390, 1977.

9. Hinkle LE, Carver ST, Argyros DC: The prognostic significance of ventricular premature contractions in healthy people and in people with coronary heart disease. *Acta Cardiol* 43:5, 1974.

10. Moss AJ, Davis HT, Decamilla J, et al: Ventricular ectopic beats and their relation to sudden and nonsudden death after myocardial infarction. *Circulation* 60:998, 1978.

11. Ruberman W, Weinblatt E, Goldberg JD, et al: Ventricular premature beats and mortality after myocardial infarction. *N Eng J Med* 297:750, 1977.

12. Goldstein S, Landis JR, Leighton R, et al: Characteristics of the resuscitated out-of-hospital cardiac arrest victim with coronary heart disease. *Circulation* 64:977, 1981.

13. Fleg JL, Kennedy HL: Cardiac arrhythmias in healthy elderly population. *Chest* 81:302, 1982.

14. Bigger JT: Antiarrhythmic treatment: An overview. *Am J Cardiol* 53:8B, 1984.

15. Meinertz T, Hoffmann T, Kasper W, et al: Significance of ventricular arrhythmias in iodiopathic dilated cardiomyopathy. *Am J Cardiol* 53:902, 1984.

16. McKenna WJ: Does treatment influence the natural history of patients with hypertrophic cardiomyopathy. *Drugs* 29:53, 1986.

17. McKenna WJ, England D, Doi YL, et al: Arrhythmia in hypertrophic cardiomyopathy I. Influence on prognosis. *Br Heart J* 46:168, 1981.

18. Schulze RA, Strauss HW, Pitt B: Sudden death in the year following myocardial infarction: Relation to ventricular premature contractions in the late hospital phase and left ventricular ejection fraction. *Am J Med* 62:192, 1977.

19. Bigger JT: Definition of benign versus malignant ventricular arrhythmias: Targets for treatment. *Am J Cardiol* 52:47c, 1983.

20. Furberg CD: Effect of antiarrhythmic drugs on mortality after myocardial infarction. *Am J Cardiol* 52:32c, 1983.

21. The CAPS Investigators: The cardiac arrhythmia pilot study. *Am J Cardiol* 57:91, 1986.

22. McKenna WJ, Harris L, Rowland E, et al: Amiodarone for long-term management of patients with hypertrophic cardiomyopathy. *Am J Cardiol* 54:802, 1984.

23. Graboys TD, Lown B, Podrid PJ, et al: Long-term survival of patients with malignant ventricular arrhythmias treated with antiarrhythmic drugs. *Am J Cardiol* 50:437, 1982.

24. Mason JW, Winkle RA: Electrode-catheter arrhythmia induction in the selection and assessment of antiarrhythmic drug therapy for recurrent ventricular tachycardia. *Circulation* 58:971, 1980.

25. Horowitz LN, Josephson ME, Kator JA: Intracardiac electrophysiologic studies as a method for the optimization of drug therapy in chronic ventricular arrhythmias. *Prog Cardiovasc Dis* 23:81, 1980.

26. Mason JW, Winkle RA: Accuracy of the ventricular tachycardia induction study for predicting long-term efficacy and inefficacy of antiarrhythmic therapy. *N Eng J Med* 303:607, 1980.

27. Rosenbaum MB, Chiale PA, Haedo A, et al: Ten years of experience with amiodarone. *Am Heart J* 106:957, 1983.

28. Heger JJ, Prystowky EN, Jackman WN, et al: Amiodarone: Clinical efficacy and electrophysiology during long term therapy for recurrent ventricular tachycardia or ventricular fibrillation. *N Eng J Med* 305:539, 1981.
29. Nademanee K, Hendrickson JA, Cannon DS, et al: Control of refractory life-threatening ventricular arrhythmias by amiodarone. *Am Heart J* 101:759, 1981.
30. Nademanee K, Hendrickson J, Kannan R, et al: Antiarrhythmic efficacy and electrophysiologic actions of amiodarone in patients with life-threatening arrhythmias. *Am Heart J* 103:950, 1982.
31. Heger JJ, Prystowsky EN, Miles WM, et al: Clinical use and pharmacology of amiodarone. *Med Clin North America* 68(5):1339, 1984.
32. Nademanee K, Singh BN, Hendrickson JA, et al: Amiodarone in refractory life-threatening ventricular arrhythmias. *Ann Intern Med* 98:577, 1983.
33. Zipes DP, Prystowsky EN, Heger JJ: Amiodarone: Electrophysiologic actions, pharmacokinetics and clinical effects. *J Am Coll Cardiol* 3:1059, 1984.
34. Cobb LA, Baum RS, Alvaez H, et al: Resuscitation from out-of-hospital ventricular fibrillation: 4 years follow-up. *Circulation* 51(III):223, 1975.
35. Weaver WB, Cobb LA, Hallstrom AP: Ambulatory arrhythmias in resuscitated victims of cardiac arrest. *Circulation* 66:212, 1982.
36. Ruskin JN, DiMarco JP, Garan H: Out of hospital cardiac arrest: Electrophysiologic observations and selection of long-term antiarrhythmic therapy. *N Eng J Med* 303:607, 1980.
37. Nademanee K, Singh BN, Cannon DS, et al: Control of sudden recurrent arrhythmic deaths: Role of amiodarone. *Am Heart J* 106:895, 1983.
38. Singh BN, Collett JT, Chew CYC: New perspectives in the pharmacologic therapy of cardiac arrhythmias. *Prog Cardiovasc Dis* 22:243, 1980.
39. Polster P, Broekhuysen J: The adrenergic antagonism of amiodarone. *Biochem Pharmacol* 25:131, 1976.
40. Lubbe WF, McFadyen ML, Muller CA, et al: Protective action of amiodarone against ventricular fibrillation in the isolated perfused rat heart. *Am J Cardiol* 43:533, 1978.
41. Mason JW: Amiodarone. *N Eng J Med* 316:455, 1987.
42. Morady F, Scheinmany M, Hess D, et al: Electrophysiologic testing in the management of survivors of out-of-hospital cardiac arrest. *Am J Cardiol* 51:85, 1982.
43. Peter CT, Hamer A, Weiss D, et al: Sudden death survivors: Long-term empiric therapy with amiodarone. (abstract) *Circulation* 66 (Suppl 2): 222, 1982.
44. Waxman HL, Groh WC, Marchlinski FE, et al: Amiodarone for control of sustained ventricular tachyarrhythmias: Clinical and electrophysiological effects in 51 patients. *Am J Cardiol* 50:1066, 1982.
45. Finerman WB Jr, Hamer A, Peter T: Electrophysiologic effects of chronic amiodarone therapy in patients with ventricular arrhythmias. *Am Heart J* 104:987, 1982.
46. Horowitz LN, Spielman SR, Greenspan AM, et al: Ventricular arrhythmias: Use of electrophysiologic studies. *Am Heart J* 106:881, 1983.

Chapter 21

# Side Effect Profile of Amiodarone and Approaches to Optimal Dosing

Louis Rakita and Nelson D. Mostow

An ideal antiarrhythmic agent should be highly effective in suppressing supraventricular and ventricular arrhythmias and should have a long elimination half-life to allow for long dosing intervals. The drug should also have a high therapeutic to toxic ratio. Although amiodarone is the most effective antiarrhythmic agent currently known and has an extremely long elimination half-life, it is similar to all available and experimental antiarrhythmic agents in having side effects. Indeed, the side effects are numerous. They range from minor reactions during the initial loading regimens or chronic maintenance therapy of the drug to major sometimes irreversible organ damage that appears to develop either as a hypersensitivity reaction or as a function of dose and duration of chronic therapy. It is clear that a detailed understanding of the pattern of adverse reactions that may develop may permit the clinician to define the risk—benefit ratio in an individual patient in whom therapy with the drug might be indicated.

In this chapter, we discuss the side effect profile of this potent but unusual antiarrhythmic agent and present a perspective on dosing that should maintain efficacy while minimizing side effects to the lowest possible.

From: *Control of Cardiac Arrhythmias by Lengthening Repolarization*, edited by Bramah N. Singh, MD, Futura Publishing Company Inc., Mount Kisco, NY, © 1988.

## Incidence and Severity of Side Effects

Since statistically controlled studies have not been conducted with the drug, the precise incidence of side effects attributable to amiodarone relative to dose, duration, and plasma drug levels (and those of its metabolite) remains unclear. However, there have been a number of attempts to assess the incidence and severity of adverse effects. The data allow an estimate of the overall toxicity associated with the chronic use of the drug in the control of cardiac arrhythmias.

Ives Laboratories[1] in its submission of data to the Food and Drug Administration (FDA) for approval of oral amiodarone for therapy of malignant ventricular arrhythmias presented side effect information from two retrospective studies as well as a summary of the world literature on this agent. The first study was a detailed review of information on 241 consecutive patients from five centers. These patients had been treated for refractory supraventricular and ventricular arrhythmias. In this carefully monitored group, 73 percent of patients experienced one or more reactions. In 14 cases, the reactions were severe enough to require discontinuation of the drug. The severe reactions included abnormal liver function tests, congestive heart failure, pulmonary infiltrates, hyperthyroidism and hypothyroidism, leg weakness with or without peripheral neuropathy, corneal microdeposits (for the most part asymptomatic), clouded vision, rash, and insomnia. There were a total of 18 severe adverse reactions in the 14 patients. Within a mean of 3 months, range 0.5 to 8 months, 17 of the adverse reactions resolved or improved. After restarting amiodarone, 2 adverse reactions recurred. The second study presented was a survey of many centers involving 4802 patients. The overall incidence of side effects in this group was not reported. The incidence of side effects severe enough to require stopping medications in this group was 8 percent. Such an incidence, however, does not include the fact that skin pigmentation develops as a function of time and after 5 years of continuous therapy occurs in most patients.

In the Ives' review of the worldwide literature in English, the proportion of patients reporting at least one side effect ranged from 20 percent in the combined Australian–New Zealand experience to 65 percent in the reports from the United Kingdom. Reports from Argentina and the United States were intermediate at 41 percent and 54 percent respectively. Some of the differences in incidence relate to the definition of side effects. For example, the incidence of corneal microdeposits is very high with chronic therapy. A center including this as a side effect would thus report a much higher frequency than one only reporting on symptomatic side effects as the vast majority of corneal microdeposits are asymptomatic. Also, with careful questioning, a history of intermittent minor appetite problems, insomnia, tremor, and ataxia can be elicited from many patients even though the patients do not volunteer these complaints. Thus, it is our impression that virtually all patients on amiodarone will experience one or more minor problems with the drug at some time during the course of therapy. For these reasons, it is clearly important to categorize adverse reactions as potentially life-threatening, as troublesome and unacceptable but not having a lethal potential, and those that are asymptomatic or tolerable.

The most important side effects are those that threaten the life of the individual. Fatal adverse reactions have been reported with pulmonary,[2] cardiac,[3] and hepatic[4] involvement. In most reported series,[1,5,6] no correlation could be demonstrated between the daily or the cumulative doses with the occurrence of adverse reactions. However, some of the complications are clearly dose related. During the early loading phases of treatment, if the dose is large enough, many individuals will develop gastrointestinal symptoms and neurologic side effects. The former consist primarily of nausea and anorexia, sometimes accompanied by vomiting and occasionally constipation, and the latter of tremor and ataxia.[7] Headaches, impairment of memory, and confusion may also occur. These early side effects may be seen the first day of therapy and can be reduced or eliminated by a reduction in the loading dose. Occasionally, even a relatively low dose is not tolerated, especially by women, and the drug requires withdrawal.

With chronic maintenance therapy the more prominent side effects involve the skin, particularly photosensitivity, flushing, and the appearance of a blue-grey discoloration of the skin. In addition, long-term side effects include the occurrence of peripheral neuropathies, pulmonary involvement and corneal infiltrates. Sanmarti et al.[8] reported a significant incidence of thyroid dysfunction with long-term therapy (see Chapter 15). Many of this multiplicity of side effects are dose and time related. Fortunately, the majority improve or subside when the dose of the drug is reduced. Leak and Eydt[9] reported a significantly higher incidence of side effects and rate of withdrawal in patients who where receiving 600 mg/day than in those receiving 200 mg/day.

In some instances the adverse effect necessitates stopping the drug. For example, Haffajee et al.[6] reported withdrawal of medication for side effects in 10 percent of their patients. Others have reported incidences varying from 0.5 to 22 percent[1,5,6,9-13] (Table 1). The reasons for withdrawal included refractory heart failure, CNS manifestations including nightmares, tremors, paresthesias and ataxia, alopecia, headache, impotence, epididymitis, bone marrow depression, thrombocytopenia, photosensitivity, pulmonary fibrosis, weakness, anorexia, cachexia, thyroid dysfunction, exacerbation of arrhythmias or heart failure, and others. It is clear from all series reported that the reduction in dose or discontinuation of the medication will stop the progression of the adverse effects, cause them to improve, or in most instances, cause them to disappear. In some cases, as with the pulmonary complication, steroid therapy may need to be initiated in order to effect reversal,[14] although the precise value of corticosteroid therapy in this setting is not clearly defined. Restarting amiodarone may not produce a recurrence of the adverse effect, particularly if lower doses are used.[14] However, in a number of patients, there have been documented recurrences of the reaction and in the case of pulmonary involvement, where amiodarone continuation has been required as life-preserving therapy, the simultaneous use of steroids and amiodarone has proven an effective combination to allow continuation of therapy while preventing the side effect.

## Specific Organ Systems Involvement and Potential Mechanisms

Almost no organ system has escaped involvement by amiodarone. However, there is considerable variation in the incidence of involvement reported by different authors (Table 1). The exact mechanism for production of each of the varied side effects in various organs is not known. However, some general observations may be cited and data that deal with individual organ systems will be discussed separately. It has been proposed that amiodarone causes a lipid storage disturbance in the lungs and liver resulting in lipoidosis.[15,16] It is speculated that the drug binds to phospholipids inhibiting their normal degradation and resulting in their accumulation in lysozomes. Similar cellular changes have been described in other tissues including skin,[17] lymph nodes, and leukocytes.[18]

An immune mechanism has been suggested as the cause of

Table 1
Frequency of Side Effects (%)

| Author | Overall Incidence | Eyes | Skin | Neurologic | G.I. | Pulmonary | Hyper-thyroid | Hypo-thyroid | Hair | Death | Meds Discontinued |
|---|---|---|---|---|---|---|---|---|---|---|---|
| Ives[1] N = 241 | 73 | 45 | 17 | 48 | 28 | 2 | —5— | | 0 | 0.5 | 8% |
| Haffajee et al[6] N = 173 | 25 | 100 | 17 | 15 | 12 | 0.5 | 2 | 2 | 0 | — | 10% |
| Greene et al[10] N = 70 | — | 95 | 46 | 51 | 80 | 7 | 0 | 4 | 0 | 1.5 | 19% |
| Raeder et al[5] N = 217 | 53 | 4 | — | 3 | — | 3.7 | 2.8 | 2.8 | 0 | 0.5 | 8% |
| Heger et al[11] N = 45 | — | 79 | 6.7 | 20 | 27 | 6.7 | 2 | 0 | 0 | 2.0 | 7% |
| Waxman et al[12] N = 51 | 56 | 71 | 8 | 10 | — | 10.0 | 2 | 0 | 4 | — | 22% |
| McKenna et al[13] N = 53 | — | — | 77 | 38 | 4 | 0 | 2 | 0 | — | — | — |
| Leak et al[9] N = 130 | 34 | 100 | 10 | 8 | 7 | 3 | 0 | 0.7 | — | 0.7 | 18% |

some of the side effects.[19] In the lung evidence to support this hypothesis has been the demonstration of a decreased $T_4-T_3$ ratio of alveolar lymphocytes in bronchial lavage specimens as well as the elevation of IgG and IgM and a high IgM−albumen ratio.[20,21] The response to steroids might support the immunologic pathogenesis of this complication, but its resolution in the presence of amiodarone in the serum and presumably in the body tissues and its occurrence in a patient while receiving steroids would not.[14]

## Ocular Complications of Amiodarone

Attention to the ocular changes was first drawn by Joseph and Rouselie in 1968.[22] It is now known that the most common "side effect" induced by amiodarone is the occurrence of corneal microdeposits. It is probably that essentially all patients, if on long-term therapy, will demonstrate the presence of these infiltrates.[3] For example, Ingram[23] studied 175 patients receiving amiodarone long term (3 months to 10 years). Of these, 103 patients examined in some detail, 98 percent were found to have developed the characteristic patterns of corneal microdeposits, which gradually increased in intensity and then stabilized at a constant dose. They did not vary until the dose was altered.

The deposits are bilateral and symmetrical; they are not visible with the naked eye and their presence can be excluded only on the basis of slit-lamp corneal microscopy. The initial changes are similar to the Hudson-Stahli line, a brown or a grey linear mark on the cornea at the junction of the lower and the middle cornea but not reaching the limbus.[23] These early changes are superseded by more granular lines radiating outward from the center toward the limbus. The final appearance, as the deposition intensifies, is that of whorl or vortex formation. In 1982, the presence of an amiodarone-associated anterior subcapsular cataract was first noted by Chew et al.[24] but this is not a common adverse reaction. More recently macular degeneration has been reported in some patients,[9] although the frequency of this reaction is rare as it was not noted in the data presented by Ives to the FDA.[1]

The precise mechanism of the ocular changes induced by amiodarone is not defined completely but does not appear to be specific to the drug. The focal abnormalities in the cornea and the lenticular opacities induced by amiodarone, chloroquine, some phenothiazines, and related compounds appear to be related to their amphiphilic, cationic nature, which predisposes to significant tissue drug and phospholipid accumulation.[25] It is likely that amiodarone induced an accumulation of intralysosomal phospholipids forming the basis for a drug-induced lipid storage disease.[26]

The incidence of symptoms due to these infiltrates, however, is low and ranges from less than 1 percent to 4 percent. Very rarely is there a blurring of vision or impairment of visual acuity. When symptoms are encountered, the most common is the development of haloes, especially at dusk, which may interfere with driving motor vehicles. The corneal changes regress in 3 to 7 months when amiodarone is withdrawn. For routine clinical practice, there does not appear to be a need for regular slit lamp examination, although we prefer to obtain one at the baseline before the patient is placed on amiodarone therapy.

## Thyroid Disorders

Amiodarone can affect thyroid function with clinical hyperthyroidism and clinical hypothyroidism as well as thyroid function tests without clinical disease. The subject has been discussed at length by Nademanee et al.[27] and by Hershman in Chapter 15. Ward et al. reported a high incidence of thyroid test abnormalities without clinical disease.[28] The effect of amiodarone in blocking the peripheral conversion of $T_4$ to $T_3$ results in an increased serum level of $T_4$ (usually above the normal range) and reverse $T_3$ and, generally, reduced levels of $T_3$. Thyroid abnormalities manifested by elevated $T_4$ and reverse $T_3$ and general decrease in $T_3$ without overt hyperthyroidism or hypothyroidism have been ascribed to the high iodine content of the drug. It has been suggested that this results in reducing deiodination of $T_4$ to $T_3$, producing a rise in $T_4$ and preferential production of reverse $T_3$.[29,30] The role of an autoimmune mechanism has been suggested by Rabinowe et al.,[31] who demonstrated the existence of a specific antigen seen in individuals with hyperthyroidism. They evaluated T-cell subsets together with thyroid function tests and antithyroid antibodies in 10 patients receiving amiodarone chronically. They found a generalized increase in a recently discovered subset of T-cells expressing a complex ganglioside antigen reacting with monoclonal antibody 3G5. Additional abnormalities of T-cells were found in two other patients, one with hyperthyroidism and the other with euthyroid Graves' opthalmopathy. It was their conclusion that these T-cell abnormalities suggested that amiodarone precipitated organ-specific autoimmunity in susceptible persons. Further studies are needed to define the incidence of these abnormalities and their significance in inducing abnormalities of thyroid function in patients during amiodarone therapy.

As with the ocular findings the occurrence of clinically evident thyroid involvement is much lower. The reported frequencies of manifest hyperthyroidism and hypothyroidism range from 0 to 5 percent for the former and 0 to 10 percent for the latter.[10,31-33] There is a geographic variation in the overall incidence of altered thyroid state during chronic administration of amiodarone. The effect is not related to the intrinsic pharmacologic properties of the drug. Rather, it appears to be due, in susceptible patients, to the iodine load resulting from in vivo drug deiodination (see Chapter 15). From the standpoint of clinical drug usage, it clearly is important to distinguish alternations in thyroid function tests without altered thyroid state from those associated with clinical hyperthyroidism or hypothyroidism. Tolerance limits for various thyroid hormone indices have been developed by Nademanee et al.[27] to facilitate this with a high degree of predictive accuracy.

## Skin Reactions

Skin reactions are common, particularly photosensitivity (encountered in about 50 percent of patients), flushing, and the appearance of a blue-grey discoloration of the skin,[17] especially in the exposed areas of the body. This discoloration is most noticeable when it occurs on the face, where cosmetically it can be quite striking. Erythema nodosum, ecchymoses, particularly of the forearms and hands, and nonspecific skin changes have also been reported.[5,34,35] It should be emphasized that the size and the numbers of ecchymoses are accentuated in patients on concomitant anticoagulant therapy.

There is evidence that the high incidence of clinical photosensi-tivity is due to a phototoxic reaction; the responsible wavelengths are within 335−460 nm ± 30 nm, and may be prevented from penetrating the skin by the use of a zinc oxide containing reflectant topical photoprotective barrier.[36] It also has been suggested that the skin reactions may be minimized by the concomitant use of pyridoxine.[37] However, there are little controlled data that address the issue of efficacy of this approach. In patients who require continuous theapy over many years, the incidence of skin pigmentation induced by amiodarone over exposed areas of the body increases as a function of time. It regresses very slowly after the drug is withdrawn. The exact mechanism of its development is not understood; it is unsettled whether it is due to the accumulation of the parent compound or the metabolites in the skin. Electronmicroscopy of skin from patients chronically treated with amiodarone revealed changes that have been found in other tissues such as the lung; they are characterized by electron-dense lamellar and paracrystalline lysosomal inclusion bodies,[17] which have been know to be produced by drugs that induce lipidoses.

## Pulmonary Toxicity

Of all the side effects, the one responsible for the most deaths has been pulmonary involvement. Rotmensch et al.[38] first called attention to the occurrence of pulmonary infiltrates and suggested a relationship with amiodarone. Numerous other investigators since have documented the occurrence of this complication, its importance, treatment, and potentially lethal outcome.[2,14,15,39] The subject recently has been reviewed in depth by Adams et al.[40] in relation to their findings from a prospective study of patients over a period of 3 years. Of the 40 cases reported in the literature that they reviewed, one-third of the patients died.

The role of pulmonary function studies is not clear. Rakita et al.[14] and Greene et al.[10] initially were unable to demonstrate changes in pulmonary function studies. However, Green et al. suggested that baseline decrease in the diffusion capacity might indicate increased likelihood of the pulmonary complication.[10] Veltri and Reid[41] have suggested that a reduction in diffusion capacity might be the first clue to the pulmonary involvement. Van Roolj et al. have reported that pulmonary gallium-67 uptake may be a sensitive indicator of amiodarone pneumonitis.[42] However, it should be emphasized that, although it is not clear whether preexisting abnormalities of pulmonary function predisposes to the development of pulmonary infiltrates, disturbances of lung function do develop during chronic therapy with amiodarone. For example, in the prospective study of lung function in 34 patients taking amiodarone, 24 showed no functional changes but 10 developed a sustained fall in CO transfer factor ($T_{LCO}$) in excess of 15 percent. As a group, these patients had been on a somewhat higher dose of the drug during the first 3 months of therapy. In 7 of the 10, there were no clinical or radiologic changes and $T_{LCO}$ improved with reduction in drug dose. The other 3 patients developed obvious clinical and radiographic evidence of amiodarone pulmonary toxicity. All 3 cases had abnormalities of $T_{LCO}$ before being placed on amiodarone. However, larger studies should be undertaken, especially in parallel with a control untreated series, to evaluate the significance of these findings.

There is no clear relationship of the pulmonary toxicity with daily dose, duration of therapy, or total dose of the drug[10,39,40] nor has there been any demonstrated relationship between the serum level and the occurrence of toxicity. However, experimental data recently have raised the issue of whether lung toxicity may be due to a particular susceptibility of the lung to high tissue uptake of the drug or its active metabolite.[43] In isolated perfused lung, Camus and Mehendale[43] showed that the amiodarone is taken up extensively by the lungs in rats and rabbits. The uptake was not saturated by raising the concentrations over a 400-fold range and desethylamiodarone (tissue–medium ratio exceeding 500) was taken up more avidly than the parent compound. The data raise the issue of whether monitoring lung toxicity by measuring desethylamiodarone serum levels might be of clinical utility. At present there are no objective data to establish or deny such a possibility.

Pulmonary toxicity due to amiodarone can develop suddenly as early as 1 month[5] or after many years of treatment.[44] It often presents as an acute respiratory distress syndrome. Its presence has been suggested as the cause for pulmonary complications in post-cardiac surgery patients.[45] It may present as a pneumonitis with fever, as an acute respiratory distress syndrome without fever, and with or without associated pleuritis; thus, it can be confused with infection. When the infiltrates are diffuse, differentiating between amiodarone pneumonitis and congestive heart failure (Fig. 1) often requires pulmonary artery catheterization. Sometimes, radiologically there is a picture of multiple nodular infiltrates with streaky densities bilaterally,[46] which may be confused with metastatic carcinoma. The other radiologic appearance seen in cases of amiodarone toxicity is a pattern of predominantly upper lobe infiltrates.[15,40,47–51] Such a pattern may be readily confused with tuberculosis and may resemble the appearance of chronic eosinophilic pneumonia. The important elements on differential diagnosis appear to be the presence of severe dyspnea and cough with little sputum, basilar dry rales with normal pulmonary capillary pressures, and negative cultures.

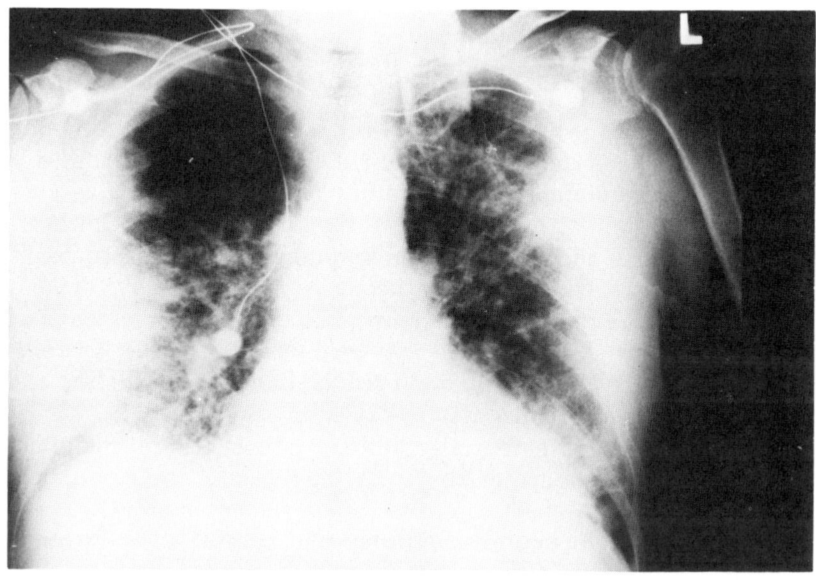

**Figure 1.** Chest radiograph of a patient with amiodarone-induced pulmonary toxicity. The appearance may be confused with pulmonary edema.

Transthoracic needle or open biopsy as well as histologic examination of autopsy specimens of the lung from a number of centers have indicated a number of distinctive changes induced by amiodarone in cases of pulmonary toxicity.[40] There usually is evidence of alveolar wall thickening, exudation associated with intra-alveolar and interstitial fibrosis with foamy macrophages. Dense infiltration with acute inflammatory cells with necrotic nodules may be found in biopsy specimens. The picture of acute necrotizing pneumonitis during amiodarone therapy also has been reported.[46] On electron microscopy, the foamy macrophages associated with amiodarone lung toxicity exhibit numerous multilamellar bodies; by energy dispersive X-ray analysis these have been shown to contain iodine.[40] It is of interest to note that Adams et al.[40] found alveolitis in patients and foamy macrophages in 6 of 8 patients who died during amiodarone therapy but without history of lung toxicity.

The precise mechanism whereby amiodarone produces pulmonary toxicity is still a matter of conjecture. It is probable, in fact, that more than one mechanism is responsible for the pulmonary manifestations, and perhaps more than one at any given time in a specific individual. Thus, it might be a toxic effect due to excess drug, a metabolic effect, or an immunologic effect. Individual reports have suggested an immunologically mediated basis. For example, findings from bronchial lavage.[42] have been consistent with a hypersensitivity reaction. Further evidence has included a positive reaction to the intradermal injection of amiodarone.[19] and lymphocyte transformation with amiodarone in in vitro studies.[19] Moreover, immunofluorescence studies of affected lung has suggested deposition of immunoglobulin or complement.[51] However, in many reports there have been immunofluorescence studies,[40] indicating that perhaps most of the cases of lung toxicity are not hypersensitivitiy reactions. D'Amico et al.[26] have suggested that since the drug is amphiphilic, it may penetrate lysozomes, accumulate as a drug-lipid complex, and produce lipidosis resembling the hereditary form of the disorder.

In view of the potentially lethal nature of the complication,[12,44,52-55] avoidance or the early diagnosis of the disorder is essential. However, apart from the timely reduction of dose to the lowest necessary to maintain efficacy and careful and continued clinical surveillance of the patient, there do not appear to be reliable methods to avoid the development of pulmonary toxicity due to amiodarone. To date, the role of serial monitoring of lung function tests,[56] chest X rays, serum drug levels, or other biochemical indices, although widely used, has not been clearly established. In cases in which the diagnosis is established or highly suggestive, it is prudent to discontinue the drug, although in a proportion of patients reduction in drug dose may allow it to be continued. In some, a rechallenge after a period of drug withdrawal has not led to a recrudescence; in others, it has. The role of corticosteroid in the management of the acute syndrome is unclear. Resolution of the clinical and radiologic findings has occurred with as well as without the use of steriods.[14,40]

## Gastrointestinal and Hepatic Toxicity

Gastrointestinal side effects include dose-related anorexia, nausea, and vomiting, constipation, and a chemical hepatitis, which usually is asymptomatic. These effects usually are encountered during the loading phase of the drug, although profound anorexia, weight loss, and other systemic reactions may be found with or without the development of thyrotoxicosis. The gastrointestinal side effects regress on dose reduction or on the discontinuation of the drug.

Although mild elevations in liver enzyme levels do occur, clinically important hepatitis[57] is unusual and the mild elevations do not require discontinuation of therapy. However, deaths due to hepatic failure have been reported. A rise in enzymes levels exceeding 2–3 times the baseline value should be an indication for considering a reduction of dose or stopping medication. The overall hepatic toxicity has been considered to be about 3 percent. It is noteworthy that concentrations of amiodarone and desethylamiodarone tend to be very high in the liver, up to 1640 mg/kg wet weight in the case of the parent compound and up to 8150 mg/kg wet weight in the case of the metabolite. The signficiance of these high drug levels in the pathogenesis of hepatic toxicity induced by amiodarone remains unclear. Radiologically, these high levels with their iodine content, lead to enhanced hepatic attenuation on CT scanning.[58]

Although biopsy of the liver is often done to assess the significance of the changes induced by amiodarone, it should be emphasized that such changes may mimic those produced by alcohol toxicity.[59] However, the periportal distribution of Mallory's hyaline may be a distinguishing feature for the drug-induced alterations evident on light microscopy. The histologic changes are those described in the lungs, skin, and nerves, being similar to those induced by drugs that produce generalized lipidoses. A case of major interest was recently reported on by Rumessen,[60] accompanied by a detailed review of the subject of hepatotoxic effects of amiodarone. His patient developed a cholestatic picture during chronic therapy with the drug. Rumessen[60] emphasized that the drug had the potential to induce serious liver disease in a few patients. The range of abnormalities included steatosis, alterations suggestive of alcoholic hepatitis, cholestatic hepatitis, and micronodular cirrhosis of the liver. The data stress the importance of regular clinical and biochemical surveillance of the patient on chronic amiodarone therapy. Persistent elevation of liver enzymes or their continued increase at a constant drug dose are indications for dosage reduction.


## Neurological Abnormalities Induced by Amiodarone

The precise incidence of neurological side effects developing during amiodarone therapy is not clearly defined. A figure as high as 74 percent has been suggested, but it is likely to be between 15 and 20 percent.[61,62] Fraser[61] recently has provided an accurate clinical perspective. Most reactions occur both during the loading phase and during chronic therapy, except for peripheral neuropathy, which develops only during protracted drug therapy.

The commonest symptoms are ataxia and tremor, which are mild and rarely necessitate drug withdrawal. Sleep disturbance, headaches, vivid dreams, and nightmares are not uncommon during the loading phase and respond to reduction in drug dosage. Less commonly, alteration in personality and temperament or impairment of memory may occur. The exact mechanisms of the CNS side effects have not been elucidated. However, it is known that large amounts of amiodarone and its metabolite cross the blood-brain barrier.

A number of cases of peripheral neuropathy has been reported.[63,64] Two features appear important in its development: large drug doses and long duration of treatment. The disorder often develops insidiously, the early symptoms including distal paresthesiae and numbness. There may be reduced temperature sensation. Weakness leads to difficulties in locomotion and the sensory loss is a progressive one culminating in a glove and stocking type of anesthesia. Nerve conduction disturbances are compatible with axonal degeneration and demyelination, being most marked in the peripheral nerves especially in the sural nerves. Histological changes are similar to those in other tissues: lamellar inclusions, with the lysosomes in the Schwann cells, fibroblasts, and vascular cells, and there is loss of myelin sheaths.[63] Although not unequivocal, the data suggests that neuropathy develops in the setting of high serum and tissue concentrations of the drug, metabolite, and iodine.[64]

Once the diagnosis of the neuropathy is established, the drug should be stopped and the patient treated by an alternative antiarrhythmic regimen. Functional recovery is protracted and may require a year or longer. Sometimes, recovery is only partial, especially if the disorder is severe and recognized late.

The available data suggests that neurological side effects are less common in children although even peripheral neuropathy has been reported to occur.


## Amiodarone and Postoperative Complications

Two reports[65,66] have suggested that amiodarone may have adverse effects in patients undergoing surgery. However, other reports have indicated that amiodarone is a relatively safe, effective agent for the treatment of postsurgical arrhythmias.[45,67,68] Recently Tuczu et al.[45] reported an increased incidence of respiratory failure leading to prolonged intubation and stay in the intensive care unit in patients on amiodarone prior to cardiac surgery. This issue needs further and more detailed evaluation.

## Proarrhythmic and Other Adverse Cardiac Effects of Amiodarone

Exacerbation of cardiac arrhythmias has been reported.[3,69–73] The reported incidence has varied between 0 and 5 percent. It is not always possible to differentiate whether the arrhythmia is a new event due to the drug or is simply a continuation or exacerbation of the underlying problem. Several types of responses have been considered to be proarrhythmic effects of amiodarone. These have included the following:

(1) A number of centers have noted that following a variable period of drug administration, in some patients, the ventricular arrhythmia may be more readily inducible (compared to the baseline condition) during programmed electrical stimulation of the heart. The inducible tachycardia may have a shorter cycle length. Although this has been considered an arrhythmogenic effect, its precise significance is not known.

(2) Mostow et al[74] reported two cases in which there appeared to be an exacerbation of the ventricular arrhythmia during the loading phase of treatment with subsequent apparent control of the abnormal rhythm by continuing amiodarone therapy. The occurrence of the phenomenon has not been reported widely but appears to have been encountered at numerous centers. The mechanism underlying the occurrence of such an effect however is not known.

(3) As with other agents that lengthen repolarization, amiodarone has been associated with torsade de pointes. It is intriguing, however, that the incidence of the disorder is lower than in the case of other drugs that prolong the $QT_c$ interval. It is of interest to note that most of the cases have occurred early during the course of therapy and have appeared to resolve within a few days of cessation of treatment.

The development of torsade, although occurring in the setting of prolonged $QT_c$ interval, cannot be related in a quantitative sense to the degree of lengthening of repolarization. The relationship to concomitant medication is not clear, since most of the reported instances of torsade de pointes or polymorphic ventricular tachycardia have occurred while the patient was on another, usually Class Ia, antiarrhythmic agent.[69] Other cases have occurred in the setting of profound hypokalemia with or without digoxin intoxication. The relationship is further confused by the demonstration that an apparent initial exacerbation may be followed by control if the medication is continued.[74] However, cases have been reported in which no other antiarrhythmic agent was used.[70]

When torsade de pointes develops in the setting of amiodarone, its electrophysiologic mechanism is likely to be simlar to that described in the case of other instances of drug-induced disorder (see Chapter 23). Its management also is similar.

At present, there have been only anecdotal reports of the potential arrhythmogenic effects of the intravenous formulation of amiodarone. For example, Sheinman and Evans[75] reported the acceleration of the ventricular rate by amiodarone in atrial fibrillation complicating the WPW syndrome.

It should be emphasized that although the effects of amiodarone are dominated by the prolongation of the action potential duration and, hence, the voltage-dependent refractoriness, it does exert potent effects on conduction especially in tissues with preexisting disease. Therefore, it is not surprising that cases of sinus arrest and other forms of conduction block during oral as well as intravenous therapy have been described.[76-80] Profound reduction in ventricular response in atrial fibrillation also is likely in patients with sick sinus syndrome and in those on concomitant therapy with drugs that block intranodal or infranodal conduction.

## Aggravation of Cardiac Failure

Although as a class, agents that lengthen cardiac repolarization are likely to be less negatively inotropic (see Chapter 6), amiodarone is unique in its pharmacologic properties. As discussed elsewhere in this book (see Chapter 14) it does exert a noncompetitive adrenergic antagonism, blocks the slow channel, and may exert a mild negative inotropic effect (see Chapter 6). Thus, although the drug is well tolerated and may be given with impunity to patients with markedly depressed ventricular ejection fraction and frank heart failure, there have been reports of cardiac failure exacerbated by the drug. However, the overall incidence is low.[81-83] The ventricular ejection fraction usually is not affected and may increase.[84-85] When heart failure appears to be aggravated late in the course of therapy, it is difficult to distinguish the effect of the drug from the progression of the underlying disease.

## Drug Interactions and Side Effects

As indicated elsewhere in this book, amiodarone has the propensity to interact with an extraordinary range of cardioactive compounds. For this reason, a number of side effects attributable to the drug might occur in the context of multiple drug therapies.

The occurrence of drug interactions with amiodarone has been well documented.[86] Specific interactions have been reported with warfarin,[87-89] digoxin,[90-92] and other antiarrhythmic medications.[93-96] Although, in general, these interactions tend to occur early and seem to be dose related, they may occur late and the responses are variable from individual to individual. Other adverse effects and drug interactions as isolated events are being reported. These include macular degeneration and corneal cysts and ulcerations,[5] extrapyramidal manifestations,[97] alopecia,[13] vasculitis and polyserositis,[98] thoracic inlet compression,[99] lens opacities,[100] hemolysis,[101] hepatitis,[60,78] interaction with lidocaine,[79] hepatotoxicity with cirrhosis,[60] intra-His block,[80] interactions with diltiazem[102] and phenytoin,[103] and epididymitis.[104] Relationship to age has been evaluated by Schneeweiss[95] who reported that, in addition to drug interactions, hypothyroidism associated with amiodarone was more common in the older group (above age 60 years) and was potentially fatal. Cutaneous lesions were less common. Others[96] have reported an increased incidence of hyper- and hypothyroidism in the elderly.

## Amiodarone Serum Concentrations and Side Effects

A number of investigators[5,105] have commented on the lack of correlation of efficacy with serum levels and on the lack of correlation of side effects with serum levels. Haffajee et al.[6] compared the incidence of side effects when serum levels were above, with the occurrence at levels below 2.5 μg/ml. It was only in relation to the decrease in CNS side effects that they were able to show a statistically significant reduction in symptoms at the lower serum level. However, they were able, as were others, to demonstrate that reduction in the dose of the medication would result in the amelioration of most side effects and a dose–serum level relationship has been reported. Although there was great overlap in the values reported, Raeder et al.[5] did show a significant, albeit weak, correlation between side effects and serum levels. The serum level of amiodarone in patients with side effects averaged 2.0 µg/ml while in those without side effects it was 1.6 µg/ml. In addition, there have been reports of a relationship between serum levels and efficacy.[106] However, it must be emphasized that, although these general relationships appear to hold, the predictability of side effects developing over a range of drug concentrations is weak. It is possible, however, that a better correlation may be found in the case of desethylamiodarone.

## Approaches to Optimal Dosing

The current understanding of optimal dosing with amiodarone has evolved both from a long clinical experience with this agent and an increasing understanding of the drug's exceedingly complex pharmacokinetic properties. It also is complicated by variable absorption rates, individual responses to the medication, and a variable half-life ranging from 20 to over 100 days. A rational approach to dosing with the drug, therefore, presupposes some understanding of its known pharmacokinetics, imperfect as it might be.

### Early Experience

When amiodarone was initially introduced in Europe in the late 1960s as an antianginal agent, the dose employed was 100–400 mg daily and side effects were uncommon. In the early 1970s, when it was discovered that amiodarone was an effective antiarrhythmic agent, the dose likewise was restricted to 100–400 mg daily, frequently with a *fenestre therapeutique* (French for "therapeutic window"), by which is meant the practice of instructing the patient to omit a daily dose of amiodarone one or more days per week. In the now classic work by Rosenbaum et al[81] in which amiodarone was reported to be highly effective against a wide variety of ventricular and supraventricular arrhythmias, amiodarone 200–800 mg daily was given for several days and then the dose was reduced as tolerated to 200–400 mg daily. Thus, the early European and South American experience with amiodarone indicated that with low doses of amiodarone, a finite delay of several days in the onset of antiarrhythmic effects during long-term therapy were very low with doses of 100–400 mg daily.

## The North American Experience

Amiodarone was first released for experimental use in the United States in 1977. Because of concern that some side effects (predominantly corneal microdeposits) had not been adequately evaluated, the drug was used primarily in the therapy of patients with refractory ventricular arrhythmias in association with an extremely high risk of sudden death. In this setting, amiodarone was found to be highly effective but a delay of several days in the onset of antiarrhythmic action presented a significant management problem. In an effort to shorten this delay and before the advent of serum concentration monitoring, Rakita and Sobol empirically increased amiodarone loading regimens from 400 mg daily to 800 mg and then 1400 mg daily.[107] They found that doses of 800–1400 mg of amiodarone daily significantly shortened the delay in onset of arrhythmia suppression from 16.9 days to 9.5 days.

While higher initial doses of amiodarone resulted in more rapid arrhythmia suppression, the continuation of doses of amiodarone of 600–800 mg daily for several months resulted in a much higher incidence of major and minor toxicity than previously had been reported. Thus, it became clear from empirical observations that, although the time required for the onset of action could be shortened by the administration of large doses, the continuation of large doses long term could result in an unfavorable side effect profile. Whether these large doses were required for continued suppression of the exceedingly malignant arrhythmias being treated was not formally evaluated, although some groups were using significantly lower doses with a clinical impression that recurrences of symptomatic arrhythmias and sudden death were being prevented.

## Pharmacokinetic Considerations Relevant to Dosing

It was not until the early 1980s that methods for the accurate determination of amiodarone concentration in serum finally were validated. This opened the way for the study of the pharmacokinetic distribution of amiodarone and the beginning of unravelling what appeared to be extremely peculiar properties of this drug, properties that in part may explain the empirical phenomena just described.

*Two-Compartment Pharmacokinetic Model*

Before discussing amiodarone's pharmacokinetic profile, a brief review of the two-compartment pharmacokinetic model used to describe the kinetic disposition of most cardiac drugs is necessary. Following an intravenous bolus, the disappearance of drugs from blood as they distribute into tissues is uniform. Furthermore, when the log of serum concentration is plotted against time, a straight line is obtained.[108] Also, the disappearance of drug from blood can be accurately described by a log-linear plot during elimination from the body via metabolism or excretion. Thus, for most drugs, the combined effects of distribution and elimination are described accurately by a two-compartment model, where blood and tissue (even though the specific tissues may not be defined) are each considered single compartments. A typical example of a drug that behaves in this fashion is lidocaine (Fig. 2).[108] In this situation, the contributions of distribution and elimination can be calculated by mathematical analysis, and the rate of distribution into tissues (distribution half-life) as well as the rate of elimination from the body (elimination half-life) can be obtained from analysis of data such as those shown in Figure 2. In this example, the distribution half-life (alpha) is 8–10 minutes and the elimination half-life (beta) is about 2 hours.

*Multicompartment Pharmacokinetic Model*

The pharmacokinetic distribution of amiodarone is more complex than the two-compartment model just described. Early studies in animals and in humans[109–111] used a two-compartment model to describe the elimination of amiodarone from blood following a single intravenous dose. The half-life of distribution was reported to be 19 minutes[72] and the half-life of elimination from 9 hours[110,111] to 21 hours.[110] These studies conflicted with reports describing the half-life of elimination of oral amiodarone from the body after long-term administration as being 1–3 months.[112,113] It subsequently was shown that distribution of amiodarone from blood into tissues was not adequately described by a two-compartment model.[114,115] In a pharmacokinetic study of 11 patients, we found an excellent fit using a four-compartment model, in which distribution was assumed to occur from blood into four compartments over a 72-hour time period.[114] The half-life of distribution into each of the four compartments was 4.2 ± 0.8 min (mean ± SD), 36.6 ± 13.9 min, 4.51 ± 2.31 h, and 33.6 ± 8.8 h.

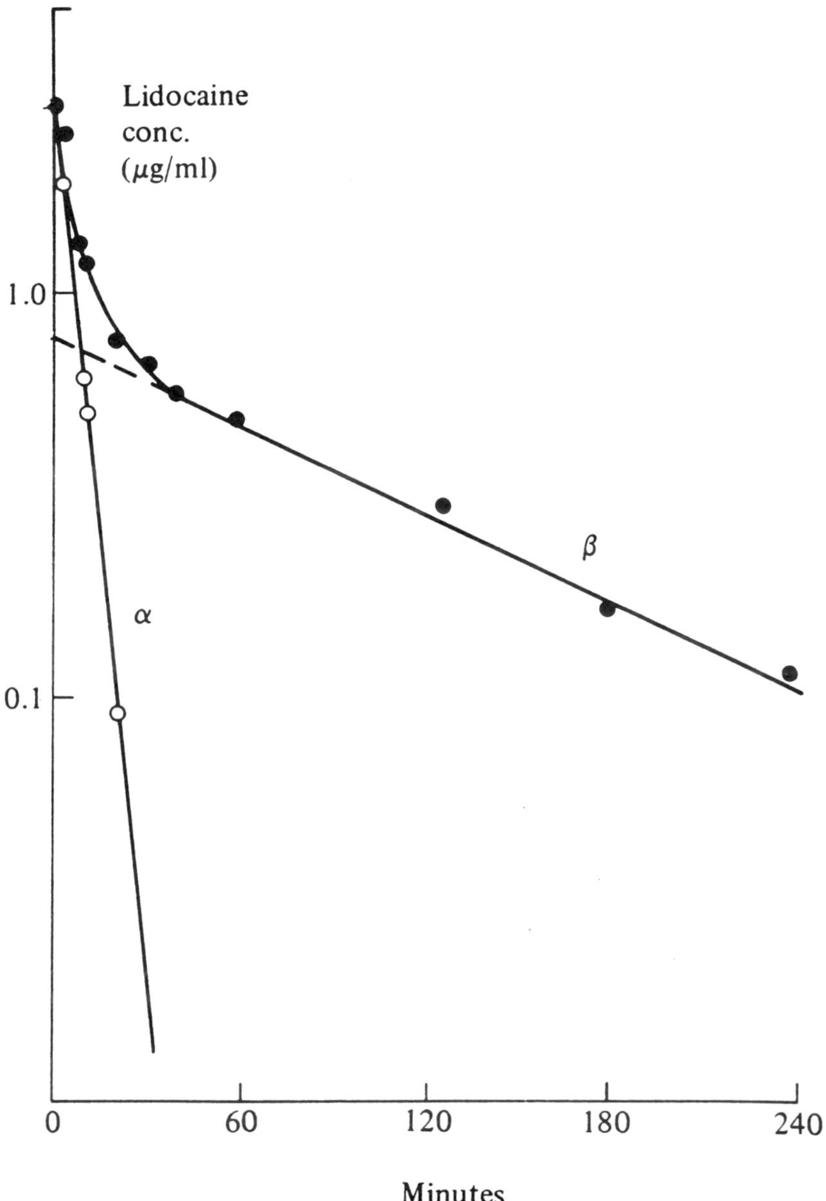


**Figure 2.** Plasma lidocaine concentration versus time after an intravenous bolus. The disappearance of lidocaine from the plasma is biphasic. The rapid distribution phase, labelled alpha, represents distribution of drug from blood into tissues and has a half-life of 8−10 minutes. The slower disappearance phase, labelled beta, represents metabolism and has a half-life of about 2 hours. (From Neis AS: Cardiovascular disorders. In KL Melman, HF Morelli (eds): *Clinical Pharmacology*. New York, Macmillan, p 240, 1978. By permission.)

Even this analysis, which demonstrated the lack of precision of a two-compartment model, was incomplete in that it described distribution into compartments over only the first 3 days and the true elimination half-life of amiodarone from the body was not defined.

To put this into descriptive rather than mathematical terms, for the first several days of amiodarone therapy, the disappearance of drug from blood represents predominantly distribution. That is, the drug that is administered goes predominantly into tissues rather than being eliminated from the body. To accurately describe the elimination of amiodarone out of the body, the tissue stores should be fully saturated, which takes at least several weeks and perhaps as long as several months. Thus, the discrepancy between the reports of elimination kinetics showing a half-life of several hours and the reports describing the half-life as being several months is explained by the improper classification of slower distribution phases after single doses in pharmacokinetic studies as elimination, whereas the reports of long half-lives after chronic oral therapy represent true elimination of drug from the body.

*Extensive Tissue Distribution of Amiodarone*

The fact that amiodarone demonstrates distribution kinetics that are better described by several different rates of distribution rather than a single rate is not surprising when the concentrations of drug as well as the rates of drug accumulation in various tissues are examined. Liver, heart, skin, muscle, fat, and other organs have been shown to have concentrations of anywhere from 10 to 1000 times that in blood.[115–119] For the liver, the accumulation of amiodarone (and metabolites) as measured by increased density on abdominal computerized tomography requires 80 days to achieve steady state.[58] On the other hand, myocardium appears to equilibrate serum within 30 minutes.[118] Thus, large tissue deposits of amiodarone exist that appear to possess individual properties both in terms of total amount of drug and rate of tissue uptake. When examined from this perspective, it is not surprising that the disappearance of drug from blood after an intravenous dose reflects a number of different distribution compartments rather than a single homogenous "tissue compartment."

## Relation of Multicompartment Analysis of Amiodarone to Dosing

The knowledge that there are large tissue deposits of amiodarone, which accumulate amiodarone at different rates, is important for the rational use of this drug, whether it be intravenously or orally. We have used this information to develop intravenous loading regimens that rapidly achieve and then maintain the serum concentration within a target range. We have shown that a two-stage intravenous loading infusion can achieve and maintain the serum concentration within a target range of 2.0–3.0 µg/ml and that this regimen resulted in significant arrhythmia suppression within 48 hours.[114] In that study, dose was individualized on the basis of the patient's pharmacokinetic profile. With the two-stage regimen, the target serum concentration range was achieved by hour 6. Subsequently, the mean infusion rates from that study were used to load an additional 19 patients requiring intravenous amiodarone for emergency arrhythmia suppression (unpublished data). For these patients, a bolus was used prior to the two-stage infusion: an initial dose of 5 mg/kg was given over 15 minutes, then an infusion of 2 mg/min for 12 hours, and then 0.7 mg/min until patients were able to take oral amiodarone. By initiating amiodarone with a bolus, the serum concentrations resulting from this regimen immediately achieved or exceeded the target range of 2.0–3.0 µg/ml. Then, by using the two-stage infusion regimen, serum concentrations were maintained in or near this target range (Fig. 3). In this case, the three-stage dosing regimen allowed for relatively constant serum concentrations as drug distributed into tissues at different rates over the first few days of therapy.

A multicompartment analysis of amiodarone's kinetics also is important for oral dosing.[119] In order to achieve serum concentrations in a target range of 2.0–3.0 µg/ml within a few days of initiating therapy large doses of oral amiodarone are required.[7] As tissue stores that rapidly take up amiodarone become saturated, less drug is required to maintain this blood level even over the first 4 days of therapy.[7]


## Recommendations for Dosing

### Practical Implications of These Pharmacologic Considerations

The major practical consideration derived from this discussion is that one cannot simply administer a "loading dose" of amiodarone and give it for a few doses, then switch to a "maintenance dose" and consider the patient in steady state. Depending on the urgency of the arrhythmia control, a high to very high dose may be

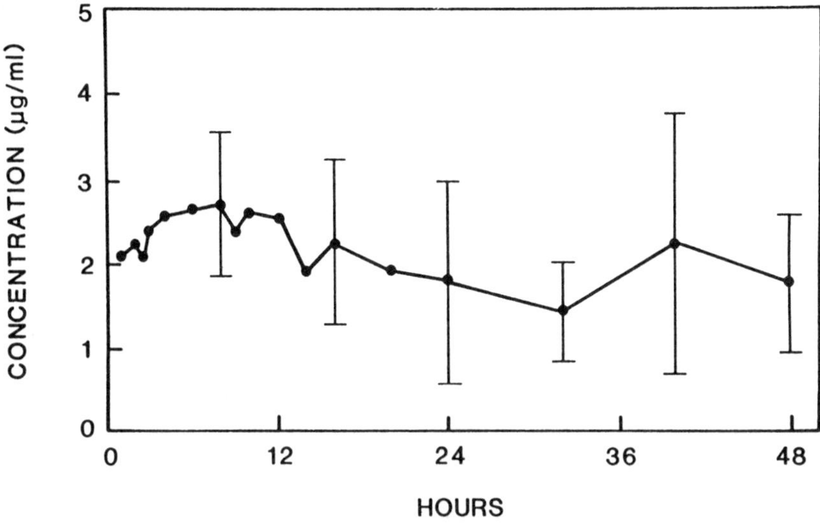


**Figure 3.** Amiodarone serum concentration (μg/ml) versus time using a three-stage intravenous loading regimen. Nineteen patients received intravenous amiodarone as follows: 5 mg/kg over 15 minutes, then 2 mg/ min for 12 hours, and then 0.7 mg/min until able to take oral medication. Data are shown as means with standard deviation bars every 8 hours for clarity.

used for 1 day, then a slightly lower dose for a few days thereafter, then a lower dose (but still high) for the next several days, then a medium dose for another few weeks, then a medium low dose for a few months, and finally, perhaps after 3–6 months, the dose can be reduced to a low amount. The goal is to maintain a relatively constant amount in the blood and, thus, presumably, at the unknown site of action while the various tissues of the body such as liver, lung, heart, fat, and brain become saturated with drug at their individual rates of drug accumulation. Finally, with all tissues saturated, the low true maintenance dose, which will usually be 400 mg or less, will represent the amount of drug eliminated from the body each day without any additional drug being accumulated by tissue.

## Factors to Be Considered in Determining Amiodarone Dose

Assuming that amiodarone therapy is reserved for refractory cases where arrhythmia control is mandatory, relatively rapid arrhythmia suppression is likely to be important. Because the risk of the early, transient side effects goes up as the initial loading dose goes up, what must be weighed is the malignancy of the arrhythmia against the desire to avoid the early, dose related side effects. Thus, a patient with a history of sustained ventricular tachycardia (VT) who has frequent short runs of VT on Holter but no sustained VT in-hospital would be treated with doses of amiodarone that might be expected to suppress the arrhythmia within several days, whereas a patient with recurrent episodes of sustained VT requiring cardioversion would receive very high doses even though nausea, vomiting, and tremor would be quite likely.

Another important consideration is the variability of absorption of drug in individual patients. Some patients will have low amiodarone serum concentrations in spite of extremely large doses and others will have high levels with lower doses. Thus, even after an initial dosage regimen has been chosen, it is imperative to assess clinical efficacy and side effects frequently. In situations where either no effect is seen when one should have happened or where side effects appear excessive for the dose, an amiodarone serum level may help determine if the problem is related to either poor or excessively good absorption or distribution. After the patient goes home, serum concentration monitoring may be useful, since the dosage must be reduced progressively to avoid long-term toxicity while maintaining efficacy.

## Specific Dosing Guidelines

With the general considerations just given, the following general guidelines are suggested. It must be stressed this schema is a general one that we have found to be effective in dosing patients for the control of arrhythmias. It is based on our experience. Others have developed somewhat differing approaches and have succeeded in suppressing recalcitrant tachyarrhythmias.

*When Rapid Arrhythmia Suppression Is Required*

    Day 1:       800 mg q 8 h with meals/snacks
    Day 2−7:     800 mg b.i.d. with meals
    Week 2−3:    400 mg b.i.d. with meals
    Week 4−6:    300 mg b.i.d. with meals
    Week 7−12:   400 mg daily with a meal
    Week 13−:    200−400 mg daily with a meal

Side effects are common, and may require dose reduction. Follow CCU monitor and Holter/EPS when no VT noted. Obtain blood levels when desired response is not seen and during dosage reduction phase. Target serum concentration: is 1.5−2.5 µg/ml.

*When Rapid Arrhythmia Suppression Is Not Required*

    Week 1:      400 mg b.i.d. with meals
    Week 2:      300 mg b.i.d. with meals
    Week 3−12: 200 mg b.i.d. with meals
    Week 13−:   200−400 mg daily

Obtain blood levels if desired response is not seen or if possible side effects are noted. During chronic therapy, maintain blood level below 2.5 µg/ml to avoid high risk of long-term toxicity.

*Highly Unstable Patients, Patients Unable to Take Oral Medications*

Intravenous amiodarone: three-stage regimen

    Stage I:   5 mg/kg in 50 cc $D_5W$ infused over 15 minutes
    Stage II:  2.0 mg/min for 12 hours
    Stage III: 0.7 mg/min thereafter until patient is able to take oral
               medication.

At present, amiodarone is not approved for intravenous use. Patients should be considered for referral for this purpose. Intravenous amiodarone should be administered via a central venous catheter to avoid phlebothrombosis.

## Summary and Conclusions

Amiodarone is an antiarrhythmic medication that is highly effective in the treatment of supraventricular and ventricular arrhythmias. Unfortunately, it is a drug that has a very high incidence of side effects, virtually 100 percent. It is helpful that most of the side effects are not serious and that they improve or disappear with dose reduction or discontinuation of the medication. Fatalities from the drug have been reported due to exacerbation of arrhythmias, pulmonary involvement, and rarely, hepatic involvement. It is probable that most of these could be avoided by early recognition of the complication and prompt dose reduction or cessation. In some instances, concomitant steroid therapy is helpful, especially in the case of pulmonary infiltrates. The occurrence of such frequent side effects and the less common, dangerous side effects warrants the admonition that the drug be used primarily in resistant arrhythmias that are either life-threatening or cause debilitating symptoms. In addition, the smallest dose of the drug that controls the arrhythmia should be utilized. Serum levels, although not helpful in accurately predicting who will develop side effects or respond to the medication, nevertheless, are helpful in assessing adequacy of absorption and compliance. Moreover, there appears to be a range of serum levels, in the stable chronic state, that are likely to yield control of the arrhythmia with a lower incidence of side effects. This range is between 1 and 2.5 µg/ml. However, this will not preclude the development of skin discoloration, corneal microdeposits, or pulmonary complications. Nor will it invarably ensure suppression of the arrhythmia. Drug interactions have been described and it is important that the physician be alert to the probability that other such reactions will occur as the drug is used more widely.

With regard to optimal dosing regimens, it is clear that the selection of the appropriate dose for any individual patient is most difficult given the variability in individual response, absorption, elimination half-life, and metabolism of the drug. In addition, the need for "loading," the severity of the arrhythmias selected for treatment and early side effects also temper the maximum dose that can be administered to a given individual. For these reasons, a target serum level that has been demonstrated to yield a significant therapeutic effect in many patients and which leads to a shortening of the time to the control of the arrhythmia while reducing the likelihood of side effects would appear to be an appropriate approach to drug dosing. We have outlined suggested modes of dosing that should lead to acceptable serum levels. Serum level determinations may provide help in establishing compliance and in developing a "therapeutic level" for the individual patient. Because of the high incidence of side effects, the lowest dose of amiodarone that achieves and maintains control with a minimum of side effects should be established for each patient. It should also be emphasized that despite the use of the pharmacokinetic approach to amiodarone dosing, a great deal of empiricism remains[120] and frequent regular clinical surveillance of the patient may still provide the best approach to the avoidance of potentially lethal side effects of the drug.

## References


1. Ives Laboratories Inc., FDA submission for NDA 18–972. April 1984.
2. Sobol SM, Rakita L: Pneumonitis and pulmonary fibrosis associated with amiodarone treatment: A possible complication of a new antiarrhythmic drug. *Circulation* 65:819, 1982.
3. Heger JJ, Prystowsky EN, Zipes DP: Clinical efficacy of amiodarone in treatment of recurrent ventricular tachycardia and ventricular and ventricular fibrillation. *Am Heart J* 106:887, 1983.
4. Lim PK, Trewby PN, Storey GCA, et al: Neuropathy and fatal hepatitis in a patient receiving amiodarone. *Br Med J* 288:1638, 1984.
5. Raeder EA, Podrid PS, Lown B: Side effects and complications of amiodarone. *Am Heart J* 109:975, 1985.
6. Haffajee EL, Love JC, Alpert G, et al: Efficacy and safety of long-term amiodarone in treatment of cardiac arrhythmias: Dosage experience. *Am Heart J* 106:935, 1983.
7. Mostow ND, Vrobel TR, Noon D, et al: Rapid suppression of complex ventricular arrhythmias with high dose oral amiodarone. *Circulation* 73:1231, 1986.
8. Sanmarti A, Permanyer-Miralda G, Castellanos JM, et al: Chronic administration of amiodarone and thyroid function: A follow up study. *Am Heart J* 108:1262, 1984.
9. Leak D, Eydt JN: Amiodarone for refractory cardiac arrhythmias. *J Can Med Assoc* 134:495, 1986.
10. Greene HL, Graham EL, Werner JA, et al: Toxic and therapeutic effects of amiodarone in the treatment of cardiac arrhythmias. *J Am Coll Cardiol* 2:1114, 1983.
11. Heger JJ, Prystowsky EN, Jackman WM, et al: Amiodarone: Clinical efficacy and electrophysiology during long term therapy for recurrent ventricular tachycardia or ventricular fibrillation. *N Eng J Med* 305:539, 1983.
12. Adams PC, Holt DW, Storey GCA, et al: Amiodarone and its desethyl metabolite: Tissue distribution and morphologic changes during long-term therapy. *Circulation* 72:1064, 1985.
13. McKenna WJ, Harris L, Rowland E, et al: Amiodarone for long term management of patients with hypertrophic cardiomyopathy. *Am J Cardiol* 54:802, 1984.
14. Rakita L, Sobol SM, Mostow ND, et al: Amiodarone pulmonary toxicity. *Am Heart J* 106:906, 1983.
15. Marchlinski FE, Gansler TS, Waxman HL, et al: Amiodarone pulmonary toxicity. *Ann Int Med* 97:839, 1982.
16. Poucell S, Ireton J, Vallencia-Mayoral P, et al: Amiodarone-associated phosopholipidosis and fibrosis of the liver. *Gastroenterology* 86:926, 1984.
17. Delge C, Legace R, Heard J: Pseudocyanotic pigmentation of the skin induced by amiodarone: A light and electron microscopic study. *Can Med Assoc J* 112:1205, 1975.
18. Dake MD, Madison JM, Montgomery CK, et al: Electron microscopic demonstration of lysosomal inclusion bodies with amiodarone pulmonary toxicity. *Am J Med* 78:507, 1985.

19. Akoun GM, Gauthier-Rahman S, Millerson BJ, et al: Amiodarone induced hypersensitivity pneumonitis: Evidence of an immunological cell-mediated mechanism. *Chest* 85:133, 1984.
20. Dake MD, Golden JA: Amiodarone and pulmonary effects. *Ann Int Med* 98:1028, 1983.
21. Sandron D, Israel Biet D, Venet A, et al: Immunoglobulin abnormalities in bronchoalveolar lavage specimens from amiodarone treated subjects. *Chest* 89:617, 1986.
22. Joseph E, Rouselie F: Round Table Seminar on amiodarone. Saltpetriere, Paris, October 1968.
23. Ingram DV: Ocular effects in long-term amiodarone therapy. *Am Heart J* 106:902, 1983.
24. Chew E, Ghosh M, McCullough C: Amiodarone-induced cornea vercillata. *Can J Opthalmol* 17:96, 1982.
25. Lullman H, Lullman-Rauch R, Wasserman O: Drug-induced phospholipidoses. *CRC Crit Rev Toxicol* 4:185, 1975.
26. D'Amico DJ, Kenyon KR, Ruskin JN: Amiodarone keratopathy: Drug-induced lipid storage disease. *Arch Opthalmol* 99:257, 1981.
27. Nademanee K, Singh BN, Callahan B, et al: Amiodarone, thyroid hormone indices and altered thyroid function: Long-term serial effects in patients with cardiac arrhythmias. *Am J Cardiol* 58:981, 1986.
28. Ward DE, Camm AS, Suprrell RAJ: Clinical antiarrhythmic effects of amiodarone in patients with resistant paroxysmal tachycardia. *Br Heart J* 44:91, 1980.
29. Burger A, Dinichert P, Nicod P, et al: Effect of amiodarone on serum triiodothyronine, reverse triiodothyronine, thyroxin and thyrotropin. *J Clin Invest* 58:255, 1976.
30. Singh BN, Nademanee K: Amiodarone and thyroid function: Clinical implications during antiarrhythmic therapy. *Am Heart J* 106:857, 1983.
31. Rabinowe SL, Larsen PR, Antman EM, et al: Amiodarone therapy and autoimmune thyroid disease: Increase in a new monoclonal antibody-defined T-cell subset. *Am J Med* 81:53, 1986.
32. Furlanello F, Inaura G, Ferrari M, et al: Amiodarone and amiodarone plus digoxin in the treatment of paroxysmal supraventricular reciprocating tachyarrhythmias. *Pharmacol Res Comm* 14:731, 1982.
33. Fogoros RN, Anderson KP, Winkle RA, et al: Amiodarone clinical efficacy and toxicity in 96 patients with recurrent, drug refractory arrhythmias. *Circulation* 68:88, 1983.
34. Peter T, Hamer A, Mandel WJ: Evaluation of amiodarone therapy in the treatment of drug-resistant cardiac arrhythmias: Long-term follow up. *Eur Heart J* 6:(Suppl D):151, 1985.
35. Marcus FL: Amiodarone in antiarrhythmic therapy. *Cardiovasc Med* 11:25, 1986.
36. Ferguson J: Amiodarone: A study of cutaneous photosensitivity. *Brit J Clin Prac* 40(4):63, 1986.
37. Kaufmann G: Pyridoxine against amiodarone-induced photosensitivity. *Lancet* 1:51, 1984.
38. Rotmensch HH, Liron M, Tupilski M, et al: Possible association of pneumonitis with amiodarone therapy. *Am Heart J* 100:412, 1980.

39. Zaher C, Hamer A, Peter T, et al: Low dose steroid therapy for prophylaxis of amiodarone-induced pulmonary infiltrates. (letter) *N Eng J Med* 308:779, 1983.

40. Adams PC, Gibson GJ, Morley AR, et al: Amiodarone pulmonary toxicity: Clinical and subclinical features. *Quart J Med* 229(9):449, 1986.

41. Veltri EP, Reid PR: Amiodarone pulmonary toxicity: Early changes in pulmonary function tests during amiodarone rechallenge. *J Am Coll Cardiol* 6:802, 1985.

42. Van Roolz WJ, Vander Meer SC, Van Royen EA: Pulmonary gallium-67 uptake in amiodarone pneumonitis. *J Nucl Med* 25:211, 1984.

43. Camus P, Mehendale HM: Pulmonary sequestration of amiodarone and desethylamiodarone. *J Pharmacol Exp Ther* 237:867, 1986.

44. Tatti V, Ramelli G: Pneumopathie interstitielle et amiodarone. *Schweiz Med Wschr* 116:377, 1986.

45. Tuczu M, Maloney JD, Sangain B, et al: Adverse effects of chronic amiodarone therapy complicating cardiac surgery. Abstract 1197, p 209. World Congress of Cardiology, Washington D.C., 1986.

46. Pollak PT, Sami M: Acute necrotizing pneumonitis and hyperglycemia after amiodarone therapy. *Amer J Med* 76:935, 1984.

47. Quyyumi AA, Omerod LP, Clarke SW, et al: Pulmonary fibrosis—A serious side effect of amiodarone therapy. *Eur Heart J* 4:521, 1983.

48. Kennedy JI, Myers JL, Plumb VJ, et al: Amiodarone pulmonary toxicity: Clinical and pathologic study of eleven cases. *Am J Clin Pathol* 87:7, 1987.

49. Leech JA, Gallestegui J, Swiryn S: Pulmonary toxicity of amiodarone. *Chest* 85:444, 1984.

50. Olson LK, Forrest JV, Friedman PJ, et al: Pneumonitis after amiodarone therapy. *Radiology* 150:327, 1984.

51. Suarez LD, Poderoso JJ, Elsner B, et al: Subacute pneumopathy during amiodarone therapy. *Chest* 83:566, 1983.

52. Venet A, Caubarrere I, Bonan G: Five cases of immune-mediated amiodarone-mediated pneumonitis. (letter) *Lancet* 1:962, 1984.

53. Costa-Jussa FR, Corrin B, Jacobs JM: Amiodarone lung toxicity: A human and experimental study. *J Pathol* 143:73, 1984.

54. Joelson J, Kluger J, Cole S, et al: Possible recurrence of amiodarone pulmonary toxicity following corticosteroid therapy. *Chest* 85:284, 1984.

55. Darmanata JI, Van Zandwijk N, Duren DR: Amiodarone pneumonitis: Three further cases and a review of published reports. *Thorax* 39:57, 1984.

56. Kudenchek PJ, Pierson DJ, Greene HL, et al: Prospective evaluation of amiodarone pulmonary toxicity. *Chest* 86:541, 1984.

57. Adams PC, Bennett MK, Holt DW: Hepatic effects of amiodarone. *Br J Clin Prac* 40(4):81, 1986.

58. Shenasa M, Vaisman U, Wojciechowski M, et al: Abnormal abdominal computerized tomography with amiodarone therapy and clinical significance. *Am Heart J* 107:929, 1984.

59. Simon JB, Manley N, Brien JF, et al: Amiodarone toxicity simulating alcoholic liver disease. *N Eng J Med* 311:167, 1984.

60. Rumessen JJ: Hepatotoxicity of amiodarone. *Acta Med Scand* 219:235, 1986.
61. Fraser AG: Neurological and pulmonary adverse effects of amiodarone. *Br J Clin Prac* 44(4):74, 1986.
62. Lustman F, Monseu G: Amiodarone and neurological side effects. (letter) *Lancet* 1:568, 1974.
63. Lemaire JF, Autret A, Bizierre K, et al: Amiodarone neuropathy: Further arguments for human drug-induced neurolipidosis. *Eur Neurol* 21:65, 1985.
64. Fraser AG, McQueen INF, Watt AH, et al: Peripheral neuropathy during high-dose amiodarone therapy. *J Neurol Neurosurg Psych* 48:576, 1985.
65. MacKinnon G, Landymore R, Marble A: Should oral amiodarone be used for sustained ventricular tachycardia in patients requiring open heart surgery? *Can J Surg* 26:355, 1983.
66. Gallagher JD, Liederman RW, Meranze J, et al: Amiodarone induced complications during coronary artery surgery. *Anesthesiology* 55:186, 1981.
67. Michat L, Cabrol C, Cabrol A, et al: Effets antiarrhythmiques de l'amiodarone injectable en reanimation de chirurgie cardiovasculaire. *Nouv Presse Med* 5:1996, 1976.
68. Installe E, Schoevaerdts JC, Gadisseux P, et al: Intravenous amiodarone in the treatment of various arrhythmias following cardiac operations. *J Thorac Cardiovasc Surg* 81:302, 1981.
69. Vestveer DC, Gadowski GA, Gordon S, et al: Amiodarone-induced ventricular tachycardia. *Ann Int Med* 97:561, 1982.
70. Sclarovsky S, Lewin RF, Kracoff O, et al: Amiodarone induced polymorphous ventricular tachycardia. *Am Heart J* 105:6, 1983.
71. McComb JM, Logan DR, Khan MM, et al: Amiodarone induced ventricular fibrillation. *Eur J Cardiol* 11:381, 1980.
72. Keren A, Tzivoni D, Gottlieb S, et al: Atypical ventricular tachycardia (torsade de pointes) induced by amiodarone. *Chest* 81:384, 1982.
73. Guanggeng C, Huang W, Urthaler F: Ventricular flutter during treatment with amiodarone. *Am J Cardiol* 51:609, 1983.
74. Mostow ND, Vrobel TR, Rakita L: Transient exacerbation followed by control of ventricular tachycardia with amiodarone. *Am Heart J* 111:178, 1986.
75. Sheinman BD, Evans T: Acceleration of ventricular rate by amiodarone in atrial fibrillation associated with Wolff-Parkinson-White syndrome. *Br Med J* 285:999, 1982.
76. Veltri EP, Reid PR: Sinus arrest with intravenous amiodarone. *Am J Cardiol* 58:1110, 1986.
77. McGovern B, Garan H, Ruskin JR: Sinus arrest during treatment with amiodarone. *Br Med J* 264:160, 1982.
78. McGovern B, Garan H, Kelly E, et al: Adverse reactions during treatment with amiodarone hydrochloride. *Br Med J* 287:175, 1983.
79. Keidar S, Grenadier E, Palanat A: Sino-atrial arrest due to lidocaine injection in sick sinus syndrome during amiodarone administration. *Am Heart J* 104:1384, 1982.
80. Kennedy EE, Batsford WP: Amiodarone-induced intra-His block. *J Am Coll Cardiol* 4:192, 1984.

81. Rosenbaum MB, Chiale PA, Halpern MS, et al: Clinical efficacy of amiodarone as an antiarrhythmic agent. *Am J Cardiol* 38:934, 1976.

82. McGovern B, Goran H, Ruskin JN: Serious adverse effects of amiodarone. Clin Cardiol 7:131, 1984.

83. Rotmensch HH, Behassen B, Ferguson RK: Amiodarone-benefits and risk in perspective. *Am Heart J* 104:1117, 1982.

84. Singh BN: Amiodarone: Historical development and pharmacologic profile. *Am Heart J* 106:788, 1983.

85. De Paola AVA, Horowitz LN, Spielman SR, et al: Amiodarone therapy in patients with sustained ventricular tachyarrhythmias: Observations on heart failure and the influences of ejection fraction. *Am J Cardiol* (in press).

86. Marcus F: Drug Interactions with amiodarone. *Am Heart J* 106:924, 1983.

87. Simpson WT: *Amiodarone in Cardiac Arrhythmias.* International Congress and Symposium Series No. 16, Royal Society of Medicine. New York, Grune and Stratton, 1979, p. 45.

88. Serlin MJ, Sibeon RG, Green GJ: Dangers of amiodarone and anticoagulant treatment. *Br Med J* 283:57, 1981.

89. Rees A, Palal JJ, Reid PG, et al: Dangers of amiodarone and anticoagulant treatment. *Br Med J* 282:1756, 1981.

90. Oetgen WJ, Sobol SM, Tri TB, et al: Amiodarone digoxin interaction: Clinical and experimental observations. *Chest* 86:75, 1984.

91. Moysey JO, Jaggarao NSV, Grundy EN, et al: Amiodarone increases plasma digoxin concentrations. *Br Med J* 282:272, 1981.

92. Nademanee K, Kannan R, Hendrickson JA, et al: Amiodarone-digoxin interaction: Clinical significance, time course of development potential pharmacokinetic mechanisms and therapeutic implications. *J Am Coll Cardiol* 4:111, 1984.

93. Tartini R, Kappenberger L, Steinbrunn W, et al: Dangerous interaction between amiodarone and quinidine. *Lancet* 1:1327, 1982.

94. Shea P, Lal R, Kim SS, et al: Flecainide and amiodarone interaction. *J Am Coll Cardiol* 7:1127, 1980.

95. Schneeweiss A: Safety profile of amiodarone in the elderly. Abstract 2831, p 488. World Congress of Cardiology, Washington, D.C., 1986.

96. Quatrini L, Raffaeli S, Andreoni A, et al: Side effects of chronic therapy with amiodrone in the elderly. Abstract 737, p 473. World Congress of Cardiology, Washington, D.C., 1986.

97. Lloveras J, Masramon J, Aubia J, et al: Amiodarone metoclopramide, and renal failure. *Lancet* 981 (May 5) 1979.

98. Staubli M, Zimmerman A, Bircher J: Amiodarone induced vasculitis and polyserositis. *Postgrad Med J* 61:245, 1985.

99. Samanta A, Jones GR, Burden AC, et al: Thoracic inlet compression due to amiodarone induced goiter. *Postgrad Med J* 61:249, 1985.

100. Flach AJ, Dolan BJ, Sudduth B, et al: Amiodarone-induced lens opacities. *Arch Ophthalmol* 101:1554, 1983.

101. Hesselman J, Huep WW, Schroder E: Lebensbedroliche alveolitis and hemolyse nach amiodarone. *Med Welt* 34:858, 1983.

102. Lee TH, Friedman PL, Goldman L, et al: Sinus arrest and hypotension with combined amiodarone-diltiazem therapy. *Am Heart J* 109:163, 1985.

103. McGovern B, Geer VR, LaRaia RJ, et al: Possible interaction between amiodarone and phenytoin. *Ann Int Med* 101:650, 1984.

104. Gasparich JP, Mason JT, Greene HL, et al: Amiodarone-associated epididymitis: Drug-related epididymitis in the absence of infection. *J Urol* 133:971, 1985.

105. Collaborative Group for Amiodarone Evaluation: Multicenter controlled observation of a low-dose regimen of amiodarone for treatment of severe ventricular arrhythmias. *Am J Cardiol* 53:1564, 1984.

106. Mostow ND, Rakita L, Vrobel TR, et al: Amiodarone: Correlation of serum concentration with suppression of complex ventricular ectopy. *Am J Cardiol* 54:569, 1984.

107. Rakita L, Sobol SM: Amiodarone in the treatment of refractory ventricular arrhythmias. Importance and safety of initial high-dose therapy. *JAMA* 250:1293, 1983.

108. Nies AS: Cardiovascular disorders. In KL Melman, HF Morelli, (eds): *Clinical Pharmacology.* New York, Macmillan, p 240, 1978.

109. Riva E, Gerna M, Latini R, et al: Pharmacokinetics of amiodarone in man. *J Cardiovasc Pharmacol* 4:264, 1982.

110. Riva E, Gerna M, Neyroz PX, et al: Pharmacokinetics of amiodarone in rats. *J Cardiovasc Pharmacol* 4:270, 1982.

111. Mostow ND, Noon DL, Myers CM, et al: Determination of amiodarone and its n-deethylated metabolite in serum by high-performance liquid chromatography. *J Chromatog* 227:229, 1983.

112. Kannan R, Nademanee K, Hendrickson JA, et al: Amiodarone kinetics after oral doses. *Clin Pharmacol Ther* 31:438, 1982.

113. Holt DW, Tucker GT, Jackson PR, et al: Amiodarone pharmacokinetics. *Am Heart J* 106:840, 1983.

114. Mostow ND, Rakita L, Vrobel TR, et al: Amiodarone: Intravenous loading for rapid suppression of complex ventricular arrhythmias. *J Am Coll Cardiol* 4:97, 1984.

115. Tucker GT, Jackson PR, Storey GCA, et al: Amiodarone disposition: Polyexponential power and gamma functions. *Eur J Clin Pharmacol* 26:655, 1984.

116. Haffajee CI, Love JC, Canada AT, et al: Clinical pharmacokinetics and efficacy of amiodarone for refractory tachyarrhythmias. *Circulation* 67:1347, 1983.

117. Goldman IS, Winkler ML, Raper SE, et al: Increased hepatic density and phospholipidosis due to amiodarone. *Am J Radiol* 144:541, 1985.

118. Connolly SJ, Latini R, Kates RE: Pharmacodynamics of intravenous amiodarone in the dog. *J Cardiovasc Pharmacol* 6:531, 1984.

119. Siddoway LA, McAllister CB, Wikinson GR, et al: Amiodarone dosing: A proposal based on its pharmacokinetics. *Am Heart J* 106:951, 1983.

120. Nademanee K, Singh BN, Hendrickson JA, et al: Amiodarone in refractory life-threatening ventricular arrhythmias. *Ann Int Med* 98:577, 1983.

# Chapter 22

# Drug Interactions with Class III Antiarrhythmic Drugs

## Frank I. Marcus

---

In recent years, an increasing plethora of cardioactive compounds has been introduced into clinical therapeutics. Antiarrhythmic agents usually are employed in patients with structural heart disease who may be treated with a diversity of agents to control cardiac failure, myocardial ischemia, hypertension, and other cardiovascular disorders. It is of interest that although cardiac glycosides and quinidine have been used concomitantly for many decades, only in the last decade has a pharmacokinetic interaction between the two compounds been identified.[1] A heightened awareness of such an interaction has led to an earlier recognition of digoxin interactions with the newer antiarrhythmic compounds. For example, a significant interaction between digoxin and verapamil recently was found and a similar interaction between amiodarone and digoxin came to light during the early evaluation of these drugs as antiarrhythmic agents.[1-7]

Drug interactions involving newer antiarrhythmic compounds are of particular significance, since many of these agents alter the kinetics and the pharmacodynamics of many drugs commonly used in cardiologic practice. The subject of this chapter is drug interactions involving compounds whose major electrophysiologic action is the prolongation of cardiac repolarization, the so-called Class III antiarrhythmic compounds. These include amiodarone, bretylium, N-acetylprocainamide, and sotalol. Melperone also is a Class III antiarrhythmic compound but neither its clinical antiarrhythmic effects or its potential for drug–drug interactions have been eval-

---

From: *Control of Cardiac Arrhythmias by Lengthening Repolarization*, edited by Bramah N. Singh, MD, Futura Publishing Company Inc., Mount Kisco, NY, © 1988.

uated systematically. In this class of agents, pharmacokinetic interactions have been documented between amiodarone and a number of concurrently administered drugs. No major drug–drug pharmacokinetic interactions have been reported with bretylium, sotalol, and N-acetylprocainamide although an interaction between N-acetylprocainamide and amiodarone during procainamide administration has been described.

## Types of Drug Interactions

Drug interactions may be classified into three main types: pharmaceutical, pharmacokinetic, and pharmacodynamic. *Pharmaceutical* interactions occur when two compounds are given together in the same infusion or when a pharmacologic agent reacts with the electrolytes in the infusion solution. An example of this is the case of amiodarone, which precipitates in infusions containing electrolytes. Another instance is the precipitation of verapamil in bicarbonate solutions.

In contrast, *pharmacokinetic* interactions, clinically perhaps the most significant, are those in which the absorption, distribution, biotransformation, and clearance of one agent is altered by another during concomitant administration. Each one of the features of disposition of one drug may be altered significantly by the overall action of another. The resultant alterations in plasma and tissue concentrations of a drug thus may lead in turn to a change in its pharmacodynamic effects that may produce unexpected and sometimes potentially lethal and deleterious clinical effects. Perhaps the best studied example of a pharmacokinetic interaction is that of digoxin and quinidine.[1]

*Pharmacodynamic* interactions are those in which two drugs given together have the same locus of action. The combined action leads to an augmentation of the pharmacologic effects that, under certain circumstances, may be of therapeutic value, as in the case of combination therapy with antiarrhythmic agents. In other situations, such an interaction may result in potentially serious adverse reactions. For example, it is well known that a combination of beta blocker and verapamil may lead to an increase in the incidence of atrioventricular nodal conduction disturbances, bradycardia, and asystole, especially in patients with preexisting conduction system disease. In the case of antiarrhythmic agents, there appear to be two major consequences of pharmacodynamic interactions. The first is the electrophysiologic interaction in which the effects of the two agents summate and produce an exaggerated response with deleterious consequences. The second is a hemodynamic interaction. In such a case, the negative inotropic effects of two agents (e.g., beta blockers and disopyramide), might be additive with a marked net depressant effect on ventricular performance.

The most significant pharmacokinetic and pharmacodynamic interactions involving Class III antiarrhythmic agents have been in the case of amiodarone. The remainder of this chapter deals with the known interactions involving this compound. References to the effects of the other Class III compounds will be made only for completeness.

## Pharmacokinetic Interactions Involving Amiodarone

The almost ubiquitous nature of interaction between amiodarone and other cardioactive compounds now increasingly is recognized.[2] A central feature to such an action may be the depressant effect of the drug on the activity of the hepatic oxidative metabolizing enzymes. For example, Grech-Berlanger[8] found that when 50–100 mg/kg of amiodarone were given daily to rats, there was a significant reduction of aniline, the O- and N-demethylations of p-nitroanisole and aminopyrine, respectively, and the level of cytochrome P-450. Testosterone hydroxylation also was depressed by amiodarone at the higher dose. Cytochrome $b_5$ content and lipid peroxidation were depressed significantly with smaller doses of amiodarone. The inhibitory effect of amiodarone also was shown in vivo by an increase in the elimination half-life and a decrease in the clearance of antipyrine. We consider that these overall effects, in part, explain the drug interactions induced by amiodarone. However, further investigations are needed to delineate the precise fundamental nature of the interactions between amiodarone and other cardioactive compounds.

## Digoxin and Amiodarone Interaction

In 1981, Moysey, et al.[4] showed that digoxin serum concentrations increased nearly 100 percent when patients who were being treated with digoxin were given amiodarone. This phenomenon has been confirmed in a number of studies. It has been found that the steady-state serum level of digoxin increases (Fig. 1) as a function of time at a constant dose of amiodarone during the loading phase of therapy (Fig. 2). It has been found that the increases in the serum levels of digoxin have been most striking during high-dose drug administration.

A number of investigators have attempted to define the mechanisms to account for the interactions between amiodarone and digoxin. For example, Koren[9] and Venkatesh et al.[10] recently confirmed the increases in serum digoxin levels induced by amiodarone in rats in vivo. Koren[9] reported that in vitro amiodarone significantly reduced the uptake of digoxin in renal cortical slices but had no effect in cardiac muscle. Venkatesh et al.[10] found that the tissue levels of digoxin rose under the influence of chronic amiodarone administration but less in the myocardium than in brain and skeletal muscle (Fig. 3). Concomitant administration of amiodarone and digoxin increased the serum digoxin concentration by 94 percent (p < 0.001), in skeletal muscle by 172 percent (p < 0.001), and in the brain by 110 percent (p < 0.001). Of particular interest, the tissue to serum ratios of digoxin in all three tissues fell, indicating a differential displacement of the glycoside induced by amiodarone. Such an effect, also demonstrated for the metabolite, desethylamiodarone,[11] may contribute to the observed increases in the serum levels of digoxin produced by amiodarone. It also is of interest that Senholzi[12] found that amiodarone and desethylamiodarone did not displace digoxin from $Na^+/K^+$ ATPase as measured by [86] rubidium uptake by the red blood cell method.

Subsequently, the potential mechanisms of this interaction have been elucidated in normal subjects and in patients (Table 1).[5,6] Digoxin accumulation is due partly to a decrease in its nonrenal clearance. This could be the result either of a decrease in the secretion of digoxin into the gut or a decrease in biliary secretion of this drug, or both. The renal clearance of digoxin was found to be decreased in normal subjects, and there was a similar but nonsignificant trend in patients. Since creatinine clearance was unchanged, the decrease in the renal clearance of digoxin probably is due to diminished renal tubular secretion of this drug. The net effect of a decrease in renal as well as nonrenal clearance of digoxin is an increased elimination half-life and this was found to be significant in normal subjects. The magnitude of the digoxin–amiodarone interaction may be even greater in children, since renal tubular secretion of digoxin appears to be more important in children than in adults and amiodarone inhibits this mechanism of digoxin excretion.[7]

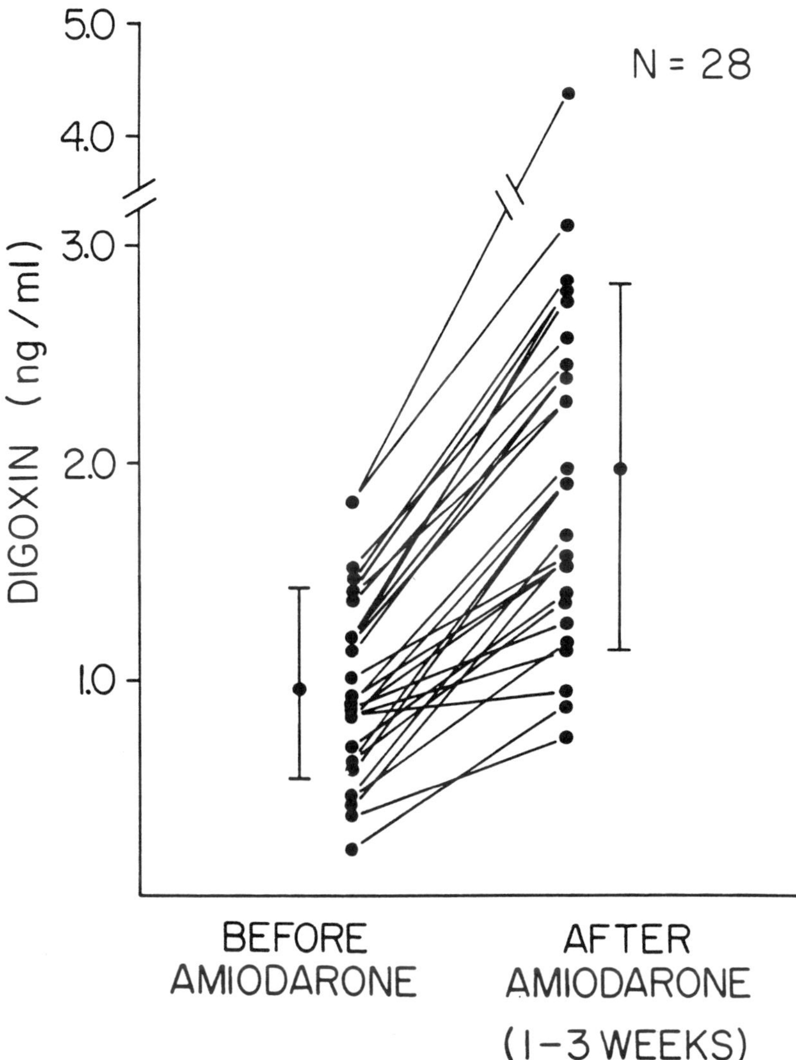


**Figure 1.**  Changes in the steady-state serum digoxin concentrations induced by the concomitant administration of amiodarone (600–1600 mg/day; mean 1251 ± 335) for 7–21 days (mean 3.3 ± 5.3). Each closed circle represents a value from one patient. The verticle bars indicate standard deviations from the mean value. Amiodarone increased digoxin levels in all patients. (From Nademanee K, Kannan R, Hendrickson J, et al: Amiodarone–digoxin interaction: Clinical significance, time course of development, potential pharmacokinetic mechanisms and therapeutic implications. *J Am Coll Cardiol* 4:111, 1984. By permission of the authors and the journal.)

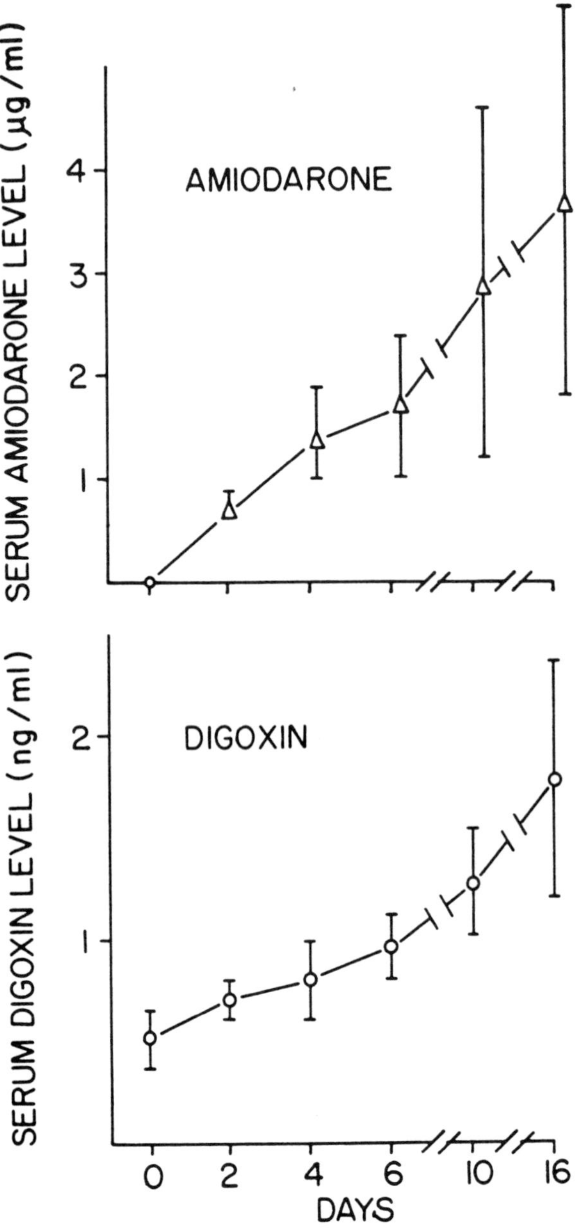



**Figure 2.** The time course of increase in serum digoxin (circles) and serum amiodarone (triangles) levels in 5 patients given fixed doses of digoxin and amiodarone for 16 days (after they had been receiving the same dose of digoxin alone for the previous 4 weeks. The data shown are mean values ± standard deviation. Despite a fixed dose of amiodarone, serum levels continue to increase over the period of observation; during this period, serum digoxin levels are augmented, the initial increment being apparent by day 2. (From Nademanee K, Kannan R, Hendrickson J, et al: Amiodarone–digoxin interaction: Clinical significance, time course of development, potential pharmacokinetic mechanisms and therapeutic implications. *J Am Coll Cardiol* 4:111, 1984. By permission of the authors and the journal.)

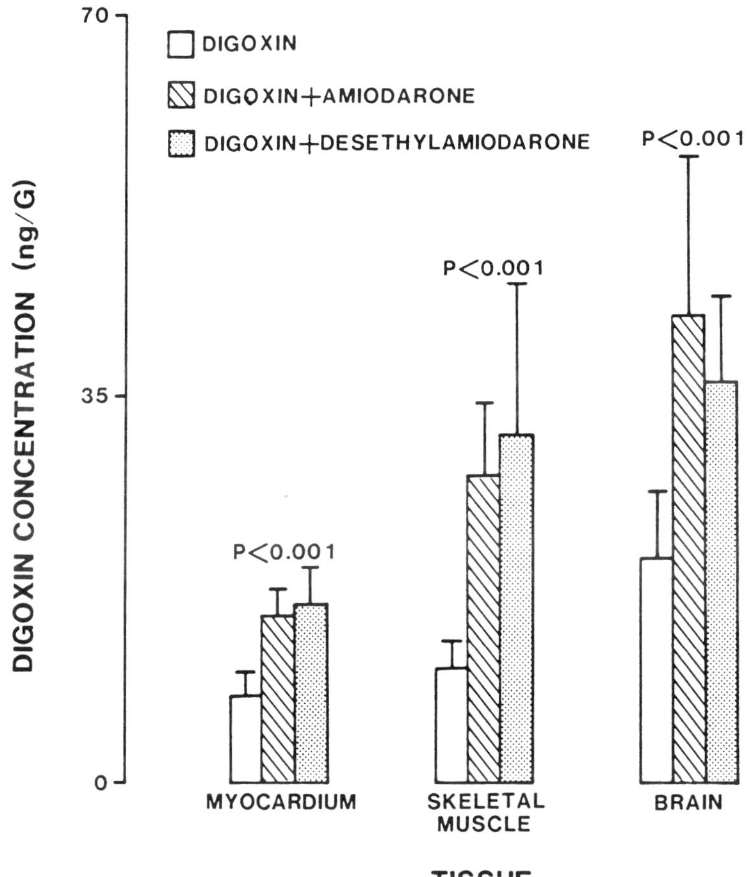


**Figure 3.** Changes observed in the digoxin concentrations in the myocardium, skeletal muscle, and brain of rats treated with digoxin alone, digoxin plus amiodarone, and digoxin plus desethylamiodarone. Combination therapies induced significant increases (p < 0.005) in tissue digoxin concentrations when compared to the levels in rats receiving digoxin alone. The apparent differences between the two groups receiving combination therapies were not statistically different. (From Vankatesh N, Singh BN, Al-Sarraf L, et al: Digoxin–desethylamiodarone interaction in the rat: Comparison with the effects of amiodarone. *J Cardiovasc Pharmacol* 8:309, 1986. By permission of the authors and the journal.)

The clinical manifestations of digitalis intoxication due to the amiodarone–digoxin interaction are due to central nervous system effects of digitalis (anorexia, nausea, vomiting, photophobia, and headaches) or due to excessive vagal stimulation or to the antiad-

Table 1
Pharmacokinetic Antiarrhythmic Drug Interactions with Amiodarone

| Concomitant Drug | Onset (days) | Interaction Magnitude | Recommended Dose Correction |
|---|---|---|---|
| Aprindine | ? | Increases serum conc. by 100% | ↓ ½ |
| Digoxin | 1 | Increases serum conc. by 100% | ↓ ½ |
| Flecainide | ? | Increases serum conc. by 100% | ↓ ⅓ |
| Phenytoin | ? | Increases serum conc. by 100% | ↓ ⅓ |
| Procainamide (PA) | 1–2 | Increases PA serum conc. by 57% and NAPA levels by 32% | ↓ ⅓ to ½ |
| Quinidine | 1–2 | Increases serum conc. by 50% | ↓ ⅓ to ½ |

NAPA = N-Acetyl Procainamide

renergic effects of digitalis (sinus bradycardia, sinoatrial block). Both the central nervous system and the cardiac effects of digoxin may summate with those of amiodarone in terms of clinical manifestations. Digitalis-induced tachyarrhythmias have not been reported with this interaction except when associated with hypokalemia.[6] The absence of digitalis-induced tachyarrhythmias may be due to the antiarrhythmic effects of amiodarone, which may suppress this manifestation of digitalis toxicity. In support of this hypothesis is the observation that amiodarone, given intravenously, has been used successfully to treat intractable ventricular tachyarrhythmias after massive digoxin overdose.[13,14]

The amiodarone digoxin interaction may be enhanced further by hypothyroidism induced by amiodarone;[15] in turn, the hypothyroid state may cause further serum elevation of digoxin by mechanisms that still are not clear. Under these circumstances, the slow heart rate induced by the accumulation of digoxin may become even slower due to the bradycardic effect of hypothyrodism and temporary pacing may be required[16] (Fig. 4).

One of the major metabolites of amiodarone is desethylamiodarone. The tissue concentration of desethylamiodarone is greater than that of amiodarone in almost all tissues except fat. This metabolite has been found to have antiarrhythmic potency (see Chapter 14). The desethylmetabolite, when given to rats also increases

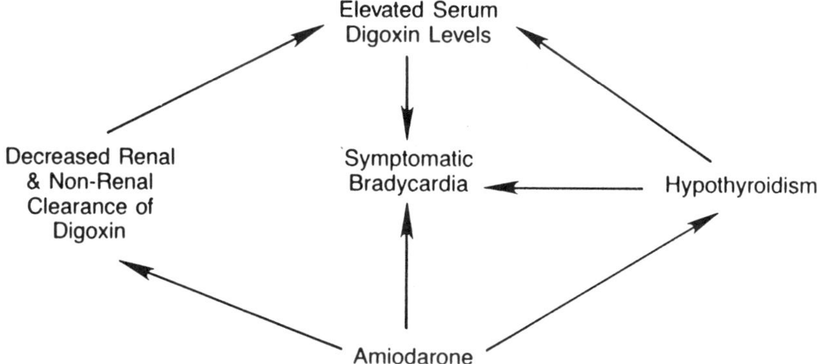


**Figure 4.** Proposed pharmacokinetic interactions leading to symptomatic bradycardia due to interaction between digoxin and amiodarone. Amiodarone may cause hypothyroidism leading to exacerbation of bradycardia by several mechanisms illustrated in this figure.

serum digoxin concentration to a similar degree (see Fig. 3), as does amiodarone.[11]

## Interactions of Amiodarone with Antiarrhythmic Compounds

Interactions between amiodarone and other anti-arrhythmic agents (Table 2) illustrates the complex interplay of pharmacokinetic and pharmacodynamic components. In considering these, it is clearly important to appreciate that the electrophysiologic effects of amiodarone encompasses all four major classes of actions (see Chapter 14) and that such actions are accentuated in the presence of preexisting disease.

When amiodarone is given concurrently with other antiarrhythmic drugs, such as aprindine,[17] flecainide,[18] phenytoin,[19,20] procainamide,[21] or quinidine,[22] the serum concentrations of these antiarrhythmic drugs are increased significantly above their steady state prior to amiodarone administration. The potential interactions between mexiletine, tocainide, or propafenone and amiodarone are poorly defined. The interaction between flecainide and amiodarone is the first one reported with the so-called Class Ic agents; such a possibility with encainide and its metabolites, indecainide, lorcainide, or recainam, has not been explored. In the case of flecainide, the magnitude of the interaction suggested a dose reduction by one-third during combination therapy and amiodarone.

Table 2

Digoxin Pharmacokinetics Before and During Amiodarone in 10
Normal Subjects and in Six Patients

|  | Digoxin Alone | Digoxin during Amiodarone | Significance (p) |
|---|---|---|---|
| Systemic Clearance ml/min | 234 (164)* | 172 (119) | <0.01 (<0.05) |
| Renal Clearance ml/min | 105 (67.4)* | 84 (50) | <0.05 (NS) |
| Nonrenal Clearance ml/min | 130 (96.7)* | 88 (66) | <0.01 (<0.05) |
| Volume of Distribution l/kg | 9.7 (7.9)* | 8.6 (7.0) | NS (NS) |
| Elimination Half-Life hours | 34 (49)* | 40 65 | <0.05 (NS) |

Data from normal subjects from Fenster P et al: *JACC* 5:108, 1985.

Data from patients from Nademanee K et al: *JACC* 4:111, 1984.[5*]

The mechanisms responsible for these pharmacokinetic interactions involving amiodarone and various antiarrhythmic compounds have not been well established. One of the dangers resulting from these interactions is the induction of torsades de pointes. This arrhythmia may occur when a Class Ia drug, such as quinidine which prolongs the QT intervals, is given together with amiodarone, which by itself will prolong the QT interval.[22] Precipitation of this arrhythmia may be further enhanced by the effect of amiodarone inducing bradycardia (see Chapter 14).

All the antiarrhythmic drugs that interact with amiodarone have linear or first-order pharmacokinetics except for phenytoin. With first order kinetics, a doubling of the administered dose would be expected to cause a twofold rise in the serum concentration of the drug. For example, with the digoxin–amiodarone interaction, a doubling of the serum concentration of digoxin due to coadministration of amiodarone is anticipated. To compensate for this expected change in serum digoxin concentration the digoxin dose should be decreased by one-half. However, the amiodarone-induced interference with phenytoin metabolism may result in an exponential rise in phenytoin serum concentration due to saturation of the hepatic metabolism of phenytoin. Steady-state serum concentrations of phenytoin four or more times higher have been observed after amiodarone has been administered to patients who have phenytoin levels in the therapeutic range prior to administration of amiodarone.[19,20] Conversely, the dose of phenytoin may need to be decreased only by one-third in patients who have phenytoin levels two or three times that which is desired.

The degree of the interaction between amiodarone and antiarrhythmic drugs is quite variable from one individual to another. In general, half the usual dose of an antiarrhythmic drug should be prescribed when combination antiarrhythmic drug therapy with amiodarone is undertaken. The drug serum concentration should be measured at appropriate intervals, and the dose adjusted. These recommendations also should apply when antiarrhythmic drugs other than those mentioned earlier are given with amiodarone. Since most antiarrhythmic drugs are excreted primarily by hepatic metabolism and since amiodarone decreases hepatic metabolic enzyme activity, it should be anticipated that most antiarrhythmic drugs may accumulate to a greater extent when given concurrently with amiodarone.

It must be emphasized that at present the precise nature of the interactions between various antiarrhythmic agents and amiodarone is understood poorly. However, given the potentially hazardous nature of such interactions, the practical implications should be appreciated because of the increasing trend to combine antiarrhythmic compounds for the control of recalcitrant arrhythmias. For example, although the use of an intravenous agent (e.g., Class I agent) to supplement the effects of amiodarone in preventing an inducible ventricular arrhythmia may produce a desirable therapeutic effect acutely, long-term therapy may lead to a deleterious outcome if the issue of drug cumulation is ignored. Thus, the use of combination therapy in this setting presupposes continued clinical and pharmacokinetic surveillance.

## Amiodarone–Warfarin Interaction

In 1979, Simpson[23] noted that amiodarone may potentiate coumadin effects and recommended close monitoring of prothrombin times during the introduction of amiodarone. Independently, Podrid and Lown[24] found considerable difficulty in controlling prothrombin times in patients receiving amiodarone and coumadin. Bleeding due to this interaction also was reported.[25,26] Hamer et al.[27] provided unequivocal evidence that amiodarone potentiates the anticoagulant effect of warfarin. They postulated that there might be a direct effect of amiodarone on metabolism of warfarin, vitamin K, or clotting factor. Further studies of the mechanism of this interaction was made by Richard et al.,[28] who found that the decrease in prothrombin activity was associated with lower serum concentrations of vitamin K coagulation factors, especially factors 7, 9, and 10. It is reasonable to assume that amiodarone decreases the metabolism of warfarin sodium, and this has been observed.[29] It is known that prothrombin time may double after amiodarone therapy in patients who have a steady-state effect on warfarin. The onset of the interaction may be as early as 3−4 days but may be delayed for 3 weeks. It also is known that following the discontinuation of amiodarone, the potentiating effect of the drug on prothrombin time may persist for weeks or even months. It is noteworthy that plasma protein binding of warfarin, determined by equilibrium dialysis is not altered by amiodarone,[4] but it is known that the effect of amiodarone on prothrombin activity influenced by warfarin is dose dependent.

## Pharmacodynamic Drug Interactions

As indicated earlier, pharmacodynamic drug interactions are those in which the action or effect of one drug is altered by another drug given concurrently and these changes are not due to alterations of the pharmacokinetics of either drug. In the case of amiodarone, pharmacokinetic and pharmacodynamic interactions may coexist. Significant examples of the effects that may involve amiodarone are listed in Table 3.

Pharmacodynamic interactions often can be predicted by knowing that the two concurrently given drugs may have similar effects, and that these effects can be additive. For example, pharmacodynamic interactions with *amiodarone* may be predicted by knowing that amiodarone is a noncompetitive beta-and alpha-adrenergic antagonist. Its beta-antagonistic effect may cause sinus bradycardia, sinus arrest, or AV block.[30,31] Drugs with similar effects, such as beta-adrenergic blocking drugs or calcium channel blocking drugs (verapamil, diltiazem), given concurrently may enhance these effects of amiodarone and cause profound symptomatic bradycardia or second or third degree AV block.[32] Infranodal block may ensue in the case of amiodarone and potent Class I agents in patients with preexisting conduction system disease.

Pharmacodynamic interactions with anesthetic agents in patients receiving chronic amiodarone therapy may be particularly

**Table 3**
Pharmacodynamic Interactions

| Drug Interaction | Consequences |
| --- | --- |
| Amiodarone – Class I anti-arrhythmic agents | Accentuation of QT prolongation (Ia agents), torsade de pointes, infranodal AV block |
| Amiodarone – beta blockers | Bradyarrhythmias, sinus arrest, AV block, sinoatrial block |
| Amiodarone – calcium antagonists (verapail and diltiazem) | Bradyarrhythmias, sinus arrest, AV block, sinoatrial block |
| Amiodarone – digoxin | Sinus arrrest, AV block (intranodal), sinoatrial block |

hazardous. An unusually high intraaortic balloon pump augmentation and a state of alpha-adrenergic block causing low systemic vascular resistance have been observed.[33] These complications may have contributed to the deaths of 3 of 12 patients who underwent cardiopulmonary bypass surgery, all of whom were receiving chronic amiodarone therapy.

*Bretylium* has antiarrhythmic properties independent of its adrenergic effects. Bretylium is taken up selectively by peripheral adrenergic nerve terminals, where it exerts two effects: an initial release of norepinephrine, producing a sympathomimetic effect and a later, inhibition of norepinephrine release producing adrenergic neuronal blockade. Under experimental conditions, bretylium can aggravate ventricular arrhythmias induced either by administration of halothane anesthesia, followed by epinephrine, or by administering ouabain until near toxicity.[34] Under these circumstances the enhancement of ventricular arrhythmias is due to release of endogenous catecholamines by bretylium following its neuronal uptake.

Orthostatic hypotension associated with prolonged bretylium administration can occur due to uptake of bretylium by the norepinephrine pump. It has been observed that tricyclic antidepressants can minimize orthostatic hypotension associated with bretylium. Tricyclic antidepressants compete with bretylium transport to peripheral adrenergic neurons; the function of the norepinephrine pump is restored and hypotension is ameliorated.[35] This is an example of a beneficial drug interaction. The antiarrhythmic effect of bretylium is not altered by the concomitant use of tricyclic antidepressants.

Since sotalol is a beta-adrenergic blocking drug, dynamic interactions should be anticipated when other drugs that cause bradycardia and/or hypotension are given concurrently. These include the beta-adrenergic blocking drugs, calcium-channel blocking drugs, or antihypertensive agents. As noted with amiodarone, administration of drugs with sotalol that cause QT prolongation may result in torsades de pointes. These drugs include Class Ia agents; in addition, hypokalemia can result in torsades when sotalol is administered.[36] The potential mechanisms underlying such interactions involving prolonged repolarization are discussed in Chapter 23.

## Conclusions

Class III antiarrhythmic compounds constitute a chemically heterogeneous group of compounds, and clinically important pharmacokinetic and pharmacodynamic interactions have been reported with these drugs. Amiodarone has an unusually high incidence of pharmacokinetic interactions, such drug interactions presumably reflecting the complex nature of its molecule and its interaction with hepatic cell metabolism. Therefore, it is advisable to decrease the dose of concurrently administered drugs and measure serum concentrations of these other drugs, particularly antiarrhythmic agents, the combination therapy with which are likely to be particularly hazardous in view of the pharmacokinetic and pharmacodynamic interactions. The interaction of amiodarone and coumadin may result in bleeding, which may be life threatening. Pharmacodynamic drug interactions usually may be predicted by an awareness of the pharmacologic effects of the drugs given concurrently. These include the hemodynamic as well as electrophysiologic properties of the two drugs that may be given concurrently. A knowledge of pharmacokinetic and pharmacodynamic drug interactions with Class III agents clearly is crucial to the safe and effective use of these drugs in the control of cardiac arrhythmias.

## References


1. Bigger JT Jr, Giardina EGV: Drug interactions in antiarrhythmic therapy. *Ann NY Acad Sci.* 427:140, 1984.
2. Marcus FI: Drug interactions with amiodarone. *Am Heart J* 106:924, 1983.

3. Marcus FI: Clinical pharmacology of amiodarone. In HM Greenberg et al. (eds): *Clinical Aspects of Life Threatening Arrhythmias.* New York, *Annals. of the New York Academy of Science*, pp 112, 1984.

4. Moysey JO, Jaggarao NSV, Grundy EN, et al: Amiodarone increases plasma digoxin concentrations. *Br Med J* 282:272, 1981.

5. Fenster PE, White NW, Jr., Hanson CD: Pharmacokinetic evaluation of the digoxin-amiodarone interaction. *J Am Coll Cardiol* 5:108, 1985.

6. Nademanee K, Kannan R, Hendrickson J, et al: Amiodarone–digoxin interaction: Clinical significance, time course of development, potential pharmacokinetic mechanisms and therapeutic implications. *J Am Coll Cardiol* 4:111, 1984.

7. Koren G, Hesslein PS, MacLeod SM: Digoxin toxicity associated with amiodarone therapy in children. *J Pediatr* 104:467, 1984.

8. Grech-Berlanger O: Depressive effect of amiodarone on hepatic drug metabolism. *Res Commun Chem Path Pharmacol* 44:15, 1984.

9. Koren G: Digoxin-amiodarone interaction: In vivo and in vitro studies in rats. *Can J Physiol Pharmacol* 61:1483, 1984.

10. Venkatesh N, Al-Sarraf L, Kannan K, et al: Tissue-serum correlates of digoxin-amiodarone pharmacokinetic interaction in rats: Evidence for selective tissue accumulation and reduced tissue-binding. *J Pharm Sci* 74:1067, 1985.

11. Venkatesh, N, Singh BN, Al-Sarraf L, et al: Digoxin–desethylamiodarone interaction in the rat: Comparison with the effects of amiodarone. *J Cardiovasc Pharmacol* 8:309, 1986.

12. Senholzi CS: The effects of amiodarone and desethylamiodarone on digoxin suppression of $^{86}$Rb red blood cell uptake in vitro. *Drug Int Chem Pharm* 17:445, 1983.

13. Maheswaran R, Bramble MG, Hardisty CA: Massive digoxin overdose: Successful treatment with intravenous amiodarone. *Br Med J* 287:392, 1983.

14. Nicholls DP, Murtagh JG, Holt DW: Use of amiodarone and digoxin specific Fab antibodies in digoxin overdosage. *Br Heart J* 53:462, 1985.

15. Ben-Chetrit E, Ackerman Z, Eliakim M: Case report: Amiodarone-associated hypothyroidism—A possible cause of digoxin intoxication. *Am J Med Sci* 289:114, 1985.

16. Marcus FI: Commentary: Digoxin–amiodarone–hypothyroidism interaction. *Am J Med Sci* 289:117, 1985.

17. Southworth W, Friday KJ, Ruffy R: Possible amiodarone–aprindine interaction. *Am Heart J* 104:323, 1982.

18. Shea P, Lal R, Kim SS, et al: Flecainide and amiodarone interaction. *J Am Coll Cardiol* 7:1127, 1986.

19. Gore JM, Haffajee CI, Alpert JS: Interaction of amiodarone and diphenylhydantoin. *Am J Cardiol* 54:1145, 1984.

20. McGovern B, Geer VR, LaRaia PJ, et al: Possible interaction between amiodarone and phenytoin. *Ann Intern Med* 101:650, 1984.

21. Saal AK, Werner JA. Greene HL, et al: Effect of amiodarone on serum quinidine and procainamide levels. *Am J Cardiol* 53:1264, 1984.

22. Tartini R, Kappenberger L, Steinbrunn W, et al: Dangerous interaction between amiodarone and quinidine. *Lancet* 2:1327, 1982.

23. Simpson W. In WT Simpson, ADS Cladwell (eds): *Amiodarone in Car-*

*diac Arrhythmias*. Royal Society of Medicine International Congress Series, No. 16. London, RSM/Academic Press/Grune and Stratton, p 50, 1979.

24. Podrid PJ, Lown B: Amiodarone therapy in symptomatic, sustained refractory atrial and ventricular tachyarrhythmias. *Am Heart J* 101:374, 1981.

25. Rees A, Dalal JJ, Reid PG, et al: Dangers of amiodarone and anticoagulant treatment. *Br Med J* 282:1756, 1981.

26. Martinowitz U, Rabinovici J. Goldfarb D, et al: Interaction between warfarin sodium and amiodarone. *N Eng J Med* 304:671, 1981.

27. Hamer A, Peter T. Mandel WJ, et al: The potentiation of warfarin anticoagulation by amiodarone. *Circulation* 65:1025, 1982.

28. Richard C, Riou B, Fournier C, et al: Suppression of vitamin K–dependent coagulation by amiodarone. (abstract) *Circulation* 68(III):278, 1983.

29. Serlin MJ, Sibeon RG: Dangers of amiodarone and anticoagulant treatment. *Br Med J* 283:58, 1981.

30. Navalgund AA, Alifimoff JK, Jakymec AJ, et al: Amiodarone-induced sinus arrest successfully treated with ephedrine and isoproterenol. *Anesth Analg* 65:414, 1985.

31. McGovern B, Garan H, Ruskin JN: Sinus arrest during treatment with amiodarone. *Br Med J* 284:160, 1982.

32. Derrida JP, Ollagnier J, Benaim R, et al: Amiodarone et propranolol: Une association dangereuse? *Nouv Press Med* 8:1429, 1979.

33. Liberman BA, Teasdale SJ: Anaesthesia and amiodarone. *Can Anaesth Soc J* 32:629, 1985.

34. Allen JD, Zaidi SA, Shanks RG, et al: The effects of bretylium on experimental cardiac dysrhythmias. *Am J Cardiol* 29:641, 1972.

35. Woosley RL, Reele SB, Roden DM, et al: Pharmacologic reversal of hypotensive effect complicating antiarrhythmic therapy with bretylium. *Clin Pharmacol Ther* 32:313, 1982.

36. Bennett JM, Gourassas J, Konstantinides S: Torsades de pointes induced by sotalol and hypokalemia. *S Afr Med J* 68:591, 1985.

# Chapter 23

# Arrhythmogenic Potential of Class III Antiarrhythmic Agents: Comparison with Class I Agents

## Dan M. Roden

Syncope following administration of quinidine has been described since the 1920s, but only in 1964 was it recognized that this potentially lethal adverse drug reaction actually was due to the induction of a morphologically distinctive ventricular tachyarrhythmia.[1] The term *torsades de pointes* was coined in 1966 to describe a similar tachyarrhythmia occurring in an elderly patient with bradyarrhythmias.[2] In addition to the slowly changing electrical axis seen in torsades de pointes, these early cases also were characterized by a striking prolongation of the QT interval of the surface electrocardiogram. Since this repolarization abnormality appears to be linked to the genesis of the arrhythmia, we and other investigators have confined our use of the term *torsades de pointes* to those cases of the morphologically distinctive ventricular tachyarrhythmias that occur in the presence of marked QT prolongation.[3,4] Others have used the term to describe a similar tachyarrhythmia occurring in the absence of QT prolongation; such arrhythmias in fact can be successfully treated by quinidinelike drugs and probably have different etiologies.

Aside from torsades de pointes, it has become apparent that, under appropriate circumstances, antiarrhythmic drugs may provoke other arrhythmias. These include profound bradyarrhyth-

From: *Control of Cardiac Arrhythmias by Lengthening Repolarization*, edited by Bramah N. Singh, MD, Futura Publishing Company Inc., Mount Kisco, NY, © 1988.

mias, supraventricular arrhythmias, incessant circus movement tachycardias, a marked increase in the frequency of isolated ventricular ectopic depolarizations and episodes of nonsustained ventricular tachycardia, the development or marked increase in episodes of sustained ventricular tachycardia, and increased difficulty in converting such arrhythmias. It is likely that these phenomena have multiple underlying etiologies. This chapter will concentrate on antiarrhythmic drug-induced torsades de pointes, describing the typical clinical features, the possible basic electrophysiological mechanisms involved, and the problems associated with individual antiarrhythmic drugs. Aspects of the propensity of the so-called Class III agents to induce torsades de pointes have been dealt with elsewhere in this book (see Chapters 4, 7, 11, and 22).

## Clinical Features of Antiarrhythmic Drug-Induced Torsades de Pointes

Several large clinical series recently have described the typical clinical features of torsades de pointes.[3,5-10] Although antiarrhythmic agents and especially quinidine constitute the single most commonly implicated cause, multiple other etiologies have been reported, including the syndromes of congenital QT prolongation (see Chapter 4) with or without deafness,[11-13] liquid protein diets,[14-16] other drugs (e.g., organophosphorus insecticides,[17] thioridazine[18]), central nervous system injury,[19] and hypokalemia,[20,21] and hypomagnesemia.[22] Interestingly, although hypothyroidism and hypocalcemia both consistently prolong QT interval, only very rare case reports have described torsades de pointes in these settings.[23] Thus, the genesis of torsades de pointes cannot be related solely to the lengthening of the action potential duration of cardiac muscle. Several clinical features however, should be emphasized: (1) Electrolyte abnormalities (hypokalemia, hypomagnesemia) are common. In our series,[3] 14 of 21 cases of quinidine-associated long QT syndrome had serum potassium concentrations under 4.0 mEq/L. This occurred most often in association with potassium-wasting diuretic drugs, although occasionally gastrointestinal disturbances can be implicated. Most patients in our series had normal serum magnesium concentrations, although others have found a high incidence of relative hypomagnesemia. (2) Although it has been stated that patients treated for ventricular arrhythmias do not develop torsades de pointes, the underlying rhythm abnormalities in our series and those of others were divided equally between patients with ventricular arrhythmias and patients with atrial fibrillation or flutter. In patients with atrial fibrillation, torsades de pointes invariably occurred after quinidine had converted the arrhythmia to sinus and not during atrial fibrillation itself. (3) A number of investigators have described typical electrocardiographic features that immediately precede the development of an episode of antiarrhythmic drug-induced torsades de pointes.[3,9,10,24] An ectopic beat or short run of tachycardia is followed by a compensatory pause that is terminated by a normal sinus beat (Fig. 1). The QT interval of this normal sinus beat is markedly prolonged and torsades de pointes arises after the peak of the TU wave. The arrhythmia itself has a cycle length of 160–230 msec. These features are fairly typical of torsades de pointes related to antiarrhythmic drugs and may be useful in establishing the diagnosis when it is unclear. In other settings, however, particularly in patients with the congenital long QT syndromes, torsades de pointes, while it develops in the presence of long QT intervals, may not be preceded by these cycle length changes. In patients with the congenital syndromes, adrenergic stimulation (e.g., in the form of treadmill exercise, sudden fright) accompanied by an increased heart rate typically precedes the development of the episode.[25] (4) The treatment of antiarrhythmic drug-induced torsades de pointes relies first on the recognition of the arrhythmia and withdrawal of the offending agent then correction of accompanying electrolyte abnormalities (potassium, magnesium). Intravenous magnesium has been advocated even in the absence of frank hypomagnesemia.[26] "Usual" antiarrhythmic therapy, such as lidocaine or bretylium, is reported effective in about 50 percent of cases, some of which might have resolved without these drugs. The rationale for the use of bretylium has not been established, although the beneficial response may result from the initial release of catecholamines. It may be argued that the subse-

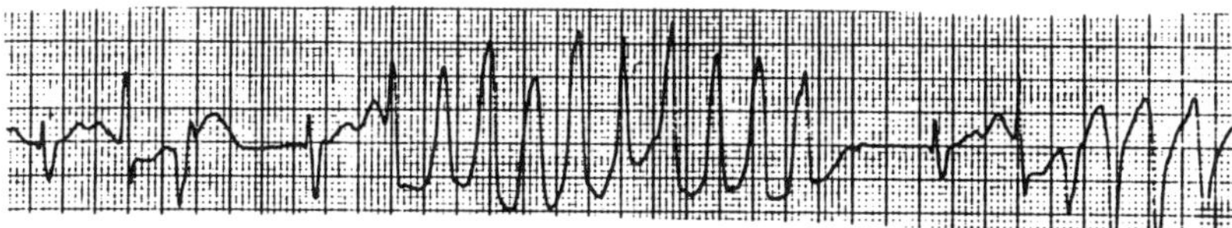

**Figure 1.** An example of torsades de pointes. Note the compensatory pause followed by a sinus beat, the QTc interval of which is markedly lengthened.

quent prolongation of the action potential duration may even be deleterious.

Measures to increase heart rate (isoproterenol, ventricular pacing) usually are effective. Our own approach is to use isoproterenol as soon as the diagnosis is made and to proceed to pacing if isoproterenol is inappropriate because of the underlying heart disease or if therapy for longer than 3–4 hours is anticipated. The chronic management of the patient with marked QT prolongation in the absence of antiarrhythmic drugs or transient electrolyte abnormalities[27-29] relies on drugs that shorten repolarization (phenytoin, high-dose beta blockers) or interventions that decrease autonomic input to the heart and reduce dispersion of repolarization (left stellate ganglion ablation).[30,31] The question of whether patients who have had an episode of torsades de pointes can later receive therapy with other drugs that prolong QT interval will be discussed further.

## Basic Electrophysiologic Mechanisms

The precise electrophysiologic mechanisms forming the basis for torsades de pointes has been controversial.[32] Purely on theoretical grounds, it has been suggested that torsades may arise as a result of focal reentrant excitation, with a changing pathway of conduction. Such a possibility is consistent with the self-termination of the arrhythmia when the impulse finally is blocked by a zone of refractoriness, deterioration into ventricular fibrillation due to the fragmentation into numerous and changing circuits, and the occasional transformation of torsades into a pattern of monomorphic ventricular tachycardia, allegedly when the circuit of reentry becomes stable.[32] However, the most recent experimental observations support the possibility of triggered automaticity due to early afterdepolarizations (EADs) as the likely mechanism of torsades in the setting of delayed cardiac repolarization.

Since abrupt increases in cycle length and hypokalemia are common clinical features of antiarrhythmic drug-induced torsades de pointes, studies of the electrophysiologic effects of antiarrhythmic drugs under these conditions are desirable. When we examined the effects of quinidine on action potentials from canine Purkinje fibers, we found marked action potential prolongation by even low concentrations of quinidine when extracellular potassium was lowered to 2.7 mM and stimulation cycle length increased above 2000 msec.[33] Under these conditions, early afterdepolarizations (EADs) interrupting the terminal phase of repolarization (phase 3) were elicited consistently (Fig. 2). The striking parallels between these EADs and the clinical syndrome of torsades de pointes (potassium dependency, rate dependency, timing of arrhythmia development) strongly suggest that EADs may play a role in some cases of antiarrhythmic drug-induced torsades de pointes. Alternatively, dispersion of repolarization within the ventricle, which can be increased by factors such as hypokalemia, slow stimulation rates, and autonomic imbalance, may be increased further by antiarrhythmic drug administration to the point that reentrant arrhythmias are elicited. Dessertenne,[2] who first coined the term *torsades de pointes*, felt that the distinctive morphology of the arrhythmia was due to two or more automatic foci that drove the heart at slightly different rates. While the torsades de pointes morphology can be reproduced experimentally using stimulation at different rates,[34] this by no means proves Dessertenne's contention. It also is possible that both abnormal automaticity in the form of EADs and dispersion of repolarization are required to generate and maintain torsades de pointes.

Other interventions that have been associated with either clinical or experimental torsades de pointes also have been reported to

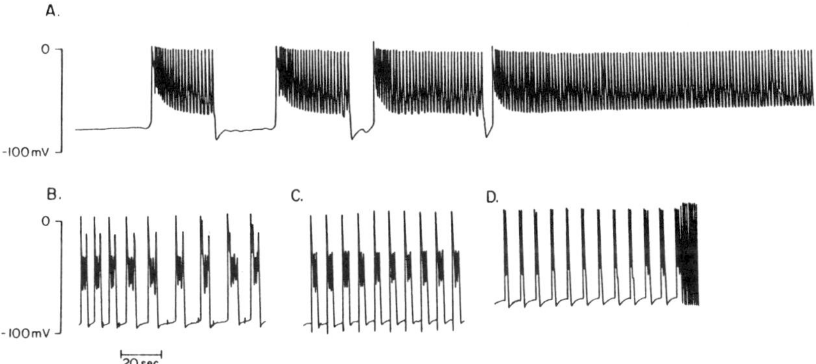

**Figure 2.**   Early afterdepolarizations in four different preparations in low [K$^+$]o and 10 μM quinidine at slow rates of depolarization (either spontaneous, panels A and B, or stimulated at a cycle length of 8000 msec, panels C and D). (From Roden DM, Hoffman BF: Action potential prolongation and induction of abnormal automaticity by low quinidine concentrations in canine Purkinje fibers: Relationship to potassium and cycle length. *Card Res* 56:857, 1985. By permission of the authors and of the American Heart Association.)

cause EADs in canine Purkinje fibers. These include the antiarrhythmic agents N-acetylprocainamide (NAPA)[35] and sotalol,[36] which have predominant Class III activity, and the potassium blocker cesium.[37] Recent in vivo studies with cesium have documented striking abnormalities in monophasic action potential alteration preceding and accompanying episodes of torsades de pointes-like arrhythmia, further supporting a role for afterdepolarizations in the genesis of the arrhythmia.[38] In this study, monophasic action potentials were recorded in the endocardium and epicardium in the left ventricle simultaneously with the surface electrocardiogram. Cesium chloride was given intravenously to prolong the time course of repolarization. Afterdepolarizations were identified in each of the 8 dogs and were similar to the early afterdepolarizations in vitro. They occurred during phase 3 of the monophasic action potential and could be attenuated by overdrive pacing. There was a close temporal relationship between such afterdepolarizations and ventricular arrhythmias (Fig. 3). The data provide reasonably convincing evidence for the possibility that torsades de pointes in the setting of prolonged QT interval may arise on the basis of early afterdepolarization. Other workers have demonstrated that EADs generated under a variety of experimental conditions can be propagated into apparently normal adjacent Purkinje fibers or myocardial tissue.[39,40] These findings have not only suggested a role for EADs in the genesis of arrhythmias related to prolonged repolarization but also have raised the possibility that similar abnormalities of repolarization may play a role in arrhythmias in other settings, such as acute ischemia.

The ionic currents reponsible for the striking changes in action potential configuration and the genesis of EADs are not known with certainty. Although definitive conclusions with respect to these phenomena will require voltage-clamp studies, limited inferences based on already available data obtained in Purkinje fibers can be made. First, action potential prolongation must be due to either an increase in inward current or a decrease in outward current. Agents that delay or block sodium current inactivation prolong action potential and have been associated with afterdepolarizations (veratradine, aconitine, batrachotoxin).[41–43] On the other hand, the antiarrhythmic drugs associated with QT prolongation and induction of torsades de pointes either do not alter cardiac sodium channels or depress the sodium current; these include quinidine, NAPA,[35,44–46] sotalol,[36,47–49] amiodarone,[50,51] procainamide,[52] and disopyramide,[6] as well as cesium, which is not used clinically. Moreover, a number of these interventions have been

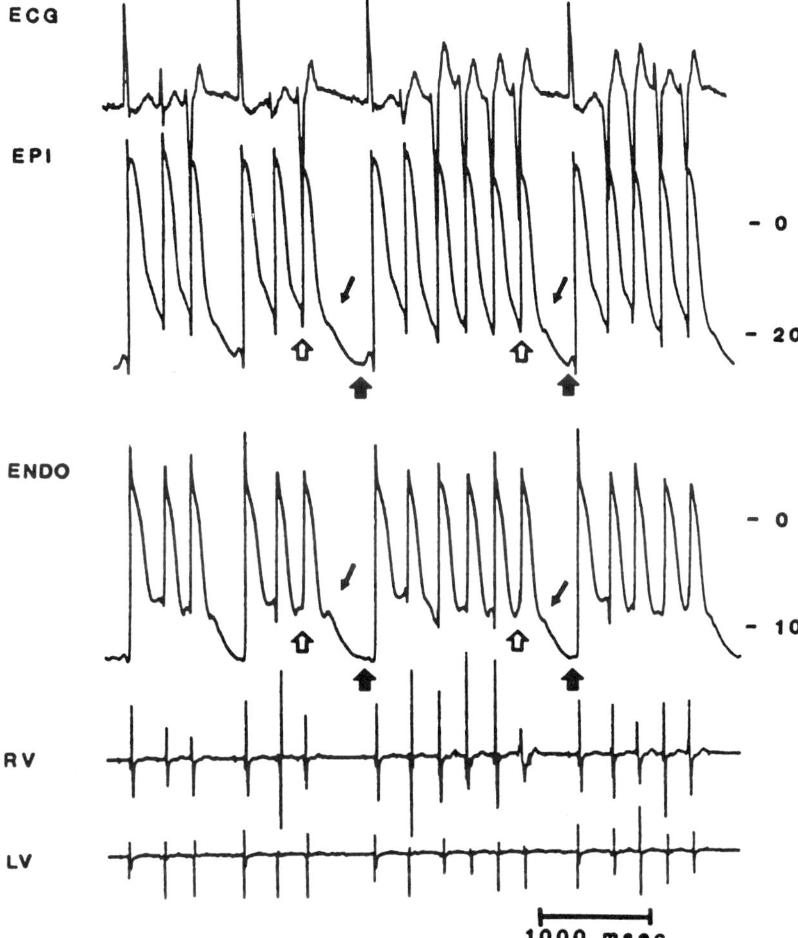


**Figure 3.**    An example of an analog recording in which frequent salvos of nonsustained ventricular tachycardia developed after administration of cesium. An electrocardiogram (ECG), an epicardial MAP (EPI), an endocardial MAP (ENDO), and a left (LV) and a right (RV) ventricular bipolar electrogram are shown. Note that afterdepolarizations are present in both the endocardial and epicardical MAPs (small arrows), that their amplitude is related to the take off potential of the ectopic beats (hollow arrow), that they are of the same polarity and relative magnitude, and that their coupling interval is related to the compling interval of the ectopic beats present in the tracing. Note also that the baseline resting potential of the supraventricular beats is relatively constant (large arrow), implying a stable recording. (From Levine HJ, Spear JF, Guarnieri T, et al: Cesium, chloride-induced long QT syndrome: Demonstration of afterdepolarization and triggered activity in vivo. *Circulation* 72:1092, 1985. By permission of the authors and of the American Heart Association.)

demonstrated to block outward potassium currents (quinidine,[52] sotalol,[53] cesium[54]). Therefore, it is likely that action potential prolongation by currently available antiarrhythmic agents reflects potassium current blockade rather than augmentation of inward currents. Whereas it could be argued that quinidine, because it is a sodium channel blocker, should shorten action potential duration, this effect is smaller at long cycle lengths[33] (due to the well known frequency dependence of sodium channel blockade by drugs such as quinidine), so that the action potential prolonging effect due to potassium current blockade predominates.

The specific ionic current responsible for the genesis of EADs also is not known with certainty. It has been demonstrated that depolarization-induced automaticity developing upon current injection can be blocked by either sodium-channel or calcium-channel blocking drugs, depending upon the voltage range over which the depolarization-induced automaticity is elicited.[56] It has been shown that the calcium-channel blocker, $D_{600}$, blocks cesium-induced EADs but does not shorten action potential duration.[57] Similarly, we have demonstrated that the calcium channel blocking drugs, bepridil and lidoflazine, which prolong QT interval and have been associated with torsades de pointes, also cause marked abnormalities of repolarization in Purkinje fibers but rarely induce EADs unless epinephrine is added. We attribute this finding to their calcium-channel blocking properties, which may be antagonized by catecholamines.[58] These findings also suggest that catecholamines, which are used commonly in the treatment of drug-induced torsades de pointes, actually may generate arrhythmias when repolarization is markedly abnormal. This would explain the apparent paradox that patients with the congenital long QT syndromes frequently develop torsades de pointes with adrenergic stimulation.

Sodium channel blockade by tetrodotoxin shortens action potential duration and abolishes EADs.[35-37] Thus, it is not certain whether this effect of tetrodotoxin reflects blockade of the inward current responsible for EADs or merely shortening of the action potential that then is associated with abolition of EADs. Lidocaine[33] and mexiletine[59] also block quinidine-induced EADs while shortening action potential duration. Another current that could contribute to EADs is the transient inward current, implicated in digitalis-induced delayed afterdepolarizations (DADs). Unlike EADs, DADs occur during phase 4 and are augmented by rapid drive. Despite these differences, it is still conceivable that trains of EADs actually represent a single EAD followed by multiple delayed afterdepolarizations, which do arise during phase 4 of the EAD.[60]

In summary, currently available evidence implicates early afterdepolarizations in the genesis of torsades de pointes, and a facilitatory role for dispersion of repolarization appears possible. Action potential prolongation by interventions used clinically probably is related to blockade of outward potassium currents, while the current responsible for the genesis of EADs may be the fast inward sodium current, the slow inward (calcium) current, or the transient inward current.

## Torsades de Pointes During Therapy with Agents with Predominantly "Class I" Actions

These drugs have as their major electrophysiologic action blockade of the fast inward sodium current. Subclassification based on either the kinetics of drug interaction with cardiac sodium channels (rapid, intermediate, or slow) or on ancillary effects on repolarization (shortened, lengthened, no change) have been proposed (see Chapter 3). Interestingly, the two approaches yield similar subgroupings. Drugs with lidocainelike electrophysiology (Class Ib: lidocaine, mexiletine, tocainide) can be shown to associate with and dissociate from cardiac sodium channels fairly quickly and, under most conditions, shorten repolarization. None of these drugs has been reported to cause long QT-associated torsades de pointes, although sporadic case reports of polymorphic ventricular tachycardia (without QT prolongation) have been reported. As outlined earlier, drugs of this type are occasionally useful in the management of long QT-associated arrhythmias. Class Ic antiarrhythmics, including flecainide and encainide, are very potent sodium channel blockers, with slow kinetics of interaction with cardiac sodium channels and generally very little effect on cardiac repolarization. While arrhythmia aggravation can be a problem during therapy with these agents, particularly in patients with severe left ventricular dysfunction and a history of sustained ventricular tachycardia, typical long QT-associated torsades de pointes is unusual. However, sporadic cases have been described. In the case of encainide, it is possible that prolongation of repolarization is due to the effects of a metabolite, 3-methoxy -desmethyl encainide, which we have recently demonstrated to prolong QT interval in humans.[61]

Class Ia sodium-channel blocking drugs, including quinidine, disopyramide, and procainamide, have intermediate kinetics of interaction with cardiac sodium channels and also prolong repolarization under most in vitro, experimental, and clinical conditions. The only drug for which even modestly reliable figures on the incidence of torsades de pointes are available is quinidine, presumably reflecting the fact that quinidine, at least until very recently, was the most commonly prescribed antiarrhythmic agent in the world. Reports on quinidine syncope or death following initiation of quinidine therapy estimate the incidence at $0.5-8.5$ percent.[3,62-64] In our own series, the estimated incidence was $2-3$ percent per year. Although most cases in our and others' series occurred within 48-hours of institution of quinidine therapy, approximately one-quarter developed during chronic quinidine therapy, usually when hypokalemia and/or bradyarrhythmias supervened. High plasma concentrations of quinidine are not necessary to initiate torsades de pointes. In fact, in our series, over one-half of the concentrations were below the usual lower limit of the so-called "therapeutic" range of concentrations. While it is possible that unmeasured metabolites might accumulate excessively and account for torsades de pointes in some of these patients, we do not think this is likely for two reasons. First, we have evaluated the electrophysiologic effects of the four major known quinidine metabolites as well as those of the commonly found commercial impurity dihydroquinidine and have found that, while each of the test substances produces electrophysiologic changes quantitatively similar to those of quinidine, including the occasional development of EADs, none was more active than quinidine.[65] Second, when we compared plasma concentrations of quinidine, its metabolites, and dihydroquinidine in patients who developed torsades de pointes to those in patients who tolerated quinidine therapy without developing torsades de pointes, no differences were found in distributions between the two groups for any of the test substances.[66] Therefore, it is likely that in most cases, low concentrations of quinidine in a patient "sensitized" by abnormalities in such factors as electrolyte concentrations or autonomic tone are responsible. The incidence of torsades de pointes during disopyramide or procainamide therapy is not known, although, in one series, disopyramide was a more commonly implicated drug than was quinidine.[6] Differences in local prescribing habits (of diuretic drugs as well as antiarrhythmics) obviously will have a major impact on observed differences between drugs, as well as the incidence with each drug.

Bepridil and lidoflazine are experimental antiarrhythmic

agents with a multiplicity of electrophysiologic actions: they act as slow inward current blockers (as outlined earlier); they depress the fast inward sodium current; and they prolong repolarization. Each agent has been associated with torsades de pointes. Again, while the incidence is unknown for each drug, individual small series suggest that this is not a trivial problem.[67-69] One group of investigators reported on a series of 9 cases of bepridil-associated torsades de pointes,[68] but gave no denominator to estimate the true incidence. The arrhythmia developed weeks to months after the initiation of bepridil with 2 of 9 patients being hypokalemic. Plasma concentrations, available in 3 patients, were all elevated. Among 15 patients being treated with lidoflazine for a variety of supraventricular and ventricular arrhythmias, 4 died suddenly.[69] Another patient reported by the same group developed torsades de pointes during lidoflazine therapy (despite high potassium concentrations) and redeveloped torsades de pointes after being switched to quinidine. Thus, although the exact incidence is not known from large series, a potential for torsades de pointes clearly exists in therapy with both these agents.

## Torsades de Pointes During Therapy with Agents with Predominantly Class III Action

Agents of this type have as their major electrophysiologic effect prolongation of repolarization. No systematic data are available, but the potential for arrhythmia aggravation in the form of torsades de pointes appears to vary widely among drugs with this class of action. NAPA, the major metabolite of procainamide, does not block cardiac sodium channels (unlike the parent drug).[35] It produces EADs in canine Purkinje fibers and bradycardia-dependent ventricular tachyarrhythmias in dogs with slow heart rates.[35] Accumulation of high concentrations of NAPA during procainamide therapy has been strongly implicated as a cause of torsades de pointes,[44,45] and therapy with NAPA itself has also been associated with torsades de pointes.[46] Again, the incidence is not known. In our own experience with NAPA therapy of variable duration in 40 patients, we observed 1 unexpected death and 1 patient who developed torsades de pointes shortly after a NAPA dose increase.

Sotalol is an agent with both beta-blocking (Class II) and Class III properties.[36,70] QT-interval prolongation during sotalol therapy appears generally to be dose- and plasma-concentration related.[71,72] EADs during in vitro testing of sotalol were described in the late 1960s,[36] and marked bradycardia and QT interval prolongation with torsades de pointes is a ubiquitous finding during sotalol overdose.[73] At more usual dosages, sotalol clearly can cause torsades de pointes, particularly in the presence of hypokalemia.[47-49] A large series of such cases was reported from South Africa, where the drug combination sotazide (sotalol plus thiazide) was used for hypertension.[49] Both the NAPA and sotalol data suggest, but by no means prove, that torsades de pointes with these agents, unlike the situation with quinidine, generally is related to elevated plasma drug concentrations.

Amiodarone also has prominent Class III activity but, in addition to its pharmacokinetic and toxicologic characteristics, appears to be somewhat different from the other agents with Class III activity in its potential to induce arrhythmias. It is an impression of many investigators that, despite marked QT prolongation which is the hallmark of amiodarone therapy in many patients, torsades de pointes is unusual. There however is no question that it can occur and, because of amiodarone's long elimination half-life, prolonged treatment with isoproterenol or pacing may be required. In one series of 5 patients,[51] hypokalemia was present in 2 but the arrhythmia persisted for days to weeks after correction of the electrolyte abnormality.

In addition to its Class III action, amiodarone also blocks cardiac sodium channels in the inactivated state (i.e., during phases 2 and 3 of the action potential),[50] blocks the slow inward calcium current, and has antiadrenergic properties. It also is a very potent blocker of depolarization-induced automaticity arising at both negative and depolarized membrane potentials (i.e., both sodium and calcium channel dependent).[50] Moreover, amiodarone may decrease dispersion of repolarization, particularly between Purkinje network and ventricular muscle sites. Thus, amiodarone possesses a multiplicity of ancillary electrophysiologic properties, each of which might reverse the basic electrophysiologic abnormalities producing torsades de pointes.


## Comparisons Among Drugs

The incidence of torsades de pointes with each of the agents described earlier, with the possible exception of quinidine, is not well known. In the case of quinidine, the incidence appears to be 0.5—8.5 percent, and fairly clearly the reaction is not related to high plasma concentrations. On the other hand, in the cases of NAPA and sotalol, high plasma concentrations appear to contribute to the problem. For quinidine and sotalol, even mild hypokalemia and possibly hypomagnesemia in the setting of diuretic therapy is a potent exacerbating factor.

If a patient develops torsades de pointes during therapy with one action-potential prolonging drug, it is not known whether therapy with other agents possessing this property will be equally dangerous. In our own series of quinidine-induced cases, 3 patients were treated with disopyramide and procainamide for "ventricular tachycardia resistant to quinidine" and torsades de pointes persisted. Scattered reports and small series[9,10,69,74] from other groups similarly suggest that a rechallenge with a different action-potential prolonging drug after an episode of antiarrhythmic drug-induced torsades de pointes frequently results in recurrence of the arrhythmia. This issue is not well studied in the case of amiodarone, although very small numbers suggest that the risk may be present.

Chronic antiarrhythmic management in patients who have developed torsades de pointes while receiving a repolarization-prolonging drug is uncertain. Our own bias is to avoid other drugs with this electrophysiologic property even if a clearcut exacerbating factor such as hypokalemia or bradyarrhythmia[75,76] was present and had been corrected. Our reasoning is that, although repolarization-prolonging antiarrhythmic drugs may be tolerated in the short term, the occurrence of torsades de pointes identifies a patient "at risk" and should any exacerbating factor redevelop, the arrhythmia may recur. Similarly, although basic electrophysiologic studies suggest that combinations of drugs such as quinidine plus mexiletine do not prolong QT interval to the same extent as quinidine alone[77] and mexiletine reverses quinidine-induced EADs in vitro,[58] therapy with such drug combinations in patients who have had torsades de pointes remains risky.[9] The occurrence of torsades de pointes should prompt an overall reevaluation of the specific indication for antiarrhythmic therapy and the risk—benefit ratio in a particular patient.

Studies of torsades de pointes have not only helped raise the level of awareness of this distinctive adverse drug reaction in the general cardiologic and medical communities but also have pointed the way for electrophysiologic research on the fundamental mechanisms of this distinctive arrhythmia. Studies are required to further identify factors that may render a particular patient at risk for these arrhythmias and that may exacerbate the corresponding rhythm abnormalities in vitro.

## Conclusions

Torsades de pointes as a complication of antiarrhythmic therapy with agents that prolong cardiac repolarization is a distinct electrophysiologic entity. However, the precise mechanism that underlies this abnormality still is not understood completely, although the evidence in support of early afterdepolarization is reasonably compelling. However, a facilitatory role for dispersion of repolarization is not excluded. It appears that simple lengthening of the $QT_c$ does not always predispose to torsades de pointes, and antiarrhythmic compounds producing a similar degree of $QT_c$ lengthening appear to exhibit differing propensities to induce torsades. Factors such as bradycardia and electrolyte abnormalities in the setting of prolonged cardiac repolarization predispose to the development of torsades de pointes. An appreciation of the setting in which torsades de pointes occurs as a complication of antiarrhythmic therapy allows the institution of appropriate management. Although ionic currents mediating the genesis of this arrhythmia have not been defined, it is clear that torsades de pointes is a distinct clinical and electrophysiologic entity most frequently induced by antiarrhythmic agents that prolong cardiac repolarization.

*The research behind this chapter was supported in part by a grant from the United States Public Health Service (HL32694).*

## References

1. Selzer A, Wray HW: Quindine syncope: Paroxysmal ventricular fibrillation occurring during treatment of chronic atrial arrhythmias. *Circulation* 30:17, 1964.
2. Dessertenne F: La tachycardie ventriculaire a deux foyers opposes variables. *Arch des Mal du Courer* 59:263, 1966.
3. Roden DM, Woosley RL, Primm RK: Incidence and clinical features of the quinidine-associated long QT syndrome: Implications for patient care. *Am Heart J* 111:1088, 1986.

4. Tzivoni D, Keren A, Stern S: Torsades de pointes versus polymorphous ventricular tachycardia. *Am J Cardiol* 52:639, 1983.
5. Sclarovsky S, Strasberg B, Lewin RF, et al: Polymorphous ventricular tachycardia: Clinical features and treatment. *Am J Cardiol* 44:339, 1979.
6. Keren A, Tzivoni D, Gavish D, et al: Etiology warning signs and therapy of torsades de pointes. *Circulation* 64:1167, 1981.
7. Khan MM, Logan KR, McComb JM, et al: Management of recurrent ventricular tachyarrhythmias associated with QT prolongation. *Am J Cardiol* 47:1301, 1981.
8. Schweitzer P, Mark H: Delayed repolarization syndrome. *Am J Med* 75:393, 1983.
9. Kay GN, Plumb VJ, Arciniegas JG, et al: Torsades de pointes: The long-short initiating sequence and other clinicial features: Observations in 32 patients. *J Am Coll Cardiol* 2:806, 1983.
10. Bauman JL, Bauernfeind RA, Hoff JV, et al: Torsades de pointes due to quinidine: Observations in 31 patients. *Am Heart J* 54:59, 1957.
11. Jervell A, Lange-Nielsen F: Congential deaf-mutism, functional heart disease with prolongation of the QT interval and sudden death. *Am Heart J* 56:59, 1957.
12. Romano C, Genrme G, Pongiglione R: Artimie cardiache rare dell'eta pediatrica. *Clin Pediatr* 45:656, 1963.
13. Ward OC: A new familial cardiac syndrome in children. *J Irish Med Assoc* 54:103, 1964.
14. Isner JM, Sours HE, Paris AL, et al: Sudden, unexpected death in avid dieters using the liquid-protein–modified-fast diet. *Circulation* 60:1401, 1979.
15. Siegel RJ, Cabeen WR Jr, Roberts WC: Prolonged QT interval–ventricular tachycardia syndrome from massive rapid weight loss utilizing the liquid-protein–modified-fast diet: Sudden death with sinus node ganglionitis and neuritis. *Am Heart J* 102:121, 1981.
16. Isner JM, Roberts WC, Heymsfield SB, et al: Anorexia nervosa and sudden death. *Ann Int Med* 102:49–52, 1985.
17. Ludomirsky A, Klein HO, Sarelli P, et al: QT prolongation and polymorphous ("Torsades de pointes") ventricular arrhythmias associated with organophosphorus insecticide poisoning. *Am J Cardiol* 49:1654, 1982.
18. Kemper AJ, Dunlap R, Pietro DA: Thioridazine-induced torsades de pointes: Successful therapy with isoproterenol. *J Am Med Assoc* 249:2931, 1983.
19. Hust, MH, Nitsche K, Hohnloser S, et al: QT prolongation and torsades de pointes in a patient with subarachnoid hemorrhage. *Clin Cardiol* 7:44, 1984.
20. Redleaf PD, Lerner IJ: Thiazide-induced hypokalemia with associated major ventricular arrhythmias: Report of a case and comment on therapeutic use of bretylium. *JAMA* 608:1302, 1968.
21. Curry P, Stubbs W, Fitchett D, et al: Ventricular arrhythmias and hypokalemia. *Lancet* 1:231, 1976.
22. Ramee SR, White CJ, Svinarich JT, et al: Torsade de pointe and magnesium deficiency. *Am Heart J* 109:164, 1985.
23. Fredlund BO, Olsson SB: Long QT interval and ventricular tachycar-

dia of "torsade de pointe" type in hypothyroidism. *Acta Med Scand* 213:213, 1983.

24. Denes P, Gabster A, Huang SK: Clinical, electrocardiographic and follow-up observations in patients having ventricular fibrillation during Holter monitoring. *Am J Cardiol* 48:9, 1981.

25. Schwartz PJ: Idiopathic long QT syndrome: Progress and questions. *Am Heart J* 109:399, 1985.

26. Chadda K, Ballas M, Boderheimer MM: Efficacy of magnesium replacement in patients with hypomagnesemia and cardiac arrhythmia. *Circulation* 70:II-444, 1984.

27. Vincent GM, Abildskov JA, Burgess MJ: QT-interval syndromes. *Prog Cardiovasc Dis* 6:523, 1974.

28. Warren MS, Gallagher JJ: "Les torsades de pointes": An unusual ventricular arrhythmia. *Ann Int Med* 93:578, 1980.

29. Bhandari AK, Scheinman M: The long QT syndrome. *Mod Concepts Cardiovasc Dis* 54:45, 1985.

30. Bhandari AK, Scheinman MM, Morady F, et al: Efficacy of left cardiac sympathectomy in the treatment of patients with the long QT syndrome. *Circulation* 70:1018, 1984.

31. Crampton R: Pre-eminence of the left stellate ganglion on the long QT syndrome. *Circulation* 59:769, 1979.

32. Coumel P, Leclercq J-F, Dessertenne F: Torsades de pointes. In *Tachycardias: Mechanisms, Diagnosis and Treatment*. Philadelphia, Lea and Febiger, p 325, 1984.

33. Roden DM, Hoffman BF: Action potential prolongation and induction of abnormal automaticity by low quinidine concentrations in canine Purkinje fibers: Relationship to potassium and cycle length. *Circ Res* 56:857, 1985.

34. D'Almoncourt CN, Zierhut W, Luderiz B: "Torsades de pointes" tachycardia re-entry or focal activity? *Br Heart J* 48:213, 1982.

35. Dangman KM, Hoffman BF: In vivo and in vitro antiarrhythmic and arrhythmogenic effects of N-acetylprocainamide. *J Pharmacol Exp Ther* 217:851, 1981.

36. Strauss HC, Bigger JT, Hoffman BF: Electrophysiological and beta-receptor blocking effects of MJ 1999 on dog and rabbit cardiac tissue. *Circ Res* 26:661, 1970.

37. Brachmann J, Scherlag BJ, Rosenshtraukh LV, et al: Bradycardia-dependent triggered activity: Relevance to drug-induced multiform ventricular tachycardia. *Circulation* 68:846, 1983.

38. Levine HJ, Spear JF, Guarnierei T, et al: Cesium chloride-induced long QT syndrome: Demonstration of afterdepolarization and triggered activity in vivo. *Circulation* 72:1092, 1985.

39. Kupersmith J, Hoff P: Occurrence and transmission of localized repolarization abnormalities in vitro. *J Am Coll Cardiol* 6:152, 1985.

40. Mendez C, Delmar M: Triggered activity: Its possible role in cardiac arrhythmias. In DP Zipes, J Jalife (eds): *Cardiac Electrophysiology and Arrhythmias*. Orlando, Fla., Grune and Stratton p 311, 1985.

41. Swain HH, McCarthy DA: Veratrine, protoveratrine and andromedotroxin arrhythmias in the isolated dog heart. *J Pharmacol Exp Ther* 121:379, 1957.

42. Honerjager P, Reiter R: The relation between the effects of veratridine on action potential and contraction in mammalian ventricular myocardium. *Naunyn- Schmiedebergs Arch Pharmacol* 289:1, 1975.

43. Brown B: Early afterdepolarization induced by batrachotoxin: Possible involvement of a sodium current. *Fed Proc* 42:521, 1983.

44. Herre JM, Thompson JA: Polymorphic ventricular tachycardia and ventricular fibrillation due to N-acetylprocainamide. *Am J Cardiol* 55:227, 1985.

45. Stratmann HG, Walter KE, Kennedy HL: Torsades de pointes associated with elevated N-acetylprocainamide levels. *Am Heart J* 109:375, 1985.

46. Chow MJ, Piergies AA, Bowsher DJ, et al: Torsades de pointes induced by N-acetylprocainamide. *J Am Coll Cardiol* 4:621, 1984.

47. Kontopoulos A, Manoudis F, Filindris A, et al: Sotalol-induced torsades de pointes. *Postgrad Med J* 57:321, 1981.

48. Laakso M, Pentikainen PJ, Rehnberg S: Sotalol-induced prolongation of the QT-interval and attacks of unconsciousness. *Int J Clin Pharmacol Therap Toxicol* 22:487, 1984.

49. McKibbin JK, Pocock WA, Barlow JB, et al: Sotalol, hypokalaemia, syncope and torsades de pointes. *Br Heart J* 22:487, 1984.

50. Mason JW, Hondeghem LM, Katzung BG: Block of inactivated sodium channels and of depolarization-induced automaticity in guinea pig papillary muscle by amiodarone. *Circ Res* 55:277, 1984.

51. Sclarovsky S, Lewin RF, Kracoff O, et al: Amiodarone-induced polymorphous ventricular tachycardia. *Am Heart J* 105:6, 1983.

52. Strasberg B, Sclarovsky S, Erdberg A, et al: Procainamide-induced polymorphous ventricular tachycardia. *Am J Cardiol* 47:1309, 1981.

53. Coltasky TJ: Mechanisms of action of lidocaine and quinidine on action potential duration in rabbit cardiac Purkinje fibers. *Circ Res* 5017, 1981.

54. Carmeliet E: Electrophysiologic and voltage clamp analysis of the effects of sotalol on isolated cardiac muscle and Purkinje fibers. *J Pharmacol Exp Ther* 232:817, 1985.

55. Isenberg G: Cardiac Purkinje fibers: Cesium as a tool to block inward rectifying potassium currents. *Pflueg Archiv* 365:99, 1976.

56. Katzung BG: Effects of extracellular calcium and sodium on depolarization-induced automaticity in guinea pig papillary muscle. *Circ Res* 37:118, 1975.

57. Aliot E, Szabo B, Sweiden R, et al: Prevention of torsades de pointes with calcium channel blockade in an animal model. *J Am Coll Cardiol* 5:492, 1985.

58. Campbell RM, Woosley RL, Roden DM: Lack of early afterdepolarizations despite phase 3 repolarization abnormalities due to bepridil and lidoflazine. *Circulation* 72(Suppl III): 381, 1985.

59. Roden DM, Woosley RL: Cycle length dependent interactions of quinidine and mexiletine. *J Am Coll Cardiol* 5:493, 1985.

60. Cranefield PF: Action potentials, afterpotentials, and arrhythmias. *Circ Res* 41:415, 1977.

61. Barbey JT, Thompson KA, Echt DS, et al: Plasma concentration-response relations and disposition of encainide in man. *Clin Res* 34:394A, 1986.

62. Radford MD, Evans DW: Long-term results of DC reversion of atrial fibrillation. *Br Heart J* 30:91, 1968.
63. Lown B, Wolf M: Approaches to sudden death from coronary heart disease. *Circulation* 44:130, 1971.
64. Ejvinsson G, Orinius E: Prodromal ventricular premature beats preceded by a diastolic wave. *Acta Med Scand* 208:445, 1980.
65. Thompson KA, Blair I, Woosley RL, et al: Comparative *in vitro* electrophysiology of quinidine, its metabolites and dihydroquinidine. *Clin Res* 33:298A, 1985.
66. Thompson KA, Murray JJ, Blair LA, et al: Plasma concentrations of quinidine, its major active metabolites, and dihydroquindine in patients with torsades de pointes. *Clin Res* 34:408A, 1986.
67. Leclercq JF, Kural S, Valere PE: Bepridil et torsades de pointes. *Arch Mal Coeur* 3:341, 1983.
68. Manouvrier J, Sagot M, Caron C, et al: Nine cases of torsades de pointes with bepridil administration. *Am Heart J* 111:1005, 1986.
69. Kennelly BM: Comparison of lidoflazine and quinidine in prophylactic treatment of arrhythmias. *Br Heart J* 39:540, 1977.
70. Singh BN, Vaughan Williams EM: A third class of antiarrhythmic action. Effects on atrial and ventricular intracellular potentials, and other pharmacological actions on cardiac muscle of MJ 1999 and AH 3747. *Br J Pharmacol* 39:675, 1970.
71. Neuvonen PH, Blonen E, Tanskanen A, et al: Sotalol prolongation of the QTc interval in hypertensive patients. *Clin Pharm Ther* 32:25, 1982.
72. Wang T, Bergstrand RH, Siddoway LA, et al: Concentration dependent pharmacologic properties of sotalol. *Am J Cardiol* 57:1160, 1986.
73. Neuvonen PH, Elonen E, Vuorenmaa T, et al: Prolonged QT interval and severe tachyarrhythmias, common features of sotalol intoxication. *Eur J Clin Pharmacol* 20:85, 1981.
74. Clark M, Friday K, Anderson J, et al: Drug induced torsades de pointes: High concordance rate among type IA antiarrhythmic drugs and amiodarone. *J Am Coll Cardiol* 5:450, 1985.
75. Steinbrecher UP, Fitchett DH: Torsades de pointes: A cause of syncope with atrioventricular block. *Arch Intern Med* 140:1223, 1980.
76. Fontaine G, Frank R, Lascault G, et al: Torsades de pointes favorisees par stimulations ventriculaires a rythme lent. *Arch Mal Coeur* 8:918, 1983.
77. Duff HJ, Roden DM, Primm RK, et al: Mexiletine in the treatment of resistant ventricular tachycardia: Enhancement of efficacy and reduction of dose-related side effects by combination with quinidine. *Circulation* 67:1124, 1983.

# Chapter 24

# Critique of Class III Antiarrhythmic Action: Past Experience and Future Directions

## E. M. Vaughan Williams

## Historical Background

Lewis et al., in their early studies of quinidine, established that the drug reduced the maximum frequency at which cardiac muscle could respond to pacing stimuli.[1] Microelectrodes for intracellular recording were not introduced until 28 years later, so that attempts to analyze electrophysiologic mechanisms inevitably were somewhat primitive. Nevertheless Love, using an ingenious double interpolated stimulus technique,[2] concluded that the "absolute" refractory period of cardiac muscle measured by the method was not prolonged by quinidine; and many years later Wedd et al.[3], estimating action potential duration (APD) from differential surface records, observed no prolongation of APD in the presence of quinidine. In contrast, West[4,5] maintained that the antiarrhythmic effect of quinidine was due to delayed repolarization. West et al. employed very low heart rates, however; and in 1958, I was able to show that, at pacing frequencies close to those occurring in vivo, restriction of depolarizing current (Class I action) was the primary effect of quinidine. Both West and I were in agreement, however, that if a drug were able to delay repolarization it would prolong refractory period and should be antiarrhythmic. Thus, the idea

From: *Control of Cardiac Arrhythmias by Lengthening Repolarization*, edited by Bramah N. Singh, MD, Futura Publishing Company Inc., Mount Kisco, NY, © 1988.

that prolongation of APD would constitute a distinct class of anti-arrhythmic action long preceded the discovery of a drug with a potent effect of this kind.

The idea was strongly supported by the finding that thyroidectomy had just such an effect.[6] A. S. Freedberg long had been interested, as a clinical cardiologist, in the influence of differences in thyroid state in his patients, and, in 1968, came to work in my laboratory with the specific intention of discovering why atrial fibrillation was so common in hyperthyroidism,whereas arrhythmias of any kind were rare in the hypothyroid state.

Amiodarone was produced a quarter of a century ago as an antianginal drug, but one of a series of benzofurans, which were vasodilators, chosen because it was believed at that time that coronary artery dilatation was required for the treatment of angina pectoris. The beta blockers were introduced in the early 1960s (pronethalol in 1962, propranolol in 1964) and were antianginal but not coronary vasodilators. The Labaz group, however, considered that it would be preferable to induce only a partial antagonism to adrenergic stimulation, for fear of compromising a possible vital sympathetic support. Thus, amiodarone was selected because it was both a vasodilator and reduced by about a third effects mediated by both alpha and beta receptors, partly by a noncompetitive antagonism,[7] partly by diminishing release of noradrenaline from sympathetic nerve endings.[8] Charlier discovered that amiodarone was antiarrhythmic in several standard laboratory models of arrhythmias, such as those induced by aconitine, calcium chloride, chloroform, and coronary ligation, but it apparently was not very potent, having about one-sixth the activity of quinidine, and its mode of action was unclear. Was the antiarrhythmic effect simply a reflection of sympathetic antagonism (Class II action) or was some other property involved?

I was approached by Labaz to undertake an electrophysiologic study and, at about this time, Bramah Singh joined me as a doctoral student. When we found that amiodarone prolonged APD in both atria and ventricles,[9] I suggested that this might indeed represent the "third class" of antiarrhythmic action, which had been the subject of such controversy in relation to quinidine so many years before. We confirmed the antiarrhythmic action of amiodarone, in this case, in providing protection against digitalis-induced arrhythmias in guinea pigs. The two major findings that made amiodarone qualitatively different from other drugs were, first, that an action on repolarization was observed with hardly any effect on depolarization; and, second, that the effect was progressive, increasing over several weeks. Clinical studies were instituted by Labaz, now reported in the comprehensive review of Harris and Roncucci,[10] but it was not easy to persuade clinical colleagues to take the antiarrhythmic action seriously because the prolongation of ventricular APD produced a lengthening of QT interval, which was received as bad news (see Chapter 4).

## The QT Interval

The importance of measuring the QT interval as a guide to prognosis is controversial (see Chapter 4) and much has been written that need not be reviewed here. Two aspects need to be highlighted, however: cancellation of vectors and corrections for heart rate.

Any drug that induces a uniform delay of ventricular repolarization, of course, will prolong the QT interval. If there is no change in width of the QRS complex, then the lengthening of QT will be due exclusively to the prolongation of the JT interval. There are many other reasons why the QT interval may be prolonged, however. The Class Ic antiarrhythmic drugs widen the QRS, but have little effect on the JT. The new compound cibenzoline, for example, prolongs QT by precisely the number of milliseconds by which the QRS is widened. Another possibility is dispersion of repolarization times, not necessarily because of differences in APD but through dispersion of onsets of depolarization by impaired conduction. Furthermore, the end of the T wave may not signal the end of electrical activity in the ventricle because oppositely-oriented late repolarization vectors may mutually cancel each other, rendering the surface EKG electrically silent.

The latter phenomenon is well illustrated in the long QT syndrome (LQTS), usually treated by beta blockade or high left thoracic sympathectomy (see Chapter 4). Both long-term beta blockade and sympathetic denervation induce an adaptational response in cardiac cells that delays repolarization. The adaptation to beta blockade takes several days to develop, persists long after cessation of therapy, and has been demonstrated in animals with intracellular electrodes[11] and in humans with monophasic action potential recording.[12] The effect is not caused by the bradycardia associated with beta blockade, because sustained treatment with alinidine, a clonidine analog, which produces a more profound bradycardia, does not induce prolongation of APD.[13] In the LQTS, it is believed that there is a deficiency of sympathetic innervation from the right stellate ganglion,[14] which normally innervates predominantly the sinoatrial node (SAN) and the anterior wall of the heart, especially the right ventricular (RV) free wall. Children with LQTS have a lower resting heart rate (HR) than normal, and in exercise HR does not increase as much as would be expected. From experimental evidence cited earlier, it would be expected that cells deprived of their sympathetic innervation would adapt by prolonging their APD (hence, the long QT). Abildskov et al. demonstrated that in LQTS patients repolarization of the anterior wall in fact was delayed.[15]

Arrhythmias in the LQTS occur in response to exercise or emotion, in association with intense left-sided sympathetic activity, partly compensatory, partly, perhaps, because an inhibitory influence is lost from afferent nerves normally traveling with the right sympathetic.[14] Excitation of beta receptors shortens APD, beta$_1$ receptors by increasing potassium conductance, beta$_2$ receptors by activating the NaK pump, which is electrogenic, transferring one net negative (repolarizing) charge to the interior of the cell per cycle of the pump. In the LQTS, the APD on the right is long and cannot shorten in exercise because of the deficient sympathetic innervation, so that the shortening of APD on the left is unbalanced. At the junction between the denervated and innervated regions, there will be great dispersion of repolarization times, leading to reentry tachycardia or ventricular fibrillation (VF). Long-term beta blockade or high left thoracic sympathectomy will reduce the dispersion, not only by making the left ventricle less responsive to sympathetic drive, but also by inducing an adaptational lengthening of APD. The restored balance of APD on the two sides may lead to mutual cancellation of late repolarization vectors on the EKG, so that a lengthening of APD in the LV paradoxically may result in a shortening of QT interval. In support of this view is the finding by Yanowitz et al.[16] that QT interval was prolonged either by right stellectomy (long APD on the right) or by selective stimulation of the left stellate ganglion (short APD on the left).

The direct effect of beta-adrenoceptor stimulation in shortening APD in the LV makes it impossible to calculate reliable corrections for the QT interval to compensate for differences in heart rate. Many authors still employ the equation $QT_c = \dfrac{QT}{\sqrt{RR}}$ attributed to Bazett, in spite of many demonstrations of its lack of accuracy. Bazett's own equation, in fact, was "Systole = K/SQR cycle. The normal value for K is 0.37 for men and 0.40 for women."[17] The slope of the relation between QT and RR intervals depends upon the manner in which HR is altered. If RR is increased by pacing stimuli in a recumbent subject, the slope is less steep than if HR is raised by exertion, because in the latter event a direct catecholamine-induced shortening of APD is superimposed on the purely rate-induced effect. Conversely, the slope of the QR/RR relation is diminished after beta blockade.[18] The need for correction can be avoided by ensuring that QT is measured at the same heart rate before and after drug administration or other intervention.[19]

After a myocardial infarction (MI), not only is a block of cardiac muscle lost, but sympathetic nerves also may perish, thus, depriving the surviving neighborhood from its sympathetic control and inducing a sort of localized LQTS with consequent dispersion of repolarization times. Dispersion also may be created by conduction delay through an ischemic region or around a dead one. For various such reasons, a long QT can be an indicator of myocardial damage and dispersion of repolarization times, and a long QT has been regarded as a harbinger of sudden death.[20] Thus, a reluctance among cardiologists to accept that a drug that induced a lengthening of QT interval could be antiarrhythmic was not surprising, and even now it is not universally accepted that the Class III drugs are antiarrhythmic because they lengthen APD.

## Influence of Ischemia

Antiarrhythmic drugs that restrict fast inward sodium current (Class I) are more effective on ischemic than normal muscle, because failure of ischemic cells to repolarize fully delays the recovery of sodium channels from inactivation. In normal muscle, amiodarone has a comparatively minor Class I action, but this becomes much more prominent in ischemia.[21] Furthermore, in hypoxia and ischemia, APD is shortened because potassium conductance is increased, and this effect may reduce or abolish the ability of amiodarone to lengthen APD; that is, the ischemia induced outward current swamps the restriction of outward current induced by the drug in normoxic cells. This does not indicate, however, that lengthening of APD is not reponsible for its antiarrhythmic effect in arrhythmias associated with ischemia. Ischemic muscle makes a rapidly diminishing contribution to cardiac output,[22] so that abnormalities of conduction within it are irrelevant to survival. During an ischemic episode, cardiac output is dependent upon the proper function of the part of the heart that is still normoxic. Thus, the invasion of this remaining normal muscle by an arrhythmia is dangerous, and a lengthening of APD here may protect against abnormal excitation and so be responsible for the antiarrhythmic action. Rendering the ischemic region electrically silent, of course, is an important part of Class I action in additon to raising the threshold to excitation of normal muscle, and this Class I action of amiodarone in ischemia well may contribute additionally to its overall antiarrhythmic potency.

In the normal heart, the fibers that depolarize last repolarize first, perhaps to prevent backfiring or "reflection" of action potentials from the terminal region. APD is shorter in the epicardium than the endocardium, and at the apex than at the base, so that current flows in the same direction during depolarization and repolarization of the LV, rendering R and T waves concordant. If the epicardium is ischemic, epicardial APD becomes shorter still, giving the concordant T wave a higher peak. If the endocardium is ischemic, in contrast, the T wave is flattened or may even be inverted. Shifts of the ST segment are more difficult to interpret because, if cell membranes in the ischemic zone fail to repolarize fully, current continues to flow during diastole and shifts the reference baseline.[23] Heterogeneous adrenergic stimulation also can cause localized shortening of APD, resulting in T wave abnormalities and bizarre complexes, as have been observed in normal healthy people subjected to extreme emotional stress.[24] Alternations of T wave concordance and discordance are observed in the LQTS and can be reproduced by unbalanced right and left stellate stimulation.[16] The antiarrhythmic drugs that prolong APD, including beta blockers on long-term administration, may protect against arrhythmias as much by reducing disparities of repolarization times in neighboring regions as by the absolute lengthening of APD.

## Future Directions and Conclusions

Clinicians in general are concerned mainly with the question "whether" a particular therapeutic regimen is effective, whereas basic medical scientists attempt to answer the question of "how" the therapeutic effect is achieved, by elucidating the mechanisms by which an abnormality is induced and corrected. Thus, although it may appear evident from laboratory studies that delayed repolarization must prolong refractory period, and so, provided the effect is uniform and homogeneous, should be antiarrhythmic, only the clinician can prove by stringently controlled trials whether this is so by assessing the efficacy of Class III drugs in patients. Since the introduction of amiodarone, many other compounds have been observed to delay repolarization and have proved to be antiarrhythmic, which can hardly be a coincidence. Sotalol, although a Class II agent, was shown to have antiarrhythmic activity more potent than could be accounted for by beta blockade;[25] and it would be reasonable to attribute this additional potency to its Class III effect, as it also prolongs QT interval. Bretylium, although not lengthening APD in atrial muscle, does so in the ventricle and is sometimes remarkably effective in controlling ventricular arrhythmias. N-acetylprocainamide, melperone, clofilium . . . the list of compounds that delay repolarization continues to grow, but much remains to be done in defining the types of arrhythmia in which Class III agents might be most efficacious, and it is certainly not the province of a laboratory investigator like myself to predict the result.

Nevertheless, one may, perhaps, suggest some general principles. Arrhythmias are multifactorial in origin, and it would be logical to adopt a multifaceted approach in attempting to control them. Most normal people have occasional extrasystoles, and ambulatory monitoring of the EKG of healthy subjects has demonstrated that episodes of arrhythmia are quite common yet do not cause symptoms or disability.[26] Why, then, do such arrhythmic events, innocuous in the normal population, progress to serious, even life-threatening, situations in cardiac patients? It is reasonable to conclude that in the latter additional factors, such as local ischemia, sympathetic imbalance, or congenital abnormality, provide a pathway for reentry. In some conditions, especially pre-excitation arrhythmias of the Wolff-Parkinson-White type or as sequel to a previous pathological lesion, the presence of an anatomical substratum for reentry can be demonstrated by electrophysiologic study and may even be susceptible to surgical removal. In others, ventricular fibrillation may occur without previous evidence of cardiac disease, yet it is reasonable to assume that some additional factor, such as localized ischemia too small to be apparent on the EKG, must be present to permit a precipitating event to progress to reentry tachycardia or VF.

If several factors contribute to arrhythmias, more than one type of antiarrhythmic action may be necessary to control them. Indeed, it is remarkable that some of the most effective, recently introduced antiarrhythmic drugs possess more than one class of action. Amiodarone, in addition to its Class III action, is antisympathetic and has a substantial Class I effect in ischemic muscle. Propafenone, though primarily a Class Ic compound, is a beta blocker and also has some calcium antagonist activity. This is not to suggest that it is desirable to seek drugs with multiple actions, but that multiple actions may be necessary to treat intractable arrhythmias. Multiple actions could be exhibited in a more controlled manner by combinations of drugs with different classes of action than by combinations of actions in a single drug. Thus, the main value of a "pure" Class III agent, such as d-sotalol, could be as an adjunct to therapy with another drug. For example, an atrial flutter that was slowed in frequency but not abolished by a Class I compound might be delivered the coup de grace by the addition of "a touch of Class III."

# References


1. Lewis T, Drury AN, Iliescu CC, et al: Observations relating to the action of quinidine upon the dog's heart: With special reference to its action on clinical fibrillation of the auricles. *Heart* 9:55, 1921.
2. Love WS: The effect of quinidine and strophanthin upon the refractory period of the tortoise ventricle. *Heart* 13:87, 1926.
3. Wedd AM, Blair HA, Gosselin RE: The action of quinidine on the cold-blooded heart. *J Pharmacol Exp Ther* 75:251, 1942.
4. West TC: Mode of action of quinidine in heart muscle. *Fed Proc* 14:393, 1955.
5. West TC, Amory DW: Single fiber recording of the effects of quinidine at atrial and pacemaker sites in the isolated right atrium of the rabbit. *J Pharmacol Exp Ther* 130:183, 1960.
6. Freedberg AS, Papp JGY, Vaughan Williams EM: The effect of altered thyroid state on atrial intracellular potentials. *J Physiol* (London) 207:357, 1970.
7. Charlier R: A new antagonist of adrenergic excitation not producing competitive receptor blockade. *Br J Pharmacol* 39:668, 1970.
8. Bacq ZM, Blakeley AGH, Summers RJ: The effects of amiodarone, an alpha and beta receptor antagonist, on adrenergic transmission in the cat spleen. *Biochem Pharmacol* 25:1195, 1976.
9. Singh BN, Vaughan Williams EM: The effect of amiodarone, a new anti-anginal drug on cardiac muscle. *Br J Pharmacol* 39:657, 1970.
10. Harris L, Roncucci R: Amiodarone. *Med Sci Int* (Paris) 1986.
11. Vaughan Williams EM, Raine AEG, Cabrera AA, et al: The effect of

prolonged beta adrenoceptor blockade on heart weight and intracellular potentials in rabbits. *Cardiovasc Res* 9:579, 1975.

12. Olsson SB: Atrial repolarization in man: Effect of beta receptor blockade. *Br Heart J* 36:806, 1974.

13. Vaughan Williams EM, Dennis PD, Garnham C: Circadian rhythm of heart rate in the rabbit: Prolongation of action potential duration by sustained beta adrenoceptor blockade is not due to associated bradycardia. *Cardiovasc Res* 20:528, 1986.

14. Schwartz PJ, Locati E: The idiopathic long QT syndrome: Pathogenic mechanisms and therapy. *Eur Heart J* 6(Suppl D):103, 1985.

15. Abildskov JA, Vincent GM, Evan AK, et al: Distribution of body surface ECG potentials in familial QT interval prolongation. *Am J Cardiol* 47:480, 1981.

16. Yanowitz R, Preston JB, Abildskov JA: Functional distribution of right and left stellate innervation to the ventricles: Production of neurogenic electrocardiographic changes by unilateral alternation of sympathetic tone. *Circ Res* 18:416, 1966.

17. Bazett HC: An analysis of the time-relations of electrocardiograms. *Heart* (London) 7:353, 1920.

18. Vaughan Williams EM, Hassan MO, Floras JS, et al: Adaptation of hypertensives to treatment with cardioselective and nonselective beta blockers. Absence of correlation between bradycardia and blood pressure control, and reduction in slope of the QT/RR relation. *Br Heart J* 44:473, 1980.

19. Birkhead JS, Vaughan Williams EM, Gwilt DJ, et al: Heart rate and QT interval in subjects adapted to beta-blockade: Bradycardia and hypotension as uncorrelated adaptations. *Cardiovasc Res* 17:649, 1983.

20. Schwartz PJ, Wolf S: QT interval prolongation as predictor of sudden death in patients with myocardial infarction. *Circulation* 49:1074, 1978.

21. Cobbe SM, Manley BS: Cellular electrophysiology of amiodarone in cardiac ischemia. *Br J Clin Prac* 40(Suppl 44): 104, 1986.

22. Gibson D, Mehmet H, Schwartz F, et al: Asynchronous left ventricular wall motion early after coronary thrombosis. *Br Heart J* 55:4, 1986.

23. Wittig J, Vaughan Williams EM: Mechanism of ST elevation during the three phases of ischemia. *Circulation* 48(Abs Suppl 3):55, 1977.

24. Taggart P, Carruthers M, Somerville W: Intense emotional stress: Effect of oxprenolol on the electrocardiogram, plasma catecholamines and lipids. In DM Burley (ed): *New Perspectives in Beta Blockade.* Horsham, England, CIBA, p 287, 1972.

25. Nathan AW, Hellestrand KJ, Bexton RS, et al: Electrophysiological effects of sotalol—Just another beta blocker? *Br Heart J* 47:521, 1982.

26. Clarke JM, Hamer NAJ, Shelton JR, et al: The rhythm of the normal human heart. *Br Heart J* 38:882, 1976.